FUNGICIDES: CHEMISTRY, ENVIRONMENTAL IMPACT AND HEALTH EFFECTS

FUNGICIDES: CHEMISTRY, ENVIRONMENTAL IMPACT AND HEALTH EFFECTS

PAUL DE COSTA
AND
PETER BEZERRA
EDITORS

Nova Biomedical Books
New York

For permission to use material from this book please contact us:
Telephone 631-231-7269; Fax 631-231-8175
Web Site: http://www.novapublishers.com

LIBRARY OF CONGRESS CATALOGING-IN-PUBLICATION DATA

Fungicides : chemistry, environmental impact, and health effects / [edited by] Paul De Costa and Peter Bezerra.
p. ; cm.
Includes bibliographical references and index.
ISBN 978-1-60692-631-4 (hardcover)
1. Fungicides--Toxicology. 2. Fungicides--Environmental aspects. I. De Costa, Paul. II. Bezerra, Peter.
[DNLM: 1. Anti-Infective Agents--poisoning. 2. Pesticide Residues--poisoning. 3. Environmental Pollutants--adverse effects. 4. Food Contamination--analysis. QV 250 F981 2009]
RA1270.F86F86 2009
363.19'2--dc22 2008053483

Published by Nova Science Publishers, Inc. ✢ New York

CONTENTS

PREFACE

Antimicrobial agents, called fungicides, sporicides or biocides have long been used to control, prevent and remediate microbial growth. Currently public concern about the impact of pesticides, including fungicides, on human health is greater than ever before. Pesticides are essential in agricultural production, but they constitute a potential risk to humans who are exposed to them directly through various ways and indirectly through diet. In vitro techniques used to study in vitro metabolism and interactions are briefly described in this book, summarizing the metabolic and kinetic properties of selected fungicides. Different analytical methods are reported in the literature for the analysis of fungicides. Developments in the methods devoted to fungicide analysis in environmental samples over the past 15 years are also looked at. In addition, biological contaminants, especially mold in buildings, which are known to act as sources of indoor air pollution, discomfort, asthma and pulmonary disease in building occupants and antimicrobial treatments of indoor mold and bacteria are reviewed. This book shows the current situation of the analysis of fungicide residues in environmental, biological and food samples, describing the analytical methods used for their determination. Finally, this book skoes the current research on adaptation and resistance to agricultural fungicides.

Short Communications A - 4,5,6,7-Tetrachlorophthalide (phthalide) is a common fungicide mainly applied to paddy fields against rice blast, which is one of the most destructive diseases of rice. The behavior of phthalide in the air, water and soil after aerial application to paddy fields was reviewed. First, the distribution of phthalide in the air and water environment is summarized. The phthalide concentration over the paddy fields was 360 - 900 ng/m^3 during the application, and 10 - 0.54 % of the applied phthalide drifted 0 - 50 m from the applied area. Phthalide was detected in the river water in the range of 0.08 - 3.9 μg/L, and was predominantly detected from July to August. Second, the phthalide runoff from the paddy fields into the water environment is described. The maximum concentration in the paddy water was 10.2 – 33.8 μg/L, and <0.01 μg/L within 14 days after the application. Occasional increases in the phthalide concentrations in the drainage channel and river waters were caused by rainfalls. Third, the phthalide behavior in the paddy fields is discussed. The maximum percentile ratios of phthalide in the paddy soil and water were 83 - 96 % and 1.7 - 9.6 %, respectively. The half-life of the phthalide in the paddy soil was 20 - 31 days. Finally, the runoff ratio of phthalide from the paddy fields to into the drainage channel is mentioned. The runoff ratio was 0.3 - 10.3 %.

Short Communications B - Many yeasts secrete glycolipids into the medium. Among these compounds, sophorolipids, cellobiose lipids, and mannosylerythritols are best studied. Cellobiose lipids differ in their structures, including the number of OH-groups in fatty acid residue and number and structures of O-substituents in cellobiose residue. For example, *Cryptococcus humicola* secretes mainly 16-(tetra-O-acetyl-β-cellobiosyloxy)-2-hydroxyhexadecanoic acid, while *Pseudozyma fusiformata* and *Pseudozyma graminicola* secrete mainly 16-[6-O-acetyl-2'-O-(3-hydroxyhexanoyl)-β-cellobiosyloxy)]-2,15-dihydroxyhexadecanoic acid. Recently it has been found that these compounds, known as surfactants, are highly active against many species of ascomycetous and basidiomycetous yeast and mycelial fungi. They exhibit maximal activity at pH ~ 4.0. The effective concentrations against basidiomycetes (*Filobasidiella neoformans*) and ascomycetes (*Candida* spp.) are 0.03 mM and 0.1-0.4 mM, respectively. The mechanism of action of cellobiose lipids on yeast cells is based on enhancement of nonspecific permeability of the cytoplasmic membrane, which results in the rapid leakage of ATP and potassium ions from the yeast cells treated with these compounds. The broad spectrum of activity, pH and temperature stability allow one to consider cellobiose lipids as promising natural biocontrol agents of yeast and mycelial fungi.

Chapter I - Currently public concern about the impact of pesticides, including fungicides, on human health is greater than ever before. Pesticides are essential in agricultural production, but they constitute a potential risk to humans who are exposed to them directly through various ways and indirectly through the diet. Accordingly, the health risk assessment of pesticides is of utmost importance for the protection of human health. Risk assessment needs reliable scientific information and one source of information is the characterization of the metabolic factors and toxicokinetics. Indeed, quantitative toxicokinetic data in humans are needed for human risk assessment to make reliable comparisons between individuals or between species. Because humans cannot be used as study subjects except in occasional circumstances, the authors have to rely upon in vitro experiments, human-derived techniques and in vitro – in vivo predictions as well. In the usual course of events, the more known about pesticides in terms of their metabolic characteristic in vitro, the better the extrapolation of in vitro and animal studies into human risk assessment will be.

Cytochrome P450 enzymes are important in the metabolism of various endogenous substrates as well as a wide range of xenobiotics. The metabolism may results in activation and/or detoxification reactions. Basically, metabolic factors such as metabolic routes, identification of the major and minor metabolites, metabolite stability, metabolizing enzymes, interindividual variability, interspecies differences and the inhibitory interactions are providing important quantitative data for chemical risk assessment.

In this review the authors will briefly describe the in vitro techniques used to study in vitro metabolism and interactions, summarize the metabolic and kinetic properties of selected fungicides and provide an example from our own studies about how to apply current techniques to obtain relevant data for risk assessment.

Chapter II - During the last decade, the use of many chemical substances without any control and studies about their behaviour in the environment has become a focus of interest for the European Union (EU). Pesticides which are widely used through Europe, entered into the environment and contaminate waters and soils with potential risks for wildlife and human health due to the proved or suspected toxicity of these compounds. Very few interests targeted on fungicides while they represent a major part of all type of pesticides used (herbicides, insecticides, rodenticides…). Nevertheless, pesticides are already regulated by the european directive 91/414/EEC which target to reduce their impact on human health and the environment. Concerning foodstuffs for human and animal consumption, pesticides residues have to not exceed the Maximum Residue Limits (MRLs) indicated in different directives (76/895/EEC, 86/362/EEC, 86/363/EEC, 90/642/EEC, 2005/396/EEC) regulating their concentration respectively in fruits and vegetables, in cereals, in foodstuffs of animal origin, and in products of vegetable origin and honey. In addition, REACH (for Regulation Evaluation and Authorization of Chemicals), the new regulation system which target to improve the protection of human health and the environment from the risks that can be posed by unknown chemicals give a focus on pollution brought by major diffusion of chemicals like pesticides and consequently fungicides. It implements directive 91/414/EEC concerning the placing of plant products on the European market [1]. In this context, sensitive, reliable and undoubtedly analytical methods for monitoring fungicides in the environment are really necessary to set up their control by the future european regulations and directives.

In this chapter, the authors will first present a quick overview of the different analytical methods reported in the literature for the analysis of fungicides. Then, the authors focus on the new methodology the authors develop to detect and quantify 33 substances suspected to interfere with the hormonal system or/and have a toxicity on human and wildlife at very low concentrations ($ng.L^{-1}$ and $\mu g.kg^{-1}$), and particularly 8 fungicides:

- 2-imidazolidinethione or ethylenethiourea, principal metabolite of many dithiocarbamates fungicides (mancozeb, ziram, propineb)
- Tebuconazole (triazole fungicide)
- Hexaconazole (triazole fungicide)
- Tetraconazole (triazole fungicide)
- Fluquinconazole (triazole fungicide)
- Bromuconazole (triazole fungicide)
- Dimethomorph (morpholine fungicide)
- Pyridaben (pyridazinone fungicide)

The optimisation of all the method steps from the extraction to the quantification by chromatography coupled with mass spectrometry as well as the method validation done by chemiometric approach, complete to be normalized for legislation rules applications and ready to be applied for toxicity studies will be discussed. Lastly, we will conclude with the application of our new methodology to real environmental samples (wastewaters, groundwater and surface waters and sediments, mud puddle, atmospheric fallout and sludge) confirming major occurrence of several compounds in the environment of the Rhône-Alpes region, France.

Chapter III - Plant endophytic fungi, microorganisms that reside in the internal tissues of living plants without causing any immediate overt negative effects, have been found in every plant species examined to date and recognized as potential sources of novel natural products for exploitation in agriculture, medicine, and food industry. This chapter describes published research on antimicrobial compounds produced by plant endophytic fungi as sources of new antimicrobials. Literature was reviewed based on our personal experience, reported antimicrobial activity against plant, human and animal pathogens, novel chemical structures of the antimicrobials from the endophytic fungi. The future prospects for these antimicrobials to control important plant and animal diseases will also be discussed.

Chapter IV - Dichlofluanid is a halogenated sulfonamide derivative from the group of aryl (dichlorofluoromethyltio) fungicides. It was used as a fungicide and acaricide in approved agricultural pesticides from 1965. Nowadays it is not included in any of the lists for European re-assessment of active ingredients under Directive 91/414/EEC. On the other hand, it has been used in aquaculture and as a booster biocide in antifouling products, especially tin-free products, to control the growth of algal, weed and animal fouling on moving or stati objects in water. Furthermore, following the review of dichlofluanid in Product type 8 (Wood preservatives) under the Biocidal Products Directive 98/8/EC, the European Commission has agreed that this active substance will enter into Annex I of the Directive on 1 March 2009.

In this regard exposure to dichlofluanid is possible during its application, but it is also detected in harbours and marinas in many European countries.

In this chapter the toxic effects of dichlofluanid to humans and animals are summarized.

Chapter V - Micronucleus assay is a widely used test in evaluating the genotoxic consequences of exposures to environmental and occupational contaminants. In this study a fungicide tolylfluanid was investigated for its ability to induce micronuclei *in vitro* using sheep peripheral lymphocytes. Lymphocyte cultures from three donors were exposed to three different concentrations of fungicide (1×10^{-4}, 1×10^{-5} and 1×10^{-6} M/L) for 48 h. At the lowest concentration (1×10^{-6} M/L) the frequency of micronuclei was not significantly different (32.33 ± 3.51/1000 binucleated cells at this concentration versus 30.33 ± 2.82/1000 binucleated cells in DMSO control, $P = 0.44$). Higher concentrations of fungicide (1×10^{-4} and 1×10^{-5} M/L) resulted in a significant dose dependent increase in the number of micronuclei in comparison with control (74.0 ± 13.0/1000 binucleated cells and 52.67 ± 10.12/1000 binucleated cells versus 30.33 ± 2.82/1000 binucleated cells in DMSO control, $P =$ 0.005 and 0.020, respectively, Anova test). Many of the treated cells also possessed multiple micronuclei. Tolylfluanid did not affect nuclear division index (NDI) at all treatment concentrations. Our results thus demonstrate a weak genotoxic effect of tolylfluanid in sheep peripheral lymphocytes *in vitro*.

Chapter VI - Biological contaminants especially mold in buildings are known to act as sources of indoor air pollution, discomfort, asthma and pulmonary disease in building occupants. Sick buildings are evidence of extremely problematic indoor air quality (IAQ), often resulting from unacceptable concentrations of biological contaminants, particulates and odors, and extreme temperatures and humidity. Biological contaminants can cause allergic, toxic, or inflammatory responses in building occupants. The risk-management approach to limiting exposure has been to implement a reduction in indoor levels of biological contamination. Antimicrobial agents, called fungicides, sporicides or biocides have long been used to control, prevent, and remediate microbial growth. The antimicrobial efficacy of EPA-

FIFRA registered chemicals and encapsulants, over the counter cleaners, and mechanical devices (such as UV irradiation) to reduce concentrations of mold and bacteria have only recently been investigated. Standard methods to test these control measures such as ASTM 6329-98, (2003) have recently been established, and now pertain to a wide set of applications.

Chapter VII - The current state of analytical methods devoted to the determination of common fungicide residues is reviewed, based on the concern of worldwide government agencies about their potential risk for human health. The review covers relevant analytical methods applied to samples of environmental interest, highlighting the analysis of natural waters and foodstuff for human consumption.

Chapter VIII - Agricultural fungicides are widely used in crop protection. However, they are potential pollutants and their accumulation in the environment can cause severe health problems. Moreover, its efficacy against a broad spectrum of phytopathogenic fungi is compromised by the emergence of multiresistant strains. Multiple drug resistance is in most cases due to the action of membrane transporters that, presumably, catalyze the extrusion of unrelated chemical compounds. The biological role and expression regulation of a number of these transporters conferring fungicide resistance in *Saccharomyces cerevisiae* and in other fungi are reviewed in this chapter.

Genome-wide analysis tools have been increasingly used to provide new insights into the mechanisms underlying organism-environment interactions. This new field of Environmental Toxigenomics may provide a better understanding of the toxicological effects of each potential environmental toxicant and on how cells are able to acquire resistance to these chemical stresses. It may also allow the identification of early and sensitive biomarkers of the toxicological response. Post-genomic experimental approaches have been applied with success to the yeast *S. cerevisiae*, a widely accepted eukaryotic model system. The knowledge gathered so far on the mechanisms underlying the toxicity of, and resistance to, agricultural fungicides in *S. cerevisiae* and in filamentous fungi based on these approaches and on more detailed analyses, is reviewed here. Emphasis is given to the systemic benzimidazole benomyl and the dithiocarbamate mancozeb.

Chapter IX - Fungicides are a group of chemicals used in agriculture to control plant diseases caused by fungal attack (fungi are the number one cause of crop loss worldwide). As a result of their widespread use and their relative persistence, fungicide residues present in waters, food, etc., can reach the consumer and may therefore represent a risk for human health. Moreover, animals can accumulate some of these substances from contaminated feed and water and also from indoor fungicide practices. All these aspects have originated the need to develop analytical methodologies that allow the determination of these compounds below their established maximum residue limits (according to current legislation) in the different countries especially in environmental and food samples. The present chapter attempts to show the current situation of the analysis of fungicide residues in environmental, biological and food samples, describing the analytical methods used for their determination.

Chapter X - Benzimidazole compounds can be used both as anthelmintic agents for the prevention and treatment of parasitic infections in animals or humans and as fungicidal agents to prevent spoilage of crops during their storage and transport. It has been repeatedly demonstrated that benzimidazole parent compounds, as well as their metabolites, are capable of reaching the edible parts of food, thus entering the trophic chain. Consequently, an increasing public concern about their massive use in recent years has led to a continuously evolving legislation that restricts their maximum residue limits (MRLs) in milk, meat or crops to a few mg/Kg. Additionally, their massive use has led to their accumulation in the environment, where a maximum contamination level of 0.1 μg/L has been legislated for ground or drinking waters.

A considerable effort has been invested in recent years in the development of new analytical methodologies for the determination of benzimidazole compounds in several kinds of samples. The present review comprises a thorough description of the currently available methodologies for the analysis of benzimidazole compounds in milk, meat, vegetables, fruits or drinking water samples.

Different extraction methodologies such as Soxhlet extraction, microwave and ultrasound assisted extraction procedures, accelerated solvent extraction and solid phase extraction will be compared. Similarly, the techniques most commonly used for the quantification of benzimidazole compounds (immunoassays, GC, HPLC or capillary electrophoresis or chemical sensors) in the aforementioned samples will be discussed in detail. Additionally, special attention will be paid to aspects such as sample clean-up and enrichment procedures.

Chapter XI - The use of fungicides on vegetable and fruit crops has reached significant levels in areas of intensive agriculture, both for consumption as fresh and those aimed at processed foods (chilled, frozen, canned, beer and wine).

From an environmental point of view, there are numerous studies in order to ascertain specific concentration levels of pesticide residues in different ecosystems, as well as their degradation, metabolism, mobility, etc. However, the field studies, designed specifically to meet their dynamics of disappearance in habitual conditions of farming, are made only for registration purposes and are less known.

The persistence of pesticides in field is directly influenced by weather conditions (temperature and solar radiation) and these are of great importance in the dissipation of residues in the case of raw vegetable ingestion. However, it should be pointed that there are manipulation and manufacturing processes that can suppose positive effects on the dissipation of pesticide residues, such as washing and blanching in the freezing process, peeling and sterilization in the can manufacture; fermentation and filtering in the beer and wine elaboration, etc.

In this chapter, the authors will present data on the field dissipation and influence of the manufacturing processes in the disappearance of fungicides belonging to different classes (penconazole, procymidone, metalaxyl, thiram, mancozeb, cyprodinil, fludioxinil, quinoxyfen, azoxystrobin, etc.) present at food agricultural products. These studies were carried out on vegetables matrices such as pepper, tomato, celery, broccoli, lettuce, apricot, peach, grape, barley, etc.

The studies analyzed show that basic processes in the manufacture of plant origin foods decrease the initial concentration in the treated crop. Thus, washing and blanching in the freezing of leafy vegetables and *Solanaceae* decrease the concentration of the fungicides studied. The peeling and thermal treatment to obtain canned stone fruit and fruit juices produce considerable elimination of the initial residues. And last, oenotechnological processes made during the wine-making manage the total elimination of fungicides residues initially present in the grapes in some cases.

The data obtained from these studies allow the determination of the so-called "transfer factor", regarded as the percentage of increase or decrease in the residue concentration in processed foods. These factors would provide significant data for inclusion in the annexes of Regulation 396/2003 of the European Union which states that when no maximum residue levels are established for processed foods, those for raw foods must be applied, considering the specific factors of concentration or dilution in the transformation processes.

Chapter XII - Fungicide resistance is an important concern to growers of horticultural crops in British Columbia, Canada. In the past, *Venturia inaequalis,* found in several orchards with an apple scab problem, were resistant to benomyl, a fungicide commonly used at the time. More recently, harvested apples decayed by *Penicillium expansum* or *Botrytis cinerea* were found to be resistant to thiabendazole. Because of this history of fungicide resistance it was decided that a survey to identify resistance to Demethylation Inhibitors (DMI-fungicides) in apple, cherry, and rose was needed now that these fungicides had been used for more than 10 years. Relative growth of 72 *V. inaequalis* isolates from 27 orchard blocks were tested for resistance to myclobutanil. Two isolates, 2445-3 and 2451-3, were found with resistance to myclobutanil at 0.05 g/L and qualify as being field resistant according to standard criteria. DMI resistance to powdery mildew fungi is difficult to quantify because conidia can only be accurately tested on living tissue of the host plant. Contamination of the host tissue and poor viability of the test fungus also makes evaluation difficult. Quantification of myclobutanil resistance by *Podosphaera leucotricha* (apple powdery mildew), *P. clandestina* (cherry powdery mildew) and *Sphaerotheca pannosa* (rose powdery mildew) were based on assaying conidia from samples collected from infected orchards and testing them for germination on leaf disks sprayed with myclobutanil. Five out of 10 apple, 13 out of 14 cherry, and 9 out of 10 rose powdery mildew samples showed some resistance to myclobutanil because the number of germinated spores on treated leaves did not differ significantly from the number of germinated spores on untreated leaves. Apple scab resistance to myclobutanil does not appear to be widespread in BC because it only occurred in one area of the provinces. On the other hand powdery mildew resistance appears to be widespread and could be responsible for ineffective control experienced by apple, cherry, and rose growers. The implications of DMI-resistance and strategies to mitigate DMI resistance are discussed.

Chapter XIII - The occurrence of filamentous fungi in drinking water has been known for many years. However, the quantity of scientific literature on the subject is only beginning to increase. Filamentous fungi have been considered only as annoying contaminants of agar plates used to count bacteria from water. There are various potential issues associated with the fungi-in-drinking-water phenomenon, including blockage of water pipes, organoleptic problems such as odour and taste, biofilm formation, spread of pathogenic fungi, and mycotoxins production. Drinking water raises issues of biosecurity in relation to mycotoxin production. This chapter presents a review of fungi in drinking water, with emphases on (a) methods of isolation, (b) fungi detected, (c) problems which occur, (d) avoidance or removal, and (e) methods to detect biochemicals such as mycotoxins. The literature on bottled will be assessed because it is being returned increasingly due to the presence of filamentous fungi.

Domestic tap water will be considered. Suggestions for future collaborative work will be made which will include the use of standardised methodology for isolation and identification of filamentous fungi, the use of "ring tests", standard biochemical analysis, and the need for international research projects. Also, sound methods for the removal and control of filamentous fungi will be devised in the longer term. It is intended that standardised methodology will be the major output of such research equivalent to those that exist for bacteria.

In: Fungicides
Editors: P. De Costa and P. Bezerra

ISBN: 978-1-60692-631-4

Short Communication A

BEHAVIOR OF AERIAL APPLIED 4,5,6,7-TETRACHLOROPHTHALIDE IN AIR, WATER AND SOIL

Kuniaki Kawata*
Faculty of Applied Life Sciences, Niigata University of Pharmacy and Applied Life Sciences, 265-1 Higashijima, Niigata 956-8603, Japan

ABSTRACT

4,5,6,7-Tetrachlorophthalide (phthalide) is a common fungicide mainly applied to paddy fields against rice blast, which is one of the most destructive diseases of rice. The behavior of phthalide in the air, water and soil after aerial application to paddy fields was reviewed. First, the distribution of phthalide in the air and water environment is summarized. The phthalide concentration over the paddy fields was 360 - 900 ng/m^3 during the application, and 10 - 0.54 % of the applied phthalide drifted 0 - 50 m from the applied area. Phthalide was detected in the river water in the range of 0.08 - 3.9 µg/L, and was predominantly detected from July to August. Second, the phthalide runoff from the paddy fields into the water environment is described. The maximum concentration in the paddy water was 10.2 – 33.8 µg/L, and <0.01 µg/L within 14 days after the application. Occasional increases in the phthalide concentrations in the drainage channel and river waters were caused by rainfalls. Third, the phthalide behavior in the paddy fields is discussed. The maximum percentile ratios of phthalide in the paddy soil and water were 83 - 96 % and 1.7 - 9.6 %, respectively. The half-life of the phthalide in the paddy soil was 20 - 31 days. Finally, the runoff ratio of phthalide from the paddy fields to into the drainage channel is mentioned. The runoff ratio was 0.3 - 10.3 %.

* E-mail: kawata@nupals.ac.jp

Introduction

Paddy rice farming plays an important role in the food production in Japan. In 2007, all the paddy fields covered an area of 2.53 million ha, and accounted for 54.4 % of the total cultivated area (4.65 million ha) in Japan [1]. In 2003, 290,458 metric tons of pesticides was sold in Japan. More than one hundred kinds of pesticides are applied to paddy fields and some of the applied pesticides occur in the drained paddy water that flow from the paddy fields into rivers and lakes through drainage channels [2-11]. Some pesticides have been aerially applied to paddy fields using helicopters or radio-controlled helicopters [9, 11-14].

Phthalide (4,5,6,7-tetrachlorophthalide) is a common fungicide in Japan. The properties of phthalide are listed in Table 1 [15, 16]. Phthalide is mainly applied to paddy fields in May through August to combat the rice blast [17], which is one of the most destructive diseases of rice. The total amount of phthalide soil in Japan was 96 metric tons in 2006. Phthalide has been detected throughout Japan in river waters [9, 11-13, 18- 22], river sediment [23], the atmosphere [14, 20, 22, 24] and rainwaters [25].

In this paper, the phthalide distribution and behavior in paddy fields and the environment are described. First, the distribution of phthalide in the air and water environment is summarized. Second, the phthalide runoff from paddy fields into the water environment is reviewed. Third, the phthalide behavior in the paddy fields is discussed. Finally, the runoff ratio of phthalide from the paddy fields into the drainage channel is mentioned.

Table 1. Properties of phthalide

IUPAC name, 4,5,6,7-tetrachlorophthalide
Common name, phthalide
CAS, 27355-22-2
Molecular formula, $C_8H_2Cl_4O_2$
Molecular weight, 271.9
log P_{OW}, 3.01 [15]
Water solubility, 2.5 mg/L at 25 °C [15]
Organic carbon normalized soil sorption coefficient (Koc), 738 [16]
Half-life (DT_{50}) in soil, 70 days [16]
Appraisal standard in air for aerial application, 200 $\mu g/m^3$

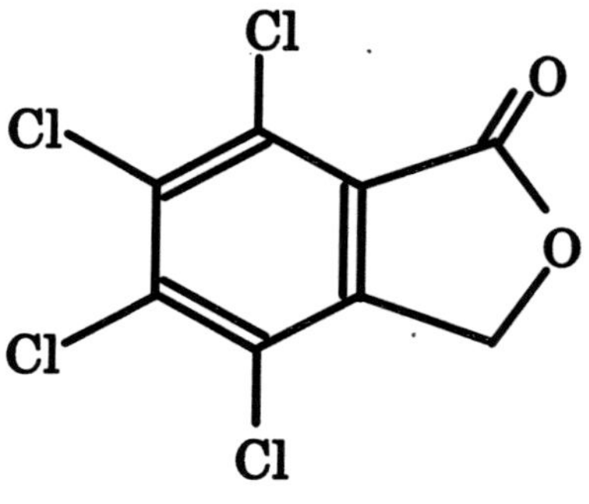

Determination

Air

Phthalide in the air was collected using solid adsorbents, such as the 2,6-diphenyl-*p*-phenylene oxide polymer [14], quartz-fiber wool and activated carbon [24], and the styrene-divinylbenzene copolymer [20], at 2-3 L/min for 60 – 90 min [14, 20]or 0.1 L/min for one week [24]. Phthalide collected on the adsorbents was eluted with organic solvents, e.g., acetone [14], acetone and toluene-ethanol (4:1, v/v), [24], and dichloromethane [20]. The eluate was reduced to a small volume under a stream of purified nitrogen for gas chromatography/mass spectrometry (GC/MS) determination. In case of requiring a cleanup, the resulting solution was treated with a silica gel cartridge [14] as described in the CLEANUP section.

Water

A water sample (50 – 500 mL) was passed through a cartridge containing the styrene-divinylbenzene copolymer [26] or octadecyl bonded silica gel [9] at 10 mL/min. After the cartridge was washed with purified water, it was dried by passing air over it. Phthalide collected on the cartridge was then eluted with acetone [9]. The obtained eluate was concentrated to 1 mL under a pure nitrogen gas stream for the GC/MS determination.

Sediment and Soil

Phthalide in the sediment samples [23] was extracted using an ultrasonically-assisted procedure, and then cleaned using reversed phase column chromatography followed by normal phase column chromatography as described in the CLEANUP section. A 10 g sediment sample with 10 mL acetone was ultrasonicated for 15 min and then shaken for 15 min. After the slurry was centrifuged, the supernatant solvent phases were filtered through a glass-fiber filter. The extraction procedure was repeated twice. The extracts were combined and evaporated to 5 mL at 30°C.

The solution was added to 250 mL of purified water and the resulting solution was passed through a cartridge containing the styrene-divinylbenzene copolymer at the flow rate of 10 mL/min. After the cartridge was washed with purified water, it was dried by passing air followed by centrifugation. Phthalide collected on the cartridge was eluted in the opposite direction of the collection with 4 mL of acetone and then 4 mL of hexane. The combined eluate was concentrated to ca 1 mL under a stream of purified nitrogen, and then 5 mL of hexane was added.

The solution was washed three times with 2 mL of purified water. After the hexane layer was dried over anhydrous sodium sulfate, 250 mg of copper powder was added to the hexane solution and the mixture was shaken to remove the sulfur interferences. The hexane solution was transferred to another container. The residual copper powder was rinsed with a minimum amount of hexane, and then the rinses were added to the hexane solution. The solution was concentrated to 1 mL under a pure nitrogen gas stream.

Phthalide in a soil sample [27] was extracted, and the resulting extract was concentrated to 1 mL. After the hexane layer was dried over anhydrous sodium sulfate, the combined eluates were concentrated to ca 1 mL under a stream of purified nitrogen, and the solution was concentrated to 1 mL for the GC/MS analysis.

Cleanup

The obtained solution was cleaned using normal phase column chromatography [22]. If the solution contained acetone, the acetone was removed as described in the SEDIMENT AND SOIL section. The obtained hexane solution was placed in the silica gel cartridge then eluted with 2 mL of hexane. The hexane eluate was later discarded. The cartridge was subsequently eluted with 4 mL of an acetone–hexane (20 : 80, v/v) solution. The eluate was concentrated to 1 mL under a pure nitrogen gas stream for the GC/MS determination.

Determination

The concentrated solution with an added internal standard, e.g., 9-bromoanthracene [9, 26], was analyzed by GC/MS. An example of the GC/MS conditions was as follows [9, 11]: column, a 30 m×0.25 mm i.d. (0.25 μm film thickness) fused-silica BPX-5 column (SGE, Ringwood, Victoria, Australia), column temperature, programmed from 100 °C (held for 1 min) to 280 °C (held for 3 min) at the rate of 20 °C/min; injector temperature, 250 °C; injection mode, splitless; helium carrier gas flow rate, 1.0 mL/min; MS transfer temperature, 290 °C; ion source temperature, 250 °C; ionization mode, electron impact; ionization energy, 70 eV; mass scan range, m/z 50–350. The quantification ions for the phthalide and 9-bromoanthracene were 243 and 256, respectively.

BEHAVIOR OF PHTHALIDE IN AIR, WATER AND SOIL

PHTHALIDE CONCENTRATIONS IN THE ENVIRONMENT

The phthalide concentrations in the air after aerial applications are summarized in Table 2. The phthalide concentration over the paddy fields was 360 - 900 ng/m^3 during the application [14, 20, 22], and decreased to 25 ng/m^3 within five days after the application [14]. The concentrations in the leeward sites of the paddy fields were 76 - 500 ng/m^3 during the application [14, 20, 22], and decreased to 20 - 360 ng/m^3 within one hour after the application [14, 20]. These concentrations were dependent on the distance from the applied area, and elapsed time after the application [14]. They could also be affected by the wind speed, wind direction and air temperature [28].

Ohara et al. evaluated the drifted phthalide amounts over the paddy fields [14]. Thirteen mg/m^2 of phthalide had deposited on the paddy fields; the deposit value was 87 % of the applied phthalide (15 mg/m^2). The phthalide amounts that drifted 0 m, 5 m and 50 m from the applied area were 1.5 mg/m^2 (10 %), 0.29 mg/m^2 (1.9 %) and 0.081 mg/m^2 (0.54 %), respectively. A stream of air generated by the helicopter rotors caused the drift. A part of the drifted phthalide could be a major source of that detected from the drainage channels immediately after the aerial applications [20].

Table 2. Phthalide concentrations in air after aerial applications

Site	Applied amount (mg/m^2)	Elapsed time [a] (h)	Concentration (ng/m^3)	Reference
Hokkaido in 2007	18 by RCH [b]			14
Paddy fields		1	93	
		21	97	
		102	25	
1- 40 m leeward		During application	76 - 240	
		1	20 - 27	
		6 - 54	<1.5 - 35	
Hyogo in 2006	15 by RCH [b]			20
Near by paddy fields		During application	360 - 450	
		1 - 2	220 - 360	
Saitama in 1998	Not reported			22
Paddy fields		-	900 (maximum)	
			200 (mean [c])	
50 m leeward		-	500 (maximum)	
			180 (mean [c])	
100 m leeward		-	<300 (maximum)	
			140 (mean [c])	
Niigata, July-August, 1993	Not reported			23
250 m from paddy fields			0.1 - 13	

[a] Elapsed time after application.
[b] Radio-controlled helicopter.
[c] Mean 5 days after application.

The phthalide concentrations in the river water and sediment are summarized in Table 3. Phthalide was detected in the river water at the range of 0.08 - 3.9 μg/L. The phthalide was predominantly detected from July to August in the rivers of Niigata Prefecture, while it decreased to below the detection limit in the middle of September [11, 12, 18]. The transport of pesticides by surface runoff during the rainfall events is a major contribution to the pesticide contamination in the rivers [29]. Distinct runoff events of phthalide were reported; they were mainly caused by the rainfall [9, 11, 18].

Phthalide was detected from the river sediment from July to August, and was at its highest concentration (11 μg/kg) in August [23]. Moreover, phthalide was not detected at the end of September. Since the variation was remarkably similar to that in the river water, it depended on the application practices of the phthalide.

Table 3. Phthalide concentrations in environmental water samples

Site	Prefecture	Month	Year	Concentration (μg/L [a] or μg/kg [b])	Reference
River water					
Anno River	Niigata	August - December	2006	<0.03 – 0.86 (0.17 mean)	11
		August	2005	0.07 – 0.68 (0.26 mean)	9
Sugihara River	Hyogo	April - February	2004-5	<0.01 – 0.17	19
Sugata River	Tochigi	April - September	1999	0.41 mean	13
Shin River	Niigata	April – September	1998	<0.01 - 1.8 (0.55 median)	12
Shin River	Niigata	April – September	1997	<0.01 - 2.1 (0.11 median)	12
Shin River	Niigata	June - September	1996	<0.01 - 3.9 (0.65 median)	12
Shinano River	Niigata	April - August	1996	0.008 – 0.99 (0.049 - 0.15 mean)	18
River sediment					
Shin River	Niigata	July - September	1999	4 – 11 (7 mean)	23

[a] Water.
[b] Sediment.

PHTHALIDE RUNOFF FROM PADDY FIELDS TO WATER ENVIRONMENT

Variations in the concentrations of phthalide aerially applied by a radio-controlled helicopter have been investigated [9, 11, 27] in a rice cultivation area in Agano City, Niigata Prefecture. The paddy fields in the prefecture occupied a total area of 121,000 ha in 2007. Phthalide was aerially sprayed at 18 mg/m^2 on the paddy fields in this area in August. Water samples and soil samples were collected from paddy fields 1 and 2 (sites A and B) covering 1470 and 1200 m^2, respectively. Water samples were also collected from drainage channels 1 and 2 at sites C and D, respectively, as well as from the Anno River at site E. The C, D and E sampling sites were located on the downstream side of the investigated paddy fields (Figure 1). The drainage areas flowing to sites C and D were 168,000 and 1,082,000 m^2, respectively. The drainage from paddy fields 1 and 2 flowed to drainage channel 1 and then to drainage channel 2. The drainage from drainage channel 2 then flowed into the Anno River.

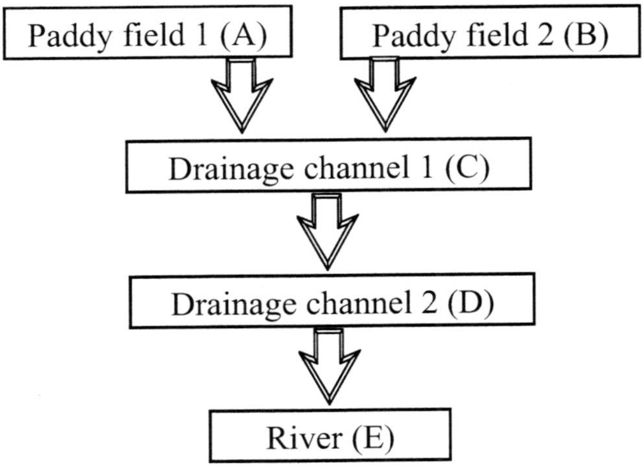

Figure 1. Diagram of water flow from investigated paddy fields to river in Niigata.

The maximum concentrations (one hour after application) in the paddy waters (sites A and B) were 10.2 – 33.8 μg/L [9, 11]. The concentrations decreased to 15 - 29 % of the maximum concentrations within 24 hours, 3.9 - 7.8 % within 48 hours, and <0.01 μg/L within 14 days after the application [11]. Narita and Nakamura reported that the phthalide concentration in the paddy water located in Saitama was 6.2 μg/L on the applied day, 10.1 μg/L on the day after the application, and 1.6 μg/L two days after the application [22]. The differences in the variations could be cause by the different in water amounts. The mean concentrations at sites A and B were 2.4 – 4.4 μg/L. The maximum concentrations in the paddy soils (sites A and B) were 309 – 320 μg/kg (dry base) on the day of application [27]. The concentrations decreased to 32 - 41 % of the maximum concentrations within 7 days, 11 - 33 % within 30 days, 5 - 14 % within 60 days, and <4μg/kg within 137 days after the application. The mean concentrations were 86 – 114 μg/kg [27].

The mean concentrations in the drainage channels (sites C and D) ranged from <0.03 to 7.5 μg/L and 0.36 – 0.97 μg/L, respectively [9, 11]. The maximum concentration in drainage channel 1 was observed within one hour after the application, and then decreased to less than 5 % of the maximum concentrations within 1 d after the application [11]. It appears that the definite increase in the phthalide within one hour after the application was caused by the aerial drifts of phthalide into the drainage channel [20].

Phthalide in the drainage channel waters was predominantly detected in August, then decreased to below the detection limit at the end of September [11]. These results are consistent with those in the river waters [12, 18]. The concentrations in the Anno River (site E) are given in Table 3 [9, 11]. For the herbicides clomeprop and oxaziclomefone, which were applied in May, their runoff events from the paddy fields occurred with the drainage of all the paddy water as well as with the overflows of the paddy water due to rainfall [7]. On the other hand, the amounts of paddy waters in August were less than those in May, and the paddy waters did not drain in August. Therefore, occasional increases in the phthalide concentrations at sites C, D and E were caused by rainfall [11], which is a major carrier of phthalide from the paddy fields to the drainage channels and river.

Phthalide Behavior in Paddy Fields

Phthalide applied to paddy fields became distributed between the soil and water in the paddy fields [27]. The phthalide amounts in the paddy soils and paddy waters in paddy fields 1 and 2 (Figure 1) in Niigata were calculated from the data obtained in the 2006 investigation [11, 27]. The percentile ratios of the phthalide amounts in the paddy soils or the paddy waters to the applied amounts are given in Figure 2. The percentile ratios of phthalide in the soils/waters of paddy fields 1 and 2 were 82.7 %/1.7 % and 95.9 %/1.7 % one hour after its application, respectively. Although the ratios in the waters were 1.7 % in the investigation, the ratios in the waters of paddy fields 1 and 2 in the previous year were determined to be 9.6 % and 5.5 %, respectively [9]. This was caused by the lower volumes of paddy waters in 2006 than those in 2005 [11]. Moreover, the lower amounts of applied phthalide could transfer to the paddy soils in 2005 compared to those in 2006. Therefore, it appears that the amounts of phthalide transferred to the paddy soils are affected by the amounts of paddy waters during/after the application.

The phthalide amounts in the paddy soils decreased to 62 - 70 % of that applied on the next day after the application, and to 33 - 34 % six days after the application. Phthalide was detected from the soils for 112 days after the application, while not detected 137 days after the application. The half-life (DT_{50}) values in the soil were reported as 20 – 31 days [27] using first-order reaction kinetics.

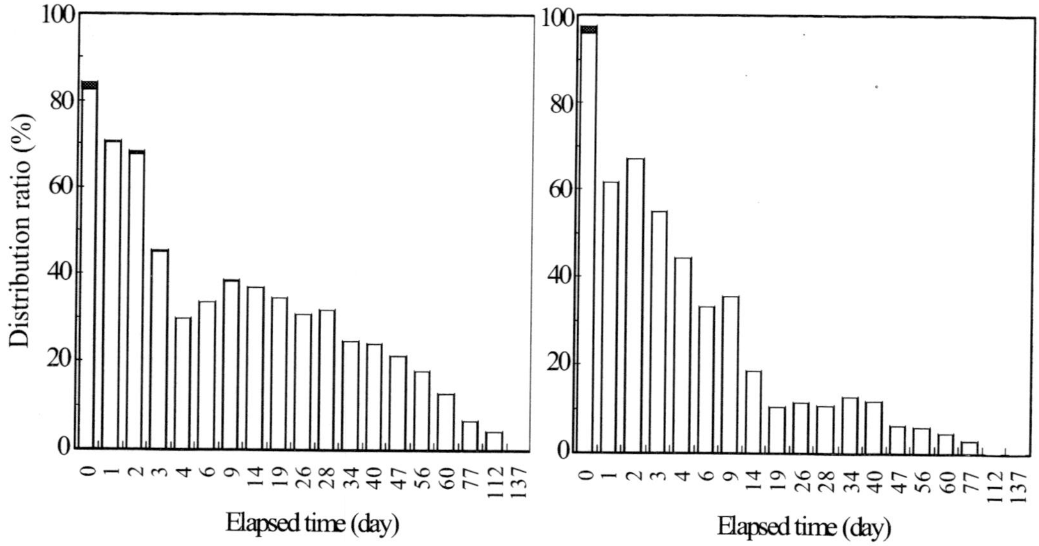

Figure 2. Distribution of phthalide in paddy soil (open bar) and paddy water (closed bar). Percentile ratios are cited or calculated from the data in the references [11, 27].

Table 4. Runoff ratio of phthalide from paddy fields in Japan

Site	Applied amount (mg/m^2)	Applied method	Year	Runoff ratio (%)	Reference
Shiga	15.1	Not reported	2006	1.5, 1.8	21
Niigata	18	Radio-controlled helicopter	2006	1.1 - 2.4	11
Niigata	18	Radio-controlled helicopter	2005	1.6, 1.7	9
Tochigi	Not reported	Helicopter	1999	0.44, 5.64	13
Tochigi	Not reported	Helicopter	1998	2.73	13
Okayama	6	Not reported	1998	6.07, 10.3	30
Saitama	Not reported	Helicopter	1998	0.3	22
Niigata	Not reported	Helicopter	1997	3.1	12
Niigata	Not reported	Helicopter	1996	1.6	12
Niigata	Not reported	Helicopter	1995	2.7	12

RUNOFF RATIO OF PHTHALIDE FROM PADDY FIELDS

Shiota et al. [9] calculated the runoff ratio of phthalide using the following equation:

Runoff ratio (%) = 100 (RR /AA)

where AR is the runoff amount of phthalide in a drainage channel and AA is the amount applied to the catchment area of the drainage channel. Mitobe et al. [12], Narita and Nakamura [24], Inao [30] and Maeda et al. [11] evaluated the runoff ratios by the same method. However, the amounts applied to the investigated areas could not be obtained in some cases. Itoh [13] estimated the amounts applied using questionnaire surveys given to farms in the area.

The reported runoff ratios of phthalide from the paddy fields to the drainage channels are listed in Table 4. The runoff ratios ranged from 0.3 % to 10.3 %. The values depended on the volumes of overflow and drained waters from the paddy fields [9, 11, 13]; as mentioned previously, rainfall was a major carrier of the phthalide from the paddy fields to the drainage [11]. The reported runoff ratios of the other fungicides from paddy fields are summarized in Table 5. The relation between the runoff ratios of fungicides and their water solubilities is given in Figure 3. The runoff ratios of herbicides from paddy fields were reported to correlate with their water solubilities [13]. However, the runoff ratios of fungicides from paddy fields did not significantly correlated with their water solubilities. Moreover, the ratios correlated with neither the P_{OW} nor K_{OC} values. This suggests that the runoff ratios are predominantly affected by the volumes of overflow and drained waters from the paddy fields as mentioned above.

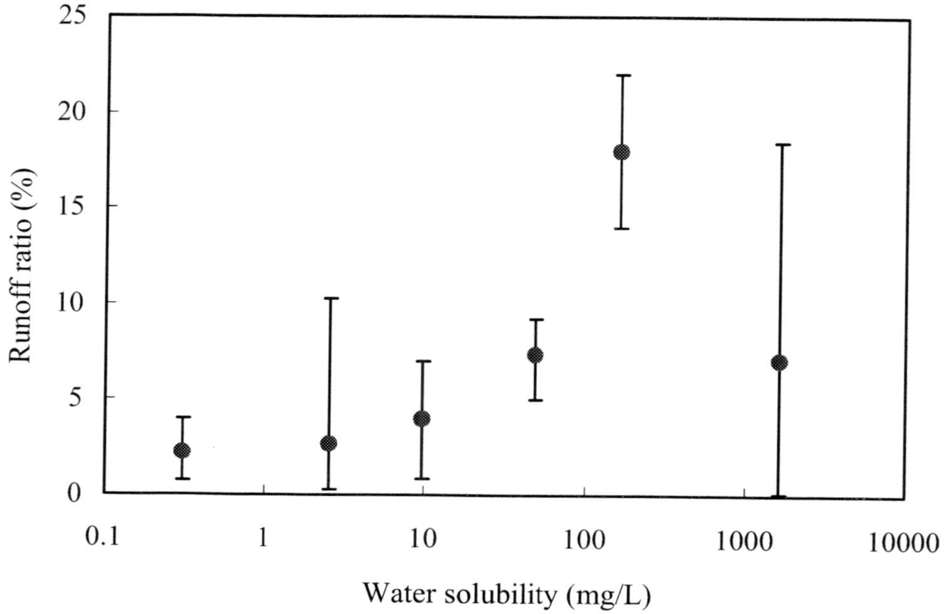

Figure 3. Reported runoff ratios of fungicides *vs*. their water solubilities. Solid circle represents mean value; the error bars mark the maximum and minimum values.

Table 5. Runoff ratio of fungicides from paddy fields

Site	Year	Fungicide	Runoff ratio (%)	Sw [a] (mg/L)	Reference
Okayama	1998	Ferimzone	14, 22	162 at 30 °C	30
Niigata	1995 - 1997	Flutolanil	0.8 - 1.8 (4.0 in mean)	9.6 at 20 °C	12
Niigata	1995 - 1997	Isoprothiolane	5.0 - 9.2 (7.4 in mean)	48 at 20 °C	12
Niigata	1995 - 1997	Pencycuron	0.7 - 4.0 (2.2 in mean)	0.3 at 20 °C	12
Niigata	1995 - 1997	Tricyclazole	0.06 - 9.4 (3.3 in mean)	1600 at 25 °C	12
Okayama	1998	Tricyclazole	18.5	1600 at 25 °C	30

[a] Water solubility [16].

References

[1] Ministry of Agriculture, Forestry and Fisheries (2008). *Monthly statistics of agriculture, forestry and fisheries*, Tokyo, Japan: Ministry of Agriculture, Forestry and Fisheries, Japan.

[2] Sudo, M., Kunimatsu, T., & Okubo, T. (2002). Concentration and loading of pesticide residues in Lake Biwa basin (Japan). *Water Research, 36*, 315 - 329.

[3] Sudo, M., Kawachi, T., Hida, Y., & Kunimatsu, T. (2004). Spatial distribution and seasonal changes of pesticides in Lake Biwa, Japan. *Limnology, 5*, 77 – 86.

[4] Nakano,Y., Miyazaki, A., Yoshida, T., Ono, K., & Inoue, T. (2004). A study on pesticide runoff from paddy fields to a river in rural region—1: field survey of pesticide runoff in the Kozakura River, Japan. *Water Research, 38*, 3017 - 3022.

[5] Ishii, Y., Inao, K., & Kobara, Y. (2004). Dissipation of some herbicides in a flooded rice field and increase of water-holding times after application of herbicides. *Bulletin of National Institute for Agro-Environmental Sciences, 23,* 15 – 25.

[6] Kawakami, T., Ishizaka, M., Ishii, Y., Eun, H., Miyazaki, J., Tamura, K., & Higashi, T. (2005). Concentration and distribution of several pesticides applied to paddy fields in water and sediment, from Sugao Marsh, Japan. *Bulletin of the Environmental Contamination and Toxicology, 74*, 954 - 961.

[7] Kawata, K., Asada, T., Tanabe, A., & Oikawa, K. (2005). Runoff of clomeprop and oxaziclomefone from a paddy field. *Bulletin of the Environmental Contamination and Toxicology, 75*, 922 - 928.

[8] Numabe, A., & Nagahora, S. (2006). Estimation of pesticide runoff from paddy fields to rural rivers. *Water Science and Technology, 53,* 139 – 146.

[9] Shiota, N., Hori, T., Nissato, K., Asada, T., Oikawa, K., & Kawata, K. (2006). Runoff of Aerially Applied Phthalide from Paddy Fields. *Bulletin of the Environmental Contamination and Toxicology,* 77, 508-515.

[10] Watanabe, H., Nguyen, M.H.T., Souphasay, K., Vu, S.H., Phong, T.K., Tournebize, J., & Ishihara, S. (2007). Effect of water management practice on pesticide behavior in paddy water. *Agricultural Water Management, 88,* 132 - 140.

[11] Maeda, T., Iwashita, M., Hori, T., Asada, T., Oikawa, K., & Kawata, K. (2008). Variation of 4,5,6,7-tetrachlorophthalide in water after aerial application to rice cultivation area. *Bulletin of the Environmental Contamination and Toxicology, 80*, 399 - 402.

[12] Mitobe, H., Ibaraki, T., Tanabe, A., Kawata, K., Sakai, M., & Kifune, I. (1999). Variation of pesticides in a river flowing through paddy fields area. *Journal of Environmental Chemistry, 9*, 311-320.

[13] Itoh, K. (2002). Runoff of Pesticides from Rice Paddy Fields and Evaluation of Runoff Estimates made using the Pesticide Paddy Field Model(PADDY). *Bulletin of Tochigi Agricultural Experiment Station, 51,* 29 - 36.

[14] Ohara, H., Iahara, R., & Otsuka, H. (2008). Fluctuation of the aerial fungicide vaporized from paddy field sprayed by radio-controlled model helicopter. *Proceedings of 17th Symposium on Environmental Chemistry*, Japanese Society for Environmental Chemistry, 764 - 765.

[15] British Crop Protection Council (2000). *The pesticide manual* (12th edition), ed by Tomlin, C.D.S., Surrey, UK: British Crop Protection Council.

[16] Kanazawa, J. (1996). *Environmental character and toxicity data of pesticides*. Tokyo: Godo-shuppan.

[17] Inoue, S., Maeda, K., Uematsu, T., & Kato, T. (1984). Comparison of tetrachlorophthalide and pentachlorobeuzy1 alcohol with chlobenthiazone and other melanin lnhibitors in the mechanism of rice blast control. *Journal of Pesticide Science, 9*, 731 - 736.

[18] Tanabe, A., Mitobe, H., Kawata, K., Yasuhara, A., & Shibamoto, T. (2001). Seasonal and spatial studies on pesticide residues in surface waters of the Shinano River in Japan. *Journal of Agricultural and Food Chemistry, 49*, 3847-2852.

[19] Yoshida, M. & Fujimori, K. (2005). The Study of Pesticide in the River Water around the Paddy Area. *Bulletin of the Hyogo Prefectural Institute of Public Health and Environmental Sciences, 2*, 28 - 36.

[20] Yoshida, M., Suzuki, M., Moriguchi, Y., & Yoshioka, M. (2007). Fluctuations of pesticide levels in the environment following aerial spraying in the paddy field. *Proceedings of 16th Symposium on Environmental Chemistry*, Japanese Society for Environmental Chemistry, pp. 576 - 577.

[21] Sudo, M., Hasukawa, H., & Shibahara, F. (2008). Effects of practicing environmental-conscious agriculture on paddy pesticide loading. *Yosui to Haisui, 50*, 54 - 62.

[22] Narita, I. & Nakamura, K. (2002). Fate of pesticides by aerial application in atmosphere and water. *Bulletin of Saitama Agricultural Experiment Station, 2,* 1 - 8.

[23] Kawata, K., Asada, T., Oikawa, K., & Tanabe, A. (2005). Multiresidue determination of pesticides in sediment by ultrasonically assisted extraction and gas chromatography/mass spectrometry. *Journal of AOAC International, 88*, 1440-1451.

[24] Kawata, K., Mukai, H., & Yasuhara, A. (1995). Monitoring of pesticides in air by gas chromatography/mass spectrometry and the use of quartz-fiber wool and activated carbon for sampling. *Journal of Chromatography A, 710*, 243-250.

[25] Suzuki, S., Otani, T., Iwasaki, S., Ito, K., Omura, H., & Tanaka, Y. (2003). Monitoring of 15 Pesticides in Rainwater in Utsunomiya, Eastern Japan, 1999-2000. J *Journal of Pesticide Science, 28*, 1-7.

[26] Tanabe, A., Mitobe, H., Kawata, K., Sakai, M., & Yasuhara, A. (2000). A new monitoring system for 90 pesticides and related compounds in river water by solid-phase extraction with gas chromatography/mass spectrometry. *Journal of AOAC International, 83*, 61-77.

[27] Iwashita, M., Maeda, T., Hori, T., Asada, T., Oikawa, K., & Kawata, K. (2008). Decrease of 4,5,6,7-Tetrachlorophthalide in Paddy Field Soil after Aerial Application. *Proceedings of 17th Symposium on Environmental Chemistry*, Japanese Society for Environmental Chemistry, 760 - 761.

[28] Kawata, K., & Yasuhara, A. (1994). Determination of Fenitrothion and Diazinon in Air. *Bulletin of the Environmental Contamination and Toxicology, 52*, 419 - 424.

[29] Fox. GA., Pulijala. SH., & Sabbagh, G.J. (2007). Influence of rainfall distribution on simulations of atrazine, metolachlor, and isoxaflutole/metabolite transport in subsurface drained fields. *Journal of Agricultural and Food Chemistry, 55*, 5399 - 5407.

[30] Inao, K. (2004). Development and validation of simulation model for predicting pesticide behavior in paddy rice environment. *Bulletin of National Institute for Agro-Environmental Sciences, 23,* 27 - 76.

In: Fungicides
Editors: P. De Costa and P. Bezerra
ISBN: 978-1-60692-631-4

Short Communication B

ANTIFUNGAL ACTIVITIES OF GLYCOLIPIDS SECRETED BY THE YEAST

Tatyana V. Kulakovskaya, Ekaterina V. Kulakovskaya, Wladyslav I. Golubev

Skryabin Institute of Biochemistry and Physiology of Microorganisms, Russian Academy of Sciences, Pushchino, Moscow Region, 142290 Russia

ABSTRACT

Many yeasts secrete glycolipids into the medium. Among these compounds, sophorolipids, cellobiose lipids, and mannosylerythritols are best studied. Cellobiose lipids differ in their structures, including the number of OH-groups in fatty acid residue and number and structures of O-substituents in cellobiose residue. For example, *Cryptococcus humicola* secretes mainly 16-(tetra-O-acetyl-β-cellobiosyloxy)-2-hydroxyhexadecanoic acid, while *Pseudozyma fusiformata* and *Pseudozyma graminicola* secrete mainly 16-[6-O-acetyl-2'-O-(3-hydroxyhexanoyl)-β-cellobiosyloxy)]-2,15-dihydroxyhexadecanoic acid. Recently it has been found that these compounds, known as surfactants, are highly active against many species of ascomycetous and basidiomycetous yeast and mycelial fungi. They exhibit maximal activity at pH ~ 4.0. The effective concentrations against basidiomycetes (*Filobasidiella neoformans*) and ascomycetes (*Candida* spp.) are 0.03 mM and 0.1-0.4 mM, respectively. The mechanism of action of cellobiose lipids on yeast cells is based on enhancement of nonspecific permeability of the cytoplasmic membrane, which results in the rapid leakage of ATP and potassium ions from the yeast cells treated with these compounds. The broad spectrum of activity, pH and temperature stability allow one to consider cellobiose lipids as promising natural biocontrol agents of yeast and mycelial fungi.

INTRODUCTION

Today, mycoses have become widespread because of mass application of antibiotics and abundance of immunodeficiency states. Their control, as well as the control of plant diseases and food spoiling caused by fungi calls forth the necessity of search for and development of novel fungicidal agents.

Quite recently, it has been revealed that extracellular glycolipids secreted by some yeast species and being biosurfactants [1-5] possess antifungal activity [6]. Glycolipids are carbohydrates in combination with long chain aliphatic acids or hydroxyl-aliphatic acids. Multiple biological activities and potential applications of extracellular yeast glycolipids are discussed in reviews [1-5]. Here, the prospects of application of biosurfactants as antimicrobial, in particular, fungicidal compounds are considered as well.

Glycolipids of various types, such as mannosylerythritols, sophorolipids, and cellobiose lipids, are produced by *Cryptococcus, Candida, Geotrichum, Kurtzmanomyces, Pseudozyma,* and *Ustilago* species [1-6]. Among them, cellobiose lipids as fungicidal compounds have been studied best of all. Cellobiose lipids were revealed as extracellular products of *Ustilago maydis* long ago [7-9]. However, their function and biological activities were obscure and the observed antibiotic activity was low [8]. It has also been shown that the yeasts *Cryptococcus humicola* [10] and *Pseudozyma fusiformata* [11] produce non-protein compounds, which inhibit the growth of a wide range of both ascomycetous and basidiomycetous yeasts, including medically important species of the genera *Filobasidiella, Malassezia,* and *Trichosporon.* Fungicidal activities were exhibited at pH 3-5 induced by thermostable compounds, insensitive to proteinases, with molecular masses below 1000 kDa [10, 11]. Cellobiose lipids that proved to be responsible for this activity were purified later from the culture liquid of these and some other yeast species [12-14]. This review pursues primarily consideration of the data on the fungicidal activity of cellobiose lipids.

CELLOBIOSE LIPID STRUCTURES

Glycolipid structures are determined by NMR spectroscopy and mass spectrometry. The known natural antifungal glycolipids contain cellobiose (1-4-β-D-glucopyranosyl-D-glucose) linked by glycoside bond to saturated fatty hydroxyl acids. However, they differ in the structures of O-substituents in the cellobiose residue and in the number of hydroxyl groups in the fatty acid residue. Figure 1 shows the structures of some cellobiose lipids. In *Cr. humicola,* 16-(tetra-O-acetyl-β-cellobiosyloxy)-2-hydroxyhexadecanoic acid (Cellobiose lipid 1, Figure 1) was structurally defined as the major product [12, 15, 16], while 16-(tetra-O-acetyl-β-cellobiosyloxy)-2,15-dihydroxyhexadecanoic acid [12, 17] and cellobiose lipids containing 2,15,16-trihydroxyoctadecanoic acid or 2,16-dihydroxyoctadecanoic acid [12] were identified as minor products. *Cr. humicola* belongs to tremellaceous yeasts, while other producers of cellobiose lipids are phylogenetically affiliated with the Ustilaginomycetes. *Sympodiomycopsis paphiopedili* was found to secrete 16-cellobiosyloxy)-2,15-dihydroxyhexadecanoic acid [13]. *Ps. fusiformata* [14] and *Ps. graminicola* [18] secretes mainly 16-[6-O-acetyl-2'-O-(3-hydroxyhexanoyl)-β-cellobiosyloxy)-2,15-dihydroxyhexadecanoic acid (Cellobiose lipid 2, Figure 1). *Pseudozyma flocculosa* secrete 16-[6-O-acetyl-2'-O-(3-hydroxyoktanoyl)-β-2-acetyl-cellobiosyloxy)-2,15-dihydroxyhexadecanoic acid (Cellobiose lipid 3, Figure 1) [19]. Cellobiose lipids similar to those produced by the yeast of the genus *Pseudozyma* have been obtained previously from the culture broth of *Ustilago maydis* [7-9].

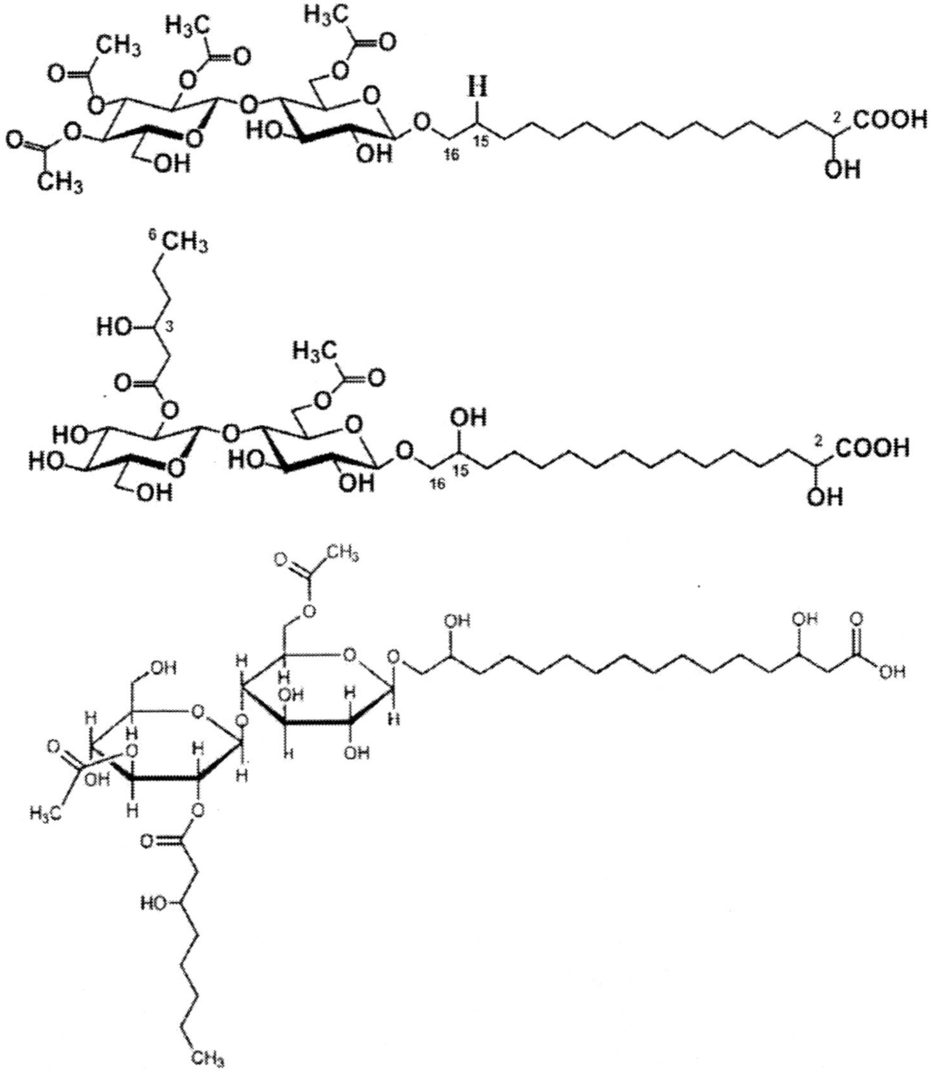

(1)

(2)

(3)

Figure 1. The structures of cellobiose lipids from culture broth of *Cryptococcus humicola* (1), *Pseudozyma fusiformata* (2) and *Pseudozyma flocculosa* (3).

ANTIFUNGAL ACTIVITIES OF CELLOBIOSE LIPIDS

The killer patterns of cellobiose lipids are not taxonomically specific. The "culture-to-culture" testing shows (Table 1) that *Ps. fusiformata,* a producer of these cellobiose lipids, inhibit the growth of nearly all strains of the yeast, yeast-like and filamentous fungi of about 300 species of Ascomycota and Basidiomycota. The spectrum of antifungal activity of *Ps. fusiformata* is close to that of *Cr. humicola* when tested by the same method [10]. Basidiomycetous yeasts are more sensitive to these compounds than ascomycetes.

Table 1. Yeast organisms (the number of tested strains and species) which growth is inhibited by *Pseudozyma fusiformata* VKM Y-2821 under "culture-to-culture" testing [11]

Agaricostilbum (1,1)	Mrakia (2, 3)
Arthroascus (1, 1)	Myxozyma (4, 4)
Arxula (1, 1)	Nadsonia (1, 1)
Bensingtonia (6, 6)	Pichia (1, 1)
Bullera (11, 30)	Platygloea (1, 1)
Bullerumyces (1,1)	Protomyces (1, 1)
Candida (2, 2)	Puccinia (1, 1)
Cryptococcus (33, 33)	Rhodosporidium (1, 1)
Cystofilobasidium (4, 4)	Rhodotorula (34, 43)
Debaryomyces (7, 7)	Saccharomyces (1, 1)
Dipodascus (1, 1)	Septobasidium (1, 1)
Entyloma (1, 1)	Sorosporium (1, 1)
Erythrobasidium (1, 1)	Sphacelotheca (1, 1)
Exobasidium (6, 8)	Sporidiobolus (3, 3)
Farysia (1, 1)	Sporisorium (2, 3)
Fellomyces (3, 3)	Sporobolomyces (22, 25)
Filobasidiella (1, 44)	Stephanoascus (1,1)
Filobasidium(2, 4)	Sterigmatomyces (2, 2)
Guilliermondella (1,1)	Sympodiomycopsis (1, 1)
Gymnosporangium (1, 1)	Taphrina (8, 8)
Holtermannia (1,1)	Tausonia (1, 1)
Issatchenkia (1,1)	Tilletiaria (1, 1)
Itersonilia (1,2)	Tilletiopsis (7, 9)
Kockovaella (1,1)	Torulaspora (1,1)
Kurtzmanomyces (1,1)	Trichosporon (11, 12)
Leucosporidim (2, 2)	Trimorphomyces (1,1)
Lipomyces (3, 3)	Udeniomyces (3, 12)
Lodderomyces (1,1)	Ustilago (10, 12)
Malassezia (2, 2)	Wickerhamia (1, 1)
Mastigobasidium (1, 1)	Xanthophyllomyces (1, 4)
Mastigomyces (1, 1)	Zygozyma (1, 1)
Microbotryum (4, 4)	

The number of species and strains tested is shown in the parenthesis.

Table 2. The concentrations of cellobiose lipids (1) and (2) causing complete death of the cells of test cultures after 30-min incubation (pH 4.0)

Test culture	Concentration, mM	
	Cellobiose lipid (1)	Cellobiose lipid (2)
Basidiomycetous		
Cryptococcus terreus VKM Y-2253	0.023	0.026
Filobasidiella neoformans IGC 3957	0.027	0.026
Trichosporon asahii VKM Y-803	0.06	0.09
Trichosporon faecalis VKM Y-2865	0.18	0.18
Ascomycetous		
Candida albicans JCM 1542	0.19	0.19
Candida glabrata CBS 138	0.38	0.39
Clavispora lusitaniae IGC 2705	0.19	0.13
Candida parapsilosis VKM Y-58	0.29	0.26
Candida tropicalis RBF-988	0.64	0.26
Candida viswanathii CBS 4024	0.19	0.13
Saccharomyces cerevisiae VKM Y-1173	0.38	0.39

Figure 2 shows growth inhibition activities of purified cellobiose lipids obtained from the culture broth of *Cr. humicola* and *Ps. fusiformata* against different yeast species. The dependences of the sizes of growth inhibition zones on the amounts of glycolipids under cultivation of test cultures on an agar medium were similar for compounds (1) and (2). As for the viability test, the data are presented in Table 2. Cellobiose lipids 1 and 2 inhibit the growth of a number of medically important species: *Candida albicans, Candida glabrata, Candida viswanathii, Filobasidiella neoformans, Clavispora lusitaniae* and other species. Cellobiose lipids were more efficient against basidiomycetous yeasts of the genera *Cryptococcus* and *Filobasidiella* than against ascomycetous yeasts of the genera *Saccharomyces*, *Candida*, and *Clavispora*.

The growth of mycelial fungi under study was more efficiently inhibited by cellobiose lipid (2) than cellobiose lipid (1). The amount of glycolipid (2) giving growth inhibition zones for phytopathogenic fungus *Sclerotinia sclerotiorum* was 5 times lower as compared with the amount of cellobiose lipid (1) (Figure 3). *Phomopsis helianthii* and *Mucor mucedo* were also less sensitive to the cellobiose lipid (1). Cellobiose lipid (2) with hydroxycaproic acid as O-substitute and the second hydroxyl group in the fatty acid residue is more effective against myceial fungi than cellobiose lipid (1) with only acetate groups as O-substitutes and a single OH-group in the fatty acid residue. The question of how these peculiarities affect the activity against mycelial fungi needs further investigation.

Cellobiose lipid (3) of *Pseudozyma flocculosa* was active against different strains of *C. albicans, C. glabrata, C. lusitanie,* and *Trichosporon asahii* [19]. The minimal inhibitory concentration (MIC) for all strains was 50 μg/mL at pH 5 and tenfold higher (500 μg/mL) at pH 7.0 [19]. This cellobiose lipid was also active against phytopathogeic fungi, such as *Phomopsis* sp., *Sphaerotheca fulginea,* and other species [20]. This is in agreement with the peculiarities of its structure, which is close to the structure of cellobiose lipid (2).

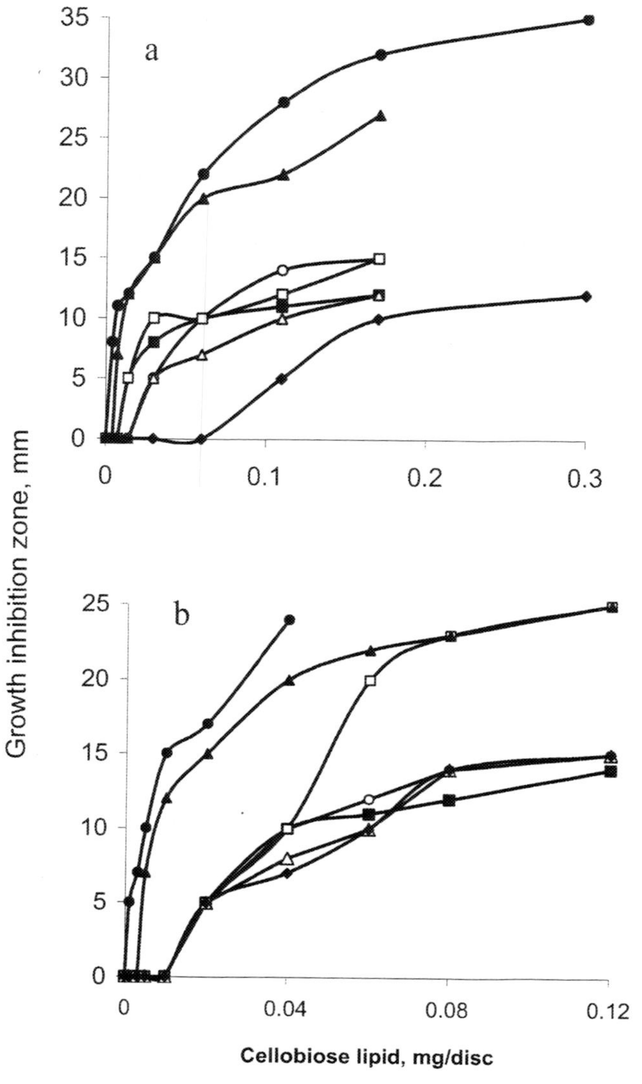

Figure 2. The inhibition of yeast growth by cellobiose lipid 1 (a) and 2 (b). The aliquots of methanol solution of cellobiose lipids were placed onto sterile 5-mm diameter glass microfiber filter discs GF/C, and after drying the disc were placed onto the surface agar medium (0.5% glucose, 0.2% yeast extract, 0.25% peptone,2% agar with citrate-phosphate buffer, pH 4.0) inoculated with a strain examined.

Fully O-deacylated analogue, namely 16-(β-cellobiosyloxy)-2-hydroxyhexadecanoic acid and synthetic compound 16-(β-cellobiosyloxy)-hexadecanoic acid did not exhibit any activities against *Saccharomyces cerevisiae*, *F. neoformans,* and *C. albicans*, while fully deacylated analogue 16-(β-cellobiosyloxy)-2,15-dihydroxyhexadecanoic acid exhibited growth inhibition zones of no more than 8-10 mm even at application of 1 mg of compound per disk [17]. Thus, the structures of the carbohydrate part and fatty acid aglycon moiety influence the fungicidal activity of cellobiose lipids under study.

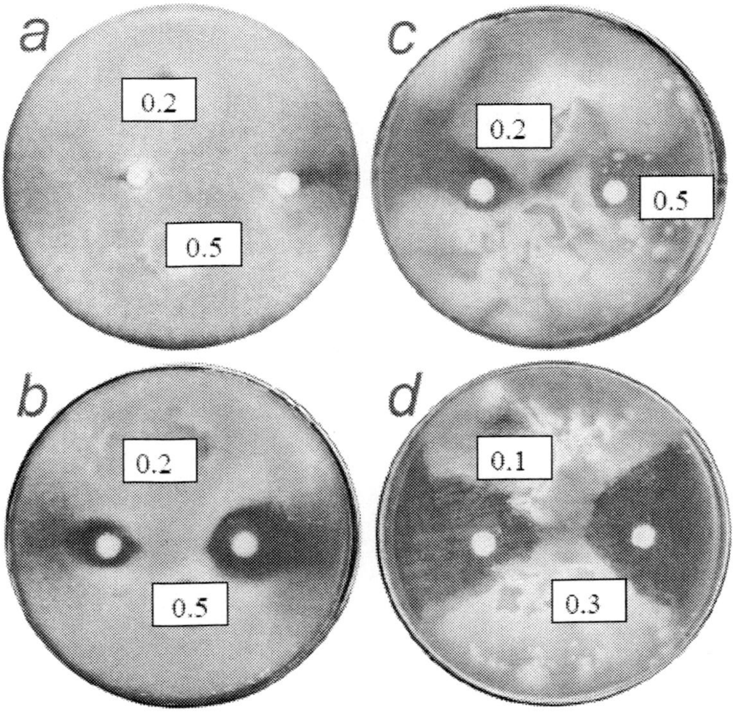

Figure 3. The inhibition of fungi growth by cellobiose lipids: a - *Sclerotinia sclerotiorum,* cellobiose lipid (1); b – *Sc. sclerotiorum,* cellobiose lipid (2); c - *Mucor mucedo* VKM F-1355, cellobiose lipid (1); d - *M. mucedo* VKM F-1355, cellobiose lipid (2) The amount of cellobiose lipids per disc in indicated by numbers.

One of characteristic features of cellobiose lipids is the pH optima of fungicide action. The antifungal activity is maximal at pH 3-4.5 [14, 15, 19] and abruptly drops at pH increase. This observation is true for the test systems including culture-to-culture growth on solid media [10, 11] and for the experiments with purified cellobiose lipids tested both on agar and in liquid media [14, 15, 16].

Temperature (25 or 37 °C) had little effect on the activity of cellobiose lipid of *Ps. flocculosa* [19]. For cellobiose lipid of *Ps. fusiformata,* the fungicidal activity was reported to increase at a temperature rise from 10 to 30°C [21].

Mechanisms of Action of Cellobiose Lipids

All of the known glycolipids are surface-active compounds reducing the surface tension of water solutions. Cellobiose lipids of *Cr. humicola* have a high surface activity comparable with that of SDS [12]. The effects of the mixture of these *Cr. humicola* cellobiose lipids on permeability of artificial planar lipid bilayers of various compositions were investigated [12]. The primary effect was current fluctuation, and only then membrane disruption was observed. The intercalation of glycolipid of *Cr. humicola* into liposomes containing diphytanoylphosphatidylcholine, ergosterol, and phosphatydilserine was demonstrated [12].

These data suggest that the mycocidal effect of cellobiose lipids is associated with its detergent-like properties. Based on these observations and on the electrical measurements on planar phospholipid bilayers, which showed glycolipid-induced membrane permeabilization, it was suggested that the cytoplasmic membrane is the primary target of cellobiose lipid activity. The ATP leakage from *Cr. terreus* cells treated by cellobiose lipid of *Cr. humicola* was demonstrated and compared with the similar effect of the known antibiotic nystatin [12].

The ATP leakage from yeast cells treated with the purified glycolipids of *Symp. paphiopedili* [13] and *Ps. fusiformata* was maximal at pH 4.0-4.5 and 20-30°C [14, 21]. The cells treated with cellobiose lipids are stained by bromocresol purple, a fluorescent dye that does not penetrate into yeast cells with the intact plasma membrane [21]. Figure 4 shows the dependence of ATP leakage on concentrations of cellobiose lipids (1) and (2) from the cells of different yeast species. Comparison of the data from Figure 4 and Table 2 demonstrates that the minimal concentrations causing the death of yeast cells and ATP leakage from them are similar for the same yeast species.

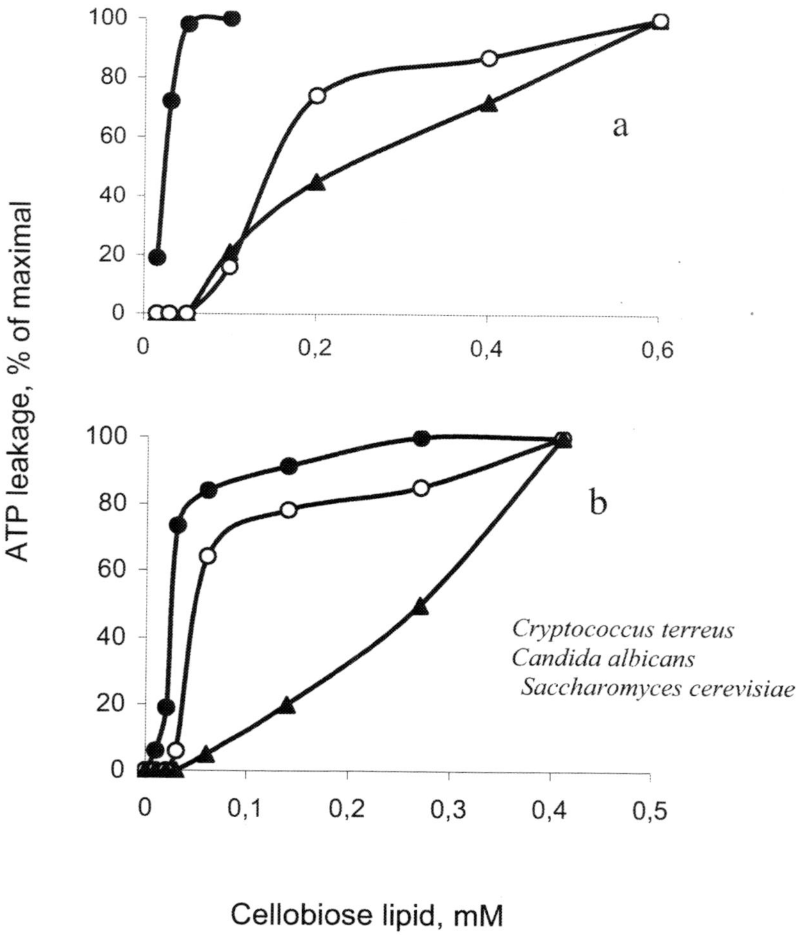

Figure 4. The effect of cellobiose lipids 1 (a) and 2 (b) on ATP leakage from yeast cells at pH 4.0 and 20°C.

The leakage of potassium ions from the cells of *S. cerevisiae* and *Cr. terreus* under the influence of cellobiose lipids from *Cr. humicola* and *Ps. fusiformata* was also shown to develop in the first 5 min of treatment, like the leakage of ATP [22]. The obtained results suggest that the primary effect induced by glycolipids is the increasing permeability of the yeast cytoplasmic membrane. The question why basidiomycetes are more sensitive to cellobiose lipids than ascomycetes is still open. Probably, it is associated both with the peculiarities of their lipid membrane composition and with the peculiarities of cell wall structure.

FUNGICIDAL ACTIVITY OF OTHER DETERGENTS AND YEAST GLYCOLIPIDS

The comparison of effective concentrations of different glycolipids, both natural and synthetic, against yeast and fungal cultures, reported by different authors [2, 12, 19, 20], is an intricate problem because of different methods used for their determination and different species and strains used as test cultures. Sometimes it is impossible to assess the antifungal efficiency of glycolipids, when experiments are performed at neutral pH values.

As regards MEL and sophorolipids, there are the data on rather low antifungal activity as compared with cellobiose lipids [2]. Well- known biosurfactent rhamnolipid altered the polypeptide profiles of cell and membrane proteins in the same way as Triton X-100 but have no effect on the growth kinetics of *S. cerevisiae* [23]. Sophorolipid and rhamnolipid were tested as antifungal agents against plant pathogenic fungi [24]. Rhamnolipid, 200 mg/L, or sophorolipid, 500 mg/L, inhibited the mycelial growth of plant pathogens (*Phytophthora* sp. and *Pythium* sp.) by 8%. The zoospore motility of Phytophthorá sp. decreased by 90% in the presence of 50 mg/L of rhamnolipid and by 80% in the presence of 100 mg/L of sophorolipid. For *Phytophthora capsici,* the 80% lysis was observed with 100 mg/l of di-rhamnolipid or lactonic sophorolipid. These results showed the potential of these biosurfactants as antifungal agents against damping-off plant pathogens [24]. There is a patent informing that sophorolipids and some of their derivatives are able to inhibit the growth of *Candida albicans* by 20-40% in the concentration of 5 mg/mL (~ 5 mM) [25].

The fatty acids of MEL have short chains and sophorolipids are lactonized in an acid medium, which may complicate incorporation into the lipid bilayer [26] and, hence, reduce the ability for cellular membrane damaging.

At consideration of the mechanism of fungicidal effect of cellobiose lipids, it should be noted that fatty acids, the residues of which are the main hydrophobic component of these compounds, are known as uncouplers that destroy the ion gradients on biological membranes. The data on the fungicidal effect of fatty acids are available in the literature. Hydroperoxy- and hydroxy-derivatives of linoleic and linolenic acids, produced by plants, are components of the system of plant protection from phytopathogenic fungi [27, 28]. It has been shown that 6-nondecanoic acid inhibits the growth of *Filobasidiella neoformans* at a concentration of about 0.004 mM but is ineffective against *Candida albicans* [29]. Antifungal activity is typical of not only unsaturated but also some saturated fatty acids. In particular, the C_{10} and C_{12} saturated fatty acids inhibit the growth of *Candida albicans* in the concentration of 2.5-5 mM [30]. For comparison, cellobiose lipids inhibit the growth of *C. albicans* in the concentration of 0.2 mM.

Since glycolipids are promising as fungicides, the studies are performed on obtaining and biological testing of various synthetic analogs. However, their fungicidal activities are often lower than those of natural cellobiose lipids. For example, alkyl 2,6-dedeoxy-L-arabino-hexopyranosides obtained synthetically and possessing the high surface activity were less active against *C. albicans* than cellobiose lipids, giving inhibition zones of no more than 10 mm at application of 0.3 mg of this compound [31].

Various strains of pathogenic species, including *Candida albicans* and *Filobasidiella neoformans,* significantly differ in sensitivity to the well-studied antifungal preparations such as nystatin and fluconasols (from 0.019 to 10 mg/L) [32]. The wide application of these preparations results in the increase of the number of resistant strains. Hence, cellobiose lipids, due to their low toxicity for human and animal cells [19], are challenging for development of novel fungicides. For cellobiose lipid of *Ps. flocculosa*, the combined application with amphotericin B was proposed with the purpose of decreasing the effective concentrations of both compounds [20]. There is a patent that describes the methods of production of *Ps. flocculosa* cellobiose lipid and its testing as a fungicidal preparation [33].

Conclusion

Cellobiose lipids of the yeast are natural detergents, which at relatively low concentrations (as compared with such compounds as SDS and other widely used synthetic detergents) can induce cell death of the yeast and mycelial fungi. This effect is conditioned by their membrane-damaging properties. The above compounds are characterized by the maximal activity at acid pH values, thermal stability, and low toxicity for animal cells. The experiments on colonization of plants by the producer of these compounds, *Ps. fusiformata,* have shown the absence of negative effect on growth and increase of resistance to fungal diseases [34]. Cellobiose lipids are interesting for development of novel antifungal preparations and for joint application with the known antibiotics for reducing their effective concentrations. Besides, these compounds can be used in laboratory practice as membrane-damaging agents.

References

[1] Spencer, JFT; Spencer, DM; Tulloch, AP. Extracellular glycolipids of yeasts. In: A. H. Rose AH editor. *Economic Microbiology*, vol. 3, Secondary Products of Metabolism, Acad. Press, London, 1979, 523-540.

[2] Kitamoto, D; Isoda, Y; Nakahara, T. Functions and potential applications of glycolipid biosurfactants – from energy-saving material to gene delivery carriers. *J. Biosci. Bioeng.*, 2002, 94, 87-201.

[3] Cameotra, SS; Makkar, RS. Recent applications of biosurfactants as biological and immunological molecules. *Cur. Opin. Microbiol.*, 2004, 7, 262-266.

[4] Van Bogaert, INA; Saerens, K; De Muynck, C; Develter, D; Soetaert, W; Vandamme, EJ. 2007. Microbial production and application of sophorolipids. *Appl. Microbiol. Biotechnol.* 2007, 76, 23-34.

[5] Rodrigues, L; Banat, IM; Teixeira, J; Oliveira, R. Biosurfactants: potential application in medicine. *J. Antimicrob. Chemother.*, 2007, 57, 609-618.

[6] Golubev, WI. Antagonistic interactions among yeast. In: *Biodiversity and Ecophysiology of the Yeasts,* Berlin Verlag, 2006, 197-219.

[7] Lemieux, RU; Thorn, JA; Brice, C; Haskins, RH Biochemistry of the ustilaginales. II. Isolation and partial characterization of ustilagic acid. *Can. J. Chem.*, 1951, 29, 409-414.

[8] Haskins, RH; Thorn, JA Biochemistry of the Ustilaginales. VII. Antibiotic activity of ustilagic acid. *Can. J. Botany*, 1951, 29, 585-592.

[9] Bhattacharjee, SS; Haskins, RH; Gorin, PAJ. Location of acyl groups on two partly acylated glycolipids from strains of *Ustilago* (smut fungi). *Carbohydr. Res.*,1970, 13, 235-246.

[10] Golubev, W; Shabalin, Y. Microcin production in *Cryptococcus humicola. FEMS Microbiol. Lett.*, 2004, 119, 105-110.

[11] Golubev, VI, Kulakovskaia, TV, Golubeva, EV. *Pseudozyma fusiformata* BKM Y-2821-a producer of antifungal glycolipid. *Mikrobiologiia,* 2001, 70, 642-646.

[12] Puchkov, EO; Zahringer, U; Lindner, B; Kulakovskaya, TV; Seydel, U; Wiese, A. Mycocidal, membrane-active complex of *Cryptococcus humicola,* is a new type of cellobiose lipid with detergent features. *Biochim. Biophys. Acta (Biomembranes),* 2002, 1558, 161-170.

[13] Kulakovskaya, TV; Shashkov, AS; Kulakovskaya, EV; Golubev, WI. Characterization of antifungal glycolipid secreted by the yeast *Sympodiomycopsis paphiopedili. FEMS Yeast Res.*, 2004, 5, 247-252.

[14] Kulakovskaya, TV; Shashkov, AS; Kulakovskaya, EV; Golubev, WI. Ustilagig acid secretion by *Pseudozyma fusiformata* strains. *FEMS Yeast Res.*, 2005, 5, 919-923.

[15] Kulakovskaya, EV; Golubev, VI; Kulaev IS. Extracellular antifungal glycolipids of *Cryptococcus humicola* yeasts. *Dokl. Biol. Sci.*, 2006, 410, 393-395.

[16] Kulakovskaya, EV; Kulakovskaya, TV; Golubev, WI; Shashkov, AS; Grachev, AA; Nifantiev, NE. Fungicidal activity of cellobiose lipids from culture broth of yeast *Cryptococcus humicola* and *Pseudozyma fusiformata. Russian J. Bioor. Chem.,* 2007, 33, 156-161.

[17] Kulakovskaya, TV; Shashkov, AS; Kulakovskaya, EV; Golubev WI; Zinin, AI; Tsvetkov, EY; Grachev, AA; Nifantiev, NE. Structures and fungicidal activities of cellobiose lipids. In: *Glycolipids: New Research.* Nova Science Publishers, Inc. 2008. pp. 171-184

[18] Golubev, WI; Kulakovskaya, TV; Shashkov, AS; Kulakovskaya, EV; Golubev NV. Antifungal cellobiose lipid secreted by the epiphytic yeast *Pseudozyma graminicola. Microbiology*, 2008, 77, 171-176.

[19] Mimee, B; Labbe, C; Pelletier, R; Belanger, RR. Antifungal activity of flocculosin, a novel glycolipid isolated from *Pseudozyma flocculosa. Antimicrob. Agents Chemother.*, 2005, 49, 1597-1599.

[20] Cheng, Y; McNally, DJ; Labbe, C; Voyer, N; Belzyle, F; Belanger, RR. Insertional mutagenesis of a fungal biocontrol agent led to a discovery of a rare cellobiose lipid with antifungal activity. *Appl. Environ. Microbiol.*, 2003, 69, 2595-2602.

[21] Kulakovskaya, TV; Kulakovskaya, EV; Golubev, WI. ATP leakage from yeast cells treated by extracellular glycolipids of *Pseudozyma fusiformata. FEMS Yeast Res.*, 2003, 3, 401-404.

[22] Kulakovskaya, EV; Ivanov, AY; Kulakovskaya, TV; Vagabov, VM; Kulaev IS. Effects of cellobiose lipid B on *Saccharomyces cerevisiae* cells: K^+ leakage and inhibition of polyphosphate accumulation *Microbiology*. 2008, 77, 288 -293.

[23] Vasileva-Tonkova, E; Galabova, D; Karoenko, E; Shulga A. Biosurfactant-rhamnolipid effects on yeast cells. *Lett. Appl. Microbiol.* 2001, 33, 280-284.

[24] Yoo Dal-Soo; Lee Baek-Seok; Kim Eun-Ki Characteristics of microbial biosurfactant as an antifungal agent against plant pathogenic fungus. *J. Microbiol. Biotechnol.*, 2005, 15, 1164-1169.

[25] Gross, RA; Shah, V. Antifungal Properties of Various Forms of Sophorolipids, United States Patent 20050164955. Publication Date:07/28/2005

[26] Nunez, A; Foglia, TA; Ashby, R. Enzymatic synthesis of a galactopyranose sophorolipid fatty acid-ester. *Biotechnol. Lett.*, 2003, 25,1291-1297.

[27] Hou, CT; Forman, R J. Growth inhibition of plant pathogenic fungi by hydroxy fatty acids. *J. Industr. Microbiol. Biotechnol.* 2000, 24, 275-276.

[28] Graner, G; Hamberg, M; Meijer, J. Screening of oxylipins for control of oilseed rape (*Brassica napus)* fungal pathogens. *Phytochemistry,* 2003, 63, 89-95.

[29] Carballeira, NM; Sanabria, D; Parang, K. Total synthesis and further scrutiny of the in vitro Antifungal activity of 6-nonadecynoic acid. *Arch Pharm (Weinheim)*. 2005, 338, 441-443.

[30] Bergsson, G; Arnfinnsson, J; Steingrimsson, O; Thormar H. In vitro killing of *Candida albicans* by fatty acids and monoglycerides. *Antimicrob Agents Chemother.*, 2001, 45, 3209-3212.

[31] Rauter, AP; Lucas, S; Almeida, T; Sacoto, D; Ribeiro, V; Justino, J; Neves, A; Silva, FV; Oliveira, MC; Ferreira, MJ; Santos, MS; Barbosa, E. Synthesis, surface active and antimicrobial properties of new alkyl 2,6-dideoxy-l-arabino-hexopyranosides. *Carbohydr. Res.*, 2005, 340, 191-201.

[32] Carrillo-Munoz, AJ; Quindos, G; Tur, C; Ruesga, MT; Miranda, Y; del Valle, O; Cossum, PA; Wallace, TJ. In-vitro antifungal activity of liposomal nystatin in comparison with nystatin, amphotericin B cholesteryl sulphate, liposomal amphotericin B, amphotericin B lipid complex, amphotericin B desoxycholate, fluconazole and itraconazole. *J. Antimicrob. Chemother.*, 1999, 44, 397-401.

[33] Belanger, R; Labbe, C; Cheng Y; McNally, D. Flocculosin-CA antimicrobial molecule. Canadian Patent CA2492666 Publication Date: 2004/01/22.

[34] Georgievskaya, EB, Zacharchenko NS; Buryanov IY; Golubew WI. (2006) The effect of yeast *Pseudozyma fusiformata* on the resistance of plants to white mould agent *Sclerotinia sclerotiorum.* Mycologia and Phytopatologya (In Russian), 2006, 40, 53-58.

In: Fungicides
Editors: P. De Costa and P. Bezerra

ISBN: 978-1-60692-631-4

Chapter I

METABOLIC AND INTERACTION PROPERTIES OF SELECTED FUNGICIDES

Khaled Abass*[*], *Petri Reponen and Olavi Pelkonen
Department of Pharmacology and Toxicology, University of Oulu, Finland
Department of Chemistry, University of Oulu, Finland

ABSTRACT

Currently public concern about the impact of pesticides, including fungicides, on human health is greater than ever before. Pesticides are essential in agricultural production, but they constitute a potential risk to humans who are exposed to them directly through various ways and indirectly through the diet. Accordingly, the health risk assessment of pesticides is of utmost importance for the protection of human health. Risk assessment needs reliable scientific information and one source of information is the characterization of the metabolic factors and toxicokinetics. Indeed, quantitative toxicokinetic data in humans are needed for human risk assessment to make reliable comparisons between individuals or between species. Because humans cannot be used as study subjects except in occasional circumstances, we have to rely upon in vitro experiments, human-derived techniques and in vitro – in vivo predictions as well. In the usual course of events, the more we know about pesticides in terms of their metabolic characteristic in vitro, the better we will be in extrapolation of in vitro and animal studies into human risk assessment.

Cytochrome P450 enzymes are important in the metabolism of various endogenous substrates as well as a wide range of xenobiotics. The metabolism may results in activation and/or detoxification reactions. Basically, metabolic factors such as metabolic routes, identification of the major and minor metabolites, metabolite stability, metabolizing enzymes, interindividual variability, interspecies differences and the

[*] Correspondence: Khaled M. Abass. Department of Pharmacology and Toxicology. Institute of Biomedicine, PO Box 5000; FIN-90014, University of Oulu, Finland. Tel +358 8 5375011; E-mail: khaled.megahed@oulu.fi; khaled.m.abass@gmail.com

inhibitory interactions are providing important quantitative data for chemical risk assessment.

In this review we will briefly describe the in vitro techniques used to study in vitro metabolism and interactions, summarize the metabolic and kinetic properties of selected fungicides and provide an example from our own studies about how to apply current techniques to obtain relevant data for risk assessment.

Keywords: Human-derived Techniques, In vitro metabolism, Risk assessment, Fungicides

INTRODUCTION

Pesticides are widely used in agriculture, sanitation and pest control. Inevitably humans are exposed to them in various ways: workers in chemical plants when manufacturing raw materials and final products, agricultural workers when using them in the fields and general public as residues in food staffs. In general, protecting public health is the primary reason why risk assessment of pesticides is of utmost importance. Risk assessment needs reliable scientific information and one source of information is the characterisation of metabolic fate and toxicokinetics of pesticides. Because humans cannot be used as study subjects except in occasional circumstances, we have to rely upon in vitro and animal experiments. We have been developing in vitro approaches to screen metabolic properties of any chemical substances, using human tissues and genetically engineered experimental systems. We have also applied these experimental systems for the metabolic characterisation of selected pesticides.

Pesticides are metabolized by many enzymes, including the cytochrome P450 enzymes, which play a key role in the metabolism of a wide variety of xenobiotics (phase I metabolism). We have to carry out studies, trying to answer some scientifically important questions: What is the metabolic stability of the compound? What kinds of metabolites are formed? What are the specific enzymes and isoforms involved? Is the reaction an activation or a detoxication reaction? Do induction and/or inhibition occur? The more we know about pesticides in terms of their metabolic fate in vitro, the better we will be in the extrapolation of in vitro and animal studies into human risk assessment.

Upon implementation of REACH legislation and in preparation for establishment of European Chemicals Agency (ECA) in Helsinki, there is a need for robust and quick methods to characterize metabolic fate and metabolic interactions of selected chemicals. One of the important groups is pesticides or in general agrochemicals. A scheme for metabolic studies has originally been developed for the screening of potential drugs at the preclinical screening phase and this scheme has been modified and applied for the study of pesticides metabolism and interactions.

1. Xenobiotic-Metabolizing Enzymes and their Role in Toxicokinetics

Xenobiotic biotransformation is the process by which lipophilic foreign compounds are detoxified through enzymatic biotransformation to hydrophilic metabolites that are eliminated directly via renal elimination or after conjugation with endogenous cofactors. These metabolic enzymes are divided into two groups, Phase I and Phase II enzymes (Figure 1) [1]. It is well recognized that these metabolic processes may lead to detoxification and/or activation reactions. Many compounds, such as organophosphorothionate, phosphorodithioate and phosphorothiloate insecticides, have been found to be activated. Bioactivation occur in these compounds via cytochrome P450 enzymes mediated desulfuration to phosphate oxon metabolites.

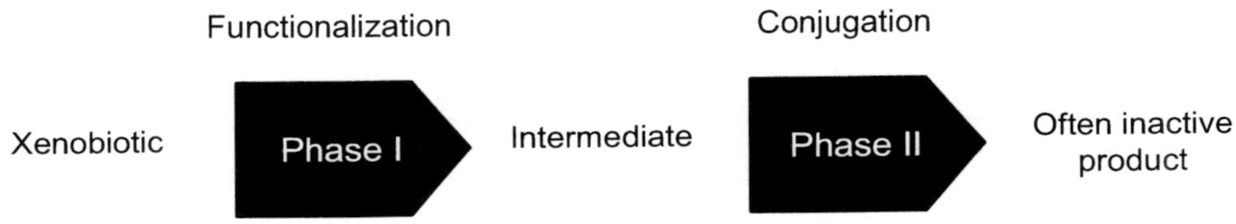

Figure 1. Xenobiotic metabolism. In general, a parent compound is converted into an intermediate metabolite which then forms conjugates, but metabolism may involve only one of these reactions. Some metabolites are more toxic than the parent compound (based on Oesch *et al.* [1]).

1.1. Phase I Enzymes and Reactions (Functionalization Reactions)

Phase I reactions, considered as functionalization reactions, add or uncover functional groups on xenobiotics with increasing polarity or nucleophilicity creating a suitable substrate for Phase II metabolism. Phase I reactions generally involve oxidation, reduction and hydrolytic reactions as well as other rarer miscellaneous reactions. Oxidation involves the enzymatic addition of oxygen, removal of hydrogen or changing the oxidative state of the xenobiotic. These reactions are mediated primarily by cytochrome P450 family of enzymes, but other enzymes (e.g. flavin monooxygenases, peroxidases, amine oxidases, dehydrogenases, xanthine oxidases) also catalyze oxidation of certain functional groups [2].

The P450 enzymes are hemoproteins with approximate molecular weight of 50,0000 Da. Theses enzymes catalyze the monooxidation of a wide variety of structurally unrelated compounds, including endogenous steroids and fatty acids and an essentially unlimited number of lipophilic xenobiotics. The cytochrome P450 enzymes are found in high concentration in the liver, but are present in a variety of other tissues, including lung [3,4], kidney [5,6] gastro intestinal tract [7,8], nasal mucosa [9,10], skin [11] and brain [12,13]. P450 enzymes are categorized into families and subfamilies by their sequence similarities. Humans have 18 families of cytochrome P450 genes and 44 subfamilies. The enzymes are thus identified by a number denoting the family, a letter denoting the subfamily and a number identifying the specific member of the subfamily. The web site, http://drnelson.utmem.

edu/CytochromeP450.html, contains more detailed classification related to the cytochrome P450 metabolizing enzymes. Human cytochrome P450 enzymes are of utmost importance because this class of metabolic enzymes are responsible for the metabolism of the majority of drugs [14,15].

Similar to the CYP family, flavin-containing monooxygenases (FMOs) are membrane bound metabolic enzymes utilizing NADPH and O_2. The microsomal FMO enzyme family is comprised of five isoforms: FMO1–FMO5 [16]. Currently there is evidence for several FMOs in human liver, but FMO3 seems to be the dominant isoform expressed in adult human liver microsomes [17].

In addition to the oxidative reactions there are different types of hydrolytic reactions catalysed by enzymes like carboxylesterases and epoxide hydrolases. Carboxylesterases are enzymes that commonly hydrolyze carboxylic, thio and phosphoric acid esters as well as amide bonds [18]. These enzymes are found in many tissues and fluids, such as liver, kidney, intestine and plasma.

Reduction reactions of certain functional groups are not as common as oxidative and hydrolytic reactions. However, reductions of ketones, nitro and azo compounds, N- and S-oxides, disulfides, quinones and alkenes as well as reductive dehalogenation have been noted in the literature.

1.2. Phase II Enzymes and Reactions (Conjugation Reactions)

Phase I products are not usually eliminated rapidly, but undergo a subsequent reaction in which an endogenous substrate such as glucuronic acid, sulfuric acid, acetic acid, or an amino acid combines with the newly established functional group to form a highly polar conjugate to make them more easily excreted. Several types of conjugation reactions are present in the body and most of them occur on heteroatoms, such as sulfur, nitrogen and oxygen. Some direct conjugations on carbon atoms can also occur. These reactions require cofactors which must be replenished through dietary sources.

Sulfation, glucuronidation and glutathione conjugation are the most prevalent classes of phase II metabolism, which may occur directly on the parent compounds that contain appropriate structural motifs, or, as is usually the case, on functional groups added or exposed by phase I oxidation. More detailed review on phase II metabolizing enzymes was published by Zamek-Gliszczynski *et al.*[19].

Glucuronidation is probably the most common form of conjugation reaction. In many ways glucuronidation complements sulfation, because conjugation with glucuronic acid occurs on many of the same molecular moieties as sulfation, but is most prevalent at higher substrate concentrations, when sulfation has become saturated either due to co-substrate depletion or enzyme saturation [19]. Uridine diphosphateglucuronosyl transferase (UGT) enzymes are subdivided into two families: UGT1 and UGT2. Isoenzymes in the UGT1A subfamily all contain a conserved C-terminal region that is responsible for UDPGA binding and attachment to the endoplasmic reticulum membrane and that is encoded by the same four exons. Glucuronidation is considered as the most prevalent form of conjugation due to the number of functional groups that can be glucuronidated, catalytic activity of the enzyme and high concentration of cofactor (UDPGA). Glucuronidation occurs by nucleophilic attack of an electron-rich heteroatom, typically oxygen, nitrogen, sulfur, and sometimes carbon.

The class of cytosolic sulfotransferases (SULT) enzymes belongs to a superfamily of enzymes that catalyze sulfation reactions. Enzymes are subdivided into three families: SULT1 [phenol sulfotransferases (PST) family], SULT2 [hydroxysteroid sulfotransferases (HST) family] and brain-specific SULT4 [20,21]. The sulfation reaction involves a high energy input from the cell because two molecules of ATP are necessary for the synthesis of one molecule of 3'-phosphoadenosine-5'-phosphosulfate (PAPS). Conjugation of hydroxyl, amino, N-oxide, and sulfhydryl groups on xenobiotics and small endobiotics with sulfate occurs in the cytosol, while sulfation of carbohydrates attached to peptides or lipids, as well as proteins occurs in the Golgi network [22].

Glutathione conjugation is catalyzed by a family of detoxification enzymes known as glutathione-*S*-transferases (GSTs). Glutathione conjugation is a reaction between the nucleophilic sulfur atom of cysteine and an electrophilic site on the xenobiotic forming a thiol ester (glutathione conjugate). A broad spectrum of diverse electrophiles can undergo glutathione conjugation. Molecular moieties amenable to glutathione conjugation include electrophilic carbon atoms as well as electrophilic nitrogen, oxygen, and sulfur atoms. Glutathione conjugates are not deconjugated in the same manner as sulfate or glucuronide metabolites. The peptide bonds in the glutathione molecule of the metabolite may be hydrolyzed sequentially to form a cysteinylglycine metabolite, which can be hydrolyzed to a cysteine metabolite, followed by N-acetylation to form a mercapturate metabolite [23].

Other phase II reactions (e.g. methylation, acetylation and amino acid conjugation) are less prevalent metabolic pathways for xenobiotics. Methylation involves the transfer of a methyl group from S-adenosylmethionine (SAM) by nucleophilic attack of an electron-rich heteroatom, such as nitrogen, oxygen, or sulphur, through an enzyme mediated reaction involving both microsomal and cytosolic methyl transferases [24-26]. Acetylation reactions are commonly found with nitrogen-containing substrates, such as aromatic and aliphatic amines, hydrazines, sulfonamides and amino acids (cysteine). Acetylation reactions are catalyzed by cytosolic enzymes termed acetyltransferases and employ the cofactor acetyl-CoA.

Methylation and, to some degree also acetylation decrease water solubility. Toxicants that undergo these reactions are retained in the body for longer periods of time. Metals such as mercury can undergo methylation to be methyl mercury, highly toxic, soluble in lipids and concentrates in neural tissue, where it may affect the structure and function of nerve cells. Nicotine, arsenic and selenium can undergo methylation while aromatic amines are primarily biotransformed by acetylation. Acetylation can either activate or deactivate aromatic amines. Activated amines can react with sensitive intracellular molecules, such as DNA causing mutations and disrupting normal cellular function. They may also interact with structural and functional proteins like enzymes [27]. Finally, amino acid conjugation is a reaction involving metabolites containing a carboxylic acid and the amino group of amino acids. The reaction involves a series of enzymes (cytosolic and mitochondrial) and cofactors (ATP and acetyl-CoA) that activate the carboxylic acid group and results in the formation of an amide bond [28].

2. In Vitro and Human-derived Techniques for Testing Xenobiotics Metabolism

In order to study metabolism and interactions of pesticides in humans we have to rely upon in vitro and human-derived techniques. Moreover, in vitro systems have become an integral part of drug metabolism throughout the drug discovery process. A scheme has originally developed for the screening of potential drugs at the preclinical screening phase. The scheme involves liver tissue preparations from either animal and human origin for the measurement of metabolic stability, metabolite identification, metabolizing enzymes recognition and enzyme inhibition [29]. However, this scheme has been modified and applied for the study of pesticides metabolism and interactions. The use of human enzyme sources and several possible applications are reviewed by Pelkonen *et al.* [30].

2.1. Subcellular Fractions

Subcellular fractions including microsomes are the most widely used in vitro systems in drug metabolism studies of new drug candidates [31]. Liver microsomes consist of vesicles of the hepatocyte endoplasmic reticulum and are prepared by standard differential ultracentrifugation [32]. Liver homogenates centrifuged at 9000g results in a supernatant (S9 fraction) rich in drug-metabolizing enzymes and a pellet containing predominately nuclei, lysosomes, peroxisomes and mitochondria. Centrifuging the S9 fraction at 100,000g results in a supernatant (cytosol) and pellet (microsomes). Liver microsomes contain almost only CYP and UGT enzymes. Microsomes can be stored at -80°C and are commercially available. Liver preparations, other than from fresh human liver, can also be used (e.g., liver slices, liver cell lines, and primary hepatocytes) for the preparation of microsomes [33,34].

Hepatic microsomes are useful for evaluation of metabolic stability, metabolite identification and quantification, and enzyme inhibition. Microsomes have many advantages including easy adaptation to higher throughput assays, easy preparation and use, good stability during storage, high CYP concentration and high rate of metabolite turnover. On the other hand, microsomes contain only phase I enzymes and UGTs while hepatic homogenates contain basically all hepatic enzymes [30,35]. Similar to microsomes, a NADPH-regenerating system is required for CYP enzymes. For the catalytic activity of phase II enzymes, addition of appropirate cofactors is necessary (e.g UDPGH, GSH and PAPS).

2.2. *c*DNA-Expressed CYPs (Single-Enzyme Systems)

Recombinant xenobiotics metabolizing enzymes (CYP, UGT) are well established and commercially available e.g. Supersomes^{TM}. Enzymes are expressed in bacterial, yeast and human lymphoblast or baculovirus infected insect cells. A NADPH-regenerating system (which consists of β-NADP, glucose 6-phosphate, and glucose 6-phosphate dehydrogenase) or NADPH is required to supply the energy demand of the CYPs [36]. For the UGT activity, uridine diphosphoglucuronic acid (UDPGA) has to be added as a cofactor.

Recombinant enzymes are easily applied for higher throughput screening and they can be used to study the role of individual CYPs in the metabolism. The disadvantage is that the effect of only one enzyme at a time can be evaluated [30,37].

2.3. Hepatocytes

Primary cultures of hepatocytes have shown good in vitro - in vivo correlations in the metabolic activity of a number of drugs and they allow a comprehensive view of whole cell metabolism since drug transporters and both phase I and II enzymes are present. Currently cultured human hepatocytes are the most recommended tools to study CYP-mediated metabolism and induction [31,38]. Hepatocytes are used to evaluate the metabolic stability of the compounds, identify the metabolizing enzymes and enzyme inhibition much like use of microsomes with the advantage of a border complement of phase I and II enzymes and transporters.

Hepatocytes in suspension are technically the easiest of all hepatocyte systems. The major limitation of use of suspensions is that hepatocytes in suspensions stay viable for a short period (up to 4 h), which prevents investigation of slowly metabolizing compounds. However, interspecies comparison seems to be more reliable with hepatocytes in suspensions than in culture due to potential damage of cytotoxic substances and variations in expression levels of drug metabolizing enzymes in cultures [39].

2.4. Liver Slices

Like the hepatocytes, as whole cell systems, the liver slices contain the whole complement of xenobiotic's metabolizing enzymes and offer a more reliable in vivo/in vitro correlation than subcellular systems [30,40]. Liver slices have begun to slowly fall out of use in the prediction of pharmacokinetic properties and drug metabolism due predominately to issues associated with drug transport into and out of the slices, lower enzyme activities and the increased use of hepatocytes to study similar reactions [41,42]. However, liver slices are still a powerful tool to study biotransformation in vitro [35].

2.5. Immortalized Cell Lines

Different human and animal cell lines are available (http://www.lgcpromochem-atcc.com). Animal cell lines are unpopular in human biotransformation research in which human systems are preferred. Human liver cell lines can be isolated from primary tumors of the liver parenchyma, seen after chronic hepatitis or cirrhosis [43]. The most common human cell lines for biotransformation studies are probably HepG2 (Hepatocellular carcinoma) [44-47], BC2 (Hepatoma) [48] and the lung-derived line A549 [49]. HepG2 is also an excellent tool to detect genotoxic properties of environmental and dietary chemicals [50]. Recently a new human hepatoma cell line, HepaRG, was derived from a hepatocellular carcinoma. The

HepaRG cells express a large panel of liver specific genes including several cytochrome P450 enzymes such as CYP1A2, CYP2B6, CYP2C9, CYP2E1 and CYP3A4, which is in contrast to the other hepatoma cell lines such as HepG2. Addition to P450 enzymes the HepaRG cells have a stable expression of phase II enzymes, transporters and nuclear transcription factors over a time period of six weeks in culture [51,52].

2.6. Organ Perfusion

Organ perfusion is the ultimate in vitro model system employed to study many aspects of metabolism or pharmacokinetics of not only the liver but also the intestine, brain, and kidney [53]. Liver perfusion is the best representation of the in vivo situation. Perfused liver has not been widely used in human biotransformation studies due to labour intensivity, poor reproducibility, handling difficulties, and availability of human liver [35].

3. In Vitro Metabolism of Pesticides

3.1. Analytical Techniques Used in Metabolite Identification

Mass Spectrometry

Determination of the structure of metabolites is most often performed either mass spectrometry or nuclear magnetic resonance (NMR) spectrometry [54]. Mass spectrometry has been the preferred technique because of its good sensitivity. Mass spectrometry is also a very robust technique and typically only protein precipitation is needed as a sample preparation method before analysis. Protein precipitation is performed by addition of denaturing solvent (acetonitrile, methanol) and is facilitated by vortexing. Finally samples are centrifuged and clear supernatant phase can be separated. Protein precipitation is ineffective at removing salts and lipids which can affect the sensitivity of the method in the long run [55].

Separation Techniques: GC vs LC

After sample preparation metabolites usually have to be separated from incubations. Earlier this was performed mostly with help of gas chromatography (GC). GC is a very good separation technique for thermally stable volatile compounds. GC is easy to connect to mass spectrometer because analytes are already in gas phase. The most common ionization technique used with GC is electron impact (EI) ionization which produces large number of fragment ions to the mass spectra. These fragmentations give valuable qualitative information which could be used in identification of analytes. There are also commercial databases (NIST/EPA/NIH Mass Spectral Library, Wiley Mass Spectral Libraries), where possible metabolites can be searched based on fragmented EI-spectra. Because metabolites are usually polar molecules they don't volatile without derivatization of analytes. Derivatization is time consuming, complex and it generates extra costs and errors to the measurements [56]. High temperature needed in GC separations could also cause labile metabolites to convert to other compounds before detection.

Better separation technique for polar metabolites is high performance liquid chromatography (HPLC). During separation analytes are in liquid phase and no derivatization is needed. Usually a basic MS compatible gradient HPLC method is suitable. For a long time connection between LC to MS was not practical until introduction of atmospheric pressure ionization (API) techniques like most commonly used electrospray ionization (ESI). Electrospray ionization is soft ionization process and mostly produce $[M \pm H]^{\pm}$ ions without fragmentation that is to say molecular weight information. Common problem for LC-MS is ion suppression. Highly concentrated matrix peaks may coelute in the separation and suppress the ionization of actual analyte.

High selectivity of mass spectrometer has decreased the importance of retention time for the identification purposes. Retention time is especially important in gas chromatography, which has a superior resolution compared to HPLC. Despite poor resolution of HPLC retention time could help to identify the metabolites if metabolite standards exist. Today's higher pressure liquid chromatographs (UPLC, RRLC etc.) and smaller particle columns have improved resolution of the HPLC to a new level.

TOF-MS for Metabolite Identification

The best mass spectrometer for screening of metabolites is the time-of-flight mass spectrometer (TOF-MS) because of its ability to detect all ionized compounds simultaneously without actual instrument scanning. This improves instrument sensitivity compared to most scanning instruments [57]. Other benefit of TOF-MS is its ability to provide accurate mass measurements (±5 ppm) which helps in identification by providing the elemental composition of the metabolites. If structures of possible metabolites have been anticipated on the basis of the parent, accurate masses give usually enough information to tentatively confirm structures of metabolites even without standards.

Triple-quadrupole MS

Other MS instruments used in identification of metabolites are triple-quadrupole mass spectrometer and quadrupole ion trap. In these instruments identification is based on fragments of metabolite molecules produced in the collision cell with the help of a collision gas such as argon (collision induced dissociation, CID). If any literature information about fragmentation of detected metabolites doesn't exist usually something about actual metabolite structure can still be concluded (e.g., which part of a molecule is changed?). To increase specificity the European Union regulatory authorities require nowadays the identification based on parent and two different MS-MS fragments [58].

Even though triple quadrupole mass spectrometers can help in structure elucidation, their best application is quantification in multiple-reaction monitoring (MRM) mode. Exceptional selectivity of MRM is based on two stage separation of metabolite, first actual metabolite and then its produced fragment ion, from the LC flow. Beside excellent selectivity also sensitivity of MS-MS experiments is good enough (usually at least 1 ng/ml). Beside triple-quadrupole mass spectrometry also other instruments could be used in quantifications with some limitations especially in dynamic range.

Because of triple quadrupole's high selectivity perfect separation of metabolites is not needed in MRM measurements. Because metabolites usually have very similar structure they can sometimes produce same fragments which can cause problems if metabolites elute at the same time. Sometimes easily fragmenting conjugated metabolites can break already during ionization which needs high voltage and temperature to operate. This so called in-source fragmentation can be a potential source of quantification error if analytes coelute or decrease sensitivity of the method. Similarities in structure can also make identification and isolation of metabolites more difficult. Even incubation samples contains little nonvolatile MS incompatible phosphate buffer at least modern instruments containing Z-spray ionization source can tolerate it sufficiently.

Nuclear Magnetic Resonance Spectroscopy

If you need to know the exact structure of a totally unknown metabolite nuclear magnetic resonance (NMR) spectroscopy is needed. Because of lower sensitivity of NMR larger amounts of a pure metabolite is needed for structure determination. However, sensitivity of NMR spectrometry has increased and modern instruments based on 950 MHz magnets are already commercially available.

The biggest problem concerning identification of metabolites in NMR spectrometry is the separation before measurements. Experiments measuring metabolites of xenobiotic directly from urine, plasma or bile sample have been published [59,60]. If simple 1D-NMR spectroscopy won't provide the answer because of overlapping signals from many metabolites or endogenous materials, modern multidimensional NMR techniques can be applied to increase resolution. However, usually resolving power required to separate several similar metabolites in sample is not adequate. For this reason more powerful separation techniques like HPLC are needed. Traditionally actual incubation samples have to be fractionated before analysis. Fortunately recent developments in NMR probe design, electronics and software has made possible to combine HPLC with NMR. Because of low levels of metabolites the most sensitive nuclei, like 1H, 19F and 31P, have to be used. Despite of this continuous-flow measurements are not usually adequate and eluent flow has to be stopped for actual NMR measurement. Nevertheless, HPLC-NMR spectroscopy has a valuable role to play in the determination of the structure of xenobiotic metabolites. [54]

Because mass spectrometry and NMR spectrometry are clearly complementary in the identification of unknown metabolites, a technique that combines mass spectrometry and HPLC-NMR has been introduced. Even there are some difficulties concerning solvent selection and ionization conditions, some metabolic studies have already been published [61-66]. In these studies eluent flow was split to the two different instruments, MS and NMR, to make the measurement more efficient and to ensure the data acquisition on the same chromatographic peak. [54]

3.2. In vitro Experiments - A General Description of Method

Metabolism and disposition of different concentrations of a pesticide as a function of incubation time were studied using several mammalian liver preparations including human and recombinant CYPs. The full description and example of our method can be found in the latest article [67].

Formation of metabolites in microsomes was studied using the standard incubation mixture containing serial concentrations of a pesticide in DMSO, 0.1 mg of pooled liver microsomal protein, and 1 mM NADPH in a final volume of 200 µl of 0.1 M phosphate buffer (pH 7.4). After 2-min incubation at +37°C in a shaking incubator block the reaction was started by addition of NADPH. The mixture was incubated at +37°C for different time points and the reaction was stopped with 200 µl of ice-cold acetonitrile containing an appropriate internal standard. After centrifugation at 10,000*g* for 15 min, the supernatant was collected and stored at -20°C until analysis.

For measuring the production of potential metabolites in human liver homogenate, incubations containing the same final pesticide concentrations as the microsomal incubations were prepared. In addition 40 µl of human liver homogenates, 5 mM uridine 5'-diphosphoglucuronic acid, 1 mM glutathione, 1.2 mM adenosine-3'-phosphate-5'-phosphosulfate and 1 mM NADPH were added in a final volume of 200 µl of 0.1 M phosphate buffer (pH 7.4). The incubations and analytical method were similar to those for the microsomal incubations.

Kinetic parameters of the metabolism were determined using a wide concentration range of parent pesticide in certain time point. The kinetic parameters V_{max} and K_m were calculated by nonlinear regression. These values were used to calculate the intrinsic clearance value (V_{max}/K_m) for all species.

Metabolism of 10 different individual human liver microsomes was measured in vitro. The specific activities of CYP isoform-catalyzed reactions in microsomes from ten human livers and their correlations with metabolite formation were studied.

To identify the human CYPs responsible for metabolism, the standard incubation mixtures (200 µl) containing 0.1 M phosphate buffer (pH 7.4), 1 mM NADPH, 100 µM pesticide and different recombinantly expressed P450 enzymes (50 pmol P450/ml) were prepared. Incubations were carried out according to the manufacturer's instructions. In brief (Supersomes™), the reaction was started by addition of recombinant enzymes to the preincubated reaction mixture (2 min at +37°C), mixed gently, and incubated for 30 min at +37°C in an incubator block without agitation. Otherwise, the incubation protocol and analytical method were similar to those for microsomal incubations. Kinetic parameters for the rCYPs were determined as with microsomal samples. Taking into account the average human hepatic microsomal protein amounts of CYPs and the actual intrinsic clearance values for various CYPs, the relative contributions of each CYP enzymes were calculated.

4. In Vitro Techniques for Testing Interactions

Induction of CYP Enzymes

CYP-xenobiotic interactions involve either induction or inhibition of metabolizing enzymes. Induction is defined as an increase in enzyme activity associated with an increase in intracellular enzyme concentration. This increase in enzymatic protein is normally (but not always) caused by an increase in transcription of the associated gene. Enzyme induction is dose independent, generally with a steep dose response relation and no clear-cut threshold of no-effect [68]. The phenomenon of induction of CYP captured the interest of pharmacologists even before the recognition of the nature of the CYP enzymes [69].

The ethical problems associated with human experiments have made the study of induction of xenobiotic-metabolising enzyme systems difficult. Many induction studies have been conducted in vitro using primary human hepatocytes, human hepatoma cell lines or cell lines derived from other human tissues [50,70-76]. Both Western blot and reverse transcription polymerase chain reaction (RT-PCR) techniques have been applied to examine pesticides-CYP induction [74-80]. However, problems in tissue availability, interindividual differences, reproducibility and ethical issues preclude the efficient large-scale use of human primary hepatocytes for induction screening. Therefore, the development of mechanism-based test systems for induction screening, based for example on in vitro pregnane X receptor/constitutive androstane receptor activation, is currently very active, and some test systems are in use as a first step for the identification of potential inducers [29].

Inhibition of CYP Enzymes

Inhibition can take place in several ways including the destruction of pre-existing enzymes, inhibition of enzyme synthesis or by complexing and thus inactivating the metabolising enzyme. Determination of the potential interactions of new chemical entity to inhibit drug-metabolizing enzymes and cause drug-drug or xenobiotic-drug interactions is very important during the development of a new chemical entity. By comparing the effects of a new chemical entity on the CYP specific-activities to the respective effects of diagnostic inhibitors, a tentative prediction of the in vivo situation can be made [30]. Inhibition interactions can be determined either by single substrate assay or cocktail assay.

4.1. Single Substrate Assay

Traditionally CYP interaction studies have been performed using specific assays for each CYP isoforms. Decrease in probe metabolite formation produced by inhibition is usually analyzed by UV-LC, LC-MS or fluorometry.

Here we will summarize our practical inhibitory interactions assays of the fungicide metalaxyl, insectisides profenofos and herbiside diuron with pooled human hepatic CYPs. In these assays metabolites of bupropion, amodiaquine, tolbutamide, omeprazole, dextromethorphan, chlorzoxazone, and midazolam were analyzed by high-performance liquid chromatography. Chromatographic methods were isocratic, except in the case of omeprazole when a linear gradient elution from 15 to 35% A in 8 min was used. Mobile phases were pumped at a flow rate of 1.0 ml/min. The injection volume used was 20 µl. The concentrations of metabolites were calculated from peak height ratios of the UV chromatograms on the basis of standard calibration curves of authentic metabolites. Metabolites of ethoxyresorufin, ethoxycoumarin, coumarin, and pentoxyresorufin were analyzed fluorometrically. All of the incubation and analysis conditions are summarized in Table 1. [81-90]A pesticide under study was added in different concentrations (final concentrations in the incubation mixture were 5–100 µM) to the incubation mixture in a small volume of DMSO as solvent. Fresh dilutions from stock solution of DMSO were used for each assay. The final amount of DMSO was 1% in incubation mixtures. For chlorzoxazone 6-hydroxylation the solvent was evaporated because of the potent inhibition effect of DMSO on CYP2E1 [14], and the residue was diluted with 10 μl of lipid solution. Lipid solution was prepared by adding 8 μl of dimethyldioctadecylammoniumbromide in chloroform (100 mg/ml) to 200 μl L-α-phosphatidylethanolamine dioleyl [C18:1 (*cis*)-9] in chloroform. This mixture was evaporated with a stream of nitrogen flow, 2 ml of water was added, and the final mixture was sonicated on an ice bath for 10 min by using 50% power. The enzyme activities in the presence of studied pesticide were compared with the control incubations into which only solvent were added. The IC_{50} values for inhibitors (concentration causing 50% reduction of control activity) were determined from triplicate incubations by linear regression analysis from the plot of the logarithm of inhibitor concentration versus percentage of the activity remaining after inhibition.

4.2. Cocktail Reactions

The dramatically increased number of new chemicals has raised a demand for efficient and rapid screening techniques to analyze inhibition interactions [91]. Modern mass spectrometers have a capability to analyze multiple compounds simultaneously. This has been applied to inhibition studies and several cocktail-type N-in-one-assays have been developed for screening of CYP inhibitions [91-95]. The most extensive of these is the LC-MS-MS assay developed by Tolonen *et al.* [96] and it contains all the nine major CYP isoforms with 13 metabolic probe reactions. In this assay ten probe substrates were added to single incubation with tested substance and metabolites were analyzed from one run using triple quadrupole instrument in MRM mode. Eventhough this method has no reference metabolites for quantitation it nevertheless provides reliable information about inhibition potencies towards various CYP-selective activities of a studied compound by comparing peak areas in cocktail samples with different inhibitor concentrations. It has to be stressed that, if detailed and more accurate information is wanted, the traditional single substrate technique would still be the recommended assay [97].

5. CYP Interactions with Fungicides

The interactions of a number of fungicides with microsomal CYP enzymes have been investigated. Fungicides can strongly interact either in vivo or in vitro leading to destruction of native enzyme or induction/inhibition of the enzyme activity. Especially in vivo, but also in vitro studies have been usually conducted in animals or tissue samples from pesticide-treated animals. However, several factors must be considered regarding fungicides and CYP interactions, including the specific compound in question, species, sex, route and duration of exposure.

Table 1. Incubation and analysis conditions for inhibition interaction assays in vitro

CYP	Substrate	Reaction	Conc. in incubation (μM)	Protein (mg/ml)	Cofactor system	Incubation Time (min)	Determination, λ (nm)	Eluent	Ref.
Multiple CYPs	7-Ethoxycoumarin	O-deethylation	10	0.2	NADPH-regenerating	10	Fluorometric, 365/454		[81]
CYP1A1/2	7-Ethoxyresorufin	O-deethylation	1	0.1	NADPH-regenerating	5	Fluorometric, 530/585		[82]
CYP2A6	Coumarin	7-hydroxylation	10	0.2	NADPH-regenerating	10	Fluorometric, 365/454		[83]
CYP2B	Pentoxyresorufin	O-deethylation	1	0.1	NADPH-regenerating	5	Fluorometric, 530/585		[82]
CYP2B6	Bupropion	Hydroxylation	50	0.4	NADPH	15	UV-HPLC, 214/204	75 % 50 mM *o*-phosphoric acid-buffer : 25 % acetonitrile	[84]
CYP2C8	Amodiaquine	N-deethylation	30	0.5	NADPH	20	UV-HPLC, 342	70 % 50 mM *o*-phosphoric acid-buffer : 30 % acetonitrile	[85]
CYP2C9	Tolbutamide	Methylhydroxyl-ation	200	0.15	NADPH-regenerating	20	UV-HPLC, 236/204	70 % 50 mM *o*-phosphoric acid-buffer : 30 % acetonitrile	[86]
CYP2C19	Omeprazole	5-hydroxylation	40	0.1	NADPH	20	UV-HPLC, 304/204	25 mM *o*-phosphoric acid-buffer (A) and acetonitrile (B)	[87]
CYP2D6	Dextromethorphan	O-demethylation	10	0.1	NADPH-regenerating	20	UV-HPLC, 204/280	75 % 50 mM *o*-phosphoric acid-buffer : 25 % acetonitrile	[88]
CYP2E1	Chlorzoxazone	6-hydroxylation	100	0.1	NADPH-regenerating	20	UV-HPLC, 282/204	70 % 50 mM *o*-phosphoric acid-buffer : 30 % acetonitrile	[89]
CYP3A4	Midazolam	1`-Hydroxylation	10	0.1	NADPH-regenerating	5	UV-HPLC, 245/204	60 % water : 40 % acetonitrile	[90]
CYP3A4	Omeprazole	Sulfoxidation	40	0.1	NADPH	20	UV-HPLC, 304/204	25 mM *o*-phosphoric acid-buffer (A) and acetonitrile (B)	[87]

Table 2. P450-fungicide interactions are species dependant

Fungicide	Chemical class	Species	Sex	Site	Enzymes	Reaction	Values	Method	Route
Propiconazole [77]	Triazole	Mice	Male	Liver	CYP1A1	7-Ethoxyresorufin-O-deethylation	1.3 fold	In vivo	Oral, multiple
		Rat					1.4 fold		
		Mice			CYP1A2	Methoxyresorufin-O-demethylation	1.5 fold		
		Rat					1.7 fold		
		Mice			CYP2B1	7-Pentoxyresorufin-O-dealkylation	5.4 fold		
		Rat					7.1 fold		
Metalaxyl [99,100]	Acylalanine	Human	Both	Liver	CYP2B	7-Pentoxyresorufin-O-dealkylation	IC_{50} =48.9 μM	In vitro	-
		Human			CYP2B6	Bupropion hydroxylation	IC_{50} =41.7 μM		
		Mice	Male		CYP2B1	7-Pentoxyresorufin-O-dealkylation	0.72 fold	In vivo	I.p, Multiple
		Mice	Both		CYP3A	Aminopyrine N-demethylation	2.8 fold		
		Human			CYP3A4	Midazolam 1-hydroxylation	IC_{50}>100 μM	In vitro	-
		Human				Omeprazole sulfoxidation	IC_{50}>100 μM		

Table 3. P450-fungicide interactions are sex and tissue dependant

Fungicide	Chemical class	Species	Sex	Site	Enzymes	Reaction	Values (fold)	Method	Route
Dithianon [101]	Quinone	Mice	Male	Liver	CYP2A	Testosterone 6α-hydroxylation	3.7 / 1.2	In vivo	I.p, single/repeated
			Female				0.7 / 1		
			Male			Testosterone 7α-hydroxylation	4.2 / 0.7		
			Female				0.85 / 1		
			Male		CYP2B1/2	Testosterone 16β-hydroxylation	2.4 / 0.4		
			Female				0.66 / 1		
			Male		CYP2C11	Testosterone 2α-hydroxylation	4.5 / 0.6		
			Female				0.87 / 1		
			Male		CYP2D9, 2B1/2	Testosterone 16α-hydroxylation	2.7 / 0.9		
			Female				0.55 / 1		
			Male		CYP3A1/2	Testosterone 6β-hydroxylase	2.8 / 0.6		
			Female				0.58 / 1		
			Male	Kidney	CYP2C11	Testosterone 2α-hydroxylation	4.5 / 3.1		
			Female				0.52 / 5.2		
			Male	Lung	CYP2D9, 2B1/2	Testosterone 16α-hydroxylation	7.1 / 1.6		
			Female				1.8 / 2.3		
Captan [102]	Phthalimide	Mice	Male	Liver	CYP1A1	7-Ethoxyresorufin-O-deethylation	0.51	In vivo	I.p, Multiple
					CYP1A2	Methoxyresorufin-O-demethylation	0.96		
						Phenacetin-O-deethylation	0.56		
					CYP3A	Aminopyrine N-demethylation	0.8		
				Kidney	CYP1A1	7-Ethoxyresorufin-O-deethylation	1.1		
					CYP1A2	Methoxyresorufin-O-demethylation	2.3		

						Phenacetin-O-deethylation	1.8		
					CYP3A	Aminopyrine N-demethylation	2.2		
				Lung	CYP1A1	7-Ethoxyresorufin-O-deethylation	0.75		
					CYP1A2	Methoxyresorufin-O-demethylation	3.0		
						Phenacetin-O-deethylation	2.1		
					CYP3A	Aminopyrine N-demethylation	1.6		
Metalaxyl [100]	Acylalanine	Mice	Male	Liver	CYP2B1	7-Pentoxyresorufin-O-dealkylation	0.72	In vivo	
			Female				1.14		
			Male		CYP3A	Aminopyrine N-demethylation	2.7		
			Female				2.8		
			Male	Kidney	CYP3A	Aminopyrine N-demethylation	4.84		
			Female				4.5		
Thiophanate-methyl [103]	Benzimid-azole	Rat	Male	Liver	CYP1A1	Ethoxyresorufin-O-deethylation	13	In vivo	I.p, multiple
			Female				18		
			Male		CYP1A2	Mehoxyresorufin-O-demethylation	3.6		
			Female				1.2		
			Male		CYP2B1	7-Pentoxyresorufin-O-dealkylation	26		
			Female				8.0		
			Male		CYP2E1	p-Nitrophenol hydroxylation	1		
			Female				2.9		
			Male		CYP3A	Aminopyrine N-demethylation	4.3		
			Female				3.3		
			Male	Kidney	CYP1A1	Ehoxyresorufin-O-deethylation	20.8		
			Female				28.2		
			Male		CYP2B1	7-Pentoxyresorufin-O-dealkylation	0.4		
			Female				4.9		

Table 3. P450-fungicide interactions are sex and tissue dependant (Continued)

Fungicide	Chemical class	Species	Sex	Site	Enzymes	Reaction	Values (fold)	Method	Route
			Male		CYP2E1	p-Nitrophenol	0.92		
			Female			hydroxylation	6.3		
			Male		CYP3A	Aminopyrine N-	1.0		
			Female			demethylation	1.0		
			Male	Lung	CYP1A1	Ethoxyresorufin-O-	4.0		
			Female			deethylation	3.3		
			Male		CYP2B1	7-Pentoxyresorufin-O-	2.9		
			Female			dealkylation	0.6		
			Male		CYP2E1	p-Nitrophenol	1.0		
			Female			hydroxylation	1.3		
			Male		CYP3A	Aminopyrine N-	2.1		
			Female			demethylation	0.7		

5.1. Cross Species Differences

Species differences are significant in terms of activities and selectivities of specific cytochrome enzyme form [98]. Comparison of several CYP-associated probe activities demonstrates that some CYP enzyme activities such as those associated with CYP1A and CYP2E1, are well preserved across species, but several of them display large quantitative, sometimes even qualitative differences. As an example of species differences regarding pesticides, in an in vivo study, Sun *et al.*, [77] compared the effects of propiconazole on hepatic P450 gene expression and activities in rats and mice under similar dosing conditions (Table 2). Male Sprague-Dawley rats and male CD-1 mice were orally administrated propiconazole daily for 14 days. Propiconazole significantly induced both 7-pentoxyresorufin-O-dealkylation (PROD) and methoxyresorufin-O-deethylation (MROD) activities (CYP2B1 and CYP1A2 markers, respectively) in livers of both species. On the other hand, mRNA levels of CYP1A2 were induced only in rat liver.

When comparing CYP specific activities in human liver with the activity profile in liver microsomes from the male mice after the treatment with metalaxyl, some induction or inhibition differences were observed (Table 2). In an extensive in vitro screening of potential CYP-based interactions, metalaxyl moderately inhibited PROD (CYP2B) and bupropion hydroxylation (CYP2B6), whereas no significant inhibitory effects towards other CYPs in human liver microsomes were observed [99]. In an animal in vivo study, Paolini *et al.* [100] treated mice with metalaxyl intraperitoneally with either single or repeated doses. There was about a threefold increase in CYP3A isoenzymes as indicated by N-demethylation of aminopyrine and a weak but significant reduction in CYP2B1 activity in male mouse liver. Although in vitro and in vivo experiments are not strictly comparable in terms of CYP activity modifications, they nevertheless demonstrate interspecies variability in the changes of CYP enzymes.

5.2. Sex and Tissue Related Differences

There are extensive sex and organ comparisons of CYP specific activity profiles in mice and rat available as is summarized in Table 3. CYP catalyzed reactions have been studied in liver, kidney and lung microsomes from male and female Swiss Albino CD-1 mice. Dithianon was able to induce or suppress various CYPs depending on sex and organ. After a single treatment, males were more responsive to induction in all organs while females were responsive to either suppression (liver and kidney) or induction (lung). On the other hand, after repeated injections, a reduction of various CYP activities in male liver and an induction of the same enzymes in kidney and lung on both sexes were observed by Pozzetti *et al.* [101].

In a CYP modulation experiment, a single intraperitoneal dose of captan did not affect CYP activities while repeated intraperitoneal administration resulted in significant increase or decrease of some CYP activities [102]. 7-Ethoxyresorufin-O-deethylation (EROD) activity (CYP1A1-associated probe activity) was significantly decreased in the liver. In the kidney, both CYP3A- and CYP1A2-associated monooxygenases were significantly induced.

Accelerated phenacetin and methoxyresorufin metabolism (CYP1A2) was also observed in the lung.

In a study of Paolini *et al.* [100] mentioned above, a gender difference in the response to metalaxyl treatment of Swiss Albino mice in vivo was also observed. Although CYP3A isoenzyme as measured by aminopyrine N-demethylation was induced in the liver and kidney of both sexes, a reduction of CYP2B1 activity only in male mice liver was observed.

Thiophanate-methyl has been associated with various changes in the activities of CYP enzymes. Treatment of male and female Sprague-Dawley rats intraperitoneally with single or repeated doses resulted in an induction or reduction in liver, kidney and lung microsomal activities. In the liver an induction in the CYP2B1 probe activity at lower dose in both sexes and an induction of CYP1A2 at the higher dose in males were observed. In the kidney an induction in the CYP1A1 and CYP2E1 activities in females receiving higher multiple administrations were detected. In the lung the CYP3A-associated activity was the most induced in males. A significant reduction of CYP2B1-linked oxidases was also observed in repeated treatment in the kidney (males) and lung (females). [103]

5.3. Comparison of Different Fungicides

Table 4 summarizes some induction and inhibition studies for various fungicides, as measured by the increased/decreased (i.e. fold) activities exposed via different routes in vivo and by the IC_{50} values in in vitro experiments. The fold changes and IC_{50} values are dependent on the compound in question, as is shown on human placental microsomes exposed to 6 different fungicides. They were demonstrated to significantly inhibit CYP19 aromatase activity in vitro. CYP19 is very important in metabolizing steroid hormones and xenobiotics [104].

The antifungal mode of action of triazoles results from binding of the azole ring moiety to the heme protein of fungal CYP51 C-14 to inhibit demethylation in ergosterol biosynthesis [105]. Consequently, the concern regarding the potential interactions within mammalian CYP enzymes have been raised. Inhibition assays to determine inhibitory interactions of fungicides with recombinant human CYP51 (lanosterol-14α-demethylase) enzyme have been reported by Trösken *et al.* [106]. The IC_{50} values of 13 fungicides for CYP51 inhibition displayed about 30-fold variation.

The inhibitory interactions of metalaxyl and carbendazim with human liver cytochrome P450 enzymes were investigated in vitro. The IC_{50} values of metalaxyl for CYP2B and CYP2B6 were 48.9 and 41.7 μM, respectively [99]. Carbendazim inhibited only CYP2D6 (IC_{50} 12 μM). All the other values were higher than 100 μM indicating very low or absent affinity (unpublished data).

Table 4. Human in vitro P450-fungicide interactions are compound dependant

Fungicide	Chemical class	Sex	Site	Enzymes	Reaction	IC_{50}-values (μM)	Ref.
Fenarimol	Pyrimidin	Female	Place-ntal	CYP19	$[^3H]_2O$ assay	37.2	[104]
Imazalil	Imidazole					0.04	
Prochloraz						0.34	
Propiconazole	Triazole					6.5	
Triadimefon						32	
Triadimenol						21	
Bitertanol	Triazole	-	Recom -binant	CYP51	Lanosterol demethy-lation	1.30	[106]
Cyproconazole						22.8	
Epoxiconazole						1.95	
Flusilazole						3.36	
Hexaconazole						15.6	
Imazalil	Imidazole					36.1	
Myclobutanil	Triazole					29.0	
Penconazole						19.3	
Prochloraz	Imidazole					5.0	
Propiconazole	Triazole					8.25	
Tebuconazole						3.61	
Triadimefon						9.95	
Triadimenol						37.2	
Metalaxyl	Acylalanine	Both	Hepa-tic	CYP2B	7-Pentoxyres-orufin-O-dealkylation	48.9	[99]
Carbendazim	Benzimidazole					>100	*
Metalaxyl	Acylalanine			CYP2B6	Bupropion hydroxylation	41.7	[99]
Carbendazim	Benzimidazole					>100	*
Metalaxyl	Acylalanine			CYP2D6	Dextromethor phan-O-demethylation	>100	[99]
Carbendazim	Benzimidazole					12	*

* Unpublished data.

6. Literature Survey on In vitro Metabolic and Kinetic Properties of Fungicides in Mammals

As already mentioned in the introduction, in vivo studies in humans with fungicides are not possible and consequently, in vitro studies have to be performed for gaining useful information for risk assessment purposes. Fortunately, human liver and other tissue preparations are available for studies and many human hepatic CYP enzymes have been isolated, characterized and are commercially available. Enzyme kinetic measurements and metabolic pathways of fungicides are important for accurate risk assessment and predictive in vivo models. During the last few years several articles on the role of P450s in the metabolism of a wide variety of pesticides have been appeared, while only few studies on in vitro metabolism and kinetics of fungicides in mammals are available. A database covering human phase I enzymes and their isoforms that metabolize pesticides and related compounds have been published [107]. Examples of fungicides, in which P450 enzymes mediate aliphatic hydroxylation (propoconazole), aromatic ring hydroxylation (metalaxyl, pentachlorophenol and *trans*-bromuconazole), and demethylation and lactone formation (metalaxyl, furametpyr) are presented in figures 2-4.

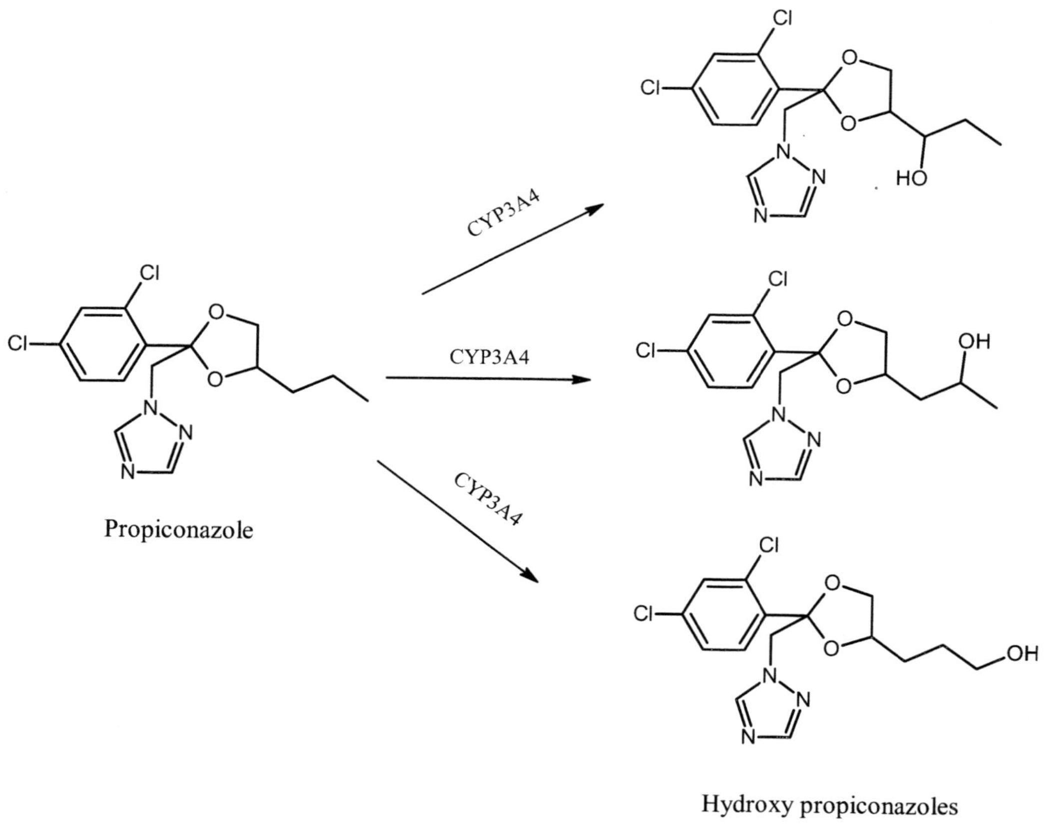

Figure 2. Aliphatic hydroxylations of propoconazole.

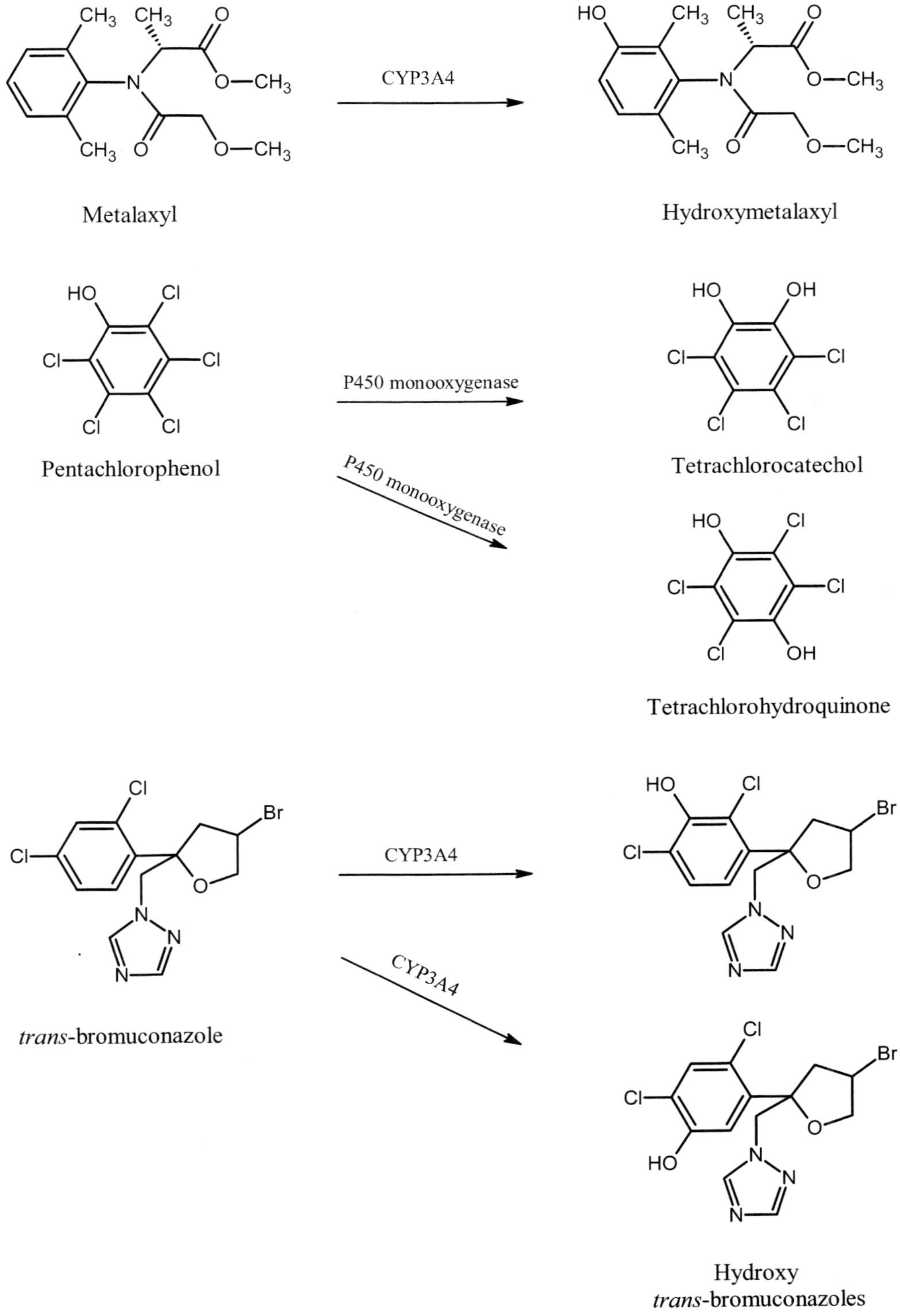

Figure 3. Aromatic ring hydroxylations of metalaxyl, pentachlorophenol and *trans*-bromuconazole.

6.1. Phenylamide Fungicides

Phenylamide oxazolidinone fungicides mode of action is to inhibit protein synthesis in fungi by interference with the synthesis of ribosomal RNA, while the mode of action for phenylamide acylalanine class is to inhibit nucleic RNA polymerase. Acylalanine class contains four different fungicides and the metabolism and interactions of one of them, metalaxyl, have been studied in vitro [99].

In this study in vitro metabolic profiles were determined in human liver microsomes and homogenates. The results showed identical metabolite profiles among human liver preparations. The biotransformation reactions were aromatic hydroxylation (Figure 3), demethylation and lactone formation (Figure 4). In human liver microsomes the predominant metabolites were two hydroxymetalaxyl derivatives or atropisomers of one of the derivatives. The hydroxylation of the phenyl ring or the aromatic methyl group was mediated by CYP3A4 and the demethylation and lactone formation reactions were mediated by both CYP3A4 and CYP2B6.

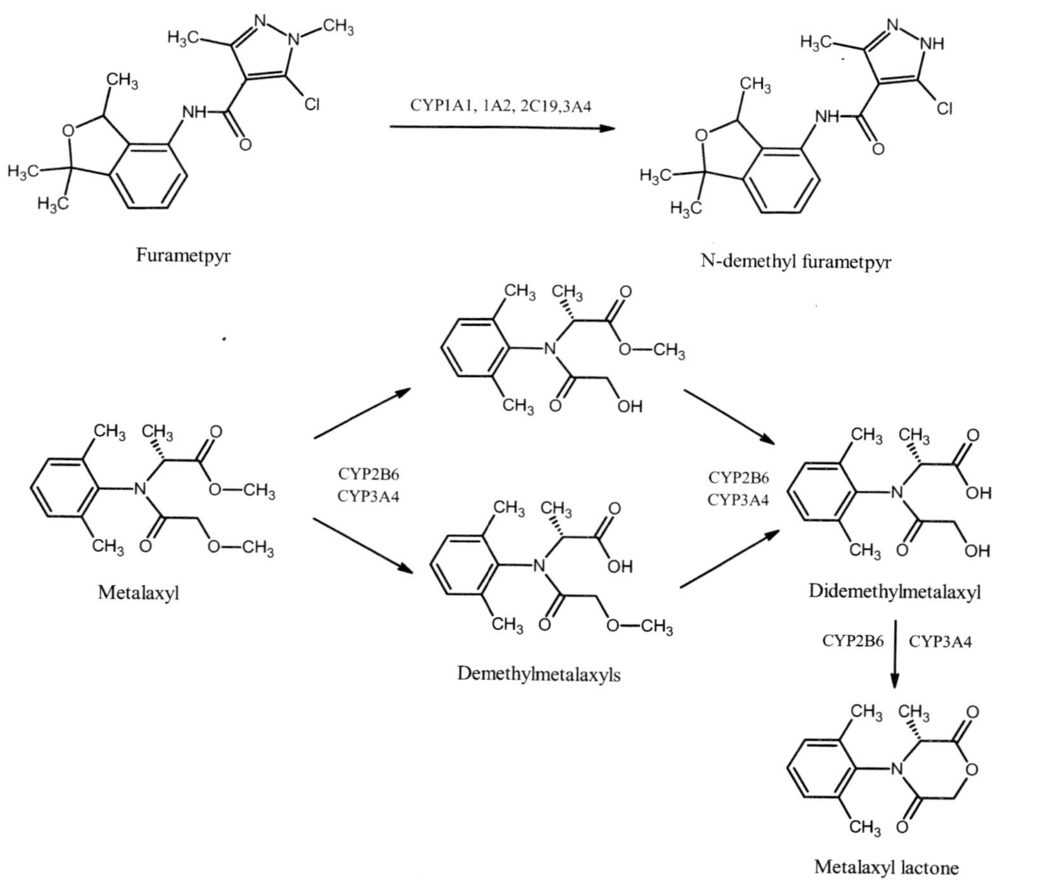

Figure 4. Demethylation and lactone formation reactions of metalaxyl and furametpyr.

6.2. Triazole Fungicides

The metabolism of 13 azoles fungicides by rat hepatic microsomes and purified human CYP3A4 has been investigated. 10 (*trans*-bromuconazole, propiconazole, triadimefon, myclobutanil, hexaconazole, triticonazole, diniconazole, fenbuconazole, uniconazole and ipconazole) out of 13 compounds tested were metabolized by rat hepatic microsomes leading to the production of both aromatic and aliphatic hydroxylations and carbonyl reduced product. As an example, aliphatic hydroxylations of propiconazole and aromatic hydroxylations of *trans*-bromuconazole are presented in figure 2 and 3. Several studies have indicated that CYP3A subfamily may play an active role in the metabolism of triazole fungicides. Nearly all metabolites detected in the rat microsomal assays were detected also in the human CYP3A4 assays, except triadimefon which underwent phase I reaction only with rat liver microsomes [105,108]. On the other hand, Barton *et al.* [109] reported that triadimefon and myclobutanil are predominantly metabolized by the CYP2C and CYP3A subfamilies.

6.3. Oxathiin Fungicides

The in vitro biotransformation of furametpyr as a member of oxathiin fungicides has been studied by human recombinant P450 isoforms. Among eleven recombinant P450 isoforms only CYP1A1, 1A2, 2C19 and 3A4 metabolized furametpyr efficiently to the N-demethylated metabolite (Figure 4). However, the furametpyr is extensively metabolized to more than 14 metabolites in rats. The major biotransformation reactions were demethylation and oxidation. It is clear that the furametpyr primarily undergoes hydroxylation of the methyl group by microsomal cytochrome P450 resulting in N-demethyl furametpyr to form the rest of metabolites [110].

6.4. Pentachlorophenol Fungicide

Pentachlorophenol, an insecticide, fungicide, and non selective pesticide, is used to control termites and, frequently, as an ester to protect wood from fungal rots and wood-boring insects [111]. The metabolism of pentachlorophenol has been studied in mammals in vitro [112,113]. The metabolic activation of pentachlorophenol to reactive quinones and semiquinones has been characterized by Tsai *et al.* [114] in rats and mice liver in vitro. Mono-S- and multi-S-substituted adducts of tetrachloro-1,4-benzoquinone, tetrachloro-1,2-benzoquinone and their corresponding semiquinones were detected in both rodent microsomes.

7. Application of In vitro Data to Help Risk Assessment of Fungicides

Risk assessment needs reliable scientific information and one source of information is the characterization of the metabolic factors and toxicokinetics. Indeed, quantitative toxicokinetic data in humans are needed for human risk assessment to make reliable comparisons between individuals or between species [115,116]. The more we know about pesticides in terms of their metabolic characteristic in vitro, the better we will be in extrapolation of in vitro and animal studies into human risk assessment.

The 100-fold uncertainty factor (UF) is used to convert a no-observed-adverse-effect level (NOEAL) from an animal toxicity study to a safe value for human intake. Furthermore, this UF has to allow for a 10-fold interspecies difference (which is subdivided into a factor of $10^{0.6}$ (4.0) for toxicokinetics and $10^{0.4}$ (2.5) for toxicodynamics) and a 10-fold interindividual variation (which is divided equally into two subfactors each of $10^{0.5}$ (3.16)) [117].

Risk assessment has to be carried out using quantitative chemical-specific data which will define the fundamental processes influencing toxicokinetics and toxicodynamics [118]. Moreover, The International Program on Chemical Safety (IPCS) proposes the use of chemical specific toxicological data instead of default assessment factors, whenever possible [119]. In vitro data may have an important contribution to chemical risk assessment by the replacement of the proposed default subdivision of the usual uncertainty factor by quantitative chemical-specific assessment factors (CSAFs). The basic idea is to replace one or more of these subfactors with chemical-specific factors that can be derived from studies that demonstrate differences in toxicokinetics or toxicodynamics. The assessment factor may either increase or decrease and the differences may be considerable.

Practical examples of using in vitro techniques to replace proposed toxicokinetics subdivisions of the usual uncertainty factor for two pesticides (profenofos, as an organophosphorothioate insecticide and diuron, as one of the phenylurea herbicide) have been published [67,120]. In vitro biotransformations and dispositions were studied in human hepatic homogenates, different types of mammalian hepatic microsomes including human and cDNA-expressed human P450 enzymes. Metabolites were identified by LC-TOF and quantified by triple quadrupole mass spectrometry.

For profenofos, two metabolites, desthiopropylprofenofos (active metabolite) and hydroxyprofenofos (alternative metabolite), were detected. The rank order of desthiopropylprofenofos formation in liver microsomes based on intrinsic clearances (V_{max}/K_m) was mouse > human > rat, while for profenofos hydroxylation it was mouse > rat > human. In view of the ratio between desthiopropylation and hydroxylation intrinsic clearance rates, human liver microsomes were most active in profenofos bioactivation. The animal to human efficiency comparison revealed that mouse liver microsomes activated profenofos 1.3-fold more than human liver microsomes, whereas the rat liver microsomes had the smallest value (0.3-fold). On the other hand, interspecies comparison for profenofos hydroxylation showed 9-fold biotransformation variability for mouse and 6.3-fold for rat indicating the need of using quantitative chemical-specific assessment factors. Human interindividual variations in both profenofos metabolites formations were within range of the default uncertainty/safety factors for chemical risk assessment.

In the in vitro biotransformation of diuron the only metabolic pathway detected in seven mammalian hepatic microsomes was demethylation at the terminal nitrogen atom. An animal to human efficiency comparison revealed that dog liver microsomes metabolized diuron more efficiently (2.3 Fold), whereas the rat liver microsomes had the smallest value (0.43-fold). The interspecies differences in *N*-demethyldiuron formation as a function of time correlated with the variations in kinetic parameters. The rank order of *N*-demethyldiuron formation in liver microsomes based on intrinsic clearance (V_{max}/K_m) was dog > monkey > rabbit > mouse > human > minipig > rat.

According to the previous data, the uncertainty factor for animal to human differences in toxicokinetics (AK_{UF}) was 2.3-fold. In addition, the uncertainty factor for human variability in toxicokinetics (HK_{UF}) was 1.5-fold, as defined by Renwick and Lazarus [117] as a variation between the mean and the highest value. It has to be stressed here that we measured only the hepatic metabolism of diuron, from which the above factors have been derived. On the other hand, metabolism is usually the most important factor contributing to interindividual and interspecies differences in toxicokinetics and thus, as a default, one could conclude that interspecies extrapolation with respect to diuron does not pose extraordinary uncertainties.

Differences in efficiencies between rat, minipig and human liver microsomes have been reported by Lang *et al.* [121] in the metabolism of triazine herbicides such as atrazine and ametryn. Also with other pesticides, such as chlorpyrifos (organophosphorus insecticide) and carbofuran (carbamate insecticide), human liver microsomes showed lower rates of metabolism than mouse and rat liver microsomes [122,123].

In our practical experiences with human derived and quantitative chemical-specific data, although restricted to metabolic data by human and animal liver preparations, the uncertainty factors for animal to human differences and for human variability in toxicokinetics were within the range of the toxicokinetics default uncertainty/safety factors for chemical risk assessment for profenofos desthiopropylation and diuron demethylation.

8. CONCLUSION

It is apparent from this chapter that there is a large number of enzymes capable of metabolising pesticides to many different products. Moreover, both phase I and phase II xenobiotic metabolism pathways cannot be considered in isolation, but rather as part of a coupled, interactive system, interfacing directly with many endogenous metabolic pathways. Human-derived techniques for testing xenobiotics metabolism have been established for many different cell types and organs. For metabolism studies, the enzyme systems used at present (liver microsomes, recombinant enzymes, liver homogenates, liver slices and hepatocytes) clearly give reliable results, if their inherent restrictions are taken into consideration [29]. However, the classical view of xenobiotic metabolism being a means for detoxification is no longer entirely true. Each of the in vitro techniques can provide important information on the mechanisms of xenobiotic detoxification as well as bioactivation. It should be also emphasised that the CYP mediated reactions principally covered here are not a complete list of possible reactions for fungicides. It would be very difficult to cover all potential reactions and interactions for all fungicides.

CYP-xenobiotic interactions involve either induction or inhibition. Induction of human CYP enzymes is difficult to study because there are no human liver cell lines that either express the full complement of CYP enzymes or reproduce the induction observed in vivo. Quite contrary, in vitro inhibition screens are widely used in the drug industry, and there is a general consensus that they are providing relatively reliable information about the potential of a compound to cause interactions in vivo [29].

There have been hundreds of articles on the subject of in vitro metabolism of pesticides and other chemicals used in agriculture and public health. In these publications, experimental animals, usually rodents have been utilized while only few studies of in vitro human metabolism have been published. However, with the realization of the fact that human data are needed to improve human risk assessment, performing investigations with human-derived in vitro model systems to predict metabolic clearance, metabolites and metabolic pattern, metabolizing enzymes and interactions are of utmost importance. Together with the advantage of novel analytical techniques (LC/TOF-MS; LC/MS-MS and HPLC-NMR) for metabolite identification and quantification the development of quantitative chemical-specific assessment factors can be achieved. Hopefully this chapter has given some insight into the usefulness of fungicide metabolism measurements in human derived techniques and its contributions to the development of human risk assessment data.

Acknowledgments

This work was funded by the Ministry of Education-supported position from Finnish Graduate School in Toxicology (ToxGS) and by a DRUG2000 grant from Finnish Funding Agency for Technology (TEKES).

References

[1] Oesch, F., Herrero, M. E., Hengstler, J. G., Lohmann, M. & Arand, M. (2000). Metabolic Detoxification: Implications for Thresholds. *Toxicologic Pathology, 28,* 382-387.

[2] Low, L. K. (1998). Metabolic changes of drugs and related organic compounds. In J. N. Delgado & W. A. Remers (Eds.), *Wilson and Gisvold's textbook of organic medicinal and pharmaceutical chemistry* (10th ed., pp. 43–122). Philadelphia: Lippincott-Raven.

[3] Lawton, M., Gasser, R., Tynes, R., Hodgson, E. & Philpot, R. (1990). The flavin-containing monooxygenase enzymes expressed in rabbit liver and lung are products of related but distinctly different genes. *Journal of Biological Chemistry, 265,* 5855-5861.

[4] Gasser, R. & Philpot, R. (1989). Primary structures of cytochrome P-450 isozyme 5 from rabbit and rat and regulation of species-dependent expression and induction in

lung and liver: identification of cytochrome P-450 gene subfamily IVB. *Molecular Pharmacology, 35,* 617-625.

[5] Hjelle, J., Hazelton, G., Klaassen, C. & Hjelle, J. (1986). Glucuronidation and sulfation in rabbit kidney. *Journal of Pharmacology And Experimental Therapeutics, 236,* 150-156.

[6] Tremaine, L. M., Diamond, G. L. & Quebbemann, A. J. (1985). Quantitative determination of organ contribution to excretory metabolism. *Journal of Pharmacological Methods, 13,* 9-35.

[7] Dutcher, J. S. & Boyd, M. R. (1979). Species and strain differences in target organ alkylation and toxicity by 4-ipomeanol: Predictive value of covalent binding in studies of target organ toxicities by reactive metabolites. *Biochemical Pharmacology, 28,* 3367-3372.

[8] Peters, W. H. M. & Kremers, P. G. (1989). Cytochromes P-450 in the intestinal mucosa of man. *Biochemical Pharmacology, 38,* 1535-1538.

[9] Adams, D. R., Jones, A. M., Plopper, C. G., Serabjit-Singh, C. J. & Philpot, R. M. (1991). Distribution of cytochrome P-450 monoxygenase enzymes in the nasal mucosa of hamster and rat. *American Journal of Anatomy, 190,* 291-298.

[10] Eriksson, C. & Brittebo, E. B. (1991). Metabolic activation of the herbicide dichlobenil in the olfactory mucosa of mice and rats. *Chemico-Biological Interactions, 79,* 165-177.

[11] Khan, W. A., Park, S. S., Gelboin, H. V., Bickers, D. R. & Mukhtar, H. (1989). Monoclonal antibodies directed characterization of epidermal and hepatic cytochrome P-450 isozymes induced by skin application of therapeutic crude coal tar. *Journal of Investigative Dermatology, 93,* 40-45.

[12] Dhawan, A., Parmar, D., Das, M. & Seth, P. K. (1990). Cytochrome P-450 dependent monooxygenases in neuronal and glial cells: Inducibility and specificity. *Biochemical and Biophysical Research Communications, 170,* 441-447.

[13] Bergh, A. F. & Strobel, H. W. (1992). Reconstitution of the Brain Mixed Function Oxidase System: Purification of NADPH-Cytochrome P450 Reductase and Partial Purification of Cytochrome P450 from Whole Rat Brain. *Journal of neurochemistry, 59,* 575-581.

[14] Pelkonen, O., Maenpaa, J., Taavitsainen, P., Rautio, A. & Raunio, H. (1998). Inhibition and induction of human cytochrome P450 (CYP) enzymes. *Xenobiotica, 28,* 1203-1253.

[15] Rendic, S. & Di Carlo, F. J. (1997). Human cytochrome P450 enzymes: A status report summarizing their reactions, substrates, inducers, and inhibitors. *Drug Metabolism Reviews, 29,* 413-580.

[16] Lawton, M. P., Cashman, J. R., Cresteil, T., Dolphin, C. T., Elfarra, A. A., Hines, R. N., Hodgson, E., Kimura, T., Ozols, J., Phillips, I. R., Philpot, R. M., Poulsen, L. L., Rettie, A. E., Shephard, E. A., Williams, D. E. & Ziegler, D. M. (1994). A Nomenclature for the Mammalian Flavin-Containing Monooxygenase Gene Family Based on Amino Acid Sequence Identities. *Archives of Biochemistry and Biophysics, 308,* 254-257.

[17] Dolphin, C. T., Cullingford, T. E., Shephard, E. A., Smith, R. L. & Phillips, I. R. (1996). Differential development and tissue-specific regulation of expression of the genes encoding three members of the flavin-containing monooxygenase family of man, FMO1, FMO3 and FMO4. *European Journal of Biochemistry, 235,* 683-689.

[18] Satoh, T. & Hosokawa, M. (1998). The Mammalian Carboxylesterases: from Molecules to Functions. *Annual Review of Pharmacology & Toxicology, 38,* 257.

[19] Zamek-Gliszczynski, M. J., Hoffmaster, K. A., Nezasa, K., Tallman, M. N. & Brouwer, K. L. R. (2006). Integration of hepatic drug transporters and phase II metabolizing enzymes: Mechanisms of hepatic excretion of sulfate, glucuronide, and glutathione metabolites. *European Journal of Pharmaceutical Sciences, 27,* 447-486.

[20] Falany, C. N., Xie, X., Wang, J., Ferrer, J. & Falany, J. L. (2000). Molecular cloning and expression of novel sulphotransferase-like cDNAs from human and rat brain. *Biochemical Journal, 346,* 857-864.

[21] Weinshilboum, R. M., Otterness, D. M., Aksoy, I. A., Wood, T. C., Her, C. & Raftogianis, R. B. (1997). Sulfation and sulfotransferases 1: Sulfotransferase molecular biology: cDNAs and genes. *The FASEB journal : official publication of the Federation of American Societies for Experimental Biology, 11,* 3-14.

[22] Strott, C. A. (2002). Sulfonation and molecular action. *Endocrine Reviews, 23,* 703-732.

[23] Parkinson, A. (2001). Biotransformation of xenobiotics. In C. D. Klaassen (Eds.), *Casarett and Doull's toxicology : the basic science of poisons* (6th ed., pp. 113–186). New York ; London: McGraw-Hill Medical Pub. Division.

[24] Ansher, S. S., Jakoby, W. B. (1990). N-Methyltransferases. In G. J. Mulder (Eds.), *Conjugation reactions in drug metabolism : an integrated approach* pp. 193-232). London: Taylor and Francis.

[25] Stevens, J. L., Bakke, J. E. (1990). S-Methylation. In G. J. Mulder (Eds.), *Conjugation reactions in drug metabolism : an integrated approach* pp. 251-272). London: Taylor and Francis.

[26] Pacifici, G. M., Santerini, S., Giuliani, L. & Rane, A. (1991). Thiol methyltransferase in humans: development and tissue distribution. *Developmental Pharmacology & Therapeutics, 17,* 8-15.

[27] Kent, C.,Ph.D. (1998). *Basics of toxicology.* New York ; Chichester: Wiley.

[28] Kanazu, T. & Yamaguchi, T. (1997). Comparison of in Vitro Carnitine and Glycine Conjugation with Branched-Side Chain and Cyclic Side Chain Carboxylic Acids in Rats. *Drug Metabolism and Disposition, 25,* 149-153.

[29] Pelkonen, O. & Raunio, H. (2005). In vitro screening of drug metabolism during drug development: can we trust the predictions? *Expert Opinion on Drug Metabolism & Toxicology, 1,* 49-59.

[30] Pelkonen, O., Turpeinen, M., Uusitalo, J., Rautio, A. & Raunio, H. (2005). Prediction of Drug Metabolism and Interactions on the Basis of in vitro Investigations. *Basic & Clinical Pharmacology & Toxicology, 96,* 167-175.

[31] Ekins, S., Ring, B. J., Grace, J., McRobie-Belle, D. J. & Wrighton, S. A. (2000). Present and future in vitro approaches for drug metabolism. *Journal of Pharmacological and Toxicological Methods, 44,* 313-324.

[32] Pelkonen, O., Kaltiala, E. H., Larmi, T. K. I. & Karki, N. T. (1974). Cytochrome P 450 linked monooxygenase system and drug induced spectral interactions in human liver microsomes. *Chemico-Biological Interactions, 9,* 205-216.

[33] Olsen, A. K., Hansen, K. T. & Friis, C. (1997). Pig hepatocytes as an in vitro model to study the regulation of human CYP3A4: Prediction of drug-drug interactions with 17α-ethynylestradiol. *Chemico-Biological Interactions, 107,* 93-108.

[34] Skaanild, M. T. & Friis, C. (2000). Expression changes of CYP2A and CYP3A in microsomes from pig liver and cultured hepatocytes. *Pharmacology and Toxicology, 87,* 174-178.

[35] Brandon, E. F. A., Raap, C. D., Meijerman, I., Beijnen, J. H. & Schellens, J. H. M. (2003). An update on in vitro test methods in human hepatic drug biotransformation research: pros and cons. *Toxicology and Applied Pharmacology, 189,* 233-246.

[36] Taavitsainen, P., Anttila, M., Nyman, L., Karnani, H., Salonen, J. S. & Pelkonen, O. (2000). Selegiline metabolism and cytochrome P450 enzymes: In vitro study in human liver microsomes. *Pharmacology and Toxicology, 86,* 215-221.

[37] Moody, G. C., Griffin, S. J., Mather, A. N., Mcginnity, D. F. & Riley, R. J. (1999). Fully automated analysis of activities catalysed by the major human liver cytochrome P450 (CYP) enzymes: assessment of human CYP inhibition potential. *Xenobiotica, 29,* 53-75.

[38] Pelkonen, O. & Turpeinen, M. (2007). In vitro–in vivo extrapolation of hepatic clearance: Biological tools, scaling factors, model assumptions and correct concentrations. *Xenobiotica, 37,* 1066-1089.

[39] Gebhardt, R., Hengstler, J., Müller, D., Glöckner, R., Buenning, P., Laube, B., Schmelzer, E., Ullrich, M., Utesch, D., Hewitt, N., Ringel, M., Hilz, B., Bader, A., Langsch, A., Koose, T., Burger, H., Maas, J. & Oesch, F. (2003). New Hepatocyte In Vitro Systems for Drug Metabolism: Metabolic Capacity and Recommendations for Application in Basic Research and Drug Development, Standard Operation Procedures. *Drug metabolism reviews, 35,* 145-213.

[40] Gómez-Lechón, M. J., Donato, M. T., Castell, J. V. & Jover, R. (2004). Human Hepatocytes in Primary Culture: The Choice to Investigate Drug Metabolism in Man. *Current Drug Metabolism, 5,* 443-462.

[41] Olinga, P., Meijer, D. K. F., Slooff, M. J. H. & Groothuis, G. M. M. (1998). Liver Slices in In Vitro Pharmacotoxicology with Special Reference to the Use of Human Liver Tissue. *Toxicology in Vitro, 12,* 77-100.

[42] Carlile, D. J., Hakooz, N. & Houston, J. B. (1999). Kinetics of Drug Metabolism in Rat Liver Slices: IV. Comparison of Ethoxycoumarin Clearance by Liver Slices, Isolated Hepatocytes, and Hepatic Microsomes from Rats Pretreated with Known Modifiers of Cytochrome P-450 Activity. *Drug Metabolism and Disposition, 27,* 526-532.

[43] Crommelin, D. J. A. & Sindelar, R. D. (1997). *Pharmaceutical biotechnology : an introduction for pharmacists and pharmaceutical scientists.* Australia;United Kingdom: Harwood Academic.

[44] Galijatovic, A., Otake, Y., Walle, U. K. & Walle, T. (1999). Extensive metabolism of the flavonoid chrysin by human Caco-2 and Hep G2 cells. *Xenobiotica, 29,* 1241-1256.

[45] Urani, C., Doldi, M., Crippa, S. & Camatini, M. (1998). Human-derived cell lines to study xenobiotic metabolism. *Chemosphere, 37,* 2785-2795.

[46] Walle, T., Otake, Y., Galijatovic, A., Ritter, J. K. & Walle, U. K. (2000). Induction of UDP-glucuronosyltransferase UGT1A1 by the flavonoid chrysin in the human hepatoma cell line Hep G2. *Drug Metabolism and Disposition, 28,* 1077-1082.

[47] Yoshitomi, S., Ikemoto, K., Takahashi, J., Miki, H., Namba, M. & Asahi, S. (2001). Establishment of the transformants expressing human cytochrome P450 subtypes in HepG2, and their applications on drug metabolism and toxicology. *Toxicology in Vitro, 15,* 245-256.

[48] Gomez-Lechon, M. J., Donato, T., Jover, R., Rodriguez, C., Ponsoda, X., Glaise, D., Castell, J. V. & Guguen-Guillouzo, C. (2001). Expression and induction of a large set of drug-metabolizing enzymes by the highly differentiated human hepatoma cell line BC2. *European Journal of Biochemistry, 268,* 1448-1459.

[49] Hukkanen, J., Lassila, A., Paivarinta, K., Valanne, S., Sarpo, S., Hakkola, J., Pelkonen, O. & Raunio, H. (2000). Induction and Regulation of Xenobiotic-Metabolizing Cytochrome P450s in the Human A549 Lung Adenocarcinoma Cell Line. *American Journal of Respiratory Cell and Molecular Biology, 22,* 360-366.

[50] Knasmüller, S., Mersch-Sundermann, V., Kevekordes, S., Darroudi, F., Huber, W. W., Hoelzl, C., Bichler, J. & Majer, B. J. (2004). Use of human-derived liver cell lines for the detection of environmental and dietary genotoxicants; current state of knowledge. *Toxicology, 198,* 315-328.

[51] Aninat, C., Piton, A., Glaise, D., Le Charpentier, T., Langouet, S., Morel, F., Guguen-Guillouzo, C. & Guillouzo, A. (2006). Expression of Cytochromes P450, Conjugating Enzymes and Nuclear Receptors in Human Hepatoma HepaRG Cells. *Drug Metabolism and Disposition, 34,* 75-83.

[52] Kanebratt, K. P. & Andersson, T. B. (2008). Evaluation of HepaRG cells as an in vitro model for human drug metabolism studies. *Drug Metabolism Disposition, 36,* 1444-1452.

[53] Sinz, M. W., Podoll, T. (2002). The Mass Spectrometer in Drug Metabolism. In D. T. Rossi & M. W. Sinz (Eds.), *Mass spectrometry in drug discovery* pp. 271-335). New York: Marcel Dekker.

[54] Wilson, I. D., Nicholson, J. K. & Lindon, J. C. (1999). The Role of Nuclear Magnetic Resonance Spectroscopy in Drug Metabolism. In T. F. Woolf (Eds.), *Handbook of drug metabolism* pp. 523-550). New York NY: Marcel Dekker.

[55] Rossi, D. T. (2002). Sample Preparation and Handling for LC/MS in Drug Discovery. In D. T. Rossi & M. W. Sinz (Eds.), *Mass spectrometry in drug discovery* pp. 171-214). New York: Marcel Dekker.

[56] Sheehan, T. L. (2002). The best MS option: GC-MS and LC-MS. *American laboratory, 34,* 40-43.

[57] Fountain, S. T. (2002). A Mass Spectrometry Primer. In D. T. Rossi & M. W. Sinz (Eds.), *Mass spectrometry in drug discovery* pp. 25-84). New York: Marcel Dekker.

[58] EU. (2002). Commission Directive 2002/657/EC implementing Council Directive 96/23/EC concerning the performance of analytical methods and interpretation of results. *Official Journal of European Communities, 45,* 8-36.

[59] Nicholson, J. K. & Wilson, I. D. (1985). High resolution nuclear magnetic spectroscopy of biological fluids as an aid to drug development. *Progress in Drug Research, 31,* 427-479.

[60] Malet-Martino, M. C. & Martino, R. (1989). The application of nuclear magnetic resonance spectroscopy to drug metabolism studies. *Xenobiotica, 19,* 583-607.

[61] Shockcor, J. P., Unger, S. H., Wilson, I. D., Foxall, P. J. D., Nicholson, J. K. & Lindon, J. C. (1996). Combined HPLC, NMR Spectroscopy, and Ion-Trap Mass Spectrometry with Application to the Detection and Characterization of Xenobiotic and Endogenous Metabolites in Human Urine. *Analytical Chemistry, 68,* 4431-4435.

[62] Dear, G. J., Plumb, R. S., Sweatman, B. C., Ayrton, J., Lindon, J. C., Nicholson, J. K. & Ismail, I. M. (2000). Mass directed peak selection, an efficient method of drug metabolite identification using directly coupled liquid chromatography-mass spectrometry-nuclear magnetic resonance spectroscopy. *Journal of Chromatography, B: Biomedical Sciences and Applications, 748,* 281-293.

[63] Sidelmann, U. G., Bjornsdottir, I., Shockcor, J. P., Hansen, S. H., Lindon, J. C. & Nicholson, J. K. (2001). Directly coupled HPLC-NMR and HPLC-MS approaches for the rapid characterization of drug metabolites in urine: application to the human metabolism of naproxen. *Journal of pharmaceutical and biomedical analysis, 24,* 569-579.

[64] Corcoran, O. & Spraul, M. (2003). LC-NMR-MS in drug discovery. *Drug discovery today, 8,* 624-631.

[65] Spraul, M., Freund, A. S., Nast, R. E., Withers, R. S., Maas, W. E. & Corcoran, O. (2003). Advancing NMR Sensitivity for LC-NMR-MS Using a Cryoflow Probe: Application to the Analysis of Acetaminophen Metabolites in Urine. *Analytical Chemistry, 75,* 1536-1541.

[66] Godejohann, M., Tseng, L., Braumann, U., Fuchser, J. & Spraul, M. (2004). Characterization of a paracetamol metabolite using on-line LC-SPE-NMR-MS and a cryogenic NMR probe. *Journal of Chromatography, A, 1058,* 191-196.

[67] Abass, K., Reponen, P., Turpeinen, M., Jalonen, J. & Pelkonen, O. (2007). Characterization of Diuron N-Demethylation by Mammalian Hepatic Microsomes and cDNA-Expressed Human Cytochrome P450 Enzymes. *Drug Metabolism and Disposition, 35,* 1634-1641.

[68] Price, D. E., Mehta, A., Park, B. K., Hay, A. & Feely, M. P. (1986). The effect of low-dose phenobarbitone on three indexes of hepatic microsomal enzyme induction. *British Journal of Clinical Pharmacology., 22,* 744-747.

[69] Okey, A. B. (1990). Enzyme induction in the cytochrome P-450 system. *Pharmacology & Therapeutics, 45,* 241-298.

[70] Dierickx, P. J. (1999). CYP1/2 Activation and Glutathione-dependent Cytotoxicity of Four Pesticides in Hep G2 and Fa32 Cells. *Toxicology in Vitro, 13,* 779-783.

[71] Delescluse, C., Ledirac, N., Li, R., Piechocki, M. P., Hines, R. N., Gidrol, X. & Rahmani, R. (2001). Induction of cytochrome P450 1A1 gene expression, oxidative stress, and genotoxicity by carbaryl and thiabendazole in transfected human HepG2 and lymphoblastoid cells. *Biochemical Pharmacology, 61,* 399-407.

[72] Coumoul, X., Diry, M. & Barouki, R. (2002). PXR-dependent induction of human CYP3A4 gene expression by organochlorine pesticides. *Biochemical Pharmacology, 64,* 1513-1519.

[73] Sanderson, J. T., Boerma, J., Lansbergen, G. W. A. & van den Berg, M. (2002). Induction and Inhibition of Aromatase (CYP19) Activity by Various Classes of Pesticides in H295R Human Adrenocortical Carcinoma Cells. *Toxicology and Applied Pharmacology, 182,* 44-54.

[74] Wyde, M. E., Bartolucci, E., Ueda, A., Zhang, H., Yan, B., Negishi, M. & You, L. (2003). The Environmental Pollutant 1,1-Dichloro-2,2-bis (p-chlorophenyl)ethylene Induces Rat Hepatic Cytochrome P450 2B and 3A Expression through the Constitutive Androstane Receptor and Pregnane X Receptor. *Molecular Pharmacology, 64,* 474-481.

[75] Lemaire, G., de Sousa, G. & Rahmani, R. (2004). A PXR reporter gene assay in a stable cell culture system: CYP3A4 and CYP2B6 induction by pesticides. *Biochemical Pharmacology, 68,* 2347-2358.

[76] Das, P. C., Cao, Y., Cherrington, N., Hodgson, E. & Rose, R. L. (2006). Fipronil induces CYP isoforms and cytotoxicity in human hepatocytes. *Chemico-Biological Interactions, 164,* 200-214.

[77] Sun, G., Thai, S., Tully, D. B., Lambert, G. R., Goetz, A. K., Wolf, D. C., Dix, D. J. & Nesnow, S. (2005). Propiconazole-induced cytochrome P450 gene expression and enzymatic activities in rat and mouse liver. *Toxicology Letters, 155,* 277-287.

[78] Goetz, A. K., Bao, W., Ren, H., Schmid, J. E., Tully, D. B., Wood, C., Rockett, J. C., Narotsky, M. G., Sun, G., Lambert, G. R., Thai, S., Wolf, D. C., Nesnow, S. & Dix, D. J. (2006). Gene expression profiling in the liver of CD-1 mice to characterize the hepatotoxicity of triazole fungicides. *Toxicology and Applied Pharmacology, 215,* 274-284.

[79] Johri, A., Yadav, S., Dhawan, A. & Parmar, D. (2007). Overexpression of cerebral and hepatic cytochrome P450s alters behavioral activity of rat offspring following prenatal exposure to lindane. *Toxicology and Applied Pharmacology, 225,* 278-292.

[80] Barber, D. S., McNally, A. J., Garcia-Reyero, N. & Denslow, N. D. (2007). Exposure to p,p′-DDE or dieldrin during the reproductive season alters hepatic CYP expression in largemouth bass (Micropterus salmoides). *Aquatic Toxicology, 81,* 27-35.

[81] Greenlee, W. F. & Poland, A. (1978). An improved assay of 7-ethoxycoumarin O-deethylase activity: induction of hepatic enzyme activity in C57BL/6J and DBA/2J mice by phenobarbital, 3-methylcholanthrene and 2,3,7,8-tetrachlorodibenzo-p-dioxin. *The Journal Of Pharmacology And Experimental Therapeutics, 205,* 596-605.

[82] Burke, M. D., Prough, R. A. & Mayer, R. T. (1977). Characteristics of a microsomal cytochrome P-448-mediated reaction. Ethoxyresorufin O-de-ethylation. *Drug Metabolism And Disposition, 5,* 1-8.

[83] Raunio, H., Valtonen, J., Honkakoski, P., Lang, M. A., Stahlberg, M., Kairaluoma, M. A., Rautio, A., Pasanen, M. & Pelkonen, O. (1990). Immunochemical detection of human liver cytochrome P450 forms related to phenobarbital-inducible forms in the mouse. *Biochemical Pharmacology, 40,* 2503-2509.

[84] Turpeinen, M., Nieminen, R., Juntunen, T., Taavitsainen, P., Raunio, H. & Pelkonen, O. (2004). Selective inhibition of CYP2B6-catalyzed bupropion hydroxylation in human liver microsomes in vitro. *Drug Metabolism and Disposition, 32,* 626-631.

[85] Li, X., Bjorkman, A., Andersson, T. B., Ridderstrom, M. & Masimirembwa, C. M. (2002). Amodiaquine Clearance and Its Metabolism to N-Desethylamodiaquine Is Mediated by CYP2C8: A New High Affinity and Turnover Enzyme-Specific Probe Substrate. *Journal of Pharmacology And Experimental Therapeutics, 300,* 399-407.

[86] Sullivan-Klose, T. H., Ghanayem, B. I., Bell, D. A., Zhang, Z. Y., Kaminsky, L. S., Shenfield, G. M., Miners, J. O., Birkett, D. J. & Goldstein, J. A. (1996). The role of the CYP2C9-Leu359 allelic variant in the tolbutamide polymorphism. *Pharmacogenetics, 6,* 341-349.

[87] Abelo, A., Andersson, T. B., Antonsson, M., Naudot, A. K., Skanberg, I. & Weidolf, L. (2000). Stereoselective metabolism of omeprazole by human cytochrome P450 enzymes. *Drug Metabolism And Disposition: The Biological Fate Of Chemicals, 28,* 966-972.

[88] Kronbach, T., Mathys, D., Gut, J., Catin, T. & Meyer, U. A. (1987). High-performance liquid chromatographic assays for bufuralol 1'-hydroxylase, debrisoquine 4-hydroxylase, and dextromethorphan O-demethylase in microsomes and purified cytochrome P-450 isozymes of human liver. *Analytical Biochemistry, 162,* 24-32.

[89] Peter, R., Bocker, R., Beaune, P. H., Iwasaki, M., Guengerich, F. P. & Yang, C. S. (1990). Hydroxylation of chlorzoxazone as a specific probe for human liver cytochrome P-450IIE1. *Chemical Research In Toxicology, 3,* 566-573.

[90] Kronbach, T., Mathys, D., Umeno, M., Gonzalez, F. J. & Meyer, U. A. (1989). Oxidation of midazolam and triazolam by human liver cytochrome P450IIIA4. *Molecular Pharmacology, 36,* 89-96.

[91] Turpeinen, M., Jouko, U., Jorma, J. & Olavi, P. (2005). Multiple P450 substrates in a single run: rapid and comprehensive in vitro interaction assay. *European Journal of Pharmaceutical Sciences, 24,* 123-132.

[92] Weaver, R., Graham, K. S., Beattie, I. G. & Riley, R. J. (2003). Cytochrome P450 inhibition using recombinant proteins and mass spectrometry/multiple reaction monitoring technology in a cassette incubation. *Drug Metabolism and Disposition, 31,* 955-966.

[93] Dierks, E. A., Stams, K. R., Lim, H., Cornelius, G., Zhang, H. & Ball, S. E. (2001). A Method for the Simultaneous Evaluation of the Activities of Seven Major Human Drug-Metabolizing Cytochrome P450s Using an in Vitro Cocktail of Probe Substrates and Fast Gradient Liquid Chromatography Tandem Mass Spectrometry. *Drug Metabolism and Disposition, 29,* 23-29.

[94] Testino, S. A. & Patonay, G. (2003). High-throughput inhibition screening of major human cytochrome P450 enzymes using an in vitro cocktail and liquid chromatography–tandem mass spectrometry. *Journal of Pharmaceutical and Biomedical Analysis, 30,* 1459-1467.

[95] Kim, M., Kim, H., Cha, I., Park, J., Shon, J., Liu, K. & Shin, J. (2005). High-throughput screening of inhibitory potential of nine cytochrome P450 enzymes *in vitro*

using liquid chromatography/tandem mass spectrometry. *Rapid Communications in Mass Spectrometry, 19,* 2651-2658.

[96] Tolonen, A., Petsalo, A., Turpeinen, M., Uusitalo, J. & Pelkonen, O. (2007). In vitro interaction cocktail assay for nine major cytochrome P450 enzymes with 13 probe reactions and a single LC/MSMS run: analytical validation and testing with monoclonal anti-CYP antibodies. *Journal of Mass Spectrometry, 42,* 960-966.

[97] Turpeinen, M., Korhonen, L. E., Tolonen, A., Uusitalo, J., Juvonen, R., Raunio, H. & Pelkonen, O. (2006). Cytochrome P450 (CYP) inhibition screening: Comparison of three tests. *European Journal of Pharmaceutical Sciences, 29,* 130-138.

[98] Turpeinen, M., Ghiciuc, C., Opritoui, M., Tursas, L., Pelkonen, O. & Pasanen, M. (2007). Predictive value of animal models for human cytochrome P450 (CYP)-mediated metabolism: A comparative study in vitro. *Xenobiotica, 37,* 1367-1377.

[99] Abass, K., Reponen, P., Jalonen, J. & Pelkonen, O. (2007). In vitro metabolism and interactions of the fungicide metalaxyl in human liver preparations. *Environmental Toxicology and Pharmacology, 23,* 39-47.

[100] Paolini, M., Mesirca, R., Pozzetti, L., Sapone, A. & Cantelli-Forti, G. (1996). Biomarkers of effect in evaluating metalaxyl cocarcinogenesis selective induction of murine CYP 3A isoform. *Mutation Research/Environmental Mutagenesis and Related Subjects, 361,* 157-164.

[101] Pozzetti, L., Paolini, M., Barillari, J. & Cantelli-Forti, G. (1999). Induction and suppression of murine CYP-mediated biotransformation by dithianon: organ- and sex-related differences. *Cancer Letters, 141,* 47-56.

[102] Paolini, M., Barillari, J., Trespidi, S., Valgimigli, L., Pedulli, G. F. & Cantelli-Forti, G. (1999). Captan impairs CYP-catalyzed drug metabolism in the mouse. *Chemico-Biological Interactions, 123,* 149-170.

[103] Paolini, M., Pozzetti, L., Perocco, P., Mazzullo, M. & Cantelli-Forti, G. (1999). Molecular non-genetic biomarkers of effect related to methyl thiophanate cocarcinogenesis: organ- and sex-specific cytochrome P450 induction in the rat. *Cancer Letters, 135,* 203-213.

[104] Vinggaard, A. M., Hnida, C., Breinholt, V. & Larsen, J. C. (2000). Screening of selected pesticides for inhibition of CYP19 aromatase activity in vitro. *Toxicology in Vitro, 14,* 227-234.

[105] Mazur, C. S. & Kenneke, J. F. (2008). Cross-Species Comparison of Conazole Fungicide Metabolites Using Rat and Rainbow Trout (Onchorhynchus mykiss) Hepatic Microsomes and Purified Human CYP 3A4. *Environmental Science & Technology, 42,* 947-954.

[106] Trösken, E. R., Adamska, M., Arand, M., Zarn, J. A., Patten, C., Völkel, W. & Lutz, W. K. (2006). Comparison of lanosterol-14α-demethylase (CYP51) of human and Candida albicans for inhibition by different antifungal azoles. *Toxicology, 228,* 24-32.

[107] Hodgson, E. (2003). In vitro human phase I metabolism of xenobiotics I: Pesticides and related compounds used in agriculture and public health, may 2003. *Journal of Biochemical and Molecular Toxicology, 17,* 201-206.

[108] Mazur, C. S., Kenneke, J. F., Tebes-Stevens, C., Okino, M. S. & Lipscomb, J. C. (2007). In Vitro Metabolism of the Fungicide and Environmental Contaminant trans-

bromuconazole and Implications for Risk Assessment. *Journal of Toxicology & Environmental Health: Part A, 70,* 1241-1250.

[109] Barton, H. A., Tang, J., Sey, Y. M., Stanko, J. P., Murrell, R. N., Rockett, J. C. & Dix, D. J. (2006). Metabolism of myclobutanil and triadimefon by human and rat cytochrome P450 enzymes and liver microsomes. *Xenobiotica, 36,* 793-806.

[110] Nagahori, H., Yoshino, H., Tomigahara, Y., Isobe, N., Kaneko, H. & Nakatsuka, I. (2000). Metabolism of Furametpyr. 1. Identification of Metabolites and in Vitro Biotransformation in Rats and Humans. *Journal of Agricultural and Food Chemistry, 48,* 5754-5759.

[111] Tomlin, C. (2000). *The Pesticide Manual, 12th ed.* Berkshire, UK: BCPC Publications.

[112] Ahlborg, U. G., Larsson, K. & Thunberg, T. (1978). Metabolism of pentachlorophenol in vivo and in vitro. *Archives of Toxicology, 40,* 45-53.

[113] Juhl, U., Witte, I. & Butte, W. (1985). Metabolism of pentachlorophenol to tetrachlorohydroquinone by human liver homogenate. *Bulletin of Environmental Contamination and Toxicology, 35,* 596-601.

[114] Tsai, C., Lin, P., Waidyanatha, S. & Rappaport, S. M. (2001). Characterization of metabolic activation of pentachlorophenol to quinones and semiquinones in rodent liver. *Chemico-Biological Interactions, 134,* 55-71.

[115] Paine, A. J. (1996). Validity and reliability of in vitro systems in safety evaluation. *Environmental Toxicology and Pharmacology, 2,* 207-212.

[116] Falk-Filipsson, A., Hanberg, A., Victorin, K., Warholm, M. & Wallén, M. (2007). Assessment factors—Applications in health risk assessment of chemicals. *Environmental Research, 104,* 108-127.

[117] Renwick, A. G. & Lazarus, N. R. (1998). Human Variability and Noncancer Risk Assessment— An Analysis of the Default Uncertainty Factor. *Regulatory Toxicology and Pharmacology, 27,* 3-20.

[118] Walton, K., Dorne, J. L. & Renwick, A. G. (2001). Uncertainty factors for chemical risk assessment: interspecies differences in the in vivo pharmacokinetics and metabolism of human CYP1A2 substrates. *Food and Chemical Toxicology, 39,* 667-680.

[119] WHO/IPCS. (2005). *Chemical-specific adjustment factors for interspecies differences and human variability: guidance document for use of data in dose/concentration-response assessment.* Geneva: World Health Organization.

[120] Abass, K., Reponen, P., Jalonen, J. & Pelkonen, O. (2007). In vitro metabolism and interaction of profenofos by human, mouse and rat liver preparations. *Pesticide Biochemistry and Physiology, 87,* 238-247.

[121] Lang, D., Criegee, D., Grothusen, A., Saalfrank, R. & Bocker, R. (1996). In vitro metabolism of atrazine, terbuthylazine, ametryne, and terbutryne in rats, pigs, and humans. *Drug Metabolism and Disposition, 24,* 859-865.

[122] Tang, J., Cao, Y., Rose, R. L., Brimfield, A. A., Dai, D., Goldstein, J. A. & Hodgson, E. (2001). Metabolism of Chlorpyrifos by Human Cytochrome P450 Isoforms and Human, Mouse, and Rat Liver Microsomes. *Drug Metabolism and Disposition, 29,* 1201-1204.

[123] Usmani, K. A., Hodgson, E. & Rose, R. L. (2004). In vitro metabolism of carbofuran by human, mouse, and rat cytochrome P450 and interactions with chlorpyrifos, testosterone, and estradiol. *Chemico-Biological Interactions, 150,* 221-232.

In: Fungicides
Editors: P. De Costa and P. Bezerra

ISBN: 978-1-60692-631-4

Chapter II

Analytical Methodology for Ultra-trace Detection and Quantification of Fungicides and other Priority Substances Concerned by European Regulations in Environmental Parts

***Jean-Baptiste Baugros*[1], *Cécile Cren-Olivé*[1,2], *Pierre Lantéri*[2], *Marie-Florence Grenier-Loustalot*[1]**

[1]Service Central d'Analyse du CNRS USR 059, Chemin du Canal, 69360 Solaize, France
[2]Laboratoire de Sciences Analytiques, Université de Lyon, Université LyonA, CNRS UMR 5180 43 Bd du 11 novembre 1918, Bat. 308 D, 69622 Villeurbanne, France

Abstract

During the last decade, the use of many chemical substances without any control and studies about their behaviour in the environment has become a focus of interest for the European Union (EU). Pesticides which are widely used through Europe, entered into the environment and contaminate waters and soils with potential risks for wildlife and human health due to the proved or suspected toxicity of these compounds. Very few interests targeted on fungicides while they represent a major part of all type of pesticides used (herbicides, insecticides, rodenticides…). Nevertheless, pesticides are already regulated by the european directive 91/414/EEC which target to reduce their impact on human health and the environment. Concerning foodstuffs for human and animal consumption, pesticides residues have to not exceed the Maximum Residue Limits (MRLs) indicated in different directives (76/895/EEC, 86/362/EEC, 86/363/EEC, 90/642/EEC, 2005/396/EEC) regulating their concentration respectively in fruits and vegetables, in cereals, in foodstuffs of animal origin, and in products of vegetable origin and honey. In addition, REACH (for Regulation Evaluation and Authorization of Chemicals), the new regulation system which target to improve the protection of human health and the environment from the risks that can be posed by unknown chemicals give a focus on pollution brought by major diffusion of chemicals like pesticides and consequently fungicides. It implements directive 91/414/EEC concerning the placing of plant products on the European market [1]. In this context, sensitive, reliable and undoubtedly analytical methods for monitoring fungicides in the environment are really necessary to set up their control by the future european regulations and directives.

In this chapter, we will first present a quick overview of the different analytical methods reported in the literature for the analysis of fungicides. Then, we will focus on the new methodology we develop to detect and quantify 33 substances suspected to interfere with the hormonal system or/and have a toxicity on human and wildlife at very low concentrations (ng.L^{-1} and μg.kg^{-1}), and particularly 8 fungicides:

- 2-imidazolidinethione or ethylenethiourea, principal metabolite of many dithiocarbamates fungicides (mancozeb, ziram, propineb)
- Tebuconazole (triazole fungicide)
- Hexaconazole (triazole fungicide)
- Tetraconazole (triazole fungicide)
- Fluquinconazole (triazole fungicide)
- Bromuconazole (triazole fungicide)
- Dimethomorph (morpholine fungicide)
- Pyridaben (pyridazinone fungicide)

The optimisation of all the method steps from the extraction to the quantification by chromatography coupled with mass spectrometry as well as the method validation done by chemiometric approach, complete to be normalized for legislation rules applications and ready to be applied for toxicity studies will be discussed. Lastly, we will conclude with the application of our new methodology to real environmental samples (wastewaters, groundwater and surface waters and sediments, mud puddle, atmospheric fallout and sludge) confirming major occurrence of several compounds in the environment of the Rhône-Alpes region, France.

INTRODUCTION

Since many years, intensive agriculture has led to a large scale use of herbicides, insecticides and fungicides in developed countries. The application of these compounds has greatly improved the productivity worldwide without thinking about their fate and the occurrence of substances in the environment. Fungicides are a special group of pesticides which are used all along the cultivation to control plant diseases from the sowing to the protection of seed after the crop [2]. More than 300 000 tonnes of pesticides are sold in Europe, 108 000 tonnes are used as fungicides [3]. During the application, formulated aqueous solution, solids or powder, up to 30-50% of the total dose never attains the wanted area [4]. Agricultural activity is closely related to the applications calendar and as results of their widespread, many of them entered into the environment from the application area by the air and water depending of the weather and the period. Water is the principal vehicle contaminating groundwaters by infiltration and surface waters by irrigation water, collected wastewaters by rainwater streaming the cultivated fields. Therefore, it is very important to develop Environmental Risk Assessment (ERA) methods to determine a priority list of substances necessary to be monitored in drinking water. Fungicides must be included into it.

The European Chemical Bureau (ECB) for the European Community [5] and the Environmental Protection Agency (EPA) for the US [6] have both developed substances evaluation database, assessment methods and environmental quality standards to protect the quality of life and the health of citizens. In addition, all their agencies must provide sufficient information for industrial decision with the utilisation or no of chemicals. REACH (Registration, Evaluation and Authorisation of Chemicals), the new European Chemicals legislation, propose to improve the ERA process by including available, reliable and ecotoxicological test methods and strategies. To perform the major objectives of REACH, scientifically justified and efficient testing system and risk assessment are required [7].

Undeniably, the recent government interest to the environmental fate of unknown chemicals and the setting up of such system need to be based on solid, robust and sensitive analytical methods for the detection and the quantification of fungicides in environmental parts.

Firstly, we will present a summary of the previous analytical methods for the analysis of fungicides in environment. Then, we will focus on our new and high performance methodology developed to detect and quantify 33 substances including 8 fungicides at very low concentrations. Finally, we will give results obtained for real environmental samples.

1. Overview of the Different Analytical Methods Reported in the Literature for the Analysis of Fungicides

Even if cultivators start to spread quantities of pesticides linked to the need of plants, pesticides are chemicals manufactured specifically to be toxic to living species and are released into the environment. A great number of published papers about the development and application of multiresidue environmental analysis has increased since pesticides have caused contamination of the hydrological system, principle origin of drinking water. The European Community directive 98/83 concerning the quality of water intended for human consumption establishes the maximum admissible concentration of each individual pesticide at 0.1 $\mu g.L^{-1}$ and the total amount of pesticides at 0.5 $\mu g.L^{-1}$ [8]. Fungicides are a part of "pesticides" legal term group.

Consequently, since a decade, several publications have been proposed about the analysis of pesticides and more specifically about fungicides in foodstuffs, particularly in fruits and vegetables [9-12]. Very few publications have been given about analytical methods of fungicides in waters [13-18] or solids environmental parts [19-22]. Other methods for the determination of fungicides have been performed on animals which can play a key role as an indicator of air/soil/water pollution, like honeybees [23], earthworms [24] or trout [25].

Table 1. Analytical procedures for the determination of fungicides in fruits and vegetables

Author	Compounds	Type of samples	Sample preparation	Analytical techniques	LOD	LOQ
Garcinuno [9]	Ethylenethiourea, Ethylenebis[isothio cyanate] sulphide	Fruits (Almond)	SPE	LC-DAD UV	NC	0.05-0.07 μg.kg^{-1}
Van Lishaut [10]	5 dithiocarbamate fungicides	Fruits and vegetables	LSE	LC-DAD UV ECD	4-8 μg CS_2.kg^{-1}	8-18 μg CS_2.kg^{-1}
Schermerhorn [11]	14 parent triazole fungicides and 8 metabolites	Apples, peaches, flour and water	LSE SPE	LC-ESI-MS/MS	0.003-9.0 μg.kg^{-1}	0.010-28 μg.kg^{-1}
Gonzales-Rodriguez [12]	11 fungicides (2 aniline-pyrimidine, 1 phenylpyrrole, 3 dicarboximide, 1 phenylamide, 4 triazole)	Leafy vegetables	LSE SPE	GC-MS	<1- 5 μg.kg^{-1}	1- 10 μg.kg^{-1}
Sannino [28]	24 new residues pesticides (3 strobilurin, 7 triazole, 1 hydroxyanilide, 1 morpholine)	Fruits and vegetables	LLE	LC-ESI-MS/MS	NC	1-20 μg.kg^{-1}
Navarro [29]	8 fungicides	Fruits and vegetables	SPE	GC-MS	3-30 μg.kg^{-1}	10-100 μg.kg^{-1}
Kumar [31]	Hexaconazole	Tea (leaves, infusion)	LSE + Clean-up flash chro-matorgaphy	GC-NPD	50 μg.kg^{-1}	100 μg.kg^{-1}
Millan [30]	6 organochlorine fungicides	Wine	SPME	LC-DAD UV	4-27 μg.L^{-1}	NC

SPE, Solid-Phase Extraction; LLE, Liquid-Liquid Extraction; LSE, Liquid-Solid Extraction; SPME, Solid-Phase MicroExtraction; ElectroChemical Detection, ECD; NC, Not Communicated.

All phases of analytical procedures allowing the quantification of fungicides are assessed, including sampling and storage, sample preparation and analysis and validation of methods but unfortunately only few give attractive applications to real samples [14-16, 18, 22].

A state of the art is listed in three tables concerning fruits and vegetables (table 1), animals (bioindicators, table 2) and environmental parts (table 3).

1.1. Occurrence of Fungicides in Fruits and Vegetables

Pesticides are efficient if they reach the infested target. Fungi can develop on plants all along its life and treatments are necessary. Furthermore, plants metabolise them and fungicides circulate into them. As a result, substances can attain each part, roots, stems, branches and fruits or vegetables. So fruits and vegetables, which human may eat, are a potential part of the plant where fungicides may accumulate. Consequently, vegetables garden and orchard treated can contaminate humans themselves by their own chemicals. Table 1 presents recent analytical methods for the determination of fungicides in fruits and vegetables.

We noticed that several authors have paid attention to dithiocarbamate and triazole fungicides as new generation of pesticides. Garcinuno and al. published an analytical protocol to the determination of two metabolites of ethylene bisdithiocarbamate pesticides which are among the most widely used fungicides to control a broad spectrum of fungi. We can list Maneb, Zineb, Mancozeb, Metiram, Nabam as commercialised formulated compounds. The instability of these active substances leads to the formation of ethylenethiourea (ETU) and ethylenebis(isocyanate)sulphide by hydrolysis and photolysis during the environmental fate. Both metabolites are considered to be the main responsible for the toxic effects of this pesticide group. It has been proved that ETU can cause teratogenic, carcinogenic, immunotoxic and mutagenic effects [26, 27]. In addition, dithiocarbamates are used as antioxydants in rubber, where ETU is a major degradation by-product and can contaminate waters and fields. For all this reasons, ETU is a key metabolite of fungicides without enough studies about it in environmental parts.

Generally, the first step of the vegetables and fruits preparation is to get analytes in organic solvent. Frequently, the sample is crushed and blended with organic solvent [10-12, 28] or solid phase [9, 29] and so ready for extractions; techniques often used are liquid-liquid or solid phase extractions. Millan and al. used solid microextraction to extract fungicides from wine, since this is a simple technique to hold out fungicides which are already in a liquid matrix [30].

Preferential analytical techniques are liquid chromatography coupled with ultraviolet detection since several fungicides present conjugated systems in their chemical structure. Most specifically, electrochemical detection is used by Van Lishaut and al. allowing the quantification of a single family of fungicides, dithiocarbamates by the determination of carbon disulfide total amount [10]. Most recently, universal and specific detection system like mass spectrometry is applied too. As GC-MS is an ordinary machine in an analytical department other methods are based on it and seems to give satisfy detection limits. But finally, LC-MS/MS gives the best sensibility on extracted fungicides from apples, peaches, flour and water [11]. The procedures summarised in table 1 show very low Limits Of Detection and Quantification (LOD and LOQ) depending on the considered matrices. They are in the range of low $\mu g.kg^{-1}$ to high hundred of $\mu g.kg^{-1}$.

The regulation about pesticides authorises a Maximum Residue Limit (MRL) of 10 $\mu g.kg^{-1}$ in fruits and vegetables (regulation 2005/396/EEC, 91/414/EEC, 76/895/EEC and 90/642/EEC). The results found by Kumar and al were very high just after treatment by hexaconazole but substance was not detected after 11 days in tea leaves [31]. More dramatically, a lot of samples analysed by Navarro and al. found concentration of fungicides in the range of 0.15 to 1.64 mg.kg^{-1} of fungicides in apples, carrot, courgette, orange and tomato with highest level of captan and tebuconazole [29]. Recently, Gonzalez-Rodriguez detected concentrations of fungicides higher than LMRs in swiss chards, lettuces and spinachs [12].

1.2. Occurrence of Fungicides in Contaminated Animals

Fungicides are directly applied onto fields, giving the possibility to animals to be in contact or feed substances. Fungicides are not directly toxic to mammals or insects but they can induce chronic toxicity and increase the seriousness of the exposure if chemicals are combined with others. Table 2 presents three analytical procedures for determination of fungicides and insecticides metabolised by animals which live in possibly polluted environment like honeybees, earthworms and trout. As toxicology data are or will be required according to legislation [1, 3, 6], studies about the bioaccumulation of fungicides in animal tissues can be critical in risk assessment process. Fungicides studied by these authors were:

- triamedinol, imazalil, flusilazol, prochloraz and difenoconazole [23]
- folpet, metalaxyl and fostyl-Al [24],
- bromuconazole, metconazole and tetraconazole [25],
- cyproconazole, myclobutanil, triadimefon, penconazole, propiconazole and tebuconazole [23, 25]
- mycobutanil [23-25]

Honeybees are known as indicators of environmental pollution. Number of suspected poisoning of honeybees by pesticides have been reported [32]. All along the growing of the plant, pesticides can be metabolised by it and chemicals can reach the flower, make the contaminated pollen ready to be consumed by honeybees. Even if the fungicides are not entirely responsible of the death, they can act in synergism with other insecticides (pyrethroid, neonicotinoid) [23]. Charlton et al. proposed a very sensitive analytical method to determine the impact of 11 fungicides on the behaviour and the health of honeybees by GC-MS. The listed results show fungicides residues and pyrethroid insecticide also.

Fungicides are spread on fields in aqueous formulated solution during the seed germination or as coating of the seed contaminating soil, micro organisms and earthworms. Schreck and al. built up a high performance method to detect 4 fungicides in artificial contaminated earthworms and soils where they can live. The sample preparation was based on PLE and analytical method on GC-MS technique. They illustrated that earthworms are not really affected by pesticides and seem to metabolise rapidly chemicals. The authors suggested a potential role of earthworms in soil detoxification. Nevertheless, earthworms suffer physiological disturbances after two weeks exposure but any trace of pesticides remain in their tissues.

Table 2. Analytical procedures for the determination of fungicides in three animals

Author	Compounds	Type of samples	Sample preparation	Analytical techniques	LOD
Charlton [23]	11 fungicides	Honeybees	Soxhlet + GPC + SPE	GC-MS	1-5 ng/bee
Schreck [24]	4 fungicides and 2 insecticides	Earthworm, soil	PLE (ASE)	GC-MS	0.55 - 12.5 $ng.g^{-1}$
Konwick [25]	9 triazole fungicides and α-HCH	Rainbow trout	LSE + clean-up GPC	GC-MS	30 – 50 $ng.g^{-1}$

GPC, Gel Permeation Chromatography; SPE, Solid-Phase Extraction; PLE, Pressured Liquid Extraction (ASE, Accelerated Solvent Extraction); LSE, Liquid-Solid Extraction.

The possible harmful effects on fishes, aquatic organisms or batrachians must be evaluated. Konwick and al. assessed the bioaccumulation and biotransformation of 9 triazole fungicides in tissue of rainbow trout [25]. The total method determines the half-lives persistence of fungicides in the tissue comprises between 1 to 2.5 days. Difficulties about conjugate metabolite have been examined and give the analytical procedure really complex.

All methods in table 2 were based on GC-MS analytical techniques with very low LODs, in the $ng.g^{-1}$ range.

1.3. Occurrence of Fungicides in Environment

Many ways can help fungicides to attain hydrological system: infiltration, leaching or streaming on soils (figure 1). Despite of the integrated farming, it can expose the aquatic ecosystem to persistent and perpetual pesticides concentrations. They depend on the amount of frequency of precipitation or irrigation, the depth to the water, soil properties (permeability, available water capacity, organic carbon content) and land management practices such as the use of subsurface drains, irrigation or conservation tillage.

As a consequence of the environmental origin of drinking water, the occurrence of pesticides in water and solid bodies can also cause potential adverse public and environmental health effects.

As far as fate of fungicides is concerned and despite of the crude environmental conditions, particularly sun UVs and bacteria, persistent fungicides reach waters as surface waters (river, lake, pond), groundwaters and wastewaters. Nevertheless, according to their chemical structures, fungicides may offer more affinity to solid parts like soils, compost, sediments and sludge from wastewater treatment plants. Thus, they can attain soils by direct applications on them, by infiltration of contaminated waters and dispersion into sediments. Another real problem was recently posed by the production of high volume of sludge coming from wastewaters treatment plant (WWTP). The answer to it was to spread sludge on fields as fertilizer. However, rainwater percolation on contaminated sludge can disperse pollutants into groundwaters.

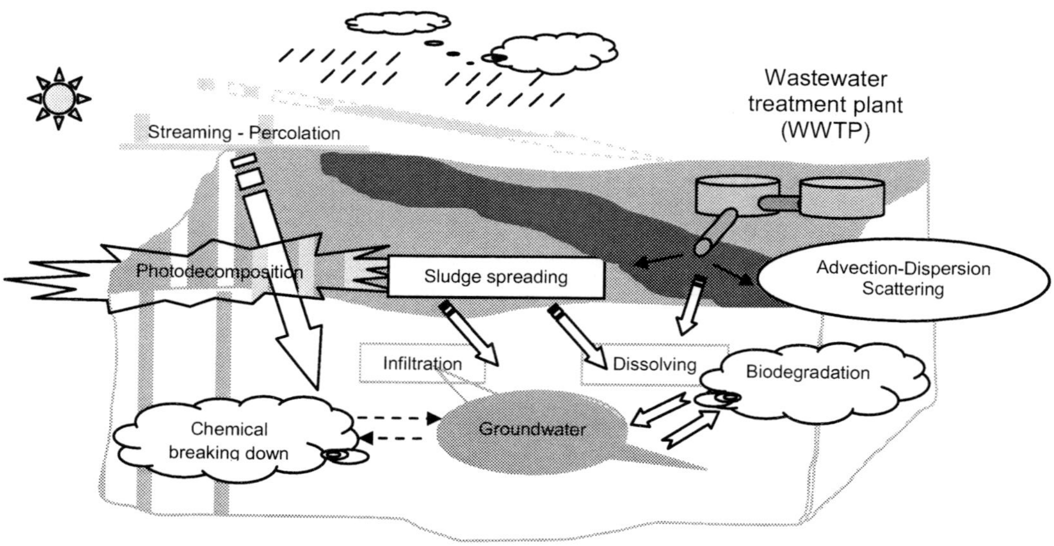

Figure 1. Possible pathways for the mobility of pollutants into the environment.

Table 3 reports the most up-to-date publications about analytical methods of fungicides in environment parts.

All these results show a great disparity in the levels of fungicides. Generally, concentrations were ranged from 0.01 to 3.35 $\mu g.L^{-1}$ in waters and 3 to 1124 $\mu g.kg^{-1}$ in solids. The difference of levels between both the matrices may be explained by the weak solubility in water of fungicides (roughly around ten of $mg.L^{-1}$ at 20°C) in regard with their partition coefficient, log P > 3. This physicochemical parameter estimates the bioaccumulation capacity of molecule on sediments or in lipid tissues of living organisms and indicates the repartition of molecules between waters and solids. When log P ≥ 3, partitioning of the fungicide is in favour of the part bound to soils than in sediments.

High concentrations have been found in soils at the vicinity of vineyards [19]. This is due to the seasonal treatment of the cultivation. The total fungicide median in soils was 82 $\mu g.kg^{-1}$, not so high if we compare it with extreme value like 1124 $\mu g.kg^{-1}$. Some fungicides are detected at the same time during the year and an ANOVA experimental design proves that they are both combined in the commercial fungicide formulation. Total fungicide concentrations found in the sediments are around 20 to 25 times lower than those in soils. This may be caused by a dilution process but their persistence is related to their high affinity to organic matter in good agreement with their log P. Eventually, all reported studies demonstrate the presence of fungicides in the environment despite of the integrating farming.

Table 3. Analytical procedures for the determination of fungicides in environmental parts

Author	Compounds	Type of samples	Sample preparation	Analytical techniques	LOD	LOQ
Salau [13]	8 fungicides	Environmental waters	Solid-Phase Disk	LC-DAD UV	0.005-0.1 µg.L^{-1}	0.01-0.1
	5 fungicides			LC-MS		
	3 fungicides			GC-ECD		
	6 fungicides			GC-MS		
Pan [14]	6 fungicides	Waters	HF-LPME	GC-ECD	4-25 ng.L^{-1}	NC
Zhou [15]	5 fungicides	Waters	SPE	LC-DAD UV	2.99-6.94 ng.L^{-1}	0.05-80 µg.L^{-1}
Balinova [17]	17 fungicides	Plants and water	SPE	TLC	0.005 - >2 µg	NC
Bermudez-Couso [19]	6 fungicides	Soils, sediments	LSE + LLE	GC-MS	1-3 µg.kg^{-1}	4-6 µg.kg^{-1}
Kawata [21, 22]	14 pesticides (2 fungicides) [21] 85 pesticides (13 fungicides) [22]	Compost [21] Sediments [22]	PLE + SPE [21] LSE + SPE [22]	GC-MS	< 20-40 µg.kg^{-1} 2-10 µg.kg^{-1}	NC NC
Hayama [33]	polycarbamate fungicides	Waters (tap water, rivers)	SPE	LC-APCI-MS/MS	0.032-0.061 µg.L^{-1}	0.11-0.20 µg.L^{-1}
Fernandez-Alba [34]	56 insecticides and fungicides	Ground waters	LLE-SPE	GC-MS	0.01-0.30 µg.L^{-1}	NC
	20 insecticides and fungicides	Ground waters	On line SPE	LC-DAD UV LC-APCI-MS	0.01-0.50 µg.L^{-1}	NC
Vanni [35]	3,5 DiChloroAniline and 4 fungicides	Compost	LSE	LC-DAD UV	15-145 µg.kg^{-1}	NC
Inam [36]	Triflumizole	Formulation, soil and waters	LSE (soil), dissolution (formulation) any preparation (waters)	pulse polarography	0.72-1.21 µmol.L^{-1}	2.39-4.10 µmol.L^{-1}

SPE, Solid-Phase Extraction; LLE, Liquid-Liquid Extraction; LSE, Liquid-Solid Extraction; HF-LPME, Hallow Fiber - liquid-Phase MicroExtraction; PLE, Pressure Liquid Extraction; LC-DAD UV, Liquid Chromatography – Diode Array Detector Ultra Violet; LC-APCI-MS, Liquid Chromatorgaphy – Atmospheric Pressure Chemical Ionisation – Mass Spectrometry; GC-ECD, Gas Chromatography – Electron Capture Detector; TLC, Thin Layer Chromatography; NC, Not Communicated.

Table 4. Concentrations of fungicides detected in environmental part

Author	Real sample	Detected compouds	Concentration
Pan [14]	Farm water (Taichung, Tawaïn)	Hexaconazole	3.35 ±0.14 $\mu g.L^{-1}$
Bermudez-Couso [19]	River sediments, vineyard soils (Galicia, Spain)	Metalaxyl, cyprodinil, penconazole, procymidone, fludioxonil	3-1124 $\mu g.kg^{-1}$ in soils 3-57 $\mu g.kg^{-1}$ in sediments
Kawata [21, 22]	Compost [21] Sediments [22]	imazalil and isoprothiolane 13 fungicides	< 0.02-210 $\mu g.kg^{-1}$ 3-69 $\mu g.kg^{-1}$
Hayama [33]	Chikugo river (Japan)	Polycarbamate fungicides	0.144-0.453 $\mu g.L^{-1}$
Fernandez-Alba [34]	Water wells (Almeria, Spain)	Chlorthalonil, vinolozolin, endosulfan, tetradifon, malathion and procymidone	0.01-0.35 $\mu g.L^{-1}$
Vanni [35]	Commercial composts	3,5-DCA, iprodione, procymidone, vinclozolin, chlozolinate	18.0-200.0 $\mu g.kg^{-1}$

2. High-Performance Analytical Methodology

2.1. Selection of Fungicides

In 2004, more than 18 000 tonnes of fungicides have been sold in France, 3 400 tonnes in Rhône-Alpes region. This area is well-known for its fruits and vegetables as well as cereal production. According to a report of the regional health organism, 19% and 13% of the pesticides detected respectively in superficial waters and in groundwaters are fungicides [37]. In this context, analytical procedure of fungicides in environment has to be developed. The proposed work has been done in a regional situation in order to offer a multiresidue analytical procedure of several priority chemicals. Alkylphenols and alkylphenols ethoxylates were the first studied compounds with phthalates-plasticizers (Diethylhexylphthalate, dibutylphthalate and bisphenol A). Then we selected pesticides, 2 organophosphorus and 8 organochlorine pesticides and 2 carbamates. Finally, considering the high potential of contamination of regional environmental coming from fungicides, we have selected 7 fungicides, bromuconazole, fluquinconazole, hexaconazole, tebuconazole, tetraconazole, pyridaben, dimethomorph (5 triazole, one morpholine and one pyridazinone) and a major metabolite of several dithiocarbamate fungicides, ethylenethiourea (ETU). The selection was based on their occurrence in the environment, their toxicity, their persistence and their possible and future regulation by Europe [8]. The whole analytical method allows the detection and the quantification of 33 regulated substances in environment. Eventually, 8 fungicide compounds of the method are listed in the table 5 and 25 other priority pollutants have been evaluated too [16].

As the table 5 shows, the hydrolysis half-life degradation time of molecules occurs after more of 20 days and 6 compounds are considered as very persistent (hydrolysis half-life >60 days). The solubility in water is in the range of ten μg.L^{-1} to around 200 mg.L^{-1}, except for ETU which is very soluble in water at 20 g.L^{-1}. In concordance with solubility, the partition coefficient is negative for ETU and roughly superior to 3 for the rest of analytes. This indicates us that it would be necessary to give our interest on both the environment parts (water and solid). Initially, all the analytical procedure was developed on samples coming from wastewater treatment plants, effluents and sludge. We will start the discussion with the optimisation of the preparation and concentration of water samples and we will present their application for solid samples. We will end this part by the optimisation of the analytical measurement.

Table 5. Physicochemical properties and environmental data of studied fungicides [38, 39]

Compounds	Fungicide chemical type	Solubility in water (mg.L^{-1}) @ 20°C	log P	Ecotoxicology (LD50 Oral Rats in mg/kg)	Hydrolysis half life in water days @ 20°C
Bromuconazole	Triazole	50	3.24	2150	very persistent
Fluquinconazole	Triazole	1.15	3.24	112	22
Hexaconazole	Triazole	18	3.90	2189	30
Tebuconazole	Triazole	32	3.70	5000	very persistent
Tetraconazole	Triazole	189.8	3.56	1248	very persistent
Pyridaben	Pyridazinone	0.012	6.37	820	very persistent
Dimethomorph	Morpholine	29	2.68	3900	70
Ethylenethiourea	Residue dithiocarbamates	20000	-0.66	1832	> 90

2.2. Methodology Extraction Optimisation

2.2.1. Aqueous Sample Pre-treatment and Analyte Extraction

Firstly, we have developed the preparation and the concentration steps required for ultra-trace determination of pollutants. It means that we have to select careful and precise techniques to keep target analytes and to eliminate coarse interferents. Environmental waters can contain particles and solid matters in suspension, particularly wastewaters. In addition, it is an active bacteriological matrix. For all of these reasons, we decided to filtrate and then to acidify the aqueous sample before extraction by SPE. All the steps of the optimisation were performed with spiked wastewater as the behaviour of pure water is not representative of the real environmental samples.

Waters were filtered using a Millipore YT30 142 HW device under nitrogen pressure. This step is essential to avoid clogging SPE cartridges by suspending matter. Tests have been carried out in order to check that the filter materials did not retain any compounds or bring pollutions by comparing the recovery of a mixture of standards after the whole filtration in the same conditions. At this step, we have evaluated SPE technique for our concentration step. Many difficulties can occur during the extraction of target compounds inducing low adsorption or incomplete desorption of strongly retained compounds on the sorbents. Therefore, all the SPE parameters (sample volume, sorbent, solvent elution, volumes, flow-rates ...) have to be carefully optimised to get the best recoveries. SPE was firstly carried out on different SPE materials, testing the following cartridges: Envi-Carb (200mg,3cc, Supelco), polymeric Starta-X (200mg,3cc, Phenomenex) and 3 identical base sorbent C-18 coming from three different providers, LC-18 (500mg,3cc, Supelco), Bond Elut (500mg,3cc, Varian) and Strata-C-18 (500mg,3cc, Phenomenex) and the performances were compared. For this step, wastewaters samples were spiked prior to the extraction with standard mixtures of target analytes at 500 ng.L^{-1}. This part of our SPE optimisation was firstly carried out on the main priority substances of REACH, alkylphenols and alkylphenols ethoxyaltes (APs) which are dispersant agents used in solid and liquid formulation fungicides. Low recoveries of these compounds were estimated from carbon graphite black and polymeric cartridges, Strata C-18 solid phase gave the best recovery rates, for all APs. Strata C-18 was finally selected since good recovery rates of fungicides were superior to 86%.

An evaluation of the pH adjustment, prior to extraction, was performed with formic acid (acid compatible with the chromatographic techniques). For this purpose, pH was adjusted from 3.8 to 6 and recovery rates were compared with the ones obtained without any pH adjustment (~7.5-8 for wastewaters). On the one hand, at wastewaters natural pH, ETU give recoveries below 26 %. On the other hand, none fundamental losses of analytes were found for a pH range of 3.8 to 5.7. So, pH was adjusted to 3.8 because of the lower RSD obtained, results are shown on figure 2. This may be explicated by the buffering role of this acid at its pKa value (3.75).

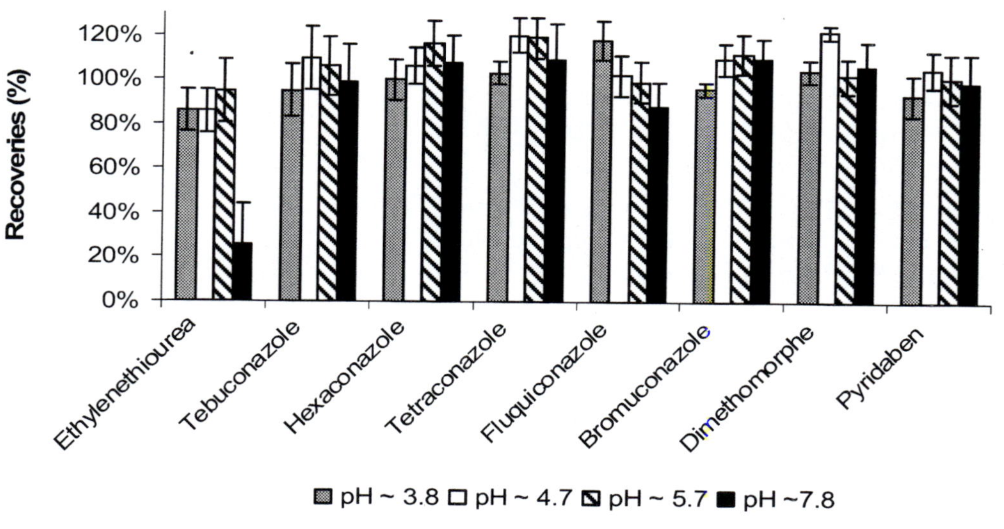

Figure 2. Influence of pH adjustment on the recoveries obtained using Strata-C18 cartridges.

As we used formic acid as preservative to stop the possible degradation of the target compounds too, we evaluated the progress of the compounds levels during 10 days for a pH adjusted spiked wastewater sample at 500 ng.L^{-1}. This experiment shows no major degradation, even after 10 days, 100% of fungicides are still present at the same concentration in the sample. This is a key point of the method since we can support that a sample could be extracted and analysed again after less than 10 days in case of legal procedure against suspected pollutants.

Then, load flow-rate was evaluated to determine its impact on the kinetic of the extraction. This part was completed with APs and the rest of the pesticides selected for the study. The results obtained show a loss of analytes with a low load flow rate, this significant loss can be due to the slow and continuous solubilities of compounds in the sample during the loading process in the same time that the solid phase is retaining them. We opted for a flow of 4 $mL.min^{-1}$. Results are shown in the publication of Baugros and Al. [16].

To estimate the capacity of saturation of the solid phase we tried to load tow volumes of sample on it, 300 mL and 500 mL, the recovery rates indicate higher recovers with a load volume of 300 mL, which can indicate a saturation of the used solid phase when passing more than 300 mL of environmental water. Finally, as our ultimate analytical method was fund on compounds with wide ranges of chemical and physical properties, elution solvents were selected by analysing the collection of the first fraction of a standard aqueous solution extraction with ethyl acetate, acetone, methanol, acetonitrile, dichloromethane. We note that methanol, dichloromethane and acetonitrile did not allow the complete elution of all target pesticides. Finally, elution solvents were selected by testing the collection of the first fraction with ethyl acetate, acetone, methanol, acetonitrile, dichloromethane. The solvents which gave the best recoveries for all compounds were acetone and ethyle acetate and were chosen for the final procedure.

To finish the concentration step, the fractions were evaporated to dryness and loss of analytes was observed. In order to prevent it, we tested different keeper solvents like dimethylsulfoxide, glycerol, n-dodecane, dimethylformamide. The easier solvent to handle and the best compatibility with the solvent chosen for the final extract, tetrahydrofurane (THF), was glycerol. THF was selected according to other pesticides analysed with the same protocol [16].

Finally, 300 mL of sample was load on SPE cartridges packed with 500 mg of Strata-C-18. The condition step was done successively with 5 mL of methanol, 5 mL of methanol/water 50/50 then 5 mL of UltraPure water (UP water). Water samples were loaded at a flow rate of 4 $mL.min^{-1}$. Firstly, the analytes were eluted with 10 mL of acetone, secondly with 10 mL of ethyl acetate.

Afterwards, the eluates were collected, combined and reduced to less than 1 mL under a gentle stream of nitrogen. In order to eliminate a maximum of interferents, we cleaned up the extract on a silica cartridge preconditioned with 3 mL heptane–acetone (30/70, v/v) as proposed by Vuillet and al [40]. The sorbent retaining the interferents, the fraction was directly collected and 50 μL of glycerol/water (50/50, w/w) was added. The final volume was taken gently to dryness under nitrogen stream and reconstituted in a total volume of 250 μL with 175 μL of THF and 25 μL of UP water.

All this selected parameters give a SPE protocol with final recoveries shown in table 6. LOD and LOQ of the method for water samples are listed in the same table.

Table 6. Recovery rates, Residual Standard Deviation (RSD), LOD and LOQ of the analytical method for aqueous samples

Compounds	Recovery (%)	RSD (n=6)	LOD ($ng.L^{-1}$)	LOQ ($ng.L^{-1}$)
Bromuconazole	96%	3.0%	4.6	15.3
Fluquiconazole	118%	8.7%	4.1	13.7
Hexaconazole	100%	9.2%	0.4	1.3
Tebuconazole	95%	12%	0.5	1.7
Tetraconazole	103%	5.1%	1.5	5.0
Pyridaben	93%	9.1%	0.9	3.0
Dimethomorph	104%	4.9%	12.3	41
Ethylenethiourea	86%	9.6%	88.9	296

2.2.2. Solid Sample Pre-treatment and Analyte Extraction [41]

Solid samples, and particularly sludge, are collected with high moisture content. To eliminate water which can grow the weight of the sample and interfere with the PLE extraction by modifying solvent mixture injected in the cellule, we have dried freeze samples during 24 hours. In addition, we sieved it at 200 μm to get a homogeneous sample.

Extraction of fungicides from solid matrices was done by PLE using a solvent mixture selected from prior works about the other targeted molecules (APs and pesticides) and from an observation of a series of experiments. 5 solvents were evaluated for the extraction of fungicides from sludge: ethyl acetate, acetone, acetonitrile, isopropanol and methanol. Methanol, acetone and ethyl acetate gave extracts with high brown colour. Acetonitrile and isopropanol gave less coloured extract supposing low extraction of humic substances and lipids from the sample. We choice a mixture of 1/1 of acetonitrile/isopropanol in volume.

Experimental Design for Extraction Approach [41]

The simultaneous extraction of multiresidue compounds is not an easy task. As a consequence, it is useful to define an optimised extraction method using experimental design in order to get the maximum recovers in one time for all compounds. We perform a four-variables full factorial design on pressure, temperature, duration and number of cycles of extractions achieved on PLE machine, ASE 200 from Dionex. We set it up on 20 experiments with 4 repetitions of the central point. The low, medium and high levels are listed in table 7. Fine range of temperature was selected cause of thermal degradation occurring for other targeted compounds like carbamate pesticides.

The full-factorial design carried out on the PLE gave significant coefficients of first-order terms, the effects of the screening model (recovery = $b_1X_1+b_2X_2+b_3X_3+b_4X_4$) are presented in figure 3. Dimethomorph 1 and 2, and bromuconazole 1 and 2 are different stereoisomers. The higher the absolute value of the coefficient (b_1,b_2,b_3,b_4), the higher the influence of the corresponding variables on the recovery. As the figure 3 shows, pressure and temperature have the strongest effect on the extraction yield. For the reason that plus or minus sign of the coefficient is directly linked to the sign of the measured response, recoveries increase when pressure increases and temperature decreases. this can demonstrate the thermolability of the selected fungicides, high pressure helping the solvent to penetrate into all porous of sludge particles which allow to disrupt the strong solute-matrix interactions caused by van der Walls forces, hydrogen bonding and dipole attractions. The duration has not strong impact on recoveries, 5 minutes were satisfied. Number of cycles gives negative effect on several compounds (ETU, tetraconazole, bromuconazole 2, tebuconazole, hexaconazole and pyridaben). Cycles have proven to be useful for sample types with a very high concentration of analyse, or samples with difficult to penetrate matrices, it is not the case in our study.

Table 7. Levels chosen for the experimental design

Parameters of PLE	Low level (-1)	Medium level (0)	High level (+1)
Pressure (bars), X_1	40	80	120
Temperature (°C), X_2	40	60	80
Duration (minutes), X_3	5	10	15
Number of cycles, X_4	1	2	3

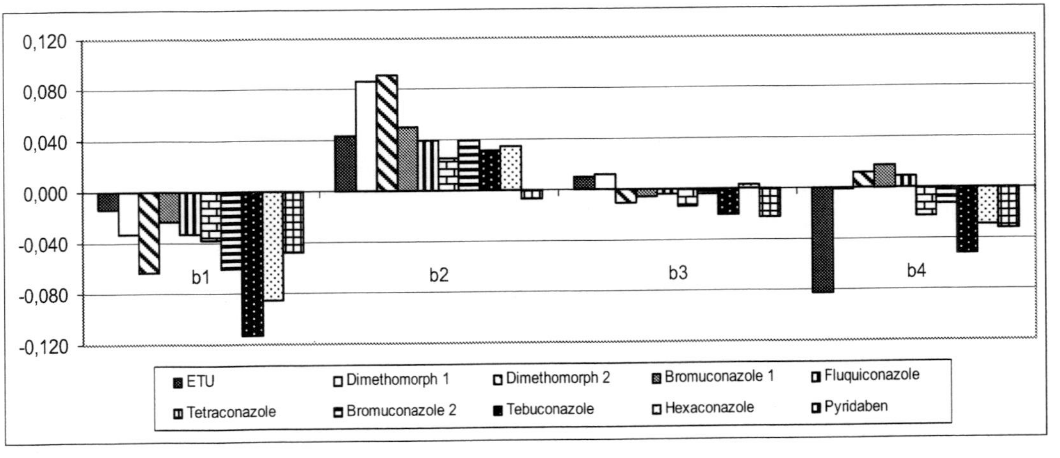

Figure 3. Coefficients of first-order terms, b_1 pressure, b_2 temperature, b_3 duration of extraction, b_4 number of cycles.

Table 8. Recovery rates, Residual Standard Deviation (RSD), LOD and LOQ of the analytical method for solid samples

Compounds	Recovery (%)	RSD (n=4)	LOD ($\mu g.kg^{-1}$)	LOQ ($\mu g.kg^{-1}$)
Bromuconazole	102%	9%	0.96	3.20
Fluquinconazole	99%	6%	0.61	2.03
Hexaconazole	97%	13%	7.55	25.17
Tebuconazole	110%	17%	0.64	2.15
Tetraconazole	107%	12%	31.5	105
Pyridaben	105%	17%	0.57	1.88
Dimethomorph	107%	9%	5.71	19.04
Ethylenethiourea	98%	7%	183.6	612

Consequently, pressure was set at 40 bars, temperature at 80°C and one cycle was sufficient. Duration was adopted for 5 minutes which minimize the total time of the PLE extraction. The final efficiency of the PLE procedure was determined and recoveries present in table 8.

Finally, the results obtained show low limits of detection which are adjusted to environmental regulations requirements in the range of $\mu g.kg^{-1}$.

2.3. Analytical Part

2.3.1. Chromatographic Optimisation

The optimisation of the chromatographic separation was performed by a serial of preliminary experiments, testing different mobile phase composed of methanol or acetonitrile as an organic phase and water with different mobile phase additives, such as acetic acid and ammonium acetate at various concentrations. Ammonium acetate in water was preferred in order to enhance and stabilise the formation of ammonium adducts of other certain target molecules (particularly APs), $[M+NH_4]^+$ against the sodium adduct, $[M+Na]^+$, during the electrospray process. The column was chosen among a large range of different stationary phases and manufacturers. The optimal separation of 22 compounds, 8 of them are studied fungicides, was achieved using 1.5 mM of NH_4Ac in aqueous mobile phase and methanol as organic phase.

As far as the final analytical method is concerned, analyses of the extract were performed on a Waters 2695 series Alliance HPLC (Waters, Milford, MA) equipped with a reversed phase column Uptispher C_{18} 3HDO (3 μm, 100 x 2.0 mm i.d.) preceded by a guard column (10 x 2.0 mm i.d. 3 μm) both from Interchim (Montluçon, France). The column was kept at 40°C and the sample injection volume was set at 10.0 μL. Simplified chromatogram is presented on the figure 4 with the single presence of fungicides peaks.

2.3.2. Mass Spectrometry Detection Optimisation

The detection was achieved on a triple quadrupole mass spectrometer Quattro LC from Micromass (Manchester, UK) equipped with a Z-spray electrospray interface. The optimisation of MS parameters was completed by Flow Injection Analysis (FIA) for each compound. Fungicides were more sensitive in positive ionization mode. For each compounds, the precursor ion was selected by acquiring in full scan and the best cone voltage was choosen for high production of the parent ion. Then collision energies were tested to give the maximum of intensity for the fragment ions. Three different transitions were monitored per compound when the fragmentation was appropriate: the first and the more abundant ion was used for quantification and the second for confirmation (ratio of quantity of signal of this two transitions in ranged of +/- 10% of a standard), the third was acquired in compliance with the UE regulation [42].

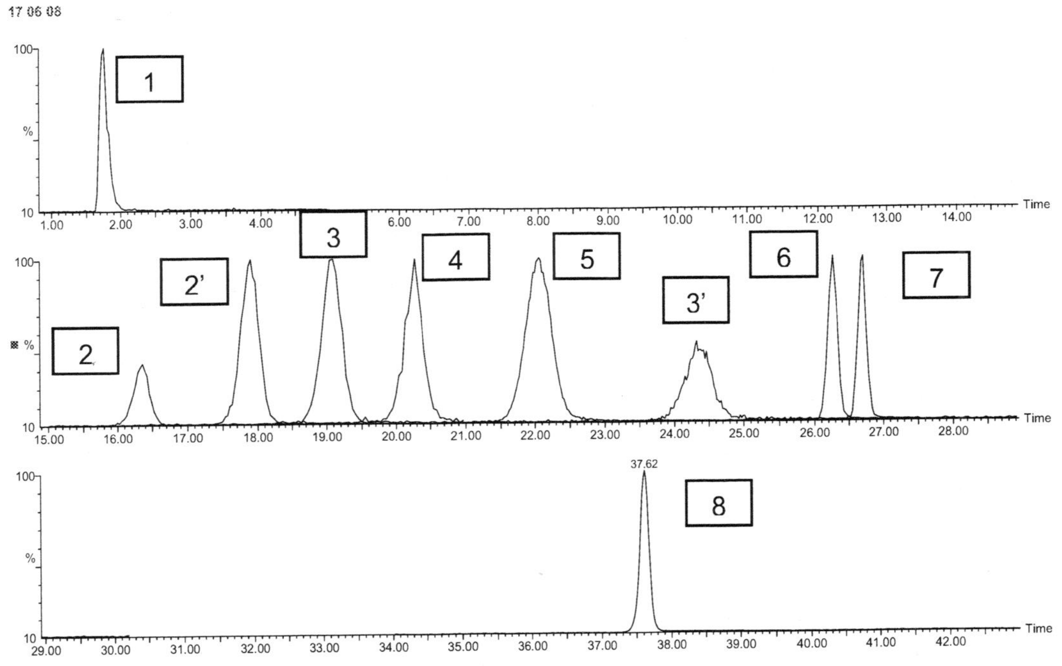

Figure 4. LC chromatogram of target fungicides (injection of a standard mixture).

For each compound, cone voltage and collision energies of the main transitions were optimised from a continuous flow of a standard injection (1 $\mu g.L^{-1}$ solution at 20 $\mu L.min^{-1}$) to obtain the maximum intensities. Parameters of liquid chromatography coupled with mass spectrometry are specified in table 9.

Optimisation of the concentration of ammonium acetate in aqueous phase was experimented in order to see the impact on the mass spectrometric signals. We have tested 5 concentrations since the analysts used to employ salts in reversed phasae LC in the range of 1 to 15 mM, results are listed in the table 10.

These results clearly show that low concentration give the highest signal. High salt concentration can reduce considerably the signal by increasing the charges of the drop during electrospray process. In addition, for salt concentrations superior to 10^{-3} M, the diameter of the spray grew which can reduce the transmission efficiency of ions to the spectrometer. As a conclusion for this aspect of the analytical optimisation we opted for 1.5 mM of ammonium acetate, since last optimised step has lead us to better reproducibility of signal quantities with this level of salt in aqueous than 1 mM.

Other target molecules, 4 pesticides and 10 endocrine disrupting compounds, were analysed during the same run and the last 11 compounds, organochlorine pesticides and phthalates, were analysed by GC-MS [16].

Table 9. LC-MS/MS conditions (retention time, ES mode used, transitions selected, Cone voltage and Collision energy)

Compounds (a)	Rt (min)	Mode	Transitions	Cone Voltage (V)	Collision energy (eV)
Ethylenethiourea (1)	1.8	ES+	103.3 → 43.8 103.3 → 69.9 103.3 → 86.0	30 30 30	30 30 30
Dimethomorph (2 and 2') (b)	16.4-17.9	ES+	388.2 → 139.0 388.2 → 165.0 388.2 → 300.9	10 10 10	30 30 20
Bromuconazole (3 and 3')(b)	19.1-24.5	ES+	378.0 → 159.0 378.0 → 160.9 378.0 → 173.0	20 20 20	30 30 30
Fluquinconazole (4)	20.3	ES+	376.0 → 272.0 376.0 → 306.8 376.0 → 348.8	20 20 20	30 20 20
Tetraconazole (5)	22.1	ES+	372.0 → 159.0 372.0 → 205.0	25 25	25 15
Tebuconazole (6)	26.3	ES+	308.2 → 70.0 308.2 → 125.1 308.2 → 151.0	28 28 28	22 22 22
Hexaconazole (7)	26.7	ES+	314.2 → 69.8 314.2 → 159.0	20 20	20 20
Pyridaben (8)	37.6	ES+	365.2 → 147.1 365.2 → 308.9	10 10	20 15

[a] Numerotation of compounds cf figure 4.
[b] Stereoisomers.

Table 10. Percentages of the mass spectrometric signal compared with the reference considered at 1 mM

	Ammonium acetate concentrations				
Compounds	1 mM	2.5 mM	5 mM	10 mM	15 mM
Ethylenethiourea	100%	85%	63%	55%	47%
Dimethomorph	100%	85%	72%	55%	44%
Bromuconazole	100%	93%	83%	61%	52%
Fluquiconazole	100%	96%	78%	54%	44%
Tetraconazole	100%	90%	73%	59%	51%
Tebuconazole	100%	89%	74%	59%	51%
Hexaconazole	100%	92%	76%	59%	51%
Pyridaben	100%	98%	91%	72%	60%

2.3.3. Evaluation of Matrix Effect and Quantitation Strategies

The major problem, in quantitative analysis of environmental samples is the impact on the analyte signals in the presence of matrix components. Matrix effect was evaluated to fix the best approach to quantify the analytes. Because matrix effect like enhancement or suppression can severely compromise quantitative analysis of environmental samples. This effect was evaluated from the equation below.

$$\textit{Signal suppression (\%)} = \left[1 - \frac{(Is - Ix)}{Id}\right] \times 100$$

Equation 1

Calculation for evaluation of signal due to matrix effect.

I_s is the analyte peak area for spiked effluent extract, I_x is the analyte peak area for an unspiked effluent extract and I_d is the analyte peak area for a standard solution.

Results showed no effect on fungicides signals but high enhancement for others compounds. This may be explained because environmental matrix contains many products which can affect the analytical signal, and because of the low detection limits required to determine some of the compounds at their biologically active concentrations.

Thus, tandem mass spectrometry is a specific and precise identification technique which can explain the absence or low matrix effect; fungicides are detected by this system. Nevertheless, we overcome this aspect by choosing standard addition as the most suitable quantification method for compensating matrix effects. Even if this quantification method presents time-consuming and laborious aspects, the results showed significant matrix effects on samples coming from wastewater treatment plant and proofed that the best and reliable method of quantification is the standard addition. Above all, this allows accurate quantification which is essential in the application of European directives [43, 44].

External calibration was selected for the quantification of compounds in solid parts since all target molecules were detected by tandem mass spectrometry, giving high specificity of the detection.

2.4. Validation Studies of the Analytical Method

Validation of the developed method was evaluated by estimation of the sensitivity, linearity, precision, recoveries and the study of the matrix effects. Thus, the quantification was based on standard addition for aqueous samples and external calibration for solid extracts. Five-point calibration plots were constructed using a least-square linear regression analysis. Good linearity was observed with correlation coefficients superior to 0.98.

The overall method repeatability, calculated as the relative standard deviation (RSD) of replicate (n=6) analysis of spiked WWTP effluents at 500 ng.L^{-1}, was satisfactory with RSD values ranging between 3 and 12% (table 6). The LOD and LOQ of the method were estimated for each analyte from the analysis of at least three replicates of wastewater and sludge spiked with a standard mixture of the analytes at the minimum detectable amount using a signal-to-noise ratio of 3 (table 6 and 8). These LOD were comprised between 0.4

and 88.9 ng.L^{-1} for fungicides detected in water samples and between 0.57 and 183.6 µg.kg^{-1} in solid matrice. In these conditions, recoveries achieved for all target compounds ranged from 86 % to 118 % were very satisfactory whatever the environmental sample.

All the analytical method for the determination of fungicides in environmental parts underwent validation procedure and passed successfully all steps. After 5 injections of 5 series of standards with concentrations ranged from 32 µg.L^{-1} to 1.06 mg.L^{-1}, calibration was calculated from linear regression. 10 injections of standard solution with levels of fungicides closes to the estimated LOD were done and the average concentration of them was calculated from regression. These results were compared with the theoretical concentrations in accordance with the equation 1 and the standard deviation of the 10 injections in accordance with the equation 2.

$$\left| \frac{LQv - \overline{uLQ}}{SLQ / \sqrt{n}} \right| < 10 \qquad \text{Equation 2}$$

$$LQv - 10 * SLQ > 0 \qquad \text{Equation 3}$$

LQv: theoretical concentration of standards; $\overline{uLQ}$ average of the signal (in concentration range);
SLQ: standard deviation estimated from 10 responses.

The results obtained with the equation 2 must be inferior to 10 and the results calculated with the equation 3 have to be positive (table 11). All these limits were reported to the concentration factor due the SPE step. As the calculations satisfy requirements, it is verified that 10 injections of standard solution with concentrations nearby the LOQ are correct at the LOQ levels.

All this procedure made of the all analytical protocol a method fully validated ready to be normalised or to be regularly applied to real samples.

Table 11. Results of 8 fungicides for method validation

Fungicides	Equation 2 (< 10)	Equation 3 (>0)	LOD in waters (ng.L^{-1})	LOD in solids (µg.kg^{-1})
Ethylenethiourea	3.07	0.09	88.9	183.9
Dimethomorph	2.84	0.02	12.3	5.71
Bromuconazole	6.50	0.02	4.6	0.96
Fluquiconazole	6.26	0.03	4.1	0.61
Tetraconazole	4.54	0.06	1.5	31.5
Tebuconazole	5.61	0.03	0.5	0.64
Hexaconazole	2.75	0.07	0.4	7.55
Pyridaben	9.69	0.04	0.9	0.57

3. Results of Real Samples

Generally, the concentrations found in the environment are the result of the amount spread through the environment, the relative stability, the metabolism by wildlife and the capacity to bioaccumulation. Contamination of surface water is mainly due to surface runoff and effluent from WWTP. Groundwater is primarily contaminated by release of fungicides from topsoil and further transport through the soil percolation (figure 1).

Table 12. Results got for water samples from Rhône-Alpes region in ng.L^{-1}

Compounds	WWTP 01/03/2007	WWTP 20/03/2007	WWTP 23/04/2007	WWTP 30/05/2007	WWTP 09/07/2007
Ethylenethiourea	nd	nd	nd	2287	d
Tebuconazole	10.2	5.8	43.3	14.5	2.2
Hexaconazole	d	nd	nd	nd	nd
Tetraconazole	nd	nd	nd	nd	nd
Fluquiconazole	nd	nd	nd	nd	nd
Bromuconazole	nd	nd	nd	nd	nd
Dimethomorph	nd	nd	nd	d	d
Pyridaben	nd	d	nd	nd	nd

Compounds	GW 1	GW 2	GW 3	SurW 1	SurW 2	TW 1	TW 2
Ethylenethiourea	nd	nd	nd	nd	nd	nd	nd
Tebuconazole	nd	894.7	32.9	28.9	30.0	25.8	31.6
Hexaconazole	nd	nd	nd	nd	nd	nd	nd
Tetraconazole	nd	nd	nd	nd	nd	nd	nd
Fluquiconazole	nd	nd	nd	nd	nd	nd	nd
Bromuconazole	nd	nd	nd	nd	nd	nd	nd
Dimethomorph	nd	nd	nd	nd	nd	nd	nd
Pyridaben	nd	nd	nd	nd	nd	nd	nd

GW Ground Water, SurW Surface Water, TW Treated Water, d, detected (clear gray); nd, not detected.

Table 13. Results obtained for sludge, Rhône river water and sediments, pond and mud puddle (MP) present on the roof of laboratory and atmospheric fallout

Compounds	Sludge µg.kg^{-1}	River water ng.L^{-1}	River sediments µg.kg^{-1}	Pond ng.L^{-1}	MP 1 µg.kg^{-1}	MP 2 µg.kg^{-1}	MP 3 µg.kg^{-1}	Fallout µg.kg^{-1}
Ethylenethiourea	nd	nd	nd	nd	nd	nd	nd	nd
Tebuconazole	d	19.9	12.3	12.6	17.8	13.5	17.2	95.3
Hexaconazole	nd	d	nd	d	nd	d	d	nd
Tetraconazole	nd	d	nd	nd	nd	nd	nd	nd
Fluquiconazole	nd	nd	nd	nd	nd	nd	nd	nd
Bromuconazole	nd	nd	nd	nd	nd	nd	nd	nd
Dimethomorph	nd	17.5	d	nd	d	nd	nd	nd
Pyridaben	nd	d	nd	nd	nd	nd	nd	nd

Environmental waters were collected in pre-cleaned glass bottles, WWTP effluents were a 24h-composite samples from the major plant located in Lyon (Saint. Fons) receiving both domestic and industrial waters. This WWTP has a 1 037 000 population equivalent capacity and an average daily flow rate of 333 530 m^3. Surface and ground waters were collected from March to April of 2007 in Rhône-Alpes region.

Results are presented in table 12.

As far as wastewaters are concerned, all samples contained trace of tebuconazole from spring to summer time at levels from 2.2 to 894.7 $ng.L^{-1}$. We found that tebuconazole was detected at maxium level superior to 2 $\mu g.L^{-1}$ in superficial water from Morgon to Gleizé (Rhône, France) [45] and this is a large scale fungicide used on many types of cultivation (cereals, fruits, vegetables and vineyard) [46]. It makes of this fungicide a persistent molecule which can quantify even in ground water (GW 2 and 3).

Dimethomorph, hexaconazole and pyridaben are detected under LOQs. Dimethormorph is recommended for vine application against mildiou, the results found can correspond at the beginning of the summer application in vineyard. Hexaconazole is a systemic and curative fungicide used as a single application on a large variety of cultivation and pyridaben can be used for fungicide application but as well as acaricide. ETU is detected at the end of spring and during the summer in wastewaters.

In table 13 we compare results obtained on sludge, river water/sediments and on mud puddle/pond coming from the laboratory roof. Three sampling zones were tested for mud. Shower occurred 2 days before sampling which gave us the possibility to collect water from pond. Atmospheric fallouts were collected by the experimental catchment station at Chassieu (Rhône, France), which are a part of the Field Observatory on Urban Hydrology (OTHU). Sludge were collected from the main WWTP of Lyon (downstream of Lyon, Saint Fons, France) as the final product from activated sludge process.

We quantified tebuconazole and dimethomorph in analysed samples from 12.3 to 95.3 $\mu g.kg^{-1}$ in solid samples and from 12.6 to 19.9 $ng.L^{-1}$ in aqueous ones. Hexaconazole, tetraconazole and pyridaben were detected too. If we compare water/solid elements, Rhône river contains 5 fungicides in water and 2 of them are present in sediments. No major differences are noticed between 3 sites of mud puddle samples from roof. The presence of ultra-trace of fungicides in pond and mud puddle can be explicated by the pre-treatment of the shingle or by the great resistance of these molecules all along the water cycle in showers. Analyse of atmospheric fallout revealed the presence of tebuconazole at 95.3 $\mu g.kg^{-1}$. Again the hypothesis of compound brought by rainwater was supposed since the vicinity of several area of cereal cultivation. Sludge contains tebuconazole quantity under the LOD and any other target fungicides.

Conclusion

Recent years have seen significant evolution in european and american regulation of chemicals released in the environment. Maximum levels of pesticides have been established by several directives. It has been shown that pesticides and particularly the most sold group of pesticides in the world, fungicides, enter the aquatic environment and contaminate soils or sediments. To give responses to new legal regulations, analytical methods need to be robust, exact and accurate to determine in low range from ng.L^{-1} in waters and μg.kg^{-1} in soils, sediments and sludge. The new multiresidue analytical method proposed is on a combined method, GC-MS and LC-MS/MS, allowed the ultra-trace and trace determination of 33 multiple-class substances in environmental waters around the low ng.L^{-1} and the low μg.kg^{-1} in soils, sediments and sludge. Eight fungicides and residue of fungicide were detected by LC-MS/MS and quantified in real samples. Permanent presence of tebuconazole was underlined in both matrices and explanations were supposed. Levels in water of other studied compounds, pesticides, alkylphenols and plasticizers, are presented elsewhere [16, 41] and levels in solid parts will be shortly shown [41].

Finally, the analytical method are in agreement with the environmental concentrations and the low ng.L^{-1} an μg.kg^{-1} limits providing a reliable and robust tool that can be used for routine analysis of multi-class substances in aqueous and solid environmental samples.

Acknowledgments

The authors acknowledge the Region Rhône-Alpes for its financial support and Grand Lyon for assistance on sampling.

References

[1] Council of the European Community/Official Journal L 396, 2006/12/30. Regulation (EC) No 1907/2006 of the European Parliament and of the Council of 18 December 2006 concerning the Registration, Evaluation, Authorisation and Restriction of Chemicals (REACH), establishing a European Chemicals Agency, amending Directive 1999/45/EC and repealing Council Regulation (EEC) No 793/93 and Commission Regulation (EC) No 1488/94 as well as Council Directive 76/769/EEC and Commission Directives 91/155/EEC, 93/67/EEC, 93/105/EC and 2000/21/EC. 2006, Rule number 1907/2006.

[2] Gupta, R. C. (2007). *Veterinary Toxicology Basic and Clinical Principles - Chapter 52 - Toxicity of fungicides* Academic Press.

[3] Europa - European Commission - Eurostat. The use of plant protection products in the European Union - Data 1992-2003. 2008. Available from http://epp.eurostat.ec.europa.eu/cache/ITY_OFFPUB/KS-76-06-669/EN/KS-76-06-669-EN.PDF.

[4] Coscollà, C., Yusà, V., Marti, P.& Pastor, A. (2008). Analysis of currently used pesticides in fine airborne particulate matter (PM 2.5) by pressurized liquid extraction and liquid chromatography-tandem mass spectrometry. *Journal of Chromatorgaphy A, In Press, Corrected Proof.*

[5] European Chemical Bureau. Consumer Product Safety and Quality. 2008. Available from http://ecb.jrc.it/.

[6] Environmental Protection Agency. 2008. Available from http://www.epa.gov/.

[7] Breitholtz, M., Rudén, C., Hansson, S. O.& Bengtsson, B.-E. (2006). Ten challenges for improved ecotoxicological testing in environmental risk assessment. *Ecotoxicology and Environmental Safety, 63,* 324-335.

[8] Council of the European Community/Official Journal L 330, 1998/12/05. Council Directive 98/83/EC of 3 November 1998 on the quality of water intended for human consumption 1998, Rule number 98/83/EC.

[9] Garcinuno, R. M., Ramos, L., Fernandez-Hernando, P.& Camara, C. (2004). Optimization of a matrix solid-phase dispersion method with subsequent clean-up for the determination of ethylene bisdithiocarbamate residues in almond samples. *Journal of Chromatorgaphy A, 1041,* 35-41.

[10] Van Lishaut, H.& Schwack, W. (2000). Selective trace determination of dithiocarbamate fungicides in fruits and vegetables by reversed-phase ion-pair liquid chromatography with ultraviolet and electrochemical detection. *Journal of AOAC International, 83,* 720-727.

[11] Schermerhorn, P. G.& Golden, P. E. (2005). Determination of 22 triazole compounds including parent fungicides and metabolites in apples, peaches, flour, and water by liquid chromatorgaphy/tandem mass spectrometry. *Journal of AOAC International, 88,* 1491-1502.

[12] Gonzalez-Rodriguez, R. M., Rial-Otero, R., Cancho-Grande, B.& Simal-Gandara, J. (2008). Determination of 23 pesticide residues in leafy vegetables using gas chromatography-ion trap mass spectrometry and analyte protectants. *Journal of Chromatorgaphy A, In Press, Corrected Proof.*

[13] Salau, J. S., Alonso, R., Batllo, G.& Barcelo, D. (1994). Application of solid-phase disk extraction followed by gas and liquid chromatography for the simultaneous determination of the fungicides: captan, captafol, carbadazim, chlorothalonil, ethirimol, folpet, metalaxyl and vinclozolin in environmental waters. *Analytica Chimica Acta, 293,* 109-117.

[14] Pan, H.-J.& Ho, W.-H. (2004). Determination of fungicides in water using liquid phase microextraction and gas chromatography with electron capture detection. *Analytica Chimica Acta, 257,* 61-67.

[15] Zhou, Q., Xiao, J.& Ding, Y. (2007). Sensitive determination f fungicides and prometryn in environmental samples using multiwalled carbon nanotubes solid-phase extraction cartridge. *Analytica Chimica Acta, 602,* 223-228.

[16] Baugros, J.-B., Giroud, B., Dessalces, G., Grenier-Loustalot, M.-F.& Cren-Olivé, C. (2008). Multiresidue analytical method for the ultra-trace quantification of 33 priority substances present in the list of REACH in real water samples. *Analytica Chimica Acta, 607,* 191-203.

[17] Balinova, A. (1995). Extension of the bioautograph technique for multiresidue determination of fungicide residues in plants and water. *Analytica Chimica Acta, 311,* 423-427.

[18] Jeannot, R., Sabik, H., Sauvard, E.& Genin, E. (2000). Application of liquid chromatography with mass spectrometry combined with photodiode array detection and tandem mass spectrometry for monitoring pesticides in surface waters. *Journal of Chromatorgaphy A, 879,* 51-71.

[19] Bermudez-Couso, A., Arias-Estévez, M., Novoa-Munoz, J. C., Lopez-Periago, E., Soto-Gonzalez, B.& Simal-Gandara, J. (2007). Seasonal distributions of fungicides in soils and sediments of a small river basin partially devoted to vineyards. *Water Research, 41,* 4515-4525.

[20] Halko, R., Padron-Sanz, C., Sosa-Ferrera, Z.& Santana-Rodriguez, J.-J. (2006). Determination of benzimidazole fungicides in soil samples using microwave-assisted micellar extraction and liquid chromatography with fluorescence detection. *Journal of AOAC International, 89,* 1403-1409.

[21] Kawata, K., Asada, T.& Oikawa, K. (2005). Determination of pesticides in compost by pressurized liquid extraction and gas chromatography-mass spectrometry. *Journal of Chromatorgaphy A, 1090,* 10-15.

[22] Kawata, K., Asada, T., Oikawa, K.& Tanabe, A. (2005). Multiresidue determination of pesticides in sediment by ultrasonically assisted extraction and gas chromatography/mass spectrometry. *Journal of AOAC International, 88,* 1440-1451.

[23] Charlton, A. J. A.& Jones, A. (2007). Determination of imidazole and triazole fungicide residues in honeybess using gas chromatography-mass spectrometry. *Journal of Chromatorgaphy A, 1141,* 117-122.

[24] Schreck, E., Geret, F., Gontier, L.& · Treilhou, M. (2008). Neurotoxic effect and metabolic responses induced by a mixture of six pesticides on the earthworm *Aporrectodea caliginosa nocturna. Chemosphere, 71,* 1832-1839.

[25] Konwick, B. J., Garrison, A. W., Avants, J. K.& Fish, A. T. (2006). Bioaccumulation and biotrnasformation of chiral triazole fungicides in rainbow trout (*Oncorhynchus mykiss*). *Aquatic Toxicology, 80,* 372-381.

[26] Saillenfait, A. M., Sabate, J. P., Langonne, I.& De Ceaurriz, J. (1991). Difference in the Developmental Toxicity of Ethylenethiourea and Three N,N'-Substituted Thiourea Derivatives in Rats >*Toxicological Sciences, 17,* 399-408.

[27] Houeto, P., Bindoula, G.& Hoffman, J. R. (1995). Ethylenebisdithiocarbamates and Ethylenethiourea: Possible Human Health Hazards *Environmental Health Perspectives, 103,* 568-573.

[28] Sannino, A., Bolzoni, L.& Bandini, M. (2004). Application of liquid chromatography with electrospray tandem mass spectrometry to the determination of a new generation of pesticides in processed fruits and vegetables. *Journal of Chromatorgaphy A, 1036,* 161-169.

[29] Navarro, M., Pico, Y., Marin, R.& Manes, J. (2002). Application of matrix solid-phase dispersion to the determination of a new generation of fungicides in fruits and vegetables. *Journal of Chromatorgaphy A, 968,* 201-209.

[30] Millan, S., Sampedro, M. C., Unceta, N., Goicolea, M. A., Rodriguez, E.& Barrio, R. J. (2003). Coupling solid-phase microextraction and high-performance liquid chromatorgaphy for direct and sensitive determination of halogenated fungicides in wine. *Journal of Chromatorgaphy A, 995,* 135-142.

[31] Kumar, V., Ravindranath, S. D.& Shanker, A. (2004). Fate of hexaconazole residues in tea and its behavior during brewing process. *Chemical Health and Safety, 11,* 21-25.

[32] Ladurner, E., Bosch, J., Kemp, W. P.& Maini, S. (2005). Assessing delayed and acute toxicity of five formulated fungicides to Osmia lignaria Say and Apis mellifera. *Apidologie, 36,* 449-460.

[33] Hayama, T., Yada, K., Onimaru, S., Yoshida, H., Todoroki, K., Nohta, H.& Yamaguchi, M. (2007). Simplified method for determination of polycarbamate fungicide in water samples by liquid chromatography with tandem mass spectrometry following derivatization with dimethyl sulfate. *Journal of Chromatorgaphy A, 1141,* 251-258.

[34] Fernandez-Alba, A. R., Agüera, A., Contreras, M., Peñuela, G., Ferrer, I.& Barceló, D. (1998). Comparison of various sample handling and analytical procedures for the monitoring of pesticides and metabolites in ground waters.

[35] Journal of Chromatography A, Volume 823, Issues 1-2, 9 October 1998, Pages 35-47. *Journal of Chromatorgaphy A, 823,* 35-47.

[36] Vanni, A., Gamberini, R., Calabria, A.& Pellegrino, V. (2000). Determination of presence of fungicides by their common metabolite, 3,5-DCA, in compost. *Chemosphere, 41,* 453-458.

[37] Inam, R., Gülerman, E. Z.& Sarigül, T. (2006). Dtermination of triflumizole by differential pulse polarography in formulation, soil and natural water samples. *Analytica Chimica Acta, 579,* 117-123.

[38] Organisme Régional de Santé, O. R. S. Tableau de bord de Santé-Environnement. 2008. Available from http://www.ors-rhone-alpes.org/environnement/pdf/Pesticides.pdf

[39] British Corp Protection Council (2003). *The pesticide manual.*

[40] Metzler, M. (2001). *The Handbook of Environmental Chemistry* Heidelberg, Springler-Verlag.

[41] Vuillet, E., Baugros, J.-B., Flament-Waton, M.-M.& Grenier-Loustalot, M.-F. (2007). Analytical methods for the determination of selected steroid sex hormones and corticosteriods in wastewater. *Analytical Bioanalytical Chemistry, 387,* 2143-2151.

[42] Baugros, J.-B., Cren-Olivé, C., Giroud, B., Lantéri, P.& Grenier-Loustalot, M.-F. (2008). Optimisation of pressurised liquid extraction by experimental design for multiresidue ultra-trace quantification of substances concerned by European regulations in sludge, sediments and atmospheric fallout. *Journal of Chromatorgaphy A, Submitted.*

[43] Council of the European Community/Official Journal L 221, 2002/08/12. Commission decision 2002/657 of 12 August 2002 implementing Council Directive 96/23/EC concerning the performance of analytical methods and the interpretation of results. 2002, Rule number 657/2002.

[44] Council, E. P./Official Journal of the European Union. Regulation (EC) No 1907/2006 of the European Parliament and of the Council of 18 December 2006 concerning the Registration, Evaluation, Authorisation and Restriction of Chemicals (REACH), establishing a European Chemicals Agency, amending Directive 1999/45/EC and repealing Council Regulation (EEC) No 793/93 and Commission Regulation (EC) No 1488/94 as well as Council Directive 76/769/EEC and Commission Directives

91/155/EEC, 93/67/EEC, 93/105/EC and 2000/21/EC. 2006, Rule number Regulation No 1907/2006.

[45] official Journal of the Euopean Communites Commision Decision 2002/657/EC of 12 August, implementing Council Directive 96/23/EC concerning the performance of analytical methods and the interpretation of the results. 12.08.2002, Rule number.

[46] DIREN (DIrection Régional de l'ENvironnement / Regional Agency for the Environment)/Editor (2005) Inventory of the presence of pesticides in the waters from Rhône-Alpes region - Results of 2004, Series.

[47] ACTA (Association de Coordination Technique Agricole) (2006). *Index Phytosanitaire ACTA 2006* Paris, ACTA.

In: Fungicides
Editors: P. De Costa and P. Bezerra

ISBN: 978-1-60692-631-4

Chapter III

ANTIMICROBIAL COMPOUNDS PRODUCED BY PLANT ENDOPHYTIC FUNGI

Ligang Zhou[1,*], Jianglin Zhao[1], Lijian Xu[1], Yongfu Huang[1], Zhanhong Ma[1], Jingguo Wang[2], Weibo Jiang[3]

[1]Department of Plant Pathology, College of Agronomy and Biotechnology, China Agricultural University, Beijing 100193, P. R. China

[2]Department of Plant Nutrition, College of Resources and Environmental Sciences, China Agricultural University, Beijing 100193, P. R. China

[3]Department of Food Science and Technology, College of Food Science and Nutritional Engineering, China Agricultural University, Beijing 100083, P. R. China

ABSTRACT

Plant endophytic fungi, microorganisms that reside in the internal tissues of living plants without causing any immediate overt negative effects, have been found in every plant species examined to date and recognized as potential sources of novel natural products for exploitation in agriculture, medicine, and food industry. This chapter describes published research on antimicrobial compounds produced by plant endophytic fungi as sources of new antimicrobials. Literature was reviewed based on our personal experience, reported antimicrobial activity against plant, human and animal pathogens, novel chemical structures of the antimicrobials from the endophytic fungi. The future prospects for these antimicrobials to control important plant and animal diseases will also be discussed.

[*] Corresponding author. Tel: +86 10 62731199; Fax: +86 10 62731062; E-mail: lgzhou@cau.edu.cn

1. Introduction

All plants have endophytes including endophytic bacteria and fungi (Saikkonen et al., 1998; Tan and Zou, 2001; Strobel, 2003; Zhang et al., 2006; Gimenez et al., 2007). Some endophytes are hitchhikers with no noticeable effect on their plant hosts, but others have intimate relations with their hosts and profound effects on their function and survival. Their secondary metabolism is particularly active, presumably due to metabolic interactions with their hosts. The importance of endophytes remained largely hidden until 1975, when Charles Bacon and his colleagues (Bacon et al., 1975) demonstrated that endophytes of pasture grasses caused toxic syndromes in cattle. This stimulated research in many aspects on the biology of endophytes, including basic and applied.

Synthetic antimicrobials were produced because of the ease with which these could be used. Their effectiveness and possibility of storage and use as and when needed became very powerful agents in the control of diseases in agriculture, horticulture, forestry, food conservation, and even human and animal health programs. However the extensive use of synthetic antimicrobials in crop protection programs around the world recently has resulted in disturbances of the environment, pest resurgence, pest resistance to pesticides and lethal effects on non-target organism agroecosystems in addition to direct toxicity to users. Use of natural microbial or plant products in an agroecosytem is now emerging as one of the prime means to protect crop production and the environment from pesticidal pollution, which is a global problem. Otherwise, an increase in the number of people in the world having health problems caused by certain cancers, drug-resistant bacteria, parasitic protozoans, and fungi has caused alarm. An intensive search for newer and more effective agents to deal with these problems is also now underway. Endophyte is a potential source of novel chemistry and biology to assist in helping solving not only plant disease, but human and animal health problems also (Strobel et al., 2004; Gimenez et al., 2007).

This chapter mainly describes the current state of the antimicrobial compounds produced by plant endophytic fungi which are a rich source of new biologically active natural products ranging from extracts commonly in use to compounds prospected and tested by researchers. The prospect and facing problems of isolating antimicrobial compounds from endophytic fungi are also discussed (Tan and Zou, 2001; Zhang et al., 2006).

2. Discovery of Antimicrobial Compounds from Endophytic Fungi

Almost all plant species examined to date were found to harbor endophytic fungi and/or bacteria (Saikkonen et al., 1998; Sturz et al., 2000; Arnold, 2007). As a matter of fact, endophytes are important components of microbial biodiversity. Commonly, several to hundreds of endophyte species can be isolated from a single plant, among them, at least one species showing host specificity. The symbiosis between plant and endophyte was ascertained, namely, the former protects and feeds the latter which produces 'in return' bioactive (plant growth regulatory, antibacterial, antifungal, antiviral, insecticidal, etc.) substances to enhance the growth and competitiveness of the host in nature (Carroll, 1988).

To efficiently screen antimicrobial compounds from endophytic fungi, some strategies are usually considered such as host plant selection, isolation of the endophytic fungi, primary screening of antimicrobial activity, taxonomic identification of the fungal isolates, bio-guided separation and activity evaluation of the antimicrobial compounds on which we discussed as follows in detail.

2.1. Host Plant Selection

As co-evolution between endophyte and plant, many endophytes showed their host specificity. Some perennial plants (i.e. *Ginkgo biloba*, *Artemisia annua*, *Taxus brevifolia*, *Podophyllum peltatum*, *Dioscorea zingiberensis*, *Paris polyphylla* var. *yunnanensis*) containing antimicrobial, insecticidal and other antibiotic compounds are usually selected to study antimicrobial compounds from their endophytic fungi (Liu et al., 2008; Lu et al., 2000; Stierle et al., 1993; Eyberger et al., 2006; Xu et al., 2008; Li et al., 2008; Zhao et al., 2008a). The environmental conditions under which the host is growing also affect the endophyte population, and the endophyte profile may be more diversified in tropical and subtropical areas (Strobel, 2002). For example, Arnold et al. (2000) isolated 418 endophyte morphospecies (estimated 347 genetically distinct taxa) from 83 healthy leaves of *Heisteria concinna* and *Ouratea lucens* in a lowland tropical forest of central Panama, and proposed that tropical endophytes themselves could be hyperdiverse with host preference and spatial heterogeneity. Accordingly, endophytes are presumably ubiquitous in the plant kingdom with the population being dependent on host species and location.

2.2. Isolation of the Endophytic Fungi

It is important to establish a specific protocol for the isolation of endophytes from a given plant, particularly as 90-99% of microorganisms are not readily cultivable (Amann et al., 1995). The most frequently isolated fungi are endophytes. The great majority of studies on endophytic fungi are done with surface-sterilized explants incubated on culture media. Plant pieces are usually surface-sterilized in ethanol, mercury bichloride and sodium hypochlorite solution, and incubated on a general purpose medium (e.g. potato dextrose agar, PDA) amended with antibiotics. Methods of isolation have been reviewed extensively (Schulz et al., 1993; Bayman, 2007). These methods are simple, inexpensive, and allow detection of a wide range of fungi. However, the choice of surface-sterilization method and culture medium will bias the results in favor of certain organisms. Fungi that are obligate biotrophs and do not grow on culture media will be overlooked, and weedy fungi that grow quickly on agar medium will be overrepresented. Distinctions between epiphytes and endophytes depend on the assumption that surface sterilization kills the former and not the latter. These limitations have stimulated the use of molecular techniques to identify endophytes.

Sampling strategy also has a great impact on which endophytes will grow out of leaf explants on agar medium. In general, using small leaf pieces reveals greater endphyte richness than when using large leaf explants. Because leaf-to-leaf variation is considerable, several leaves should be sampled. Many studies on endophyte diversity are not rigorous in sampling strategy, which often makes it difficult to compare the results between studies.

2.3. Taxonomic Identification of the Fungal Isolates

Some fungal isolates, which were screened to have antimicrobial activity, were further selected to have their taxonomic identification. Rigorous identification of endophytes requires microscopic examination of the host tissue and relies to a significant extent on the taxonomic expertise of the examiner. Morphological examination is performed by scrutinizing the culture, the mechanism of spore production, and the characteristics of the spores. Some endophytic fungi failed to produce spores or identifiable structures. Accordingly, fungal endophytic isolates are often identified using a combination of morphological and molecular methods (Zhang et al., 2006).

Special caution has to be taken when closely related or morphologically similar endophytic fungi are under identification. The morphological features of some fungi are usually medium-dependent, and some cultural conditions can affect substantially vegetative and sexual incompatibility. Thus, the morphological character of endophytes should be coupled with the available molecular evidence to enable significant differentiation between closely related species. For newly discovered endophytic fungi, sequence comparisons or internal transcribed spacer (ITS1 and ITS2) and 5.8S rDNA sequence examinations should be further investigated.

2.4. Antimicrobial Activity Evaluation of the Extracts and Compounds

Antimicrobial activity evaluation is necessary when the extracts from endophytic fungi have been prepared. Bioactive extracts and fractions were repeatedly chromatographed on silica gel and/or Sephadex LH-20 to afford pure compounds. The following is the brief introduction of some antimicrobial activity evaluation methods used for the extracts and compounds from endophytic fungi.

2.4.1. Mycelial Radial Growth Test

Aspects of the mycelial radial growth test method have been already described (Nuiroga et al., 2001; Zhou et al., 2008). It is suitable to screen antimicrobial activity of the crude extracts in large amounts on basis of mycelial radial growth rate of filamentous fungi. Test samples were dissolved in some an organic solvent (i.e. methanol, ethanol, acetone, DMSO) first. Each dissolved extract was poured into the assay flask containing a hot sterilized medium (i.e. PDA) at 50-60 °C. After thoroughly mixing, the treated medium was poured into a Petri dish. A disc (5-mm diameter) of the fungal mycelial culture was aseptically transferred to the center of the solidified medium in plates. After a period of inoculation at

20-30 °C in the dark, mycelial growth of the fungus was measured, and an average was taken of two measurements crosswise made on each plate. Negative control plates were treated with the same quantity of organic solvent mixed with medium. Reference fungicide (i.e. azoxystrobin, captan and carbendazim) was also needed to be compared. Antifungal activity was recorded in terms of percentage colony inhibition and calculated. Percentage (%) of mycelial growth inhibition was determined as $[(D_c-D_t)/D_c]\times100$, where D_c is the average diameter increase of fungal colony with the negative control, and D_t is the average diameter increase of a fungal colony with treatment.

2.4.2. Agar Diffusion Test

Extracts and/or compounds having a good diffusion coefficient may penetrate the agar medium even in small amounts. Agar diffusion test, which comprises paper disk and agar well methods, has been introduced elsewhere (Hadecek and Greger, 2000; Srinivasan et al., 2001; Tang et al., 2008a). The paper disk diffusion test was first developed for bacteria and later modified for filamentous fungi. Agar well diffusion tests are also similar, including the hole-plate diffusion test method and the cylinder test method. Paper disk method comprises the pacing of filter paper disks containing test compounds on agar plate surfaces previously inoculated with the test organism. The chemical then diffuses into the agar and inhibits growth of the test bacterium or fungus. The hole-plate diffusion method depends upon diffusion of the aqueous test compound solution from a vertical hole in the agar layer, while the cylinder method utilizes stainless steel or porcelain cylinders. After incubation, mean diameters of growth inhibition zones are recorded. Diffusion tests are recommended much more for polar rather than non-polar compounds. The dipping of filter paper disks into a test compound solution should be avoided. Instead, it is more accurate to dispense the compound dissolved in a small amount of organic solvent directly on to the filter paper disk. Rigorous drying of organic solvent is crucial. Negative controls should be included in order to detect solvent effects. As it is impossible to measure the amount of the test compound diffused into the agar medium, diffusion assays are less suitable to determine minimum inhibitory concentration (MIC) values for compound activity comparisons. So the absolute values of inhibition zones have only relative importance, the agar diffusion is appropriate as pre-test only (Hadacek and Greger, 2000).

2.4.3. Serial Dilution Test

Dilution test method has one major advantage over diffusion test, namely the test compound concentration in the medium is defined. This test yielded the best reproducible results, and was recommended as general standard methodology for testing natural products (Hadacek and Greger, 2000). Consequently, dilution test is regarded as the method of choice to compare MIC values. The advent of microtitre plates has led to significant reductions in test compound amounts. Furthermore, in combination with spectrophotometric of fluorometric plate readers, it is possible to scale up sample throughput enormously. However, filamentous fungi are not single-cell organisms. Their growth is not easy to quantify as with bacteria and unicellular yeasts where turbidity indicates growth. Turbidity can be assessed either visually or spectrophotometrically at wavelengths in the range of 550-650 nm (Pfaller et al., 1995).

Originally, liquid broth assay for filamentous fungi was carried out in 20 ml flasks (Weidenborner et al., 1989). After a 7-day growth period, fungal biomass was determined after filtering and drying to constant biomass. This assay had the major disadvantage of requiring large amounts of test compound. Consequently, the microtitre plate format will become the future standard test.

In addition to turbidity, various other elegant methods have been developed to quantify fungal growth colorimetrically or spectrofluorometrically. Dehydrogenases of metabolically active cells reduce 3-(4,5- dimethyl-2-thiazolyl) -2,5-diphyenyl-2H-tetrazolum bromide (MTT) and sodium 3,3′-[1-(phenylamino) carbonyl] -3,4-tetrazolium]- bis(4-methoxy-6-nitro) benzene sulfonic acid hydrate (XTT) to water soluble orange and water insoluble purple formazans, respectively (Mosmann, 1983; Stevens and Olsen, 1993; Al-Bakri and Afifi, 2007; Tan et al., 2008; Tang et al., 2008b). This method has been adapted to quantify antifungal growth. Alternatively, Espinel-Ingroff et al. (1997) and Pelloux-Prayer et al. (1998) used Alamar blue which consists of a reduction-oxidation indicator yielding a colorimetric change and fluorescent signal in response to metabolic changes (Page et al., 1993).

2.4.4. Bioautography

Agar overlay bioautography was developed as a quick and versatile method to detect antimicrobial natural products of microbial or plant origin, which allows the identification of even small amounts of antimicrobially active compounds in multi-compound mixtures such as crude extracts and fractions (Pauli, 2006). Following 1-D or 2-D development of TLC-plates by using an appropriate solvent system, the dried plates are overlayed with a 1-mm medium layer containing fungal conidia or bacteria. Active compounds were detected after a period of incubation (Wedge and Nagle, 2000; Tabanca et al., 2005). By combination TLC-bioautography and oxidation-reduction indicator (i.e. MTT), it was easy to screen the antimicrobial compounds in the mixtures (Zhao et al., 2008a).

2.4.5. Vapor Phase Activity Test

To test the antimicrobial activity in the vapor phase methods has been used that allow the determination relative values only. A frequently used method is the placing of a test compound containing cup 5 mm below an inoculated agar surface and the determination of the resulting inhibition zone (Alvarez-Castellanos et al., 2001). Other authors used two compartment Petri dishes, one of which contained the medium inoculated with fungal mycelia, whereas the second compartment contained the medium containing volatile substances. In this way, the fungi were not in direct contact with the volatile substances and any effect on growth of the mycelium could be attributed to vapor activity (Letessier et al., 2001; Zhao et al., 2008b).

2.4.6. Spore Germination Inhibition Test

Spore germination inhibition test is also a sensitive method to evaluate the antimicrobial activity of the compounds (Suzuki et al., 1996; Pelloux-Prayer et al., 1998; Kong et al., 2004). The fungi (i.e. *Magnaporthe oryzae, Botrytis cinerea*) were raised on an agar medium at 25 °C in the dark for a week, with spores collected by agitating with distilled water using a few days' cultures under fluorescent light after removal of the spores from the culture plate. The spore suspension was filtered through cheesecloth and diluted with fresh medium to 10-20 spores in a microscopic field. The filtered spore suspension (200 μl) was added into different concentrations of test material on a concave slide glass and incubated at 25 °C in a moist chamber for 12 h, and then the percentages of germinating and non-germinating spores were determined using a microscope (Kong et al., 2004). In addition to regular spore germination method, a spectrofluorometric method by combination of spore germination and oxidation-reduction indicator Alamar blue performed in a 96-well plate for kinetic evaluation of spore germination and mycelial growth of *Botrytis cinerea* in liquid culture was developed (Pelloux-Prayer et al., 1998).

3. Antimicrobial Compounds Isolated from Endophytic Fungi

Endophytes are a significant reservoir of genetic diversity, and an important source for the discovery of novel bioactive secondary metabolites. Of them, endophytic fungi are an important group to be a rich source of natural products displaying a broad spectrum of biological activities. The reported natural products from endophytes includes antibiotics, antimycotics, immunosupressants, anticancer compounds, antioxidant agents, and other biologically active substances (Tan and Zou, 2001; Strobel, 2003; Strobel et al., 2004; Zhang et al., 2006). This section describes the antimicrobial compounds which can be grouped into several categories, including alkaloids, peptides, steroids, terpenoids, phenols and phenolic acids, quinines, aliphatics, lactones, isocoumarin derivatives, benzophenones and others.

3.1. Alkaloids

Many alkaloids have been detected in the cultures of grass-associated endophytic fungi. These metabolites play an important role in inhibiting berbivores and insects. Although the alkaloids levels may be influenced by environmental factors, the types and levels of alkaloids seem to depend mostly on endophyte species, strain or genotype, and less on the host grass genotype and/or the environment (Mueller and Krauss, 2005). Some alkaloids derived from the endophytic fungi have significantly antimicrobial activity. Some examples including amides (**1-12**), amines (**13**) and indole derivatives (**14**) are shown in Table 1.

3.2. Peptides

Leucinostatin A (**15**), an oligopeptide with phytotoxic, anticancer and antifungal properties, was isolated from the culture of *Acremonium* sp., an ednophytic fungus from *Taxus baccata* (Strobel et al., 1997). This mycotoxin causes necrotic symptoms in many non-host plants presumably because they can not transform it into the much less toxic leucinostatin α-β-di-*O*-glucoside as can the host plant *T. baccata* (Strobel and Hess, 1997).

Other antimicrobial peptides mainly including cyclopeptides (**16-23**) and dipeptides (**24-26**) are shown in Table 1.

Table 1. Antimicrobial compounds from endophytic fungi

Compound class/ Compound name	Microorganism tested (F/B)	Endophytic fungus	Plant (family) derived	Reference
Alkaloids				
Phomopsichalasin (**1**)	*Bacillus subtilis* (B); *Pesudomonas* sp. (B); *Salmonella galinarum* (B); *Staphylococcus aureus* (B); *Candida albicans* (F)	*Phomopsis* sp.	*Salix gracilistyla* var.*melanostachys* (Salicaceae)	Horn et al., 1995
Cryptocin (**2**)	*Magnaporthe oryzae* (F)	*Cryptosporiopsis quercina*	*Tripterygium wilfordii* (Celastraceae)	Li et al., 2000
Altersetin (**3**); Tenuazonic acid (**4**)	Gram-positive bacteria (B)	*Alternaria* spp.	Not mentioned	Hellwig et al., 2002
Asperfumoid (**5**)	*Candida albicans* (F)	*Aspergillus fumigatus*	*Cynodon dactylon* (Graminae)	Liu et al., 2004
Neoplaether (**6**)	*Candida albicans* (F)	*Neoplaconema napellum*	*Hopea hainanensis* (Dipterocarpaceae)	Wang et al., 2006
Cerebrosides (**7, 8**)	*Bacillus subtilis* (B); *Escherichia coli* (B); *Pseudomonas fluorescens* (B)	*Fusarium* sp.	*Quercus variabilis* (Fagaceae)	Shu et al., 2004
Cercosporamide (**9**); Phomodione (**10**)	*Staphylococcus aureus* (B); *Pythium ultimum* (F); *Sclerotinia sclerotiorum* (F); *Rhizoctonia solani* (F)	*Phoma pinodella*	*Saurauia scaberrinae* (Actinidiaceae)	Hoffman et al., 2008
Pyrrocindine A (**11**); Pyrrocindine B (**12**)	*Aspergillus flavus* (F); *Fusarium verticillioides* (F)	*Acremonium zeae*	*Zea maydis* (Graminae)	Wicklow et al., 2005
7-Amino-4-methylcoumarin (**13**)	*Aeromonas hydrophila* (B); *Bibrio anguillarum* (B); *Escherichia coli* (B); *Salmonella enteritidis* (B); *Salmonella typhimurium* (B); *Shigella* sp. (B); *Vibrio parahaemolyticus* (B); *Yersinia* sp. (B); *Aspergillus niger* (F); *Candida albicans* (F); *Penicillium expansum* (F)	*Xylaria* sp.	*Ginkgo biloba* (Ginkgoaceae)	Liu et al., 2008

Table 1. Continued

Compound class/ Compound name	Microorganism tested (F/B)	Endophytic fungus	Plant (family) derived	Reference
6-Isoprenylindole-3-carboxylic acid (**14**)	*Bacillus subtilis* (B); *Pesudomonas* sp. (B); *Sarcina lutea* (B); *Staphylococcus aureus* (B); *Helminthosporium sativum* (F); *Phytophthora capisici* (F); *Rhizoctonia cerealis* (F)	*Colletotrichum* sp.	*Artemisia annua* (Compositae)	Lu et al., 2000
Peptides				
Leucinostatin A (**15**)	*Pythium ultimum* (F)	*Acremonium* sp.	*Taxus baccata* (Taxaceae)	Strobel et al., 1997
Cryptocandin (**16**)	*Candida albicans* (F); *Trichophyton mentagrophytes* (F); *Trichophyton rubrum* (F)	*Cryptosporiop sis quercina*	*Tripterigium wilfordii* (Celastraceae)	Strobel et al., 1999
Echinocandins A (**17**); B (**18**); D (**19**); H (**20**)	Yeast (F)	*Cryptosporiop sis* sp.; *Pezicula* sp.	*Pinus sylvestris* (Pinaceae); *Fagus sylvatica* (Fagaceae)	Noble et al., 1991
Enniatins A1 (**21**); B (**22**); B1 (**23**)	*Botrytis cinerea* (F)	*Fusarium proliferatum*	*Celatrus angulatus* (Celatraceae)	Ji et al., 2005
Cyclo(L-phenylalanine-trans-4-hydroxy-L-proline (**24**); Cyclo(L-leucine-trans-4-hydroxy-L-proline (**25**); Cyclo(L-alanine-trans-4-hydroxy-L-proline (**26**)	*Plasmopara viticola*	*Alternaria alternata*	*Vitis vinifera* (Vitaceae)	Musetti et al., 2007
Steroids				
3β,5α-dihydroxy-6β-acetoxy-ergosta-7,22-diene (**27**); 3β, 5α-dihydroxy-6β-phenylacetyloxy-ergosta-7, 22-diene (**28**);	*Bacillus subtilis* (B); *Staphylococcus aureus* (B); *Sarcina lutea* (B); *Pseudomonas* sp. (B); *Candida albicans* (F); *Aspergillus niger* (F)	*Colletotrichum* sp.	*Artemisia annua* (Compositae)	Lu et al., 2000

Table 1. Continued

Compound class/ Compound name	Microorganism tested (F/B)	Endophytic fungus	Plant (family) derived	Reference
3β-hydroxy-ergosta-5-ene (**29**); 3-oxo-ergosta-4, 6, 8(14), 22-tetraene (**30**); 3β-hydroxy-5α, 8α-epidioxy-ergosta-6, 22-diene (**31**)	*Bacillus subtilis* (B); *Staphylococcus aureus* (B); *Sarcina lutea* (B); *Pseudomonas* sp. (B); *Candida albicans* (F); *Aspergillus niger* (F)	*Colletotrichum* sp.	*Artemisia annua* (Compositae)	Lu et al., 2000
3β-hydroxy-5α, 8α-epidioxy-ergosta-6, 22-diene (**31**); ergosterol (**32**)	*Helicobacter pylori* (B); *Sarcina lutea* (B)	*Aspergillus* sp.	*Cynodon dactylon* (Gramineae)	Li et al., 2005
3β-hydroxy-5α, 8α-epidioxy-ergosta-6, 22-diene (**31**); ergosterol (**32**)	*Microbotryum violacerum* (F); *Septoria tritici* (F)	*Nudulisporium* sp.	*Juniperus cedre* (Cupressaceae)	Dai et al., 2006
Terpenoids				
Chokols A-G (**33-39**)	*Cladosporium phlei* (F)	*Epicholoe typhina*	*Phleum pretense* (Gramineae)	Koshino et al., 1989
Guanacasterpene (**40**)	Methicililin-resistant *Staphyloccoccus aureus* (F); Vancomycin-resistant *Enterococcus faecium* (F)	Unidentified fungus CR115	*Daphnopsis americana* (Thymelaeaceae)	Singh et al., 2000
Sordaricin (**41**)	*Candida albicans* (F)	*Xylaria* sp.	*Garcinia dulcis* (Guttiferae)	Pongcharoen et al., 2008
Phenols and Phenolic acids				
2-Hydroxy-6-methylbenzoic acid (**42**)	*Bacillus subtilis* (B); *Micrococsus luteus* (B); *Pseudomonas aeruginosa* (B); *Staphylococcus aureus* (B)	*Phoma* sp.	*Taxus wallachiana* (Taxaceae)	Yang et al., 1994
2-Methoxy-4-hydroxy-6-methoxymethyl-benzaldehyde (**43**)	*Cladosporium cucumerinum* (F)	*Pezicula* sp.	*Pinus* sp. (Pinaceae)	Schulz et al., 1995
p-Hydroxybenzoic acid (**44**); p-Hydroxyphenylacetic acid (**45**);	*Cladosporium herbarum* (F)	*Epichloe typhina*	*Phleum pretense* (Gramineae)	Koshino et al., 1988

Table 1. Continued

Compound class/ Compound name	Microorganism tested (F/B)	Endophytic fungus	Plant (family) derived	Reference
Tyrosol (**46**); *cis*-p-Coumaric acid (**47**); *trans*-p-Coumaric acid (**48**)	*Cladosporium herbarum* (F)	*Epichloe typhina*	*Phleum pretense* (Gramineae)	Koshino et al., 1988
Colletotric acid (**49**)	*Helminthosporium sativum* (F)	*Colletotrichum gloeosporioides*	*Artemisia mongolica* (Compositae)	Zou et al., 2000
Pestacin (**50**)	*Pythium ultimum* (F)	*Pestalotiopsis microspora*	*Terminalia morobensis* (Combretaceae)	Harper et al., 2003
Isopestacin (**51**)	*Pythium ultimum* (F)	*Pestalotiopsis microspora*	*Terminalia morobensis* (Combretaceae)	Strobel et al., 2002
Pestaloside (**52**)	*Rhizoctonia solani* (F); *Geotrichum candidum* (F); *Agaricus campestris* (F)	*Pestalotiopsis microspora*	*Torreya taxifolia* (Taxaceae)	Lee et al., 1995
1-(2,6-dihydroxyphenyl)-butan-1-one (**53**)	*Bacillus megaterium* (B); *Microbotryum violacerum* (F); *Septoria tritici* (F)	*Nudulisporium* sp.	*Juniperus cedre* (Cupressaceae)	Dai et al., 2006
1-(2-hydroxy-6-methoxyphenyl) butan-1-one (**54**); 5-Hydroxy 2-methyl 4H-chromen-4-one (**55**); 2,3-Dihydro-5-methoxy-2-methychromen-4-one (**57**);1,8-Dimethoxynaphthalene (**59**)	*Microbotryum violacerum* (F); *Septoria tritici* (F)	*Nudulisporium* sp.	*Juniperus cedre* (Cupressaceae)	Dai et al., 2006
2,3-Ddihydro-5-hydroxy-2-methyl chromen-4-one (**56**); 8-Methoxynaphthalen-1-ol (**58**); Nodulisporin A (**60**); Nodulisporin B (**61**)	*Microbotryum violacerum* (F)	*Nudulisporium* sp.	*Juniperus cedre* (Cupressaceae)	Dai et al., 2006

Table 1. Continued

Compound class/ Compound name	Microorganism tested (F/B)	Endophytic fungus	Plant (family) derived	Reference
Usnic acid (**62**)	*Staphylococcus aureus* (B); *Pythium ultimum* (F); *Sclerotinia sclerotiorum* (F); *Rhizoctonia solani* (F)	*Phoma pinodella*	*Saurauia scaberrinae* (Actinidiaceae)	Hoffman et al., 2008
Quinones				
Altersolanol (**63**)	*Bacillus subtilis* (B); *Micrococcus luteus* (B); *Pseudomonas aeruginosa* (B); *Staphylococcus aureus* (B)	*Phoma* sp.	*Taxus wallachiana* (Taxaceae)	Yagi et al., 1993; Yang et al., 1994
Jesterone (**64**)	*Pythium ultimum* (F)	*Pestalotiopsis jesteri*	*Fragraea bodenii* (Gentianaceae)	Li and Strobel, 2001
Hydroxyl-jesterone (**65**)	*Pythium ultimum* (F)	*Pestalotiopsis jesteri*	*Fragraea bodenii* (Gentianaceae)	Li and Strobel, 2001
Ambuic acid (**66**)	*Cephalosporium gramineum* (B);*Diplodia matelensis* (B); *Fusarium solani* (B); *Fusarium cubense* (B); *Helminthosporium sativum* (B); *Pythium ultimum* (B)	*Monochaetia* sp.	*Taxus wallachiana* (Taxaceae)	Li et al., 2001
Ambuic acid (**66**)	*Cephalosporium gramineum* (B); *Diplodia matelensis* (B); *Fusarium solani* (B); *Fusarium cubense* (B); *Helminthosporium sativum* (B); *Pythium ultimum* (B)	*Pestalotiopsis microspora*	*Dendrobium speciosum* (Orchidaceae); *Taxodium disticum* (Taxodiaceae); *Taxus baccata* (Taxaceae); *Torreya taxifolia* (Taxaceae)	Li et al., 2001
3-O-methylalaternin (**67**); Altersolanol A (**68**)	*Staphylococcus aureus* (B); *Staphylococcu epidermidis* (B); *Enterococcus faecalis* (B)	*Ampelomyces* sp.	*Urospermum picroides* (Compositae)	Aly et al., 2008
Preussomerins G-L (**69-74**)	*Bacillus megaterium* (B); *Eurotium repens* (F); *Fusarium oxysporum* (F); *Microbotryum violacerum* (F)	*Mycelia sterila*	*Atropa belladonna* (Solanaceae)	Krohn et al., 2001
Preussomerins EG_1 (**75**); EG_2 (**76**); EG_3 (**77**);Deoxypreussomerin B (**78**)	*Alternaria solani* (F); *Fusarium oxysporum* (F); *Phytophthora capsici* (F); *Phytophthora parasitica* (F)	*Edenia gomezpompae*	*Callicarpa acuminata* (Verbenaceae)	Macias-Rubalcava et al., 2008

Table 1. Continued

Compound class/ Compound name	Microorganism tested (F/B)	Endophytic fungus	Plant (family) derived	Reference
Aliphatics				
Ethyl *trans*-9,10-epoxy-11-oxoundecanoate (**79**); Ethyl 9-oxononanoate (**80**); Ethyl zaelate (**81**); Hydroxydihydrobovolide (**82**)	*Cladosporium herbarum* (F)	*Epichloe typhina*	*Phleum pretense* (Gramineae)	Koshino et al., 1989
6-Oxo-2-propenyl-3,6-dihydro-2H-pryan-3-yl ester (**83**)	*Vibrio salmonicida* (B); *Pseudomonas aeruginosa* (B); *Staphylococcus aureus* (B)	Unidentified	*Larix laricina* (Pinaceae)	Findlay et al., 1997
Lactones				
Phomol (**84**)	*Arthrobacter citreus* (B); *Corynebacterium insidiosum* (B); *Pseudomonas fluorescens* (B); *Nematospora coryli* (F); *Schizosaccharomyces octospora* (F); *Absidia glauca* (F); *Ascocyta pisi* (F); *Aspergillus ochraceus* (F); *Fusarium fujikuroi* (F); *Fusarium oxysporum* (F); *Paecilomyces variotii* (F); *Penicillium islandicum* (F); *Penicilium notatum* (F); *Zygorhynchus moelleri* (F)	*Phomopsis* sp.	*Erythrina crista-galli* (Leguminosae)	Weber et al., 2004
Pyrenophorol (**85**)	*Microbotryum violaceum* (F)	*Phoma* sp.	*Fagonia cretica* (Zygophyllaceae)	Krohn et al., 2007
Cytosporone B (**86**); Cytosporone C (**87**)	*Candida albicans* (F); *Fusarium oxysporum* (F)	*Phomopsis* sp.	*Excoecaria agallocha* (Euphorbiaceae)	Huang et al., 2008
Cytosporone D (**88**); Cytosporone E (**89**)	Bacteria (B)	*Cytospora* sp. *Diaporthe* sp.	Not mentioned	Brady et al., 2000

Table 1. Continued

Compound class/ Compound name	Microorganism tested (F/B)	Endophytic fungus	Plant (family) derived	Reference
Isocoumarin derivatives				
(R)-Mellein (**90**)	*Cladosporium cucumerinum* (F)	*Pezicula* sp.	*Pinus* sp. (Pinaceae)	Schulz et al., 1995
7-Butyl-6,8-dihydroxy-3(R)-pent-11-enylisochroman-1-one (**91**);7-But-15-enyl-6,8-dihydroxy-3(R)-pent-11-enylisochroman-1-one (**92**);7-Butyl-6,8-dihydroxy-3(R)-pentylisochroman-1-one (**93**)	*Mycobacterium tuberculosis* (B);*Candida albicans* (F)	*Geotrichum* sp.	*Crassocephalum crepidioides* (Compositae)	Kongsaeree et al., 2003
Benzophenones				
Monomethylsulchrin (**94**)	*Helicobacter pylori* (B); *Sarcina lutea* (B)	*Aspergillus* sp.	*Cynodon dactylon* (Gramineae)	Li et al., 2005
Rhizoctonic acid (**95**)	*Helicobacter pylori* (B)	*Rhizoctonia* sp.	*Cynodon dactylon* (Gramineae)	Ma et al., 2004
Isofusidienols A-D (**96-99**)	*Bacillus subtilis* (B); *Staphylococcus aureus* (B); *Escherichia coli* (B); *Candia albicans* (F)	*Chalara* sp.	*Artemisia vulgaris* (Compositae)	Losgen et al., 2008
Others				
Annulene (**100**)	*Pythium ultimum* (F); *Verticillum dahliae* (F)	*Gliocladium* sp.	*Eucryphia cordifolia* (Eucryphiaceae)	Stinson et al., 2003
Rubrofusarin B (**101**); Fonsecinone A (**102**); Asperpyrone B (**103**); Aurasperone A (**104**)	*Bacillus subitlis* (B); *Escherichia coli* (B); *Pseumomonas fluorescens* (B);*Candida albicans* (F); *Trichophyton rubrum* (F)	*Aspergillus niger*	*Cynodon dactylon* (Gramineae)	Song et al., 2004
Griseofulvin (**105**)	*Magnaporthe oryzae* (F); *Botrytis cinerea* (F); *Blumeria graminis* f.sp. *hordei* (F); *Corticium sasaki* (F); *Phytophthora infestans* (F); *Puccinia recondite* (F)	*Xylaris* sp.	*Abies holophylla* (Pinaceae)	Park et al., 2005

Note: F, fungus; B, bacterium.

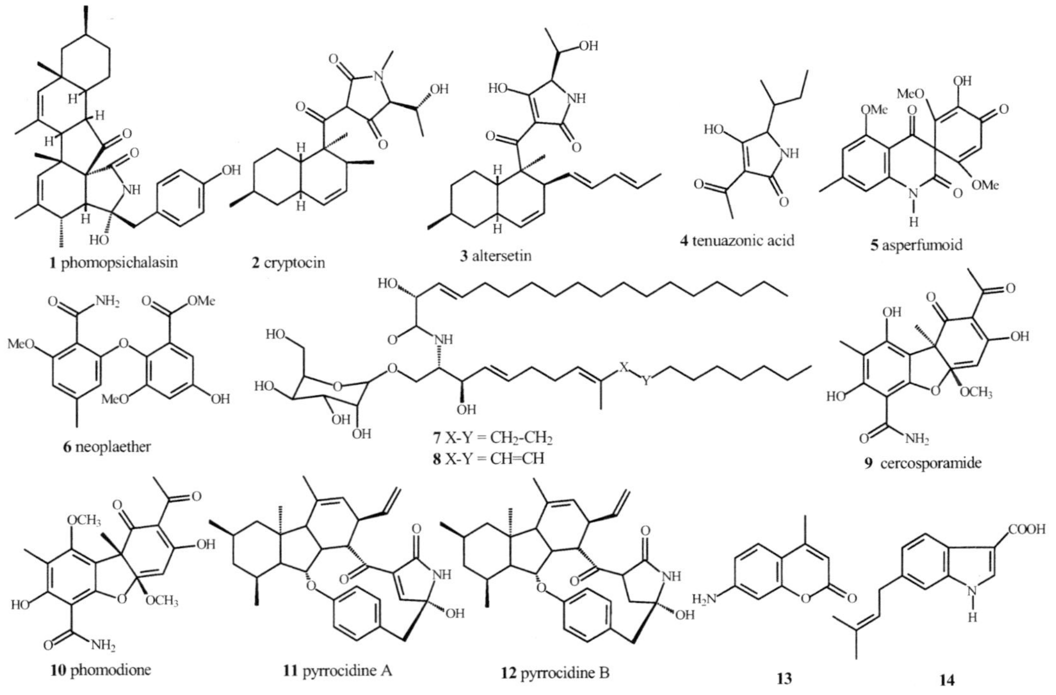

3.3. Steroids

Some steroidal metabolites from endophytic fungi have been reported. Five antimicrobial steroids 3β,5α-dihydroxy - 6β-acetoxy-ergosta-7,22-diene (**27**), 3β, 5α-dihydroxy - 6β-phenylacetyloxy - ergosta-7, 22-diene (**28**), 3β-hydroxy ergosta-5-ene (**29**), 3-oxo-ergosta-4, 6, 8(14), 22-tetraene (**30**), and 3β-hydroxy - 5α, 8α-epidioxy - ergosta-6, 22-diene (**31**) were characterized from the liquid culture of an fungal endophyte *Colletotrichum* sp. of *Artemisia annua* (Lu et al., 2000). The antimicrobial steroids from endophytic fungi are shown in Table 1.

3.4. Terpenoids

Chokols A-G (**33-39**) were the first reported sesquiterpenes isolated from stromata of *Epichloe typhina* on *Phleum pretense* and were found to be fungitoxic to the leaf sport disease pathogen *Cladosporium phlei* (Koshino et al., 1989).

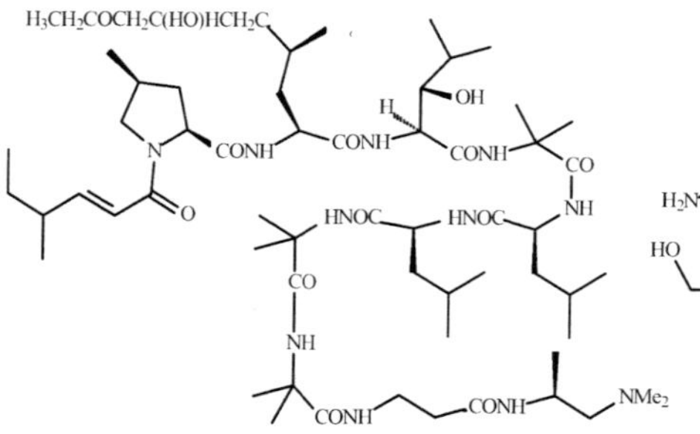

15 leucinostatin A

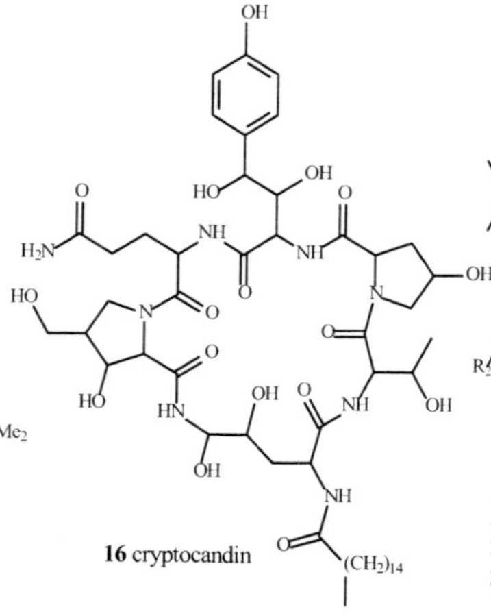

16 cryptocandin

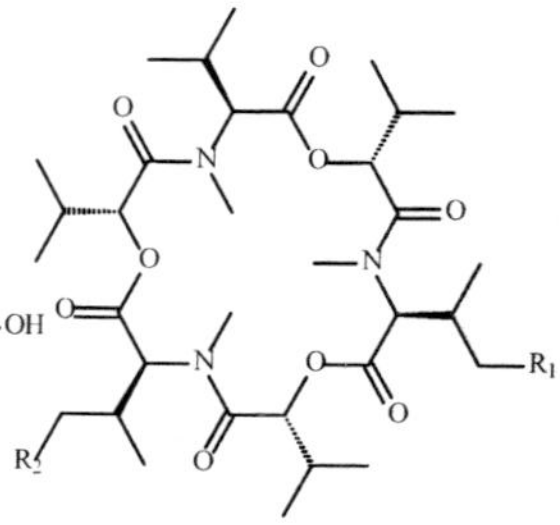

21 enniatin A1 R_1=CH_3, R_2=CH_3
22 enniatin B R_1=H, R_2=H
23 enniatin B1 R_1=CH_3, R_2=H

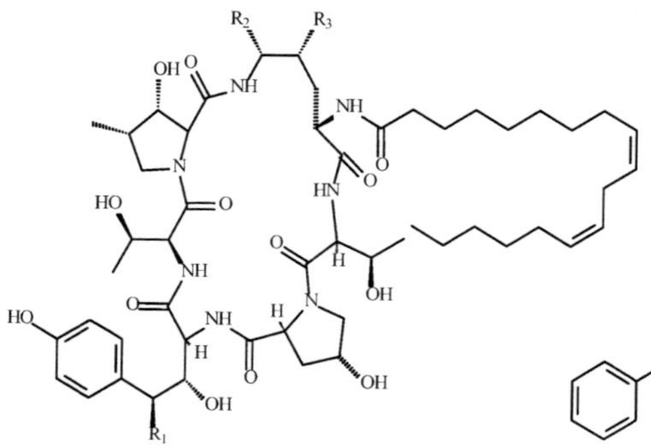

17 echinocandin A R_1=R_2=R_3=OH
18 echinocandin B R_1=H, R_2=R_3=OH
19 echinocandin D R_1=R_2=R_3=H
20 echinocandin H R_1=R_2=OH, R_3=OMe

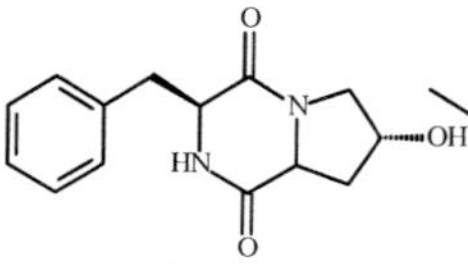

24

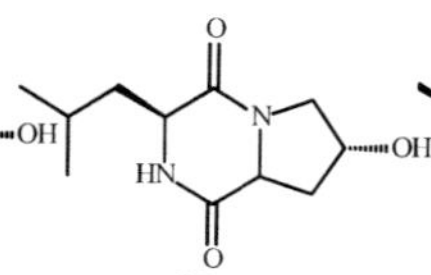

25

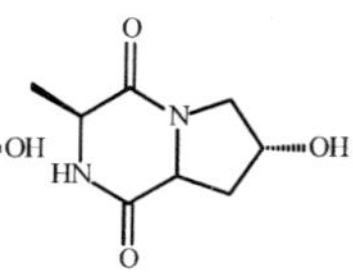

26

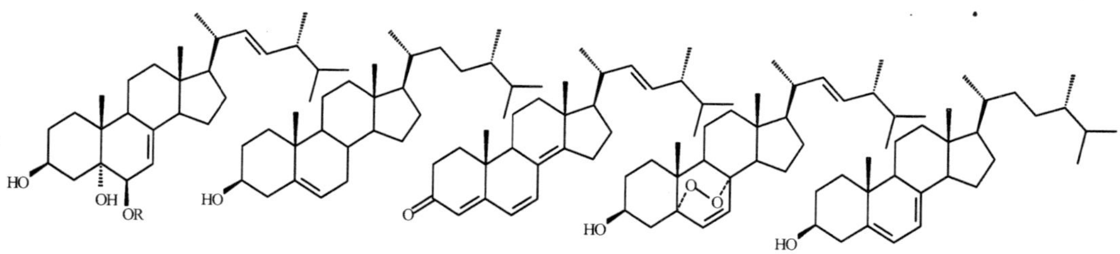

27 R=$COCH_3$
28 R=$COCH_2C_6H_5$

29

30

31

32 ergosterol

Guanacasterpene (**40**), a novel diterpenoid produced by an unidentified fungus CR115 from the branch of Daphnopsis Americana growing in Guanacaste, Costa Rica, was detected to show strong antibacterial activity against methcillin-resistant *Staphylococcus aureus* and vancomycin-resistant *Enterococcus faecium* (Singh et al., 2000). Sordaricin (**41**) from the endophytic *Xylaria* sp. PSU-D14 associated with *Garcinia dulcis* leaves was a diterpene aglycone of potent antifungal sordarins exhibiting moderate antifungal activity against *Candida albicans* with a MIC value of 32 μg/ml (Pongcharoen et al., 2008).

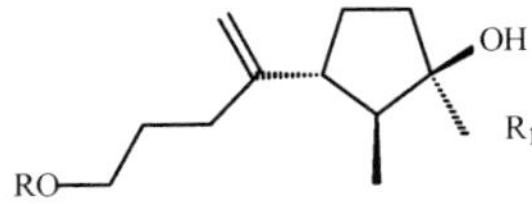

33 chokol A R = H
34 chokol F R = Ac

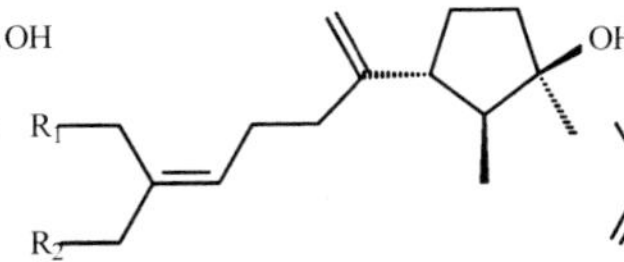

35 chokol C R_1 = H, R_2 = OH
36 chokol B R_1 = OH, R_2 = H

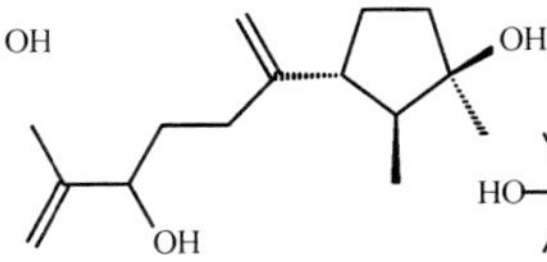

37 chokol B

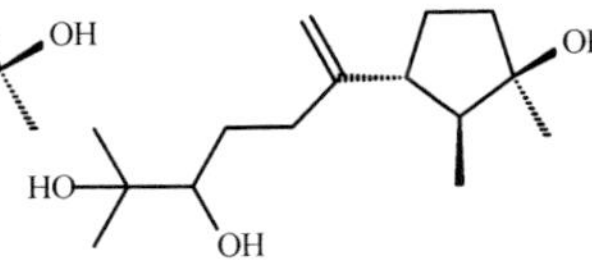

38 chokol E

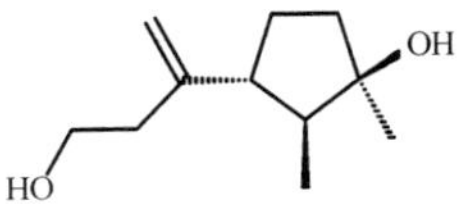

39 chokol G

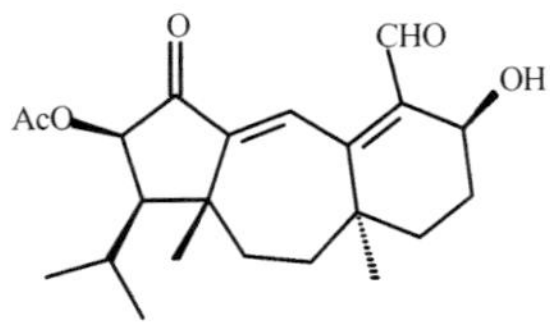

40 guanacastepene

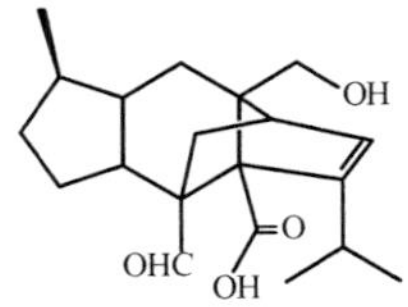

41 sardaricin

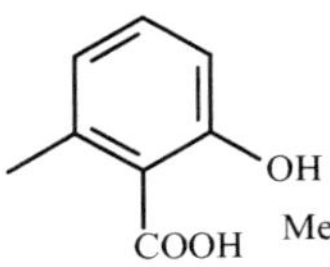

42

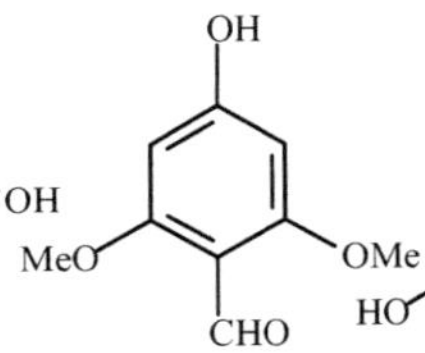

43

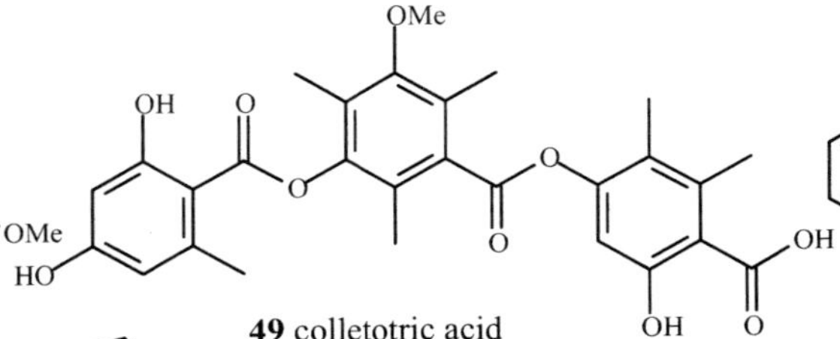

49 colletotric acid

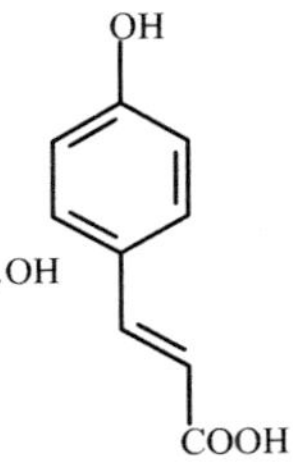

48

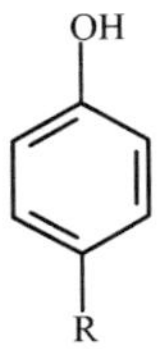

44 R = COOH
45 R = CH_2COOH
46 R = CH_2CH_2OH
47 R = CH=CHCOOH

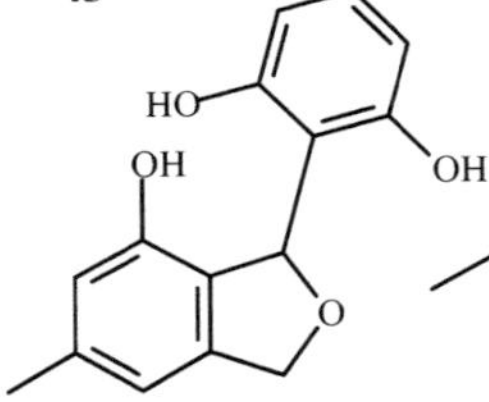

50 pestacin

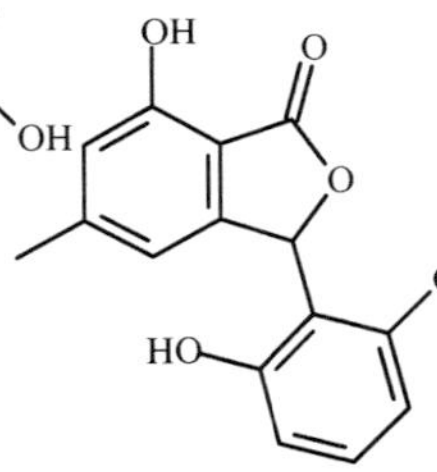

51 isopestacin

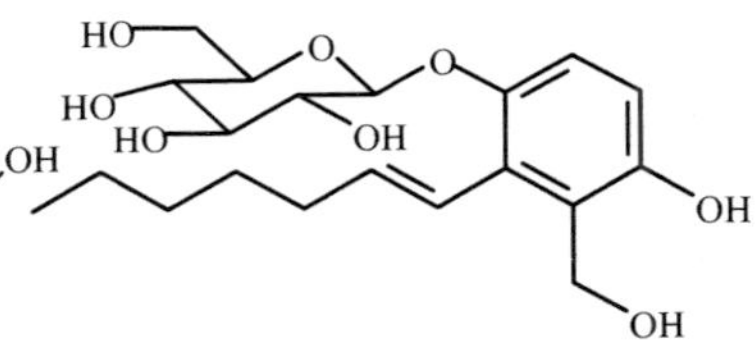

52 pestaloside

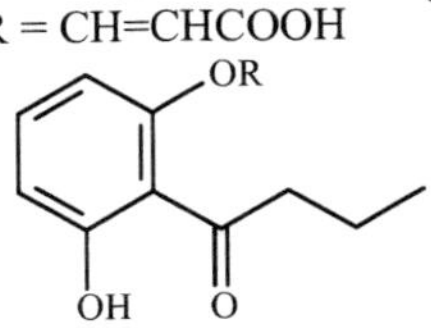

53 R = H
54 R= Me

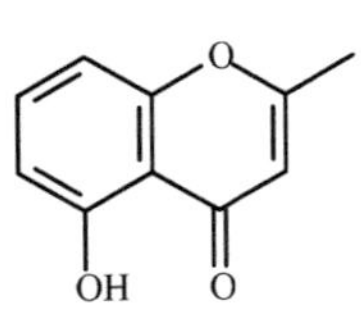

55

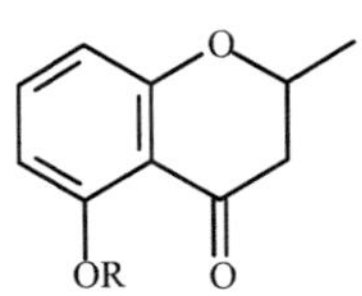

56 R = H
57 R = Me

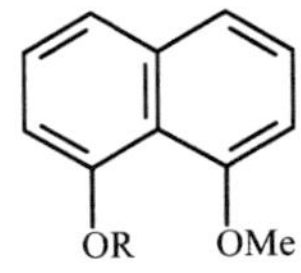

58 R = H
59 R = Me

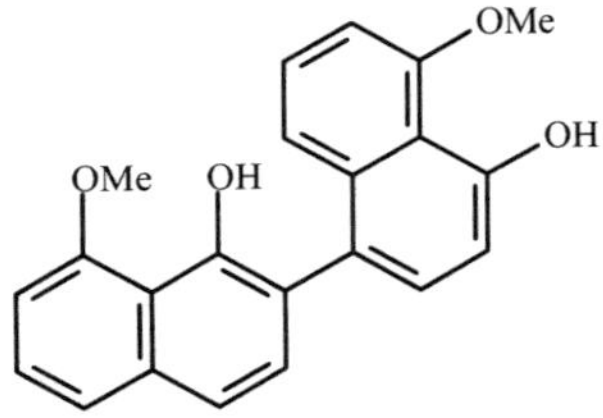

60 nodulisporin A

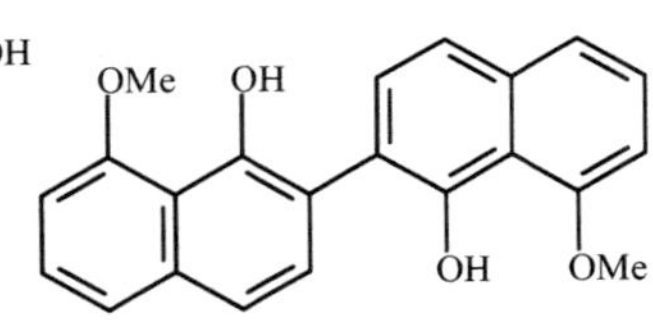

61 nodulisporin B

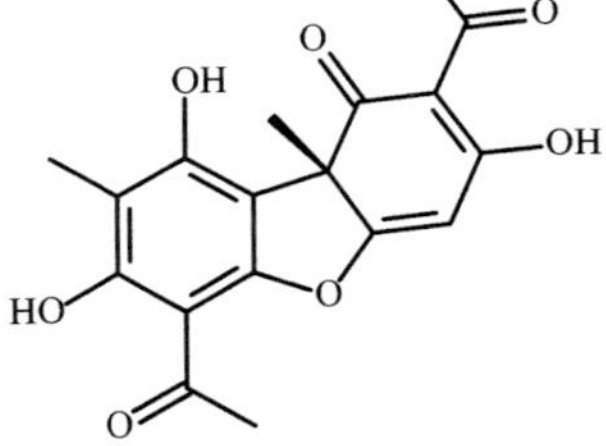

62 usnic acid

3.5. Phenols and Phenolic Acids

Phenol and phenolic acids, frequently detected in cultures of endophytic fungi, often have pronounced antimicrobial activity. Some examples are outlined in Table 1. Usnic acid (**62**), a dibenzofuran compound exhibited inhibitory activity against *Staphylococcus aureus*, *Pythium ultimum*, *Sclerotinia sclerotiorum* and *Rhizoctonia solani,* was isolated from the culture broth of *Phoma pinodella* from *Saurauia scaberrinae* (Actinidiaceae), a Guinea plant (Hoffman et al., 2008).

3.6. Quinones

A highly hydroxylated quinone altersolanol A (**63**) was isolated from an endophytic *Phoma* sp. associated with *Taxus wallachiana* (Yang et al., 1994). It had been previously isolated from a strain of tomato pathogenic *Alternaria solani* with its antibacterial activity against *Staphylococcus aureus*, *Bacillus subtilis*, *Micrococcus luteus* and *Pseudomonas aeruginosa* (Yagi et al., 1993).

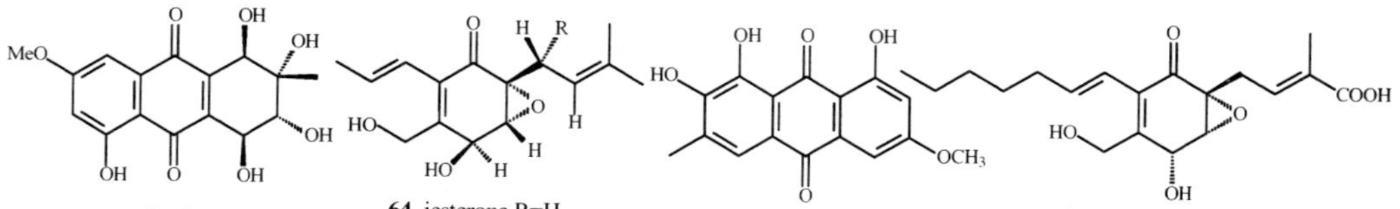

63 altersolanol A
64 jesterone R=H
65 hydroxy-jesterone R=OH
66 3-*O*-methylalaternin
67 ambuic acid

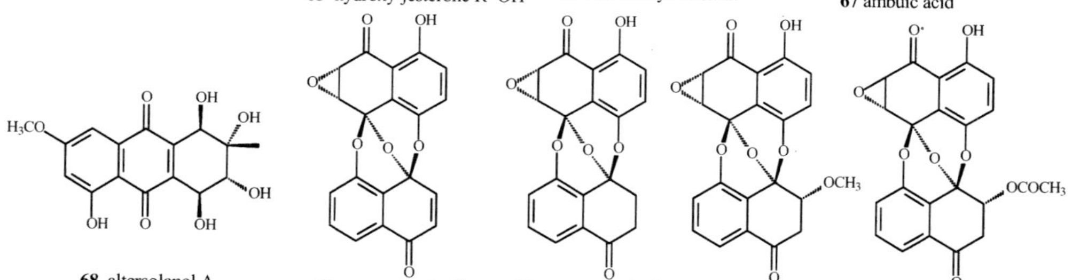

68 altersolanol A
69 preussomerin G
70 preussomerin H
71 preussomerin I
72 preussomerin J

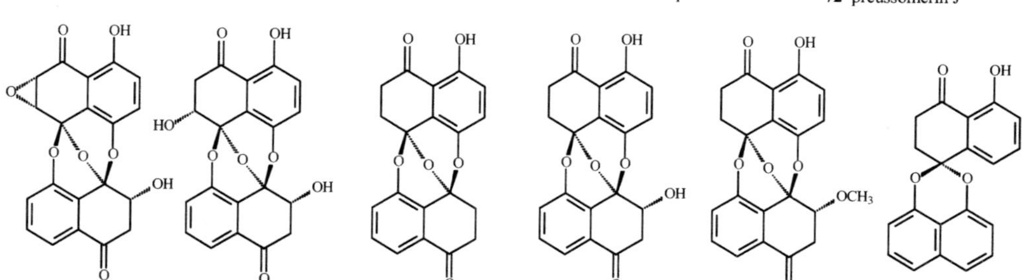

73 preussomerin K
74 preussomerin L
75 preussomerin EG$_1$
76 preussomerin EG$_2$
77 preussomerin EG$_3$
78 deoxypreussomerin B

Two antioomycete cyclohexenone epoxides jesterone (**64**) and hydroxy-jesterone (**65**) were isolated from *Pestalotipsis jeseri* by bioassay-guided fractionation using *Pythium ultimum* as the indicator organism (Li and Strobel, 2001). Another quinonoid acid ambuic acid (**66**) was isolated from *Monachaetia* sp. derived from *Taxus wallachiana*. It was also separated from other plants such as *Dendrobium speciosum*, *Taxodium disticum*, *Taxus baccata* and *Torreya taxifolia* (Li et al., 2001).

3-*O*-Methylalaternin (**67**) and altersolanol A (**68**) were anthraquinones from the endophytic fungus *Ampelomyces* sp. isolated from the medicinal plant *Urospermum picroides*. These two compounds both exhibited antimicrobial activity against the Gram-positive bacteria (i.e. *Staphylococcus aureus*, *S. epidermidis* and *Enterococcus faecalis*) (Aly et al., 2008).

Krohn et al. (2001) isolated six antimicrobial naphthoquinone spiroketal compounds preussomerins G-L (**69-74**) from endophytic fungus *Mycelia sterile* from the roots of *Atropa belladonna*. Macias-Rubalcava et al. (2008) also isolated four antifungal naphthoquinone spiroketals namely as preussomerin EG_1 (**75**), preussomerin EG_2 (**76**), preussomerin EG_3 (**77**) and deoxypreussomerin B (**78**) from a newly discovered endophytic fungus *Edenia gomezpompae* isolated from the leaves of *Callicarpa acuminata* (Verbenaceae) collected from the ecological reserve El Eden, Quintana Roo, Mexico.

3.7. Aliphatics

Four antifungal alipatics ethyl *trans*-9,10-epoxy-11-oxoundecanoate (**79**), ethyl 9-oxononanoate (**80**), ethyl zaelate (**81**) and hydroxydihydrobovolide (**82**) were isolated from the *n*-hexane soluble fraction of a 70% ethanol extract of *Epichloe typhina* by TLC bioautography with *Cladosporium herbarum* (Koshino et al., 1989). An aliphatic ester 2-methyloctanoic acid 6-oxo-2-propenyl- 3,6-dihydro-2*H*-pryan-3-yl ester (**83**) was isolated from the cultures of an unidentified endophytic fungus obtained from an eastern larch (*Larix laricina*) needles. It was active against *Vibrio salmonicida*, *Pseudomonas aeruginosa* and *Staphylococcus aureus* (Findlay et al., 1997).

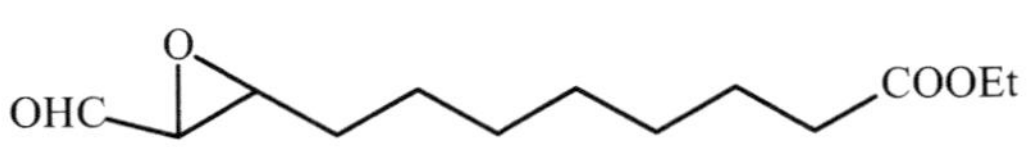

79

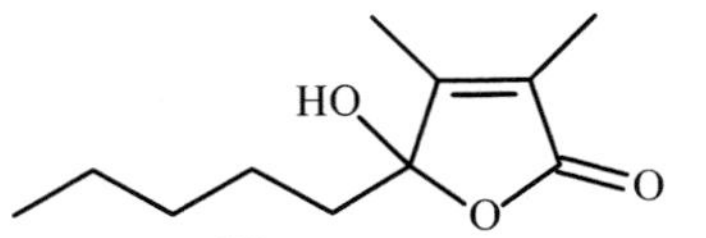

82

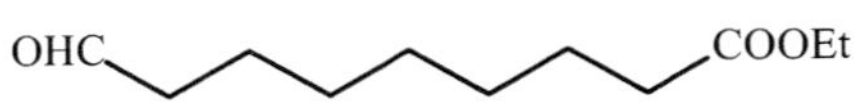

80

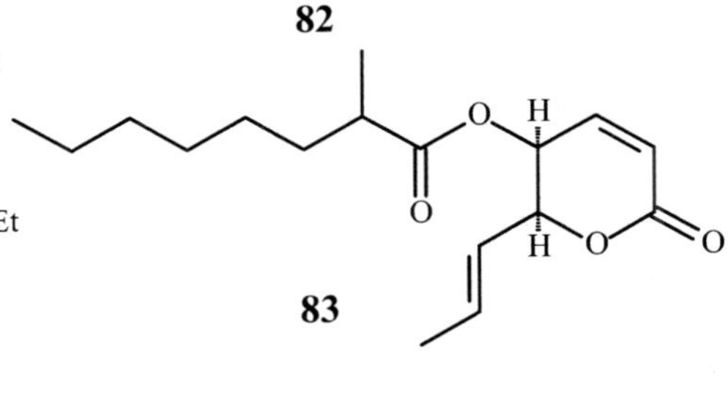

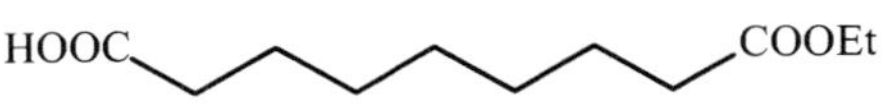

81

83

3.8. Lactones

An antimicrobial lactone named phomol (**84**) was isolated from an endophytic *Phomopsis* species present in the medicinal plant *Erythrina crista-galli* (Weber et al., 2004).

Pyrenophorol (**85**) was a lactone antibiotic from a *Phoma* species isolated from the plant *Fagonia cretica* to show its antifungal activity against *Microbotryum violaceum* (Krohn et al., 2007).

Cytosporones B (**86**) and C (**87**) were isolated from the endophytic *Phomopsis* sp. ZSU-H76 obtained from the stem of mangrove tree *Excoecaria agallocha*. They exhibited antifungal activity against *Candida albicans* and *Fusarium oxysporum* with the MIC values ranging from 32 to 64 μg/ml (Huang et al., 2008). Brady et al. (2000) isolated two antibacterial active trihydroxybenzene lactones cytosporones D (**88**) and E (**89**) from two endophytes *Cytosproa* sp. CR200 and *Diaporthe* sp. CR146, respectively (Brady et al., 2000).

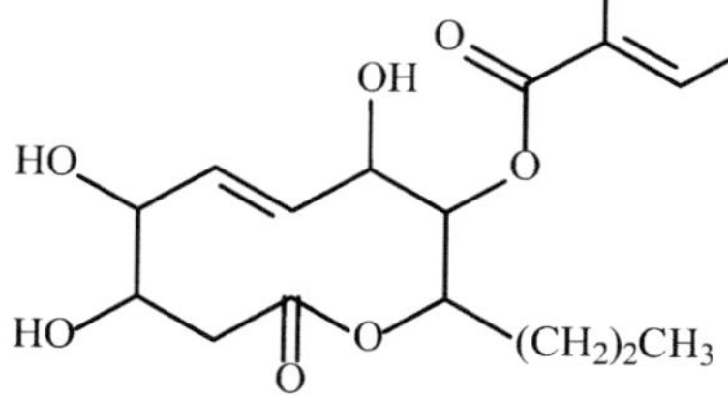

84 phomol

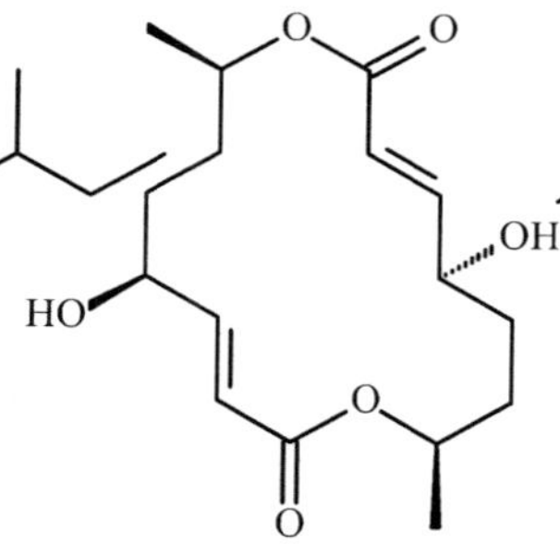

85 pyrenophorol

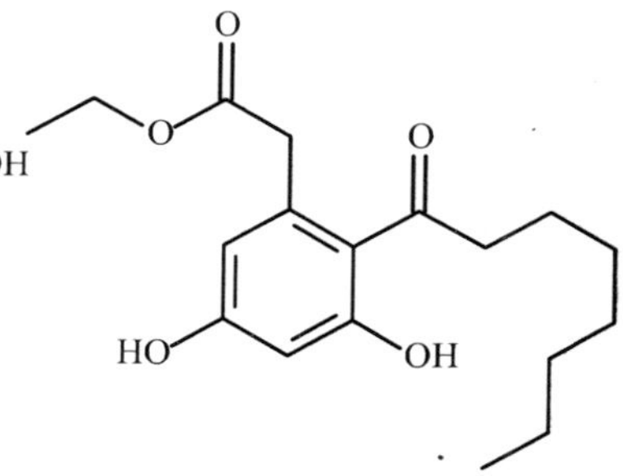

86 cytosporone B

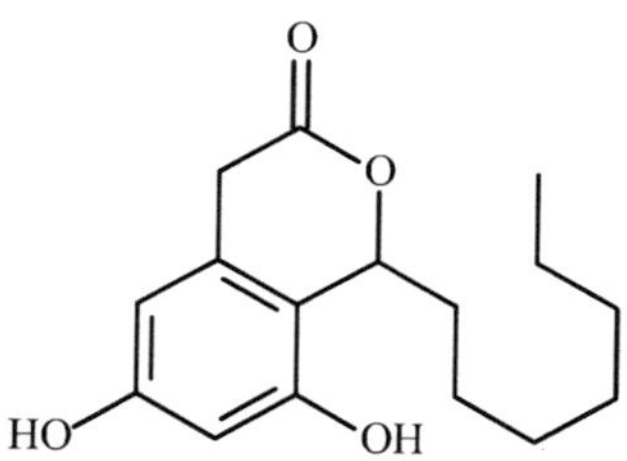

87 cytosporone C

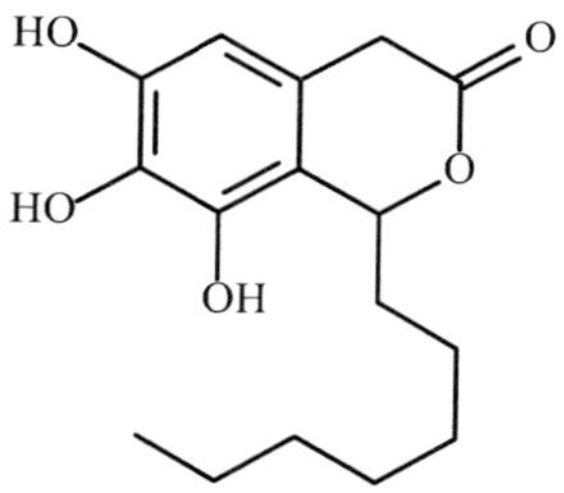

88 cytosporone D

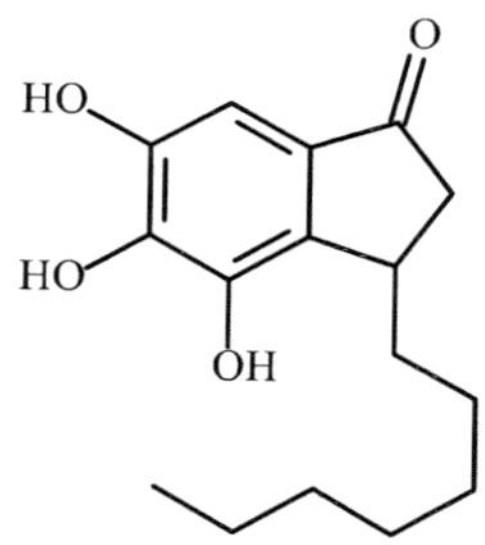

89 cytosporone E

3.9. Isocoumarin Derivatives

Some antimicrobial isocoumarin derivatives were isolated from endophytic fungi. (*R*)-Mellein (**90**) isolated from *Pezicula* sp. was screened to show the strongly fungicidal, herbicidal and algaecidal activities (Schulz et al., 1995). Three novel dihydroisocoumarin derivatives (**91-93**) with antimalarial, antituberculous, and antifungal activities have been isolated by bioassay-guided fractionation from an endophytic fungus, *Geotrichum* sp., collected from *Crassocephalum crepidioides* (Kongsaeree et al., 2003).

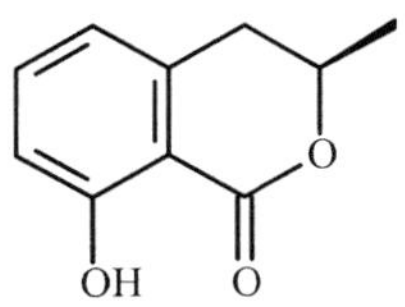

90 (*R*)-mellein

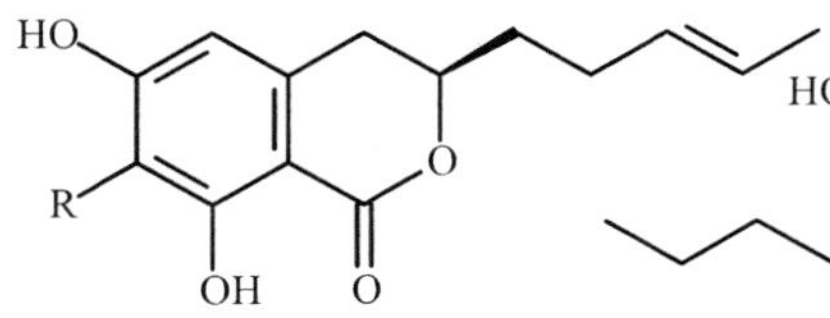

91 R = $CH_2CH_2CH_2CH_3$
92 R = $CH_2CH{=}CHCH_3$

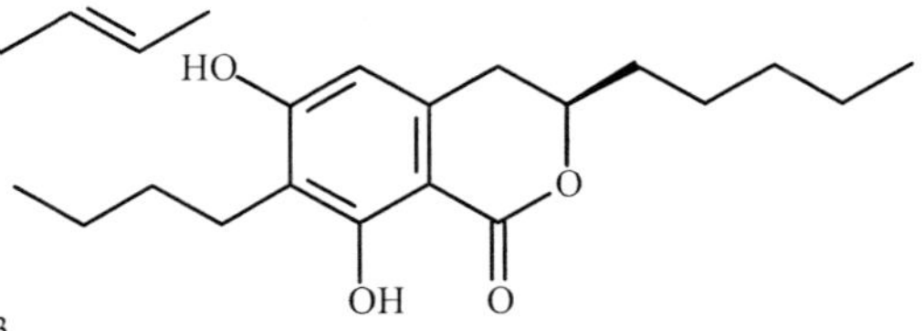

93

3.10. Benzophenones

One benzophenone monomethylsulchrin (**94**) was isolated from endophytic *Aspergillus* sp. obtained from *Cynodon dactylon*, and its MIC values against *Helicobacter pylori* and *Sarcina lutea* were 5 μg/ml and 30 μg/ml (Li et al., 2005). Another anti-*Helicobacter pylori* benzophenone rhizoctonic acid (**95**) was also isolated from endophytic *Rhizoctonia* sp. associated with the plant *C. dactylon* (Ma et al., 2004).

Four chromone-3-oxepines named isofusidienols A (**96**), B (**97**), C (**98**) and D (**99**) were produced by the endophytic fungus *Chalara* sp. that showed their antimicrobial activity on *Bacillus subtilis*, *Staphylococcus aureus*, *Escherichia coli*, and *Candida albicans* (Losgen et al., 2008).

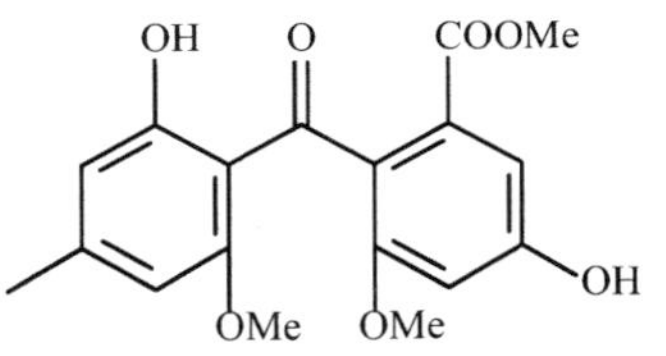

94 R=CH_3
95 R=H

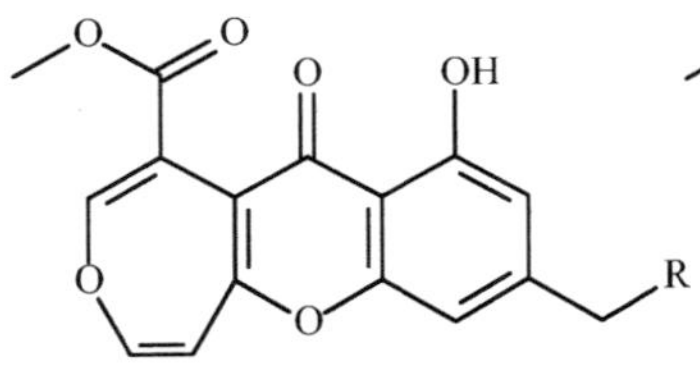

96 R=H
97 R=OH

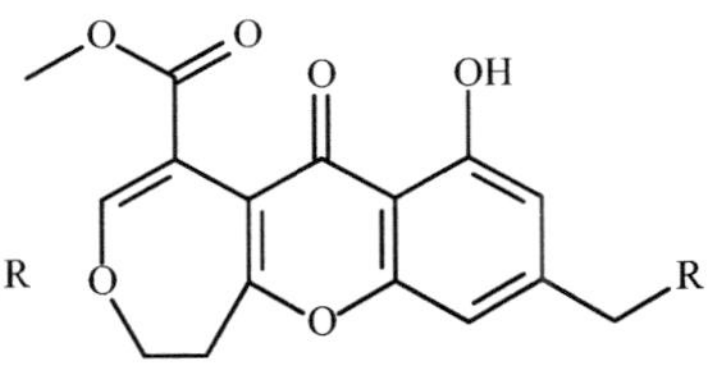

98 R=H
99 R=OH

3.11. Other Classes of Compounds

1,3,5,7-Cyclooctatetraene named annulene (**100**), which was isolated from the mixture of volatile antimicrobials from an endophytic *Gliocladium* sp. of *Eucryphia cordifolia*, effectively inhibited *Pythium utlimum* and *Verticillum dahliae* (Stinson et al., 2003). Some volatile compounds exuded by *Gliocladium* sp. such as 3-methyl-1-butanol, phenylethyl alcohol, and acetic-2-phenylethyl ether, as well as various propanoic acid esters were also produced by *Muscodor albus*, a well known volatile antimicrobial producer (Strobel et al., 2001).

Four antimicrobial naphtha-γ-pyrones, rubrofusarin B (**101**), fonsecinone A (**102**), asperpyrone B (**103**) and aurasperone A (**104**) have been identified in cultures of *Aspergillus niger* IFB-E003 obtained from *Cynodon dactylon* (Song et al., 2004). Griseofulvin (**105**), which was isolated from endophytic *Xylaria* sp. strain F0010 of *Abies holopylla*, has been detected to have strong inhibitory activity against plant fungal pathogens (i.e. *Magnaporthe* *oryzae*, *Corticium sasaki*, *Botrytis cinerea*, *Phytophthora infestans*, *Puccinia recondite*, *Blueria graminis* f.sp. *hordei*) (Park et al., 2005). Many species of *Penicillium*, such as *P. griseofulvum*, *P. patulum*, *P. urticae*, *P. nigricans*, and *P. sclerotigenum*, and *Aspergillus versicolor* and *Striptomyces albolongus* have presently been determined as typical griseofulvin (**105**) producing fungi (Kingston et al., 1976; Mantle et al., 1984).

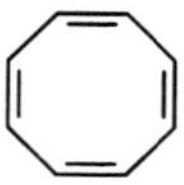

100 annulene

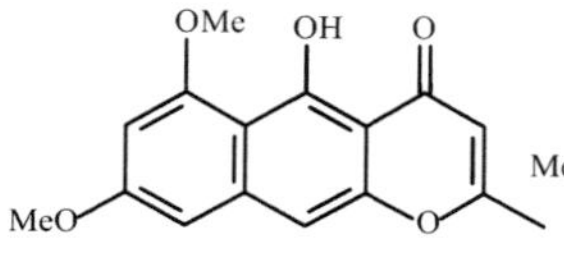

101 rubrofusarin B

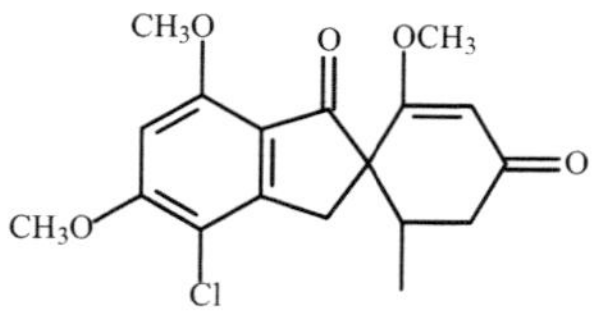

105 griseofulvin

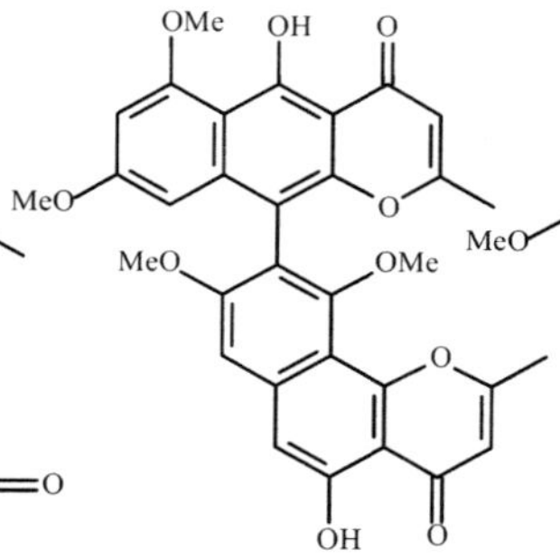

102 fonsecinone A

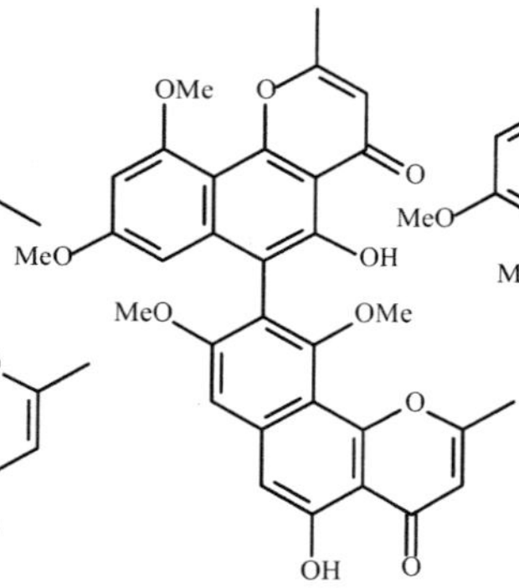

103 asperpyrone B

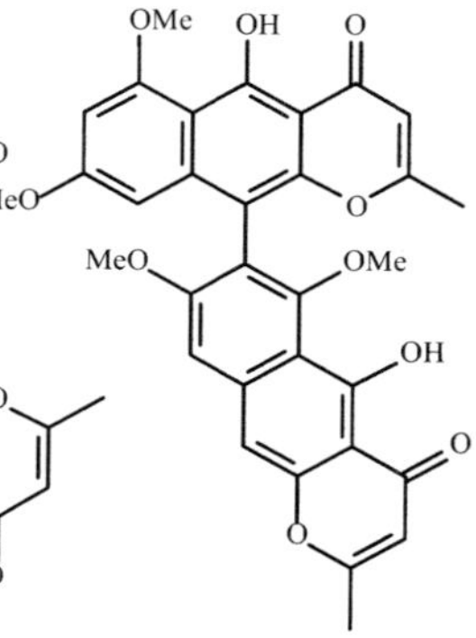

104 aurasperone A

4. Discussion

Ever since penicillin was isolated from *Penicillium notatum*, chemists have been engaged in the discovery of novel antimicrobials. Discovery and development of novel antimicrobial agents from plant endophytic fungi will provide new knowledge for use of natural products for plant protection as well as for human and animal health, and a better understanding of their physiological and ecological roles. Development of endophytic fungal metabolite-based antimicrobial agents with low mammalian and environmental toxicity will guarantee food safety, sustainability of agriculture, and ensure a safe and healthy environment (Gimenez et al., 2007).

A great progress has been achieved about discovery of the antimicrobial compounds from endophytic fungi in the last 20 years. Many reports were focused on the antimicrobial activity of the crude extracts, bioassay-guided separation of the antimicrobials, structural elucidation and activity evaluation of the compounds. Other works are still in primary such as mode of action of the active compounds, structure derivation and structural-activity relations, chemical and semi-chemical synthesis, and antimicrobial agent development from endophytic fungal compounds or extracts applying in agriculture, medicine and food process (Guo et al., 2008).

As synthetic antimicrobial agents in crop protection and medication have resulted in many problems, antimicrobial compounds derived from endophytic fungi may be an alternative means of disease control which can minimize the use of synthetic chemicals. It should be optimistic to obtain antimicrobial compounds or constituents from endophytic fungi as either lead structures of the chemical synthesis agrochemicals or antimicrobial agents to directly control bacterial and fungal pathogens of agricultural, medicinal and food industrial importance.

Acknowledgments

This work was partially supported by the grants from the Hi-Tech R&D Program of China (Nos. 2006AA10A209 and 2006AA10Z423), 11th Five-Year Key Technologies R&D Program of China (Nos. 2006BAD22B03 and 2007BAD57B02), National Natural Science Foundation of China (No. 30871662) and Natural Science Foundation of Beijing (No. 6092015).

References

Al-Bakri, AG; Afifi, FU. Evaluation of antimicrobial activity of selected plant extracts by rapid XTT colorimetry and bacterial enumeration. *Journal of Microbiological Methods*, 2007, 68(1): 19-25.

Alvarez-Castellanos, PP; Bishop, CD; Pascual-Villalobos, MJ. Antifungal activity of the essential oil of flowerheads of garland chrysanthemum (*Chrysanthemum coronarium*) against agricultural pathogens. *Phytochemistry*, 2001, 57(1): 99-102.

Aly, AH; Edrada-Ebel, R; Wray, V; Muller, WEG; Kozytska, S; Hentschel, H; Proksch, P; Ebel, R. Bioactive metabolites from the endophytic fungus *Ampelomyces* sp. isolated from the medicinal plant *Urospermum picroides*. *Phytochemistry*, 2008, 69(8): 1716-1725.

Amann, RI; Ludwig, W; Schleifer, KH. Phylogenetic identification and in situ detection of individual microbial cells without cultivation. *Microbiological Reviews*, 1995, 59(1): 143-169.

Arnold, AE. Understanding the diversity of foliar endophytic fungi: progress, challenges, and frontiers. *Fungal Biology Reviews*, 2007, 21(1): 51-66.

Arnold, AE; Maynard, Z; Glibert, GS; Coley, PD; Kursar, TA. Are tropical fungal endophytes hyperdiverse? *Ecology Letters*, 2000, 3(4): 267-274.

Bacon, CW; Porter, JK; Robbins, JD. Toxicity and occurrence of *Balansia* on grasses from toxic fescue pastures. *Applied Microbiology*, 1975, 29(4): 553-556.

Bayman, P. Fungal endophytes. In: *Environmental and Microbial Relationships, 2nd Edition, The Mycota IV* (Kubicek, CP, Druzhinina, IS. Eds.), Verlag Berlin Hedlberg: Springer, 2007: 214-227.

Brady, SF; Wangenaar, MM; Singh, MP; Janso, JE; Clardy, J. The cytosproones, new octaketide antibiotics isolated from an endophytic fungus. *Organic Letter*, 2000, 2(25): 4043-4046.

Carroll, GC. Fungal endophytes in stems and leaves: from latent pathogen to mutualistic symbiont. *Ecology*, 1988, 69(1): 2-9.

Dai, J; Krohn, K; Florke, U; Draeger, S; Schulz, B; Kiss-Szikszai, A; Antus, S; Kurtan, T; van Ree, T. Metabolites from the endophytic fungus *Nodulisporium* sp. from *Juniperus cedre*. *European Journal of Organic Chemistry*, 2006, (15): 3498-3506.

Espinel-Ingroff, A; Bartlett, M; Bowden, R; Chin, NX; Cooper, C; Fothergill, A; McGinnis, MR; Menezes, P; Messer, SA; Nelson, PW; Odds, FC; Pasarell, L; Peter, J; Pfaller, MA; Rex, JH; Rinaldi, MG; Shankland, GS; Walsh, TJ; Weizman, I. Multicenter evaluation of proposed standardized procedure for antifungal susceptibility testing of filamentous fungi. *Journal of Clinical Microbiology*, 1997, 35(1): 139-143.

Eyberger, AL; Dondapati, R; Porter, JR. Endophyte fungal isolates from *Podophyllum peltatum* produce podophyllotoxin. *Journal of Natural Products*, 2006, 69(8): 1121-1124.

Findlay, JA; Li, G; Johnson, JA. Bioactive compounds from endophytic fungus from eastern larch (*Larix laricina*) needles. *Canadian Journal of Chemistry*, 1997, 75(6): 716-719.

Gimenez, C; Cabrera, R; Reina, M; Gonzalez-Coloma, A. Fungal endophytes and their role in plant protection. *Current Organic Chemistry*, 2007, 11(8): 707-720.

Guo, B; Wang, Y; Sun, X; Tang, K. Bioactive natural products from endophytes: a review. *Applied Biochemistry and Microbiology*, 2008, 44(2): 136-142.

Hadacek, F; Greger, H. Testing of antifungal natural products: methodologies, comparability of results and assay choice. *Phytochemcial Analysis*, 2000, 11(3): 137-147.

Harper, JK; Arif, AM; Ford; EJ; Strobel, GA; Porco, JA; Tomer, DP; Oneill, KL; Heider, EM; Grant, DM. Pestacin: a 1,3-dihydro isobenzofuran from *Pestalotiopsis microspora* possessing antioxidant and antimycotic activities. *Tetrahedron*, 2003, 59(14): 2471-2476.

Hellwig, V; Grothe, T; Mayer-Bartschmid, A; Endermann, R; Geschke, F-U; Henkel, T; Stadler, M. Taxonomy, fermentation, isolation, structure and elucidation and biological activities. *The Journal of Antibiotics*, 2002, 55(10): 881-892.

Hoffman, AM; Mayer, SG; Strobel, GA; Hess, WM; Sovocool, GW; Grange, AH; Harper, JK; Arif, AM; Grant, DM; Kelley-Swift, EG. Purification, identification and activity of phomodione, a furandione from an endophytic *Phoma* species. *Phytochemistry*, 2008, 69(4): 1049-1056.

Horn, WS; Simmonds, MSJ; Schwartz, RE; Blaney WM. Phomospsichalasin, a novel antimicrobial agent from an endophytic *Phomopsis* sp.. *Tetrahedron*, 1995, 51(14): 3969-1978.

Huang, Z; Cai, X; Shao, C; She, Z; Xia, X; Chen, Y; Yang, J; Zhou, S; Lin, Y. Chemistry and Weak antimicrobial activities of phomopsins produced by mangrove endophytic fungus *Phomopsis* sp. ZSU-H76. *Phytochemistry*, 2008, 69(7): 1604-1608.

Ji, ZQ; Wu, WJ; Wang, MA; Gu, AG. Identification of fungicidal compounds from endophytic fungi *Fusarium proliferatum* in *Celastrus angulatus*. *Journal of Northwest Sci-Tech University of Agriculture and Forestry*, 2005, 33(5): 61-64.

Kingston, DG; Chen, PN; Vercellotti, JR. Metabolties of *Aspergillus versicolor*: 6,8-di-*O*-methylnidurufin, griseofulvin, dechlorogriseofluvin, and 3,8-dihydroxy-6-methoxy-1-methylxanthone. *Phytochemistry*, 15(6): 1037-1039.

Kong, C; Xu, X; Zhou, B; Hu, F; Zhang, C; Zhang, M. Two compounds from allelopathic rice accession and their inhibitory activity on weeds and fungal pathogens. *Phytochemistry*, 2004, 65(8): 1123-1128.

Kongsaeree, P; Prabpai, S; Sriubolmas, N; Vongvein, C; Wiyakrutta, S. Antimalarial dihydroisocoumarins produced by *Geotrichum* sp., an endophytic fungus of *Crassocephalum crepidioides*. *Journal of Natural Products*, 2003, 66(5): 709-711.

Koshino, H; Togiya, S; Terada, S; Yoshihara, T; Sakamura, S; Shmanuki, T; Sato, T; Tajimi, A. New fungitoxic sesquiterpenoids, chokols A-G, from stromata of *Epichloe typhina* and the absolute configuration of chokol E. *Agricultural and Biological Chemistry*, 1989, 53(3): 789-796.

Koshino, H; Yoshihara, T; Sakamura, S; Shimanuki, T; Sato, T; Tajimi A. Novel C-11 epoxy fatty acid from stroma of *Epichloe typhina* on *Pheleum pretense*. *Agricultural and Biological Chemistry*, 1989, 53(9): 2527-2528.

Krohn, K; Farooq, U; Florke, U; Schulz, B; Draeger, S; Pescitelli, G; Salvadori, P; Antus, S; Kurtan, T. Secondary metabolites isolated from an endophytic *Phoma* sp. – absolute configuration of tetrahydropyrenophorol using the solid-state TDDFT CD methodology. *European Journal of Organic Chemistry*, 2007, (19): 3206-3211.

Krohn, K; Florke, U; John, M; Root, N; Steingrove, K; Aust, H-J; Draeger, S; Schulz, B; Antus, S; Simonyi, M; Zsila, F. Biologically active metabolites from fungi. Part 16: New preussomerins J, K and L from an endophytic fungus: structure elucidation, crystal structure analysis and determination of absolute configuration by CD calculations. *Tetrahedron*, 2001, 57(20): 4343-4348.

Lee, JC; Yang, S; Schwartz, M; Strobel, G; Clardy, J. The relationship between an endangered North American tree and an endophytic fungus. *Chemistry and Biology*, 1995, 2(11): 721-727.

Letessier, MP; Svoboda, KP; Walters, DR. Antifungal activity of the essential oil of hyssop (*Hyssopus officinalis*). *Journal of Phytopathology*, 2001, 149(11-12): 673-678.

Li, J; Zhao, J; Xu, L; Zhou, L; Li, X; Wang, J. Endophytic fungi from rhizomes of *Paris polyphylla* var. *yunnanensis*. *World Journal of Microbiology and Biotechnology*, 2008, 24(5): 733-737.

Li, JY; Harper, JK; Grant, DM; Tombe, BO; Bashyal, B; Hess, WM; Strobel, GA. Ambuic acid, a highly functionalized cyclohexenone with antifungal activity from *Pestalotiopsis* spp. and *Monochaetia* sp.. *Phytochemistry*, 2001, 56(5): 463-468.

Li, JY; Strobel, GA. Jesterone and hydroxyl-jesterone antioomycete cyclohexenone epoxides from the endophytic fungus *Pestalotiopsis jesteri*. *Phytochemistry*, 2001, 57(2): 261-265.

Li, JY; Strobel, GA; Harper, J; Lobkovsky, E; Clardy, J. Cryptocin, a potent tetramic acid antimycotic from the endopytic fungus *Cryptosporiospsis* cf. *quercina*. *Organic Letters*, 2000, 2(6): 767-770.

Li, Y; Song, YC; Liu, JY; Ma, YM; Tan, RX. Anti- *Helicobacter pylori* substances from endophytic fungal cultures. *World Journal of Microbiology and Biotechnology*, 2005, 21(4): 553-558.

Liu, JY; Song, YC; Zhang, Z; Wang, L; Guo, ZJ; Zou, WX; Tan, RX. *Aspergillus fumigatus* CY018, an endophytic fungus in *Cynodon dactylon* as a versatile producer of new and bioactive metabolites. *Journal of Biotechnology*, 2004, 114(3): 279-287.

Liu, X; Dong, M; Chen, X; Jiang, M; Lv, X; Zhou, J. Antimicrobial activity of an endophytic *Xylaria* sp. YX-28 and identification of the antimicrobial compound 7-amino-4-methylcoumarin. *Applied Microbiology and Biotechnology*, 2008, 78(2): 241-247.

Losgen, S; Magull, J; Schulz, B; Draeger, S; Zeeck, A. Isofusidienols: novel chromone-3-oxepines produced by the endophytic fungus *Chalara* sp.. *European Journal of Organic Chemistry*, 2008, (4): 698-703.

Lu, H; Zou, WX; Meng, JC; Hu, J; Tan, RX. New bioactive metabolites produced by *Colletotrichum* sp., an endophytic fungus in *Artemisia annua. Plant Science*, 2000, 151(1): 67-73.

Ma, YM; Li, Y; Liu, JY; Song, YC; Tan, RX. Anti-*Helicobacter pylori* metabolites from *Rhizoctonia* sp. Cy064, an endophytic fungus in *Cyndodon dactylon. Fitoterapia*, 2004, 75(5): 451-456.

Macias-Rubalcava, ML; Hernandez-Bautista, BE; Jimenez-Estrada, M; Gonzalez, MC; Glenn, AE; Hanlin, RT; Hernandez-Ortega, S; Saucedo-Garcia, A; Muria-Gonzalez, JM; Anaya, AL. Naphthoquinone spiroketal with allelochemical activity from the newly discovered endophytic fungus *Edenia gomezpompae. Phytochemistry*, 2008, 69(5): 1185-1196.

Mantle, PG; Laws, I; Tan, MJL; Tizard M. A novel process for the production of penitrem mycotoxins by submerged fermentation of *Penicillium nigricans. Journal of General Microbiology*, 1984, 130(5): 1293-1298.

Mosmann, T. Rapid colorimetric assay for cellular growth and survival: application to proliferation and cytotoxicity assays. *Journal of Immunological Methods*, 1983, 65(1-2): 55-63.

Mueller, CB; Krauss, J. Symbiosis between grasses and asexual fungal endophytes. *Current Opinion in Plant Biology*, 2005, 8(4): 450-456.

Musetti, R; Polizzotto, R; Vecchione, A; Borselli, S; Zulini, L; D'Ambrosio, M; di Toppi, LS; Pertot, I. Antifungal activity of diketopiperazines extracted form *Alternaria alternata* against *Plasmopara viticola*: an ultrastructural study. *Micron*, 2007, 38(6): 643-650.

Noble, HM; Langley, D; Sidebottom, PJ; Lane, SJ; Fisher, PJ. An echinocandin from an endophytic *Cryptosporiopsis* sp. and *Pezicula* sp. in *Pinus sylvestris* and *Fagus sylvatica. Mycological Research*, 1991, 95(12): 1439-1440.

Page, B; Page, M; Noel, C. A new fluorometric assay for cytotoxicity measurements *in vitro. International Journal of Oncology*, 1993, 3(3): 473-476.

Park, J-H; Choi, GJ; Lee, HB; Kim, KM; Jung, HS; Lee, SW; Jang, KS; Cho, KY. Griseofulvin from *Xylaria* sp. Strain F0010, an endophytic fungus of *Abies holophylla* and its antifungal activity against plant pathogenic fungi. *Journal of Microbiology and Biotechnology*, 2005, 15(1): 112-117.

Pauli, A. Anticandidal low molecular compounds from higher plants with special reference to compounds from essential oils. *Medicinal Research reviews*, 2006, 26(2): 223-268.

Pelloux-Prayer, AL; Priem, B; Joseleau, JP. Kinetic evaluation of conidial germination of *Botrytis cinerea* by a spectrofluorometric method. *Mycological Research*, 1998, 102(3), 320-322.

Pfaller, MA; Messer, SA; Conffmann, S. Comparison of visual and spectrophotometric methods of MIC endopoint determinations by using broth microdilution methods to test five antifungal agents, including the new triazole D0870. *Journal of Clinical Microbiology*, 1995, 33(5): 1094-1097.

Pongcharoen, W; Rukachaisirikul, V; Phongpaichit, S; Kuhn, T; Pelzing, M; Sakayaroj, J; Taylor, WC. Metabolites from the endophytic fungus *Xylaria* sp. PSU-D14. *Phytochemistry*, 2008, 69(9): 1900-1902.

Quiroga, EN; Sampietro, AR; Vattuone, MA. Screening antifungal activities of selected medicinal plants. *Journal of Ethnopharmacology*, 2001, 74(1): 89-96.

Saikkonen, K; Faeth, SH; Helander, M; Sullivan, TJ. Fungal endophytes: a continuum of interactions with host plants. *Annual Review of Ecology and Systematics*, 1998, 29: 319-343.

Schulz, B; Sucker, J; Aust, HJ; Krohn, K; Ludewig, K; Jones, PG; Doering, D. Biologically active secondary metabolites of endophytic *Pezicula* species. *Mycological Research*, 1995, 99(8): 1007-1015.

Schulz, B; Wanke, U; Draeger, S; Aust, HJ. Endophytes from herbaceous plants and shrubs: effectiveness of surface sterilization methods. *Mycological Research*, 1993, 97(12): 1447-1450.

Shu, RG; Wang, FW; Yang, YM; Liu, YX; Tan, RX. Antibacterial and xanthine oxidase inhibitory cerebrosides from *Fusarium* sp. IFB-121, an endopytic fungus in *Quercus variabilis*. *Lipids*, 2004, 39(7): 667-673.

Singh, MP; Janso, JE; Luckman, SW; Brady, SF; Clardy, J; Greenstein, M; Maiese, WM. Biological activity of guanacastepene, a novel diterpenoid antibiotic produced by an unidentified fungus CR115. *Journal of Antibiotics*, 2000, 53(3): 256-261.

Song, YC; Li, H; Ye, YH; Shan, CY; Yang, YM; Tan, RX. Endophytic naphthopyrone metabolites are co-inhibitors of xanthine oxidase, SW1116 cell and some microbial growth. *FEMS Microbiology Letters*, 2004, 241(1): 67-72.

Srinivasan, D; Nathan, S; Suresh, T; Perumalsamy, PL. Antimicrobial activity of certain Indian medicinal plants used in folkloric medicine. *Journal of Ethnopharmacology*, 2001, 74(3): 217-220.

Stevens, MG; Olsen, SC. Comparative analysis of using MTT and XTT in colorimetric assays for quantitating bovine neutrophil bactericidal activity. *Journal of Immunological Methods*, 1993, 157(1-2): 225-231.

Stierle, A; Strobel, G; Stierle, D. Taxol and taxane production by *Taxomyces andreanae*, an endophytic fungus of pacific yew. *Science*, 1993, 260(5105): 214-216.

Stinson, M; Ezra, D; Hess, WM; Sears, J; Strobel, G. An endophytic *Gliocladium* sp. of *Eucryphia cordifolia* producing selective volatile antimicrobial compounds. *Plant Science*, 2003, 165(4): 913-922.

Strobel, GA; Torzynski, R; Bollon, A. *Acremonium* sp.- a leucinostatin A producing endophyte of European yew (*Taxus baccata*). *Plant Science*, 1997, 128(1): 97-108.

Strobel, GA. Endophytes as sources of bioactive products. *Microbes and Infection*, 2003, 5(6): 535-544.

Strobel, GA. Rainforest endophytes and bioactive products. *Critical Reviews in Biotechnology*, 2002, 22(4): 315-333.

Strobel, GA; Daisy, B; Castillo, U; Harper, J. Natural products from endophytic microorganisms. *Journal of Natural Products*, 2004, 67(2): 257-268.

Strobel, GA; Dirksie, E; Sears, J; Markworth, C. Volatile antimicrobials from *Muscodor albus*, a novel endophyte fungus. *Microbiology*, 2001, 147(11): 2943-2950.

Strobel, GA; Ford, E; Worapong, J; Harper, JK; Arif, AM; Grant, DM; Fung, PCW; Chau, RMW. Isopestacin, an isobenzofuranone from *Pestalotiopsis microspora*, possessing antifungal and antioxidant activities. *Phytochemistry*, 2002, 60(2): 179-183.

Strobel, GA; Hess, WM. Glucosylation of the peptide leucinostatin A. produced by an endophytic fungus of European yew, may protect the host from leucinostatin toxicity. *Chemistry and Biology*, 1997, 4(7): 529-536.

Strobel, GA; Miller, RV; Martinez, MM; Condron, MM; Teplow, DB; Hess, WM. Cryptocandin, a potent antimycotic from the endophytic fungus *Cryptosporiopsis* cf. *quercina*. *Microbiology*, 1999, 145(8): 1919-1926.

Sturz, AV; Christie, BR; Nowak, J. Bacterial endophytes: potential role in developing sustainable systems of crop production. *Critical Reviews in Plant Sciences*, 2000, 19(1): 1-30.

Suzuki, Y; Esumi, Y; Hyakutake, H; Kono, Y; Sakurai, A. Isolation of 5-(8'Z-heptadecenyl)-resorcinol from etiolated rice seedlings as an antifungal agent. *Phytochemistry*, 1996, 41(6): 1485-1489.

Tabanca, N; Bedir, E; Ferreira, D; Slade, D; Wedge, DE; Jacob, MR; Khan, SI; Kirimer, N; Baser, KHC; Khan, IA. Bioactive constituents from Turkish *Pimpinella* species. *Chemistry and Biodiversity*, 2005, 2(2): 221-232.

Tan, RX; Zou, WX. Endophytes: a rich source of functional metabolites (1987-2000). *Natural Product Reports*, 2001, 18(4): 448-459.

Tan, M; Zhou, L; Huang, Y; Wang, Y; Hao, X; Wang, J. Antimicrobial activity of globulol isolated from the fruits of *Eucalyptus globulus* Labill. *Natural Product Research*, 2008, 22(7): 569-575.

Tang, J; Zhou, L; Zhou, Y; Du, H; Liu, H; Guo, Z; Wang, J. Inhibitory effects of *Phellodendron chinense* Schneid. extracts on some phytopathogenic fungi. *Natural Product Research and Development*, 2008a, 20(3): 505-507.

Tang, J; Tan, M; Zhao, J; Wang, Y; Zhou, L. Detection of plant antibacterial components by using microplate-MTT colorimetric assay. *Natural Product Research and Development*, 2008b, 20(6): 949-952.

Wang, FW; Ye, YH; Chen, JR; Wang, XT; Zhu, HL; Song, YC; Tan, RX. Neoplaether, a new cytotoxic and antifungal endophyte metabolite from *Neoplaconema napellum* IFB-E016. *FEMS Microbiology Letters*, 2006. 261(2): 218-223.

Weber, D; Sterner, O; Anke, T; Gorzalczancy, S; Martino, V; Acevedo, C. Phomol, a new anti-inflammatory metabolite from an endophyte of the medicinal plant *Erythrina crista-galli*. *The Journal of Antibiotics*, 2004, 57(9): 559-563.

Wedge, DE; Nagle, DG. A new 2D-TLC bioautography method for the discovery of novel antifungal agents to control plant pathogens. *Journal of Natural Products*, 2000, 63(8): 1050-1054.

Weidenborner, M; Hindorf, H; Jha, HC; Tsotsonos, P; Egge, H. Antifungal activity of isoflavonoids against storage fungi of the genus *Apsergillus*. *Phytochemistry*, 1989, 28(12): 2317-3319.

Wicklow, DT; Roth, S; Deyrup, ST; Gloer JB. A protective endophyte of maize: *Acremonium zeae* antibiotics inhibitory to *Aspergillus flavus* and *Fusarium verticillioides*. *Mycological Research*, 2005, 109(5): 610-618.

Xu, L; Zhou, L; Zhao, J; Li, J; Li, X; Wang J. Fungal endophytes from *Dioscorea zingiberensis* rhizomes and their antibacterial activity. *Letters in Applied Microbiology*, 2008, 46(1): 68-72.

Yagi, A; Okamura, N; Haraguchi, H; Abo, Takahiro; Hashimoto, K. Antimicrobial tertrahydroanthraquinones from a strain of *Alternaria solani*. *Phytochemistry*, 1993, 33(1): 87-91.

Yang, X; Strobel, G; Stierle, A; Hess, WM; Lee, J; Clardy, J. A fungal endophyte-tree relationship: *Phoma* sp. in *Taxus wallachiana*. *Plant Science*, 1994, 102(1): 1-9.

Zhang, HW; Song, YC; Tan, RX. Biological and chemistry of endophytes. *Natural Product Reports*, 2006, 23(5): 753-771.

Zhao, J; Xu, L; Huang, Y; Zhou, L. Detection of antimicrobial components from extracts of the endophytic fungi associated with *Paris polyphylla* var. *yunnanensis* using TLC-bioautography-MTT assay. *Natural Product Research and Development*, 2008a, 20(1): 28-32.

Zhao, J; Huang, Y; Xu, L; Cai, X; Ma, Z; Zhou L. Composition analysis of the volatile oil from endophytic fungus *Pichia guilliermondii* from *Paris polyphyllar* var. *yunnanensis* and its antibacterial activity. *Journal of Biotechnology*, 2008b, 136(Suppl.1): S79.

Zhou, Y; Liu, H; Zhao, J; Tan, M; Sui, P; Wang, J; Zhou, L. Poplar stem blister canker and its control strategies by plant extracts. *World Journal of Microbiology and Biotechnology*, 2008, 24(8): 1579-1584.

Zou, WX; Meng, JC; Lu, H; Chen, GX; Shi, GX; Zhang, TY; Tan, RX. Metabolites of *Colletotrichum gloeosporioides*, an endophytic fungus in *Artemisia mongolica*. *Journal of Natural Products*, 2000, 63(11): 1529-1530.

In: Fungicides
Editors: P. De Costa and P. Bezerra
ISBN: 978-1-60692-631-4

Chapter IV

HEALTH AND ENVIRONMENTAL RISKS OF THE FUNGICIDE AND BIOCIDE DICHLOFLUANID (A REVIEW)

***N. Kovalkovičová*[1,*]*, I. Šutiaková*[2,†]*, J. Pistl*[1]*, J. Legáth*[1]*, V. Šutiak*[1]**

[1]University of Veterinary Medicine, Komenského 73, 041 81 Košice, Slovak Republic
[2]University of Prešov, Ul. 17. Novembra 1, 081 16 Prešov, Slovak Republic

ABSTRACT

Dichlofluanid is a halogenated sulfonamide derivative from the group of aryl (dichlorofluoromethyltio) fungicides. It was used as a fungicide and acaricide in approved agricultural pesticides from 1965. Nowadays it is not included in any of the lists for European re-assessment of active ingredients under Directive 91/414/EEC. On the other hand, it has been used in aquaculture and as a booster biocide in antifouling products, especially tin-free products, to control the growth of algal, weed and animal fouling on moving or stati objects in water. Furthermore, following the review of dichlofluanid in Product type 8 (Wood preservatives) under the Biocidal Products Directive 98/8/EC, the European Commission has agreed that this active substance will enter into Annex I of the Directive on 1 March 2009.

In this regard exposure to dichlofluanid is possible during its application, but it is also detected in harbours and marinas in many European countries.

In this chapter the toxic effects of dichlofluanid to humans and animals are summarized.

Keywords: toxicity; health; fungicide; biocide; dichlofluanid

* E-mail: kovalkovicova@uvm.sk
† E-mail: sutiakova@pobox.sk

Introduction

The hulls of ships and other artificial structures have to be protected against marine biofouling, the settlement and growth of animals and plants on submerged surfaces.

The process of biofouling has got several steps. Firstly, a freshly immersed surface rapidly adsorbs various organic molecules to form a conditioning film. This film facilitates subsequent colonisation by such micro-organisms as bacteria and diatoms, which results in the formation of a slime layer. The microfouling slime layer is subsequently succeeded by macrofouling. This can be of two types: „hard“ and „soft“ fouling. Common soft-fouling organisms include algae, sponges, tunicates and hydroids. Common hard-fouling organisms include barnacles, mussels, clams and tubeworms. Larvae of fouling organisms are more diverse and numerous in costal areas than in the open sea (U.S. Naval Institute, 1981; Clare et al., 1992).

The growth of marine fouling on underwater hulls generally has a considerable impact on ship speed, manoeuvrability, fuel consumption and economy.

The most obvious problem of growth on a ship is the eventual corrosion of the hull, leading to the ship's deterioration. Even before corrosion occurs, if left unattended, organic growth can increase the roughness of the hull, thereby decreasing its manoeuvrability and increasing drag. This domino effect continues when the ship's fuel consumption increases, in some cases by 30 %. This in turn has economic and environmental consequences, as increased fuel consumption leads to increased output of carbon dioxide pollution and other air pollutants. Economic losses are tremendous, as fuel accounts for up to 50 % of marine transportation costs. The other important problem related to biofouling is an increased risk of ecological contamination by alien species (Callow and Callow, 2002; Yebra et al., 2004; Bellas, 2006). The annual global cost due to fouling has been estimated at $5.7 billion (Rouhi, 1998).

The fish farming industry also significantly suffers from the effects of biofouling. The fouling of cages and netting, which is costly to remove, is detrimental to fish health and yield and can cause equipment failure (Braithwaite and Mc Evoy, 2005).

Once fouling has been established, the only lasting solution is an expensive docking to remove the fouling by cleanining, nutrient limitation or by the use of antifouling substances. Up to now the most effective and economic solution to prevent growth on ship has been to use an antifouling paint which releases a biocide (Kugler, 2005). One of these biocides is dichlofluanid.

Antifouling Products – Strategy of Biofouling Prevention

Use of Tributyltin Compounds in the Past

The antifouling products are approved for use on vessels of any size plus structures below the waterline. The ideal antifouling product would protect a vessel for 5 years. The period of time between repainting can however vary quite considerably depending upon the chosen antifouling product formulation, and on the environment in which it is used. Various environments will present different fouling challenges. Parameters which will influence the service time of an antifouling product include: trading patterns (coastal or deep sea, turn around time, speed of vessels etc.); fouling conditions (warm or temperate water); physico-chemical conditions of the seawater (e.g. pH and temperature) and coating type and film thickness.

Antifouling products can be broadly divided into two types; those that contain tributyltin (TBT) and those that are TBT-free.

In the past, the most effective antifouling paint system has been based on TBT, especially tributyltin oxide (TBTO). TBT or organotin compounds were introduced in the mid-1960s and were the most widely used antifouling active ingredients covering more than 70 % of the world's commercial shipping fleet for more than 30 years (Yebra et al., 2004). Besides having an excellent biocidal activity, copolymers based on TBTO show self-polishing properties and release the biocide at a constant rate over a period of five and more years. Originally, the organotin biocides were considered environmentally safe but in the late 1970s a link was established between deformities in oysters and the use of TBT-based antifouling paints (Alzieu, 2000). They also act as the endocrine disrupters in animals, inducing masculinization (imposex) in female gastropods of different species by increasing testosterone levels, e.g. sex changes in whelks and imposex in snails (ten Hallers-Tjabbes et al., 1994; Crommentuijn et al., 2000; Champ, 2000; Ramon and Amor, 2001). Besides effects on the reproductive system, as well as carcinogenic and neurotoxic effects, the most obvious effects of both various di- and tri-substituted organotins were found on the immune system of mammals, fish and other marine organisms (Krajnc et al., 1984; Vos et al., 1984, 1990; Snoeij et al., 1988; Van Loveren et al., 1990; Penninks et al., 1990; Kugler, 2005). In the 1980s it was also recognized that TBTO and other organotin antifoulants have relatively long half-lives in the environment (half-life of TBTO in seawater is more than 6 months) and tend to accumulate in marine organisms (Tanabe et al., 1998; Tanabe, 1999; Rudel, 2003; Appel, 2004).

Exposure of humans to organotin compounds can take place through consumption of contaminated fish and seafood or house dust containing harmful organotins could, however, under some conditions, become a relevant intake possibility for young children (Fromme et al., 2005). In human liver samples, mainly dibutyltin, the metabolite of TBT, could be detected indicating that organotin compounds are bioavailable after dietary exposure (Appel, 2004).

The harmful environmental effects of organotin compounds were recognized by the International Maritime Organisation (IMO) in 1989. In 1990 IMO's Marine Environment Protection Committee (MEPC) adopted a resolution which recommended that Governments adopt measures to eliminate the use of anti-fouling paint containing TBT on non-aluminium hulled vessels of less than 25 metres in length that exist in shallow coastal waters where the impacted oysters species grow; and eliminate the use of anti-fouling paints with a leaching rate of more than four microgrammes of TBT per days (d). In November 1999, the IMO adopted an Assembly resolution that called on the MEPC to develop an instrument, legally binding throughout the world, to address the harmful effects of anti-fouling systems used on ships. The resolution called for a global prohibition on the application of organotin compounds which act as biocides in anti-fouling systems on ships by 1 January 2003, and a complete prohibition by 1 January 2008 (Kugler, 2005). The present movement toward a global ban suggests that the above regulatory approach has not been sufficient in some countries. Today vessels can be painted with regulated or banned antifouling materials by boatyards in a country that does not have TBT regulations and subsequently travel in international and regulated national waters and thus bringing the impact back to the country which was trying to prevent it. Legislative policies enacted by "regulated" countries to regulate the use of TBT to protect their local marine resources have subsequently had far reaching environmental and economic impacts which have in essence transferred TBT contamination to those countries least able to deal with it. Market forces are selective for cheap labour and cheap environments. "Unregulated" countries have unknowingly accepted the environmental and human health risks to gain the economic benefits from painting TBT on ships (Champ, 2000).

As a replacement for TBT, new antifouling agents are entering the market. The use of these biocides has received increased attention due to their ecological and economic relevance.

Modern Antifouling Agents and Booster Biocides

Modern TBT-free products typically contain copper or a copper compound such as copper (I) oxide (Cu_2O), or copper (I) thiocyanate (CuSCN) as the principal biocide. For sea-faring ships copper oxide has long been a commonly used active substance of antifouling paints since the pre-1960s (Omae, 2003). Copper is also used to enhance the performance of TBT-products because organisms such as *Ectocarpus* species and *Achanthes* species are tolerant of TBTO (Callow, 1990). Such copper compounds are highly effective against sessile sea animals like barnacles, tube worms and serpulids, but some of the common marine macroalgae (e.g. *Enteromorpha* sp. and *Amphora* sp.) are tolerant towards copper. Therefore copper as an active ingredient has to be „boosted" or enhanced by the presence of one or more organic biocides (Voulvoulis et al., 2002a).

"Booster biocides" is a generic term given to a group of compounds normally found in addition to copper and occasionally triorganotin compounds. The purpose of these compounds is to enhance the product efficacy against a broader spectrum of fouling organisms than that achieved with copper alone. Booster biocides are either organic or organo-metallic compounds which have fungicidal, herbicidal or antimicrobial actions. They have been used in antifouling applications since the 1980s. Examples of these substances can be found in Table 1 (van Wezel and van Vlaardingen, 2004).

In the past the most common booster biocides were algaecides diuron and cybutryne. They inhibit the electron flow in photosystem II and are therefore toxic to many marine algae but show a low acute toxicity towards fish and other sea animals. Due to the fact that these algaecides are hardly biodegradable in seawater and moderately bioaccumulable, both compounds can accumulate in the marine environment and have recently been detected worldwide in waters and sediments from marinas and coastal sides (Okamura, 2002; Maraldo and Dahllof, 2004; Kugler, 2005).

Table 1. Substances used as booster biocides in antiflouling paints

Chemical name
2,3,5,6-tetrachloro-4-(methyl sulphonyl) pyridine – TCMS
2-methylthio-4-tertiary-butylamino-6-cyclopropylamino-*s*-triazine – Irgarol 1051
Cuprous thiocyanate
2,4,5,6-tetrachloro-*iso*-phthalo-nitrile
4,5-dichloro-2-*n*-octyl-4-isothiazol-3-one – Sea Nine 211 or DCOIT
Dichlorophenyl Dimethylurea – DCMU
Folpet
Zinc pyrithione
Copper pyrithione
4-chloro-meta-cresol
Arsenic trioxide
Maneb
Zineb
Ziram
Thiram
Cis-1-(3-chloroallyl)-3,5,7-triaza-1-azonia adamantane chloride
Chlorothalonil
2-(thiocyanomethyl thio) benzthiazole – TCMTB
Deltamethrin
Farnesol
Oxytetracycline hydrochloride
Bitumen
Dichlofluanid

van Wezel and van Vlaardingen, 2004.

Nowadays there are only three active ingredients – namely dichlofluanid, zinc pyrithione and zineb – still available for amateur use applications in European countries. For professional applications antifouling paints with the three other booster biocides DCOIT (or Sea Nine 211), copper pyrithione and zineb have been listed. Zinc pyrithione and copper pyrithione, DCOIT, dichlofluanid and tolylfluanid (a compound structurally very similar to dichlofluanid but with a better solubility in organic solvents like xylene) generally show a lower environmental persistence compared to the above mentioned photosynthesis inhibitors and organotin compounds.

Since 1993, several studies have demonstrated the presence of various biocides in European coastal environment and estuarines, particularly in marinas and harbours, as a result of their increased use. The presence of the biocides as Irgarol 1051, Sea-Nine 211, chlorothalonil, TCMS and TCMTB was also revealed in waters from Japan, United States, Singapore, Australia and Bermuda (Konstantinou and Albanis, 2004). On the other hand, in UK a removal of the previously popular booster biocides diuron and Irgarol 1051 from the market has led to a clear reduction in their water concentrations from locations where previous biocide levels were well documented (Cresswell et al., 2006). Enviromental concentrations of chlorothalonil, dichlofluanid and Sea-Nine 211 were below the limits of detection (< 1 ng/L) in all samples (Cresswell et al., 2006). Irgarol 1051 and Sea-Nine 211 have been subjected to restrictions in many EU member states because of their environmental stability and high toxicity (Ranke and Jastorff, 2000; Yebra et al., 2004).

With policies encouraging a total ban on TBT, it is expected that biocides will be used to a greater extent in the future. Their widespread use should be allowed only after research to fill the gaps in knowledge with respect to their environmental occurrence, fate, toxicity and persistence in aquatic environments (Voulvoulis et al., 2002b; van Wezel and van Vlaardingen, 2004) in which they may be released through leaching from a painted surface (Kobayashi and Okamura, 2002; Kiil et al., 2003). Decisions by regulatory authorities which were triggered by environmental risks started to change the commercial availability of booster biocides dramatically.

The objective of this chapter is to present various toxic aspects of dichlofluanid, one of the antifouling paint booster biocides, in more detail.

Dichlofluanid - The Fungicide and Booster Biocide

Use Pattern

Dichlofluanid is a halogenated sulfonamide derivative from the group of aryl (dichlorofluoromethyltio) fungicides (Hansson and Wallengren, 1995). Its general physical-chemical characteristics are summarized in Table 2 (The Pesticide Manual, 2000).

Table 2. The general physical-chemical characteristics of dichlofluanid

Common name:	Dichlofluanid
IUPAC name:	*N*-dichlorofluoromethylthio-*N'*, *N'*-dimethyl-*N*-phenylsulfamide
CAS name:	1,1-dichloro-*N*-[(dimethylamino)sulfonyl]-1-fluoro-*N*-phenylmethane-sulfenamide
CAS RN:	1085-98-9
Formula:	$C_9H_{11}Cl_2FN_2O_2S_2$
Colour:	Colourless powder
Odour:	Mild specific
Melting point:	106 °C
Molecular weight:	333.2
Log K_{ow}	3.7
Activity:	Fungicide, acaricide, wood preservative, booster biocide
Structure:	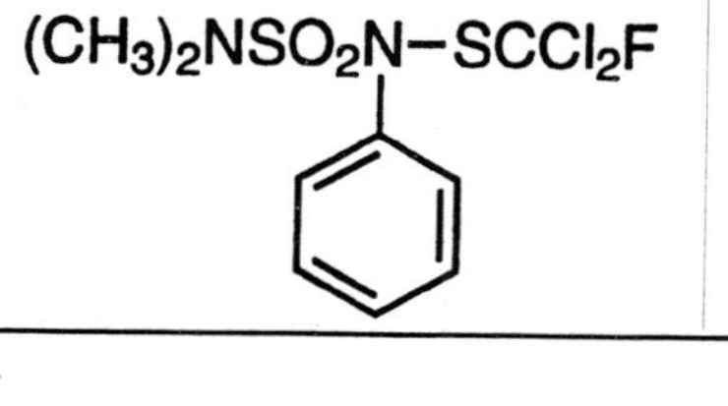

The Pesticide Manual, 2000.

Table 3. Solubility of dichlofluanid in organic dissolvents in g/L at 20 °C

Water	Dichloromethane	Toluene	Xylene	Methanol	Isopropanol	Hexane
1.3	< 200	145	70	15	10.8	2.6

The Pesticide Manual, 2000.

Dichlofluanid is slightly volatile and sensitive to light (Sedokur, 1986; Visser, 1993). It is slightly soluble in water, better in organic dissolvents (Table 3; The Pesticide Manual, 2000).

Dichlofluanid was used as a fungicide and acaricide in approved agricultural pesticides from 1965, in wood preservative products from 1978 and as a booster biocide in antifouling products from 1987. In the past it was among the world's most widely used fungicides for crop protection. It belongs to contact fungicides with protective action applicated at the time of vegetation to control scab, brown rot and storage diseases caused by *Alternaria* spp., *Clasterosporium* spp., *Peronospora* sp. and *Botrytis cinerea* on fruits, vegetables, ornamentals, and conifer seedbeds (Wojdyla, 2003; Kim et al., 2004). *In vitro* it is also effective on various kinds of moulds – *Aspergillus* and *Trichoderma* spp. (Garcia-Aguirre and Moreno-Martinez, 1987; Sas-Piotrowska and Piotrowski, 1997). Nowadays it is not included in any of the lists for European re-assessment of active ingredients under Directive 91/414/EEC. Dichlofluanid is on the EU list of hazardous substances, classified as an allergen and hazardous to the environment (Jørgensen, 2001). It is one of 320 pesticides withdrawn in 25 July 2003 as part of the European Commission new approach to the evaluation of active substances in plant protection products. This aims to improve safeguards to ensure that all such products in use are safe for the environment and human health.

However, nowadays it is used in aquaculture and as a booster biocide in antifouling products, especially tin-free products, to control the growth of algal, weed and animal fouling on moving or stati objects in water. Furthermore, following the review of dichlofluanid in Product type 8 (Wood preservatives) under the Biocidal Products Directive 98/8/EC, the European Commission has agreed that this active substance will enter into Annex I of the Directive on 1 March 2009. The maximum concentration of dichlofluanid permitted as an active ingredient within approved antifouling formulations is 10 % w/w. Products containing dichlofluanid can be used for the pre-treatment of timber against wood-staining fungi (blue stain and mould) (dipping and automated enclosed spraying by industrial, professional users) and the protective treatment of wood *in situ* by brush application (both professional and amateur users). Dichlofluanid is not recommended for treatment of wood inside housing areas (with the exception of window frames and external doors, which will usually be treated on or before installation) or for spraying manually in open systems. In EU countries wood preservatives containing dichlofluanid are marketed as e.g. "Preventol" and "Flourofolpet" or "Rentolin". "Rentolin" marketed in Denmark without a warning against indoor uses, has created a disaster. Around 200 people used Rentolin indoors and suffered serious injury. Many houses are now uninhabitable, and several people suffer from chronic diseases. Some have the diagnosis of MCS (Multiple Chemical Sensibility), meaning that they have violent reaction to all kinds of volatile chemical substances, natural and manmade as well (Jørgensen, 2001).

Dichlofluanid acts by targeting a number of metabolic processes, and thus the development of resistance in the target organism is considered to be of low risk.

Fate in the Environment

Dichlofluanid is the potential contaminant of water. For example, some research groups did report the occurrence of dichlofluanid or its metabolite dimethylsulfanilide – DMSA in harbours and marinas in Spain, Greece and the UK (Martínez et al., 2001; Albanis et al., 2002; Sakkas et al., 2002; Lambropoulou et al., 2003; Konstantinou and Albanis, 2004; Hamwijk et al., 2005). It was also detected in waste waters from farms that produce ornamentals (Sadlo and Rupak, 1991), in marine sediment (Agüera et al., 2000; Martínez et al., 2001; Harino et al., 2007). On the other hand, Thomas et al. (2002) did not detect it in water and sediment samples from various areas of boating and shipping activities in the UK.

The aquatic photochemical behaviour of dichlofluanid has been studied under natural sunlight conditions as well as under artificial solar irradiation in different types of natural waters (sea, river and lake water) as well as in distilled water and a half-life varied between 8 and 83 h, in natural seawater it was 53 h (Sakkas et al., 2001). A half-life of 18 h was reported on a bioassay method (Callow and Finlay, 1995). Dichlofluanid hydrolyzes very fast in water. The main degradation products occurred from photodegradation, hydrolysis and anaerobic degradation were dichlorofluoromethane, aniline, and DMSA (Sakkas et al., 2001; Thomas et al., 2003). DMSA is hydrolytically stable under conditions such as in natural seawater. Biodegradation of DMSA is assumed to occur slowly, although its inherent biodegradability is established. According to Jansma and Linders (1992) at pH 7.7 – 7.9 and 21 °C a DT_{50} (50 % dissipation time) of dichlofluanid in water was found of approximately 2 h. A second hydrolysis study in buffered solutions, yielded DT_{50} values of 15.3 d at pH 4, 19 h at pH 7 and < 10 min at pH 9. No parent compound could be detected at pH 9 even if analysis was performed immediately. The half-life of the parent compound is clearly depending on the pH (Jansma and Linders, 1992). In artificial seawater, it shows a half-life of approximatelly 1 h. In a water sediment system of pH 7.5 a half-life of 3 h is found whereas in a water sediment system of pH 8.1 the observed half-life is 1.2 h, which correlates well with the tests in artificial seawaters (Kugler, 2005). The persistence of dichlofluanid was increased when associated with paint particules and a half-life was determined to be 1.4 d (Thomas et al., 2003).

Due to its instability in soil, dichlofluanid is not leached into deeper soil layers. In biologically active soils it hydrolyses rapidly to DMSA with DT50 < 1 d. DMSA is further degraded and according to leached studies, is unlikely to leach into deeper soil layers (The Pesticide Manual, 2000). Leaching studies in soil showed that dichlofluanid was not mobile, whereas DMSA was shown to be mobile and susceptible to degradation with time.

The very low vapour pressure (2.15×10^{-5} Pa at 20 °C) indicates that dichlofluanid has a low tendency to volatilise, therefore air has not been considered as a compartment of concern.

In plants, dichlofluanid is metabolised to DMSA which is further demethylated or hydroxylated and conjugated. Its stability during the cryogenic sample processing of apples has been studied by Fussell et al. (2002). Losses of dichlofluanid were reduced to barely significant levels (10 %) by this processing. Residual levels and degradation rates of dichlofluanid in oranges and tomatoes were determined by Fussell et al. (2007) and in lettuce plants by Rial-Otero et al. (2005). Seven days after the last application, its levels were below the maximum allowed limit (10 mg/kg) (Rial-Otero et al., 2005). Persistence of fungicide on strawberries and in some canned products of strawberry was tested by Seifert et al. (1978). The significant decay of dichlofluanid residues occurs during the technological procedures applied. No significant differences between strawberry treated with fungicide and control has been found in flavour and taste of the canned products investigated (Davídek et al., 1981; Will and Krüger, 1999). Toxic effects of fungicide residues on the wine-producing process, in *Saccharomyces* and non-*Saccharomyces* yeasts as well as their influence on the physical, chemical and organoleptic wine properties, were described by Calhelha et al. (2006). The fungicide had a negative effect on *in vitro* yeast growth and *Zygosaccharomyces rouxii* and *Saccharomyces cerevisiae* were the most resistant yeasts while *Rhodotorula glutinis* was the most susceptible (Calhelha et al., 2006).

A fast and easy method for residue analysis was developed, e.g. in fruits and vegetables (Lehotay et al., 2005), water samples (Peñalver et al., 1999; Martínez et al., 2000; Agüera et al., 2000; Lambropoulou et al., 2000; Gimeno et al., 2001; Lambropoulou and Albanis, 2004), honey (Albero et al., 2004), wine (Soleas et al., 2000), greenhouse air (Egea González et al., 1997) and in marine sediments (Martínez and Barceló, 2001).

Toxicokinetics

In mammals, following oral administration, dichlofluanid is rapidly absorbed and excreted, mainly in the urine, with a small proportion in the faeces and via respiration. The metabolites found in urine and serum after oral administration of dichlofluanid are showed in Figure 1 (Eben and Kimmerle, 1968; Bayer, 1969). All the metabolites are excreted in the free-form and the metabolites III and IV are also excreted as glucuronides. Metabolites I and II can also be found in serum.

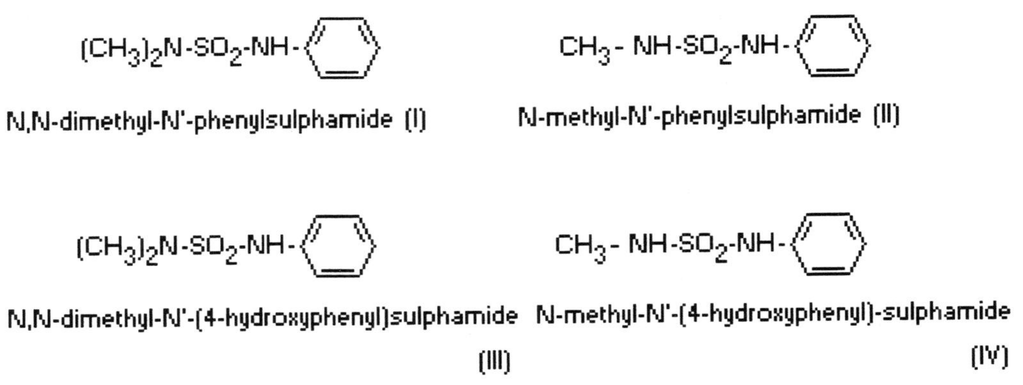

Figure 1. The metabolites found in urine and serum after oral administration of dichlofluanid (Eben and Kimmerle, 1968; Bayer, 1969).

There is no accumulation in organs and tissues. Dichlofluanid is metabolised to DMSA which is further hydroxylated or demethylated (The Pesticide Manual, 2000).

In animal organism dichlofluanid inhibits thiol enzymes, has an ability of interaction with membranes, damages mitochondrial reactions including oxidative phosphorylation and NADH oxidation (Corbertt et al., 1984).

Human Health Risk

The potential human health effects of dichlofluanid have been well investigated, almost exclusively in experimental animals. Dichlofluanid is of low acute toxicity by the oral and dermal routes of exposure, but has moderate acute toxicity by the inhalation route. It is not a skin irritant, but is an eye irritant (Pauluhn, 1982; Shiotsuka, 1986).

Median lethal doses of dichlofluanid (LD_{50}/LC_{50}) for some animal species are summarized in Table 4.

Table 4. Acute toxicity of dichlofluanid (LD_{50}/LC_{50}) for some animal species

Species	Oral LD_{50} mg/kg b.wt.	Inhalation LC_{50}	Dermal LD_{50} mg/kg b.wt.	Authors
Mouse	1850 – 2500	-	-	Sedokur (1986)
Mouse	5464 (Male) 5597 (Female)	-	-	Flucke, 1978
Rat	1850 – 2500	-	-	Sedokur (1986)
Rat	> 5000	1.2 mg/L (4 h) dust > 0.3 mg/L (4 h) aerosol	> 2000	Kroetlinger, 1990; The Pesticide Manual (2000)
Rat	-	1338 mg/m^3 (4 h, Male) 1233 mg/m^3 (4 h, Female)	-	Shiotsuka, 1986
Guinea pig	954 (Female)	-	-	Flucke, 1978
Rabbit	3 500 (Female)	-	-	Flucke, 1978

Poisoning of a puma with this fungicide described Kohout (1975).

Chronic studies indicate two critical effects: skeletal osteosclerosis and chronic nephropathy, observed in rats and dogs respectively. Following repeated oral administration of dichlofluanid, the most prominent finding was fluorosis caused by the release of fluoride from the dichlofluanid molecule during its metabolism. This resulted in skeletal osteosclerosis, observed in lifetime dietary studies in both rats and mice (Holzum, 1992; Leser, 1993a,b). Chronic nephropathy was also observed following repeated oral administration, but in dogs only (Lorke and Loeser, 1966; Christenson and Elcock, 1992). The mode of action for the nephropathy is uncertain and possible explanations include direct nephrotoxicity of the active substance or a secondary consequence of elevated systemic fluoride levels (Christenson and Elcock, 1992). In the 1-year oral study in dogs, a NOAEL of 2.5 mg/kg/d was identified for minimal to moderate chronic nephropathy (Christenson and

Elcock, 1992). In humans, prolonged environmental exposure to high levels of fluoride may cause adverse dental changes as well as skeletal changes (www.fluorideaction.org).

Few published papers are available on the cytotoxicity of dichlofluanid under *in vitro* conditions. Yamano and Morita (1993) found that it decreases viability of mitochondrie and microsomes in hepatocytes. Holovská et al. (2007) studied its *in vitro* effect on proliferative activity of various animal derived cell cultures. Suzuki et al. (1997) showed its strong cytotoxic effect in isolated rat hepatocytes. Whilst Pistl et al. (2003) observed that dichlofluanid caused significant cytotoxic effect at 10^{-1} M/L on sheep peripheral leukocytes. In spite of the fact that cytotoxicity of dichlofluanid in leukocytes was mild, the function of lymphocytes was altered. It was manifested by a significant decrease in activation of sheep lymphocytes with phytohemagglutinin (an immunotoxic effect) at the concentrations of 10^{-2} – 10^{-3} M/L of dichlofluanid (Pistl et al., 2003). The significant suppression of metabolic activity of phagocytic cells, examined by iodo-nitro-tetrazolium reductase test under *in vitro* conditions, was registered at the concentrations of 10^{-1} – 10^{-3} M/L of dichlofluanid (Pistl et al., 2002).

Dichlofluanid has been thoroughly tested for genotoxic potential in a range of *in vitro* and *in vivo* studies. It was found to be a point mutagen in studies on bacteria and cause mutations at the TK locus in eukaryotic cells (Shirasu et al., 1978; Herbold, 1984; Cifone, 1985). For example, dichlofluanid was found to be mutagenic in *Salmonella typhimurium* and *E. coli* (WP2 reversion assay); however, the mutagenic potency was rather weak and not always observed (Shirasu et al., 1978; Moriya et al., 1983; Herbold, 1984; Barrueco and de la Pena, 1988). In the EPA Gene-Tox Program 1988 dichlofluanid was classified „negative“ (*Saccharomyces cerevisiae* gene conversion) and „inconclusive“ (*Bacillus subtilis* rec assay; RTECS, 1990). In contrast to the structurally similar strong mutagens captan and folpet, dichlofluanid only gives weak and uncertain mutagenicity data in *Salmonella,* a property attributed by some authors to the high toxicity of the fluorine atom of dichlofluanid, thus preventing the detection of any possible effect in *Salmonella* (Barrueco and de la Pena, 1988). Heil et al. (1991) used seven different endpoints for detection of genotoxicity to demonstrate the DNA-altering properties of dichlofluanid. All of the seven test systems clearly showed DNA alterations, indicating significant genotoxic potential of fungicide. Their results indicate that application of dichlofluanid may be mutagenic and/or carcinogenic for exposed humans. Dichlofluanid caused gene mutations at the TK locus in mouse lymphoma cells, with or without metabolic activation (Cifone, 1985). A positive result was also obtained in an *in vitro* cytogenetics assay (Herbold, 1986a). Further *in vitro* tests, e.g. micronucleus assay in sheep lymphocyte cultures (Kovalkovičová et al., 2001) and on point mutations on the HGPRT locus in eukaryotic cells yielded negative results (Lehn, 1988a,b). Under *in vivo* conditions negative results were obtained in a mouse micronucleus and liver UDS test (Herbold, 1978; Benford, 1988). Further *in vivo* testing in a mouse spot test, a sperm cell chromosomal aberration test and a rodent dominant lethal test were all clearly negative (Herbold, 1979; 1986b; 1988). The available data indicate that dichlofluanid was not an *in vivo* somatic cell or germ cell mutagen. Overall it is unlikely to pose a genotoxicity hazard to man.

In terms of carcinogenicity, dichlofluanid induced thyroid folicular cell tumours in rats at high doses of 300 – 420 mg/kg/d, but by a mechanism not considered to be relevant for human health. These tumours occurred at a single site, were of late onset and generally benign pathology (Leser, 1993a). The results of the histopathological examination of the thyroid follicular cell tumours are consistent with a non-genotoxic aetiology. Overall, it can be concluded that dichlofluanid is a non-genotoxic rat thyroid follicular cell carcinogen. No increase in tumour incidence was observed in mice (Leser, 1993b).

Marchal-Ségault (1993) and Marchal-Ségault and Laugé (1997) studied the effect of dichlofluanid on the fertility of *Drosophila melanogaster* meigen. Effect was very strong and rapidly irreversible: the egg masses were very reduced after only one week of treatment on both treated and untreated media, and after termination of treatment there was an incomplete and temporary recuperation of the capacity to lay eggs. At the doses recommended for agricultural treatments, dichlofluanid showed high toxicity for *Drosophila* adults. On the other hand, it has a weak teratogenic properties in four generations of rats exposed to dietary doses of 1500 – 4500 mg/kg (Sedokur, 1986). In other experimental animal studies it did not affect fertility and did not cause developmental toxicity. The evidence suggests that this substance does not possess significant potential with respect to toxicity for reproduction of mammals (Holzum, 1992).

Occupational exposure during application and removal of antifouling paints containing dichlofluanid was determined by Links et al. (2007). Both primary exposure (rolling and spraying) and secondary exposure (during sand blasting) were studied. The inhalation exposure loading was 0.14 mg/m^3 during rolling, whereas the potential body exposure loading was 267 mg/h and potential hand exposure loading 277 mg/h. The study showed that the exposure loading should be considered more extensively, including applicable protective gear. In this light the findings for the potmen during sand blasting suggest that personal protective equipment should be reconsidered carefully.

Björkner et al. (1990) reported dermatitis similar to erythema multiforme in their patients and Hansson and Wallengren (1995) contact allergy after using of dichlofluanid such as wood preservative. No skin problems from use of dichlofluanid as a fungicide at low concentration on fruit and vegetables have been reported.

Environmental Risk

Dichlofluanid was found to be of low toxicity to birds. Per oral LD_{50} for Japanese quail (*Coturnix japonica*) is > 5000 mg/kg b.wt. (The Pesticide Manual, 2000). The acute oral LD_{50} of dichlofluanid to the bobwhite quail (*Colinus virginianus)* was reported to be > 2226 mg/kg b.wt. (Stubblefield, 1986a). The subacute dietary LC_{50} for two species of birds, mallard ducks (*Anas platyrhynchos*) and bobwhite quail (*Colinus virginianus*), was assumed to be > 5000 ppm. The NOEC was reported as > 5000 ppm (Stubblefield, 1986b,c).

Dichlofluanid is extremely toxic to aquatic organisms and sensitising, whereas DMSA has a low toxicity. Aquatic toxicity data for dichlofluanid are presented in Table 5.

The carps (*Cyprinus carpio*) are very susceptible to dichlofluanid exposure in which the central nervous system and the cardiovascular system are affected. Pathological effects are evident on the gill sheets where distal ends become pale due to ischaemia (Antychowicz et al., 1979).

Table 5. Aquatic toxicity data for dichlofluanid

Test species	Test duration	Ecotoxicological endpoint	Authors
Acute toxicity to freshwater organisms			
Pisces			
Lepomis macrochirus	96 h	LC_{50} = 0.025 mg/L	Swigert et al., 1986a; The Pesticide Manual (2000)
Leuciscus idus melanmotus	96 h	LC_{50} = 0.12 mg/L	Anonymous, 1980; The Pesticide Manual (2000)
Leuciscus idus melanmotus	96 h	LC_{50} = 0.12 mg/L	Jansma and Linders, 1992
Onchorhynchus mykiss	96 h	LC_{50} = 0.05 mg/L	Anonymous, 1979
Onchorhynchus mykiss	96 h	LC_{50} = 0.011 mg/L	Swigert et al., 1986b; The Pesticide Manual (2000)
Crustacea			
Daphnia magna	48 h	LC_{50} > 1.8 mg/L	Heimbach, 1983
Daphnia magna	48 h	LC_{50} = 0.37 mg/L	Frazier et al., 1986
Daphnia magna	48 h	EC_{50} = 0.42 mg/L	Forbis, 1986
Chronic toxicity to freshwater organisms			
Pisces			
Onchorhynchus mykiss	21 d	LC_{50} = 0.016 mg/L	Grau, 1989
Crustacea			
Daphnia magna	21 d	NOEC = 0.04 mg/L	Jansma and Linders, 1992
Daphnia magna	24 d	NOEC = 0.04 mg/L	Ritter, 1989

Fernandez-Alba et al. (2002) and Hernando et al. (2003) measured the toxic effects (EC_{50} value) of dichlofluanid and compared with the EC_{50} value of the pesticide mixed with methyl-tert-butyl ether (MTBE), using the *Vibrio fischeri*, *Selenastrum capricornotum* and *Daphnia magna* acute toxicity assays. MTBE, a fuel oxygenate that is added to gasoline, commonly contaminates aquatic systems, many of which are already contaminated with pesticides. Presence of MTBE enhanced the EC_{50} value of dichlofluanid (by 30 %) and the toxic response manifested more rapidly than with pure pesticide when measured with the *D. magna* assay. Castritsi-Catharios et al. (2007) determined toxicity of dichlofluanid on brine shrimp larvae (*Artemia salina*) and Bellas (2006) on embryos and larvae of three marine invertebrates, the bivalve *Mytilus edulis*, the echinoid *Paracentrotus lividus* and the ascidian *Ciona intestinalis*. The EC_{10} and EC_{50} for dichlofluanid ranged from 95 to 830 and from 244 to 4311 nM/L.

The 96 h EbC_{50} (biomass) and ErC_{50} (growth rate) values for the green alga *Scenedesmus subspicatus* were found to be > 1 mg/L (the highest concentration tested) (Heimbach, 1985).

According to the log octanol water partition coefficient (log Pow) a high bioconcentration potential of dichlofluanid could be theoretically assumed but in a fish accumulation study a low bioconcentration factor of 72 was found (Kugler, 2005).

Dichlofluanid is not toxic for bees (Sedokur, 1986).

A short term toxicity test submitted for the terrestrial toxicity endpoint demonstrates that dichlofluanid has a relatively low toxicity to earthworms. Terrestrial toxicity data for dichlofluanid are presented in Table 6 (Jansma and Linders, 1992).

The sensitivity of yeast strains of *Kluyveromyces marxianus, Pichia anomala, Candida utilis, Schizosaccharomyces pombe* and *Saccharomyces cerevisiae* to dichlofluanid was studied by Ribeiro et al. (2000).

Bonafos et al. (2008) tested the toxicity of dichlofluanid on the predatory mite *Typhlodromus pyri* Scheuten.

Table 6. Terrestrial toxicity data for dichlofluanid (Jansma and Linders, 1992)

Test species	Test duration	Ecotoxicological endpoint	
		Result test soil (mg/kg d.w.)	Result standard soil (mg/kg d.w.)
Chronic toxicity; microbial processes			
Nitrification	56 d	$EC_9 = 1.3$	$EC_9 = 9.3$
Nitrification	56 d	$EC_{21} = 13$	$EC_{21} = 92.9$
Nitrification	56 d	NOEC ≥ 1.3	NOEC ≥ 3.0
Nitrification	56 d	$EC_{13} = 13$	$EC_{13} = 29.5$
Chronic toxicity; soil organisms			
Oligochaeta			
Eisenia fetida	28 d	$LC_{50} > 1000$	-
Eisenia fetida	14 d	$LC_{50} > 913$	-
Eisenia fetida	14 d	NOEC = 288	-

CONCLUSION

Dichlofluanid is one of the pesticides that contain fluoride in their molecule and may contribute to environmental contamination with fluorides. Its potential health and environmental risks are as follows:

1. It is of low acute toxicity by the oral and dermal routes of exposure, but has moderate acute toxicity by the inhalation route. It is not a skin irritant, but is an eye irritant.
2. Its main effects in experimental animals during repeated exposure are skeletal osteosclerosis and chronic nephropathy and increased fluoride level in organism is identified.

3. The available data indicate that it was not an *in vivo* somatic or germ cell mutagen. It is unlikely to pose a genetic hazard to man.
4. It is a non-genotoxic rat thyroid follicular cell carcinogen.
5. It does not possess significant potential with respect to toxicity for reproduction of mammals.
6. It was found to be of low toxicity to birds, bees and earthworms, but it is extremely toxic to aquatic organisms.

ACKNOWLEDGMENTS

This study was supported by VEGA Grants No. 1/0545/08, 1/4375/07 and the National Reference Laboratory for Pesticides, University of Veterinary Medicine in Košice.

REFERENCES

Agüera, A., Piedra, L., Hernando, M. D. & Fernández-Alba, A. R. (2000). Multiresidue method for the analysis of five antifouling agents in marine and coastal waters by gas chromatography-mass spectrometry with large-volume injection. *J. Chromatogr. A., 889,* 1-2, 261-269.

Albanis, T. A., Lambropoulou, D. A., Sakkas, V. A. & Konstantinou, I. K. (2002). Antifouling paint booster biocide contamination in Greek marine sediments. *Chemosphere, 48,* 5, 475-485.

Albero, B., Sánchez-Brunete, C. & Tadeo, J. L. (2004). Analysis of pesticides in honey by solid-phase extraction and gas chromatography-mass spectrometry. *J. Agric. Food Chem., 52,* 19, 5828-5835.

Alzieu, C. (2000). Environmental impact of TBT: the French experience. *Sci. Total Environ., 258*, 1-2, 99-102.

Anonymous (1979). Fischtoxizität. Dichlofluanid Kü 13 032 c, Regenbogenforelle. Report No. FF-74, Bayer AG Pflanzenschutz Anwendungstechnik, Institute of Environmental Biology. Cit.: van Wezel, A. P. & van Vlaardingen, P. (2004). Environmental risk limits for antifouling substances. *Aquat. Toxicol., 66,* 4, 427-444.

Anonymous (1980). Fischtoxizität. Dichlofluanid Kü 13 032 c, Goldorfe. Report No. FO-288. Bayer AG Pflanzenschutz Anwendungstechnik, Institute of Environmental Biology. Cit.: van Wezel, A. P. & van Vlaardingen, P. (2004). Environmental risk limits for antifouling substances. *Aquat. Toxicol., 66,* 4, 427-444.

Antychowicz, J., Szymbor, E. & Roszkowsk, J. (1979). Investigations upon the effects of some pesticides on carp (*Cyprinus carpio*). *Bull. Vet. Inst. Pulawy, 23*, 124-130.

Appel, K. E. (2004). Organotin compounds: toxicokinetic aspects. *Drug Metab. Rev., 36,* 3-4, 763-786.

Barrueco, C. & De-la-Pena, E. (1988). Mutagenic evaluation of the pesticides captan, folpet, captafol, dichlofluanid and related compounds with the mutants TA 102 and TA 104 of *Salmonella typhimurium*. *Mutagenesis, 3,* 467-480.

Bayer (1969). Dichlofluanid. Unpublished Summary Report prepared and submitted by Farbenfabriken Bayer AG [online]. Available from: URL: http://www.inchem.org/documents/jmpr/jmpmono/v074pr14.htm

Bellas, J. (2006). Comparative toxicity of alternative antifouling biocides on embryos and larvae of marine invertebrates. *Sci. Total Environ., 367,* 2-3, 573-85.

Benford, D. J. (1988). *Ex vivo* hepatocyte UDS study with KUE 13032 C. The Robens Institute, University of Surrey, UK; Bayer AG. Unpublished report No. R 4593. Bayer CropScience AG [online]. Available from: URL: http://ecb.jrc.it/DOCUMENTS/Biocides/ANNEX_I/ASSESSMENT_REPORTS/AnnexI_AR_1085-98-9_PT08_en.pdf

Björkner, B., Bruze, M. & Gruvberger, B. (1990). Sensitization to dichlofluanide. *Contact Dermatitis, 23,* 246.

Bonafos, R., Auger, P., Guichou, S. & Kreiter, S. (2008). Suitability of two laboratory testing methods to evaluate the side effects of pesticides on *Typhlodromus pyri* Scheuten (Acari: Phytoseiidae). *Pest. Manag. Sci., 64*, 2, 178-184.

Braithwaite, R. A. & Mc Evoy, L. A. (2005). Marine biofouling on fish farms and its remediation. *Adv. Mar. Biol., 47,* 215-252.

Calhelha, R. C., Andrade, J. V., Ferreira, I. C. & Estevinho, L. M. (2006). Toxicity effects of fungicide residues on the wine-producing process. *Food Microbiol., 23,* 4, 393-398.

Callow, M. (1990). Ship fouling: problems and solutions. *Chem. & Ind., 5,* 123-127.

Callow, M. E. & Finlay, J. A. (1995). A simple method to evaluate the potential for degradation of antifouling biocides. *Biofouling, 9,* 239-249.

Callow, M. E. & Callow, J. A. (2002). Marine biofouling: A sticky problem. *Biologist*, *49,* 1, 10-14.

Castritsi-Catharios, J., Bourdaniotis, N. & Persoone, G. (2007). A new simple method with high precision for determining the toxicity of antifouling paints on brine shrimp larvae (Artemia): first results. *Chemosphere, 67,* 6, 1127-1132.

Champ, M. A. (2000). A review of organotin regulatory strategies, pending actions, related costs and benefits. *Sci. Total Environ., 258,*1-2, 21-71.

Christenson, W. R. & Elcock, E. L. (1992). Technical grade dichlofluanid (Euparen VM 90): Oral dosing chronic toxicity studies on the Beagle dog. Miles Inc, USA. Unpublished report No. R 5832. Bayer CropScience AG [online]. Available from: URL: http://ecb.jrc.it/DOCUMENTS/Biocides/ANNEX_I/ASSESSMENT_REPORTS/AnnexI_AR_1085-98-9_PT08_en.pdf

Cifone, M. A. (1985). Mutagenicity evaluation of KUE 13032 C (VM) - c.n. Dichlofluanid - in the mouse lymphoma forward mutations assay. Litton Bionetics, USA; Bayer AG. Unpublished report No. R 3327. Bayer CropScience AG [online]. Available from: URL: http://ecb.jrc.it/DOCUMENTS/Biocides/ANNEX_I/ASSESSMENT_REPORTS/AnnexI_AR_1085-98-9_PT08_en.pdf

Clare, A. S., Rittschof, D., Gerhart, D. J. & Maki, J. S. (1992). Molecular approaches to non-toxic antifouling. *Invertebr. Reprod. Dev., 22,* 1-3, 67-76.

Corbertt, J. R., Wright, K. & Baillie, A. C. (1984). *The biochemical mode of action of pesticides* (2nd edition). London: Academic Press. 382 p.

Cresswell, T., Richards, J. P., Glegg, G. A. & Readman, J. W. (2006). The impact of legislation on the usage and environmental concentrations of Irgarol 1051 in UK coastal waters. *Mar. Pollut. Bull., 52,* 10, 1169-1175.

Crommentuijn, T., Sijm, D., De Bruijn, J., Van Leeuwen, K. & Van de Plassche, E. (2000). Maximum permissible and negligible concentrations for some organic substances and pesticides. *J. Environ. Manage, 58,* 297-312.

Davídek, J., Hajslová, J. & Svobodová, Z. (1981). The stability of dichlofluanid and vinclozolin and their influence on the quality of strawberries. *Z. Lebensm. Unters. Forsch., 172,* 5, 368-372.

Eben, A. & Kimmerle, G. (1968). Studies on the metabolism of Bayer 47531. Unpublished Report No. 856 prepared and submitted by the Institute of Toxicology, Farbenfabriken Bayer AG [online]. Available from: URL: http://www.inchem.org/documents/jmpr/jmpmono/v074pr14.htm

Egea González, F. J., Castro Cano, M. L., Martínez Vidal, J. L. & Martínez Galera, M. (1997). Analyses of chlorothalonil and dichlofluanid in greenhouse air. *J. AOAC. Int., 80,* 5, 1091-1097.

Fernandez-Alba, A. R., Piedra, L., Mezcua, M. & Hernando, M. D. (2002). Toxicity of single and mixed contaminants in seawater measured with acute toxicity bioassays. *Sci. World J., 2,* 1115-1120.

Flucke, W. (1978). Euparen (KU 13032c): Studies for acute toxicity to rats, mice, guinea pigs, rabbits and cats. Bayer AG. Unpublished report No. 8004. Bayer CropScience AG [online]. Available from: URL: http://ecb.jrc.it/DOCUMENTS/ Biocides/ANNEX_I/ASSESSMENT_REPORTS/AnnexI_AR_1085-98-9_PT08_en.pdf

Forbis, A. D. (1986). Acute flow-through toxicity of Preventol A 4-S to *Daphnia magna.* ABC Laboratoriem Inc., USA; Bayer AG. Unpublished report No. 778. Bayer Chemicals AG [online]. Available from: URL: http://ecb.jrc.it/ DOCUMENTS/Biocides/ANNEX_I/ASSESSMENT_REPORTS/AnnexI_AR_1085-98-9_PT08_en.pdf

Frazier, S., Schoen, L. T. & Franklin, B. B. (1986). Acute flow-through toxicity of Preventol A4-S to *Daphnia magna.* Unpublished report No. 34804 (report provided by Bayer AG), Analytical Biochemistry Laboratories Inc. [online]. Available from: URL: http://ecb.jrc.it/DOCUMENTS/Biocides/ANNEX_I/ASSESSMENT_REPORTS/AnnexI_AR_1085-98-9_PT08_en.pdf

Fromme, H., Mattulat, A., Lahrz, T. & Ruden, H. (2005). Occurrence of organotin compounds in house dust in Berlin (Germany). *Chemosphere, 58,* 10, 1377-1383.

Fussell, R. J., Jackson Addie, K., Reynolds, S. L. & Wilson, M. F. (2002). Assessment of the stability of pesticides during cryogenic sample processing. 1. Apples. *J. Agric. Food Chem., 50,* 3, 441-448.

Fussell, R. J., Hetmanski, M. T., Macarthur, R., Findlay, D., Smith, F., Ambrus, A. & Brodesser, P. J. (2007). Measurement uncertainty associated with sample processing of oranges and tomatoes for pesticide residue analysis. *J. Agric. Food Chem., 55,* 4, 1062-1070.

Garcia-Aguirre, G. & Moreno-Martinez, E. (1987). The effect of fungicides *in vitro* on different species of *Aspergillus*. *Anales-del-Instituto-de-Biologia-Universidad-Nacional-Autonoma-de-Mexico-Botanica, 54,* 23-27.

Gimeno, R. A., Aguilar, C., Marcé, R. M. & Borrull, F. (2001). Monitoring of antifouling agents in water samples by on-line solid-phase extraction-liquid chromatography-atmospheric pressure chemical ionization mass spectrometry. *J. Chromatogr. A., 915,*1-2, 139-147.

Grau, R. (1989). Toxizitaït Von Dichlofluanid Techn. (VM 90) füir Regenbogenforellen (*Salmo Gairdneri*) Bei Verlaïngerter Exposition (21 Tage), pp. 15. Report no. FF-246 (report provided by Bayer AG), Bayer AG Pflanzenschutz Anwendungstechnik, Institute of Environmental Biology [online]. Available from: URL: http://ecb.jrc.it/ DOCUMENTS/Biocides/ANNEX_I/ASSESSMENT_REPORTS/AnnexI_AR_1085-989_PT08_en.pdf

Hamwijk, C., Schouten, A., Foekema, E. M., Ravensberg, J. C., Collombon, M. T., Schmidt, K. & Kugler, M. (2005). Monitoring of the booster biocide dichlofluanid in water and marine sediment of Greek marinas. *Chemosphere, 60,* 9, 1316-1324.

Hansson C. & Wallengren J. (1995). Allergic contact dermatitis from dichlofluanid. *Contact Dermatitis, 32,* 116.

Harino, H., Yamamoto, Y., Eguchi, S., Kawai, S., Kurokawa, Y., Arai, T., Ohji, M., Okamura, H. & Miyazaki, N. (2007). Concentrations of antifouling biocides in sediment and mussel samples collected from Otsuchi bay, Japan. *Arch. Environ. Contam. Toxicol., 52,* 2, 179-188.

Heil, J., Reifferscheid, G., Hellmich, D., Hergenroder, M. & Zahn, R. K. (1991). Genotoxicity of the fungicide dichlofluanid in seven assays. *Environ. Mol. Mutagen.,* 17, 20-26.

Heimbach, F. (1983). Acute toxicity of dichlofluanid (90 % Premix) to Water Fleas, pp. 7. Unpublished report No. Hb/Dm 21 (report provided by Bayer AG), Bayer AG Pflanzenschutz Anwendungstechnik, Instistitute of Environmental Biology [online]. Available from: URL: http://ecb.jrc.it/DOCUMENTS/Biocides/ANNEX_I/ ASSESSMENT_REPORTS/AnnexI_AR_1085-989_PT08_en.pdf

Heimbach, F. (1985). Growth inhibition of Green Algae (*Scenedesmus subspicatus*) by Dichlofluanid (90 % Premix). Unpublished report No. HBF/Al 13. Bayer CropScience AG [online]. Available from: URL: http://ecb.jrc.it/DOCUMENTS/ Biocides/ANNEX_I/ASSESSMENT_REPORTS/AnnexI_AR_1085-98-9_PT08_en.pdf

Herbold, B. (1978). KUE 13032 C - Micronucleus test for mutagenic effects on mice. Unpublished report No. 8027. Bayer CropScience AG [online]. Available from: URL: http://ecb.jrc.it/DOCUMENTS/Biocides/ANNEX_I/ASSESSMENT_REPORTS/AnnexI _AR_1085-98-9_PT08_en.pdf

Herbold, B. (1979). KUE 13032 C - Cytogenetic studies of spermatogoniae of Chinese hamsters to test for mutagenic effects. Unpublished Report No. 8432. Bayer CropScience AG [online]. Available from: URL: http://ecb.jrc.it/DOCUMENTS/Biocides/ ANNEX_I/ASSESSMENT_REPORTS/AnnexI_AR_1085-98-9_PT08_en.pdf

Herbold, B. (1984). KUE 13032 C - Dichlofluanid - Salmonella/microsome test to evaluate for potential point mutation. Unpublished report No. 12834 Bayer CropScience AG.

Available from: Directive 98/8/EC concerning the placing of biocidal products on the market. *Inclusion of active substances in Annex I to Directive 98/8/EC.* Assessment Report. DICHLOFLUANID. PT8. November 2006. [online]. URL: http://ecb.jrc.it/ DOCUMENTS/Biocides/ANNEX_I/ ASSESSMENT_REPORTS/AnnexI_AR_1085-98-9_PT08_en.pdf

Herbold, B. (1986a). KUE 13032 C - c.n. Dichlofluanid - *In vitro* cytogenetic study on human lymphocyte cultures to evaluate for chromosome-damaging effects. Unpublished report No. 14707. Bayer CropScience AG [online]. Available from: URL: http://ecb.jrc.it/DOCUMENTS/Biocides/ANNEX_I/ASSESSMENT_REPORTS/AnnexI_AR_1085-98-9_PT08_en.pdf

Herbold, B. (1986b). KUE 13032 C - Dichlofluanid - Dominant lethal test on the male mouse to assess for mutagenic effects. Unpublished report No. 15150. Bayer CropScience AG [online]. Available from: URL: http://ecb.jrc.it/ DOCUMENTS/Biocides/ANNEX_I/ ASSESSMENT_REPORTS/AnnexI_AR_1085-98-9_PT08_en.pdf

Herbold, B. (1988). KUE 13032 C - c.n. Dichlofluanid - Spot Test on cross-bred C57B1/6J x T stock mouse fetuses to evaluace for induced somatic changes in the genes of the coat pigment cells. Unpublished report No. 16753. Bayer CropScience AG [online]. Available from: URL: http://ecb.jrc.it/DOCUMENTS/Biocides/ANNEX_I/ASSESSMENT_REPORTS/AnnexI_AR_1085-98-9_PT08_en.pdf

Hernando, M. D., Ejerhoon, M., Fernandez-Alba, A. R. & Chisti, Y. (2003). Combined toxicity effects of MTBE and pesticides measured with *Vibrio fischeri* and *Daphnia magna* bioassays. *Water Res., 37,* 17, 4091-4098.

Holovská, V., Pistl, J. & Kovalkovičová N. (2007). *In vitro* effect of pesticides (dichlofluanid, endosulfan, simazine, tolylfluanid and triallate) on proliferative activity of animal derived cell cultures. *Acta Biol. Hung., 58,* 1, 61-74.

Holzum, B. (1992). KUE 13032 C (c.n. Dichlofluanid) - Supplementary two-generation study on rats. Unpublished report No. 21922. Bayer CropScience AG [online]. Available from: URL: http://ecb.jrc.it/DOCUMENTS/Biocides/ANNEX_I/ASSESSMENT_REPORTS/ AnnexI_AR_1085-98-9_PT08_en.pdf

Jansma, J. W. & Linders, J. (1992). Dichlofluanide. Advisory report No. 88/678801/090 (In Dutch). Cit.: van Wezel, A. P. & van Vlaardingen, P. (2004). Environmental risk limits for antifouling substances. *Aquat. Toxicol., 66,* 4, 427-444.

Jørgensen, Ch. E. (2001). Wood preservative ruined 200 homes. Chemical Awareness, 2001, Issue 17, [online]. Available from: URL: www. fluorideaction. net/pesticides/ dichlofluanid.denmark.poiso.htm - 6k -

Kiil, S., Dam-Johansen, K., Weinell, C. E., Pedersen, M. S. & Codolar, S. A. (2003). Estimation of polishing and leaching behaviour of antifouling paints using mathematical modelling: a literature review. *Biofouling, 19*, Suppl., 37-43.

Kim, Y. M., Lee, C. H., Kim, H. G. & Lee, H. S. (2004). Anthraquinones isolated from *Cassia tora* (Leguminosae) seed show an antifungal property against phytopathogenic fungi. *J. Agric. Food Chem., 52,* 20, 6096-6100.

Kobayashi, N. & Okamura, H. (2002). Effects of new antifouling compounds on the development of sea urchin. *Mar. Pollut. Bull., 44*, 8, 748-751.

Kohout, F. (1975). Poisoning of a puma with the fungicide dichlofluanid. *Zentralbl. Veterinarmed. A.*, *22*, 3, 256-259.

Konstantinou, I. K & Albanis, T. A. (2004). Worldwide occurrence and effects of antifouling paint booster biocides in the aquatic environment: a review. *Environ. Int.*, *30,* 2, 235-248.

Kovalkovičová, N., Šutiaková, I., Šulík, E., Sakalíková, A., Kačmár, P., Legáth, J., Mlynarčíková, H., Pistl, J. & Mikula, I. (2001). Induction of micronuclei in sheep lymphocyte cultures by the fungicide dichlofluanid. In: 21th International Symposium „Industrial Toxicology '01", May 30th - June 1th, 2001, Bratislava, Slovak Republic, 33-37 (ISBN 80-968011-5-5).

Krajnc, E. I., Wester, P. W., Loeber, J. G., Van Leeuwen, F. X. R., Vos, J. G., Vaessen, H. A. M. G. & Van der Heijden, C. A. (1984). Toxicity of bis(tri-n-butyltin)oxide in the rat. I. Short-term effects on general parameters and on the endocrine and lymphoid systems. *Toxicol. Appl. Pharmacol.*, *75,* 363-386.

Kroetlinger, F. (1990). KUE 13032 C 90 VM 00670/1146 B (c.n. Dichlofluanid) - Study for acute oral toxicity in rats. Bayer AG. Unpublished report No. 19247. Bayer CropScience AG [online]. Available from: URL: http://ecb.jrc.it/ DOCUMENTS/Biocides/ANNEX_I/ ASSESSMENT_REPORTS/AnnexI_AR_1085-98-9_PT08_en.pdf

Kugler, M. (2005). Booster biocides for antifouling products. Stricter environmental demands change the market. *Chemistry Today, 23,* 6, Focus on Biocides, X-XII.

Lambropoulou, D. A., Konstantinou, I. K. & Albanis, T. A. (2000). Determination of fungicides in natural waters using solid-phase microextraction and gas chromatography coupled with electron-capture and mass spectrometric detection. *J. Chromatogr. A., 893,* 1, 143-156.

Lambropoulou, D. A., Sakkas, V. A. & Albanis, T. A. (2003). Determination of antifouling compounds in marine sediments by solid-phase microextraction coupled to gas chromatography-mass spectrometry. *J. Chromatogr. A., 1010*, 1, 1-8.

Lambropoulou, D. A. & Albanis, T. A. (2004). Application of solvent microextraction in a single drop for the determination of new antifouling agents in waters. *J. Chromatogr. A., 1049*, 1-2, 17-23.

Lehn, H. (1988a). KUE 13032 C - Dichlofluanid - Mutagenicity study for the detection of induced forward mutations in the CHO-HGPRT assay *in vitro.* Unpublished report No. 17239. Bayer CropScience AG [online]. Available from: URL: http://ecb.jrc.it/ DOCUMENTS/Biocides/ANNEX_I/ASSESSMENT_ REPORTS/AnnexI_AR_1085-98-9_PT08_en.pdf

Lehn, H. (1988b). KUE 13032 C - Dichlofluanid - Mutagenicity study for the detection of induced forward mutations in the V79-HGPRT assay *in vitro.* Unpublished report No. 17127. Bayer CropScience AG [online]. Available from: URL: http://ecb.jrc.it/ DOCUMENTS/Biocides/ANNEX_I/ASSESSMENT_ REPORTS/AnnexI_AR_1085-98-9_PT08_en.pdf

Lehotay, S. J., Mastovská, K. & Lightfield, A. R. (2005). Use of buffering and other means to improve results of problematic pesticides in a fast and easy method for residue analysis of fruits and vegetables. *J. AOAC. Int., 88,* 2, 615-629.

Leser, K. H. (1993a). KUE 13032 C (Dichlofluanid) - Study on chronic toxicity and carcinogenicity in Wistar rats (administration in food over 105 weeks). Report No.

22313. Bayer CropScience AG [online]. Available from: URL: http://ecb.jrc.it/ DOCUMENTS/Biocides/ANNEX_I/ASSESSMENT_REPORTS/AnnexI_AR_1085-98-9_PT08_en.pdf

Leser, K. H. (1993b). KUE 13032 C (Dichlofluanid) - Study for oncogenicity in B6C3F1 mice (administration in feed over 2 years). Report No. 22679. Bayer CropScience AG [online]. Available from: URL: http://ecb.jrc.it/ DOCUMENTS/Biocides/ANNEX_I/ ASSESSMENT_REPORTS/AnnexI_AR_1085-98-9_PT08_en.pdf

Links, I., Van Der Jagt, K. E., Christopher, Y., Lurvink, M., Schinkel, J., Tielemans, E. & Van Hemmen, J. J. (2007). Occupational exposure during application and removal of antifouling paints. *Ann. Occup. Hyg., 51,* 2, 207-218.

Lorke, D., Loeser, E. (1966). Bayer 47531 – Subchronic toxicological study on dogs. Report from the Institute of Toxicology, Bayer CropScience AG [online]. Available from: URL: http://www.inchem.org/documents/jmpr/jmpmono/ v074pr14.htm

Maraldo, K. & Dahllof, I. (2004). Indirect estimation of degradation time for zinc pyrithione and copper pyrithione in seawater. *Mar. Pollut. Bull., 48,* 9-10, 894-901.

Marchal-Ségault, D. (1993). The effect of commercial preparations of benlate, dithane M-45, copper sulfate and dichlofluanid on the fertility of *Drosophila melanogaster* meigen. *J. Environ. Sci. Health B., 28,* 4, 397-411.

Marchal-Ségault, D. & Laugé, G. (1997). Ovarian activity of *Drosophila melanogaster* Meigen (Diptera), during a chronic intoxication with four fungicides: anatomical and cytological study. *J. Environ. Sci. Health B., 32,* 3, 411-428.

Martínez, K., Ferrer, I. & Barceló, D. (2000). Part-per-trillion level determination of antifouling pesticides and their byproducts in seawater samples by off-line solid-phase extraction followed by high-performance liquid chromatography-atmospheric pressure chemical ionization mass spectrometry. *J. Chromatogr. A., 879,* 1, 27-37.

Martínez, K. & Barceló, D. (2001). Determination of antifouling pesticides and their degradation products in marine sediments by means of ultrasonic extraction and HPLC-APCI-MS. Fresenius *J. Anal. Chem., 370*, 7, 940-945.

Martínez, K., Ferrer, I., Hernando, M. D., Fernandez-Alba, A. R., Marce, R. M., Borrull, F. & Barcelo, D. (2001). Occurrence of antifouling biocides in the Spanish Mediterranean marine environment. *Technol., 22,* 5, 543-552.

Moriya, M., Ohta, T., Watanabe, K., Miyazawa, T., Kato, K. & Shirasu, Y. (1983). Further mutagenicity studies on pesticides in bacterial reversion assay systems. *Mutat. Res., 116,* 185-216.

Okamura, H. (2002). Photodegradation of the antifouling compounds Irgarol 1051 and Diuron released from a commercial antifouling paint. *Chemosphere, 48,* 1, 43-50.

Omae I. (2003). Organotin antifouling paints and their alternatives. *Appl. Organometal. Chem., 17,* 81-105.

Pauluhn, J. (1982). KUE 13032 C (Dichlofluanid) - Studies to determine a primary irritant effect on the skin and mucous membranes. Unpublished study No: T 9010818. Bayer CropScience AG [online]. Available from: URL: http://ecb.jrc.it/DOCUMENTS/ Biocides/ANNEX_I/ASSESSMENT_REPORTS/AnnexI_AR_1085-98-9_PT08_en.pdf

Peñalver, A., Pocurull, E., Borrull, F. & Marcé, R. M. (1999). Solid-phase microextraction of the antifouling Irgarol 1051 and the fungicides dichlofluanid and 4-chloro-3-methylphenol in water samples. *J. Chromatogr. A., 839,* 1-2, 253-260.

Penninks, A. H., Snoeij, N. J., Peiters, R. H. H. & Seinen, W. (1990). Effect of organotin compounds on lymphoid organs and lymphoid functions: An overview. In: A. D. Dayan, R. F. Hertel, E. Heseltine, G. Kazantzis, E. M. Smith & M. T. Van der Venne (Eds.). *Immunotoxicity of metals and immunotoxicology* (1st edition, 191). New York: Plenum Press.

Pistl, J., Kovalkovičová, N., Legáth, J., Novotný, J., Holovská, V. & Mikula, I. (2002). Metabolic activity of sheep peripheral blood phagocytes after exposure to selected pesticides *in vitro*. *Bull. Vet. Inst. Pulawy, 46,* 247-253.

Pistl, J., Kovalkovičová, N., Holovská, V., Legáth, J. & Mikula, I. (2003). Determination of the immunotoxic potential of pesticides on functional activity of sheep leukocytes *in vitro*. *Toxicology, 188,* 1, 73-81.

Ramon, M. & Amor, M. J. (2001). Increasing imposex in populations of *Bolinus brandaris* (Gastropoda: Muricidae) in the northwestern *Mediterranean. Mar. Environ. Res., 52,* 5, 463-475.

Ranke, J. & Jastorff, B. (2000). Multidimensional risk analysis of antifouling biocides. *Environ. Sci. Pollut. R., 7,* 2, 105-114.

Rial-Otero, R., Arias-Estévez, M., López-Periago, E., Cancho-Grande, B. & Simal-Gándara, J. (2005). Variation in concentrations of the fungicides tebuconazole and dichlofluanid following successive applications to greenhouse-grown lettuces. *J. Agric. Food Chem., 53,* 11, 4471-4475.

Ribeiro, C., Veríssimo, I., Moniz, L., Cardoso, H., Sousa, M. J., Soares, A. M. V. M. & Leão, C. (2000). Yeasts as a model for assessing the toxicity of the fungicides Penconazol, Cymoxanil and Dichlofluanid. *Chemosphere, 41,* 10, 1637-1642.

Ritter, A. (1989). Influence of Dichlofluanid on the reproduction of *Daphnia magna*. RCC Umweltchemie AG, Switzerland; Bayer AG. Unpublished report No. 232841. Bayer CropScience AG [online]. Available from: URL: http://ecb.jrc.it/ DOCUMENTS/ Biocides/ANNEX_I/ASSESSMENT_REPORTS/AnnexI_AR_1085-98-9_PT08_en.pdf

Rouhi, A. M. (1998). The squeeze in tributyltins. *Chem. Eng. News, 27,* 41-42.

RTECS (1990). Registry of Toxic Effects of Chemical Substances (published by the National Institute for Occupational Safety and Health); data taken from: CHEM-BANK, CD-ROM Information System. SilverPlatter Information, Inc., Newton Lower Falls, Ma, USA, 1990.

Rudel, H. (2003). Case study: bioavailability of tin and tin compounds. *Ecotoxicol. Environ. Safety, 56,* 1, 180-189.

Sadlo, S. & Rupak, J. (1991). Study of penetration to surface waters of pesticides used for protection of greenhouse plants. *Rocz. Panstw. Zakl. Hig., 42,* 163-166.

Sakkas, V. A., Konstantinou, I. K. & Albanis, T. A. (2001). Photodegradation study of the antifouling booster biocide dichlofluanid in aqueous media by gas chromatographic techniques. *J. Chromatogr. A., 930,* 135-144.

Sakkas, V. A., Konstantinou, I. K., Lambropoulou, D. A. & Albanis, T. A. (2002). Survey for the occurrence of antifouling paint booster biocides in the aquatic environment of Greece. *Environ. Sci. Pollut. Res. Int., 9,* 5, 327-332.

Sas-Piotrowska, B. & Piotrowski, W. (1997). The reaction of *Trichoderma* spp. to synthetic and natural pesticide compounds. A. Fungicides and their compositions. *Roczniki Nauk Rolniczych, Seria E, ochrona Rostlin, 26,* 93-101.

Sedokur, L. K. (1986). No. 31 Euparen. In: A. V. Pavlova, (Eds). *Spravočnik po pesticidam. Gigijena primenenija i toksikologija* (3rd edition, pp. 53-54) (in Russian). Kiev: Urozaj.

Seifert, J., Blattný, C., Henzlerová, H. & Davídek, J. (1978). Persistence of fungicide Euparen on strawberry and/or in some canned products of strawberry. *Bull. Environ. Contam. Toxicol., 20,* 5, 702-706.

Shiotsuka, R. N. (1986). Acute inhalation toxicity study with Preventol A 4-S Dust in rats. Mobay Corp., USA. Bayer AG. Unpublished report No. 763, Bayer Chemicals AG [online]. Available from: URL: http://ecb.jrc.it/ DOCUMENTS/Biocides/ANNEX_I/ ASSESSMENT_REPORTS/AnnexI_AR_1085-98-9_PT08_en.pdf

Shirasu, Y., Moriya, M. & Watanabe, T. (1978). Mutagenicity study of Euparen on bacterial systems. Agricultural Chemicals Inst. Japan Bayer Chemicals AG [online]. Available from: URL: http://ecb.jrc.it/ DOCUMENTS/Biocides/ ANNEX_I/ASSESSMENT_ REPORTS/AnnexI_AR_1085-98-9_PT08_en.pdf

Snoeij, N. J., Penninks, A. H. & Seinen, W. (1988). Dibutyltin and tributyltin compounds induce thymic atrophy in rats due to a selective action on thymic lymphoblasts. *Int. J. Immunopharmacol., 10,* 889-891.

Soleas, G. J., Yan, J., Hom, K. & Goldberg, D. M. (2000). Multiresidue analysis of seventeen pesticides in wine by gas chromatography with mass-selective detection. *J. Chromatogr. A., 882,* 1-2, 205-212.

Stubblefield, W. A. (1986a). Acute oral LD_{50} of Preventol A4-S to Bobwhite Quail. Mobay Corp., USA; Bayer AG. Unpublished report No. 770. Bayer Chemicals AG [online]. Available from: URL: http://ecb.jrc.it/ DOCUMENTS/Biocides/ANNEX_I/ ASSESSMENT_REPORTS/AnnexI_AR_1085-98-9_PT08_en.pdf

Stubblefield, W. A. (1986b). Subacute dietary LC_{50} of Preventol A4-S to Bobwhite Quail. Mobay Corp., USA; Bayer AG. Unpublished report No. 773, Bayer Chemicals AG [online]. Available from: URL: http://ecb.jrc.it/DOCUMENTS/Biocides/ ANNEX_I/ASSESSMENT_REPORTS/AnnexI_AR_1085-98-9_PT08_en.pdf

Stubblefield, W. A. (1986c). Subacute dietary LC_{50} of Preventol A4-S to Mallard Ducks. Mobay Corp., USA. Bayer AG. Unpublished report No. 775, Bayer Chemicals AG [online]. Available from: URL: http://ecb.jrc.it/DOCUMENTS/ Biocides/ANNEX_I/ ASSESSMENT_REPORTS/AnnexI_AR_1085989_PT08_e.pdf

Suzuki, T., Komatsu, M. & Isono, H. (1997). Cytotoxicity of organochlorine pesticides and lipid peroxidation in isolated rat hepatocytes. *Biol. Pharm. Bull., 20,* 1997, 271-274.

Swigert, J., Bunch, B. & Schuster, L. (1986a). Acute flow-through toxicity of Preventol A4-S to Bluegill sunfish *(Lepomis macrochirus)*, p. 161. Report No. 34802 (report provided by Bayer AG), Analytical Biochemistry Laboratories Inc. [online]. Available from: URL: http://ecb.jrc.it/DOCUMENTS/Biocides/ANNEX_I/ASSESSMENT_REPORTS/AnnexI _AR_1085-98-9_PT08_en.pdf

Swigert, J., Bunch, B. & Schuster, L. (1986b). Acute flow-through toxicity of Preventol A4-S to Rainbow trout (*Salmo gairdneri*), p. 119. Report No. 34803 (report provided by Bayer AG), Analytical Biochemistry Laboratories Inc. [online]. Available from: URL: http://ecb.jrc.it/DOCUMENTS/Biocides/ANNEX_I/ASSESSMENT_REPORTS/AnnexI_AR_1085-98-9_PT08_en.pdf

Tanabe, S., Prudente, M., Mizuno, T., Hasegawa, J., Iwata, H. & Miyazaki, N. (1998). Butyltin contamination in marine mammals from North Pacific and Asian coastal waters. *Environ. Sci. Technol., 32*, 2, 193-198.

Tanabe, S. (1999). Butyltin contamination in marine mammals - A review. *Mar. Pollut. Bull., 39*, 62-72.

ten Hallers-Tjabbes, C., Kemp, J. F. & Boon, J. P. (1994). Imposex in whelks (*Buccinum undatum*) from the open North Sea: Relation to shipping traffic intensities. *Mar. Pollut. Bull., 28*, 311-313.

The Pesticide Manual (2000). Berkshire, UK: C.D.S. Tomlin, BCPC Publications, 1276 p. ISBN 1-901396-12-6.

Thomas, K. V., McHugh, M. & Waldock, M. (2002). Antifouling paint booster biocides in UK coastal waters: inputs, occurrence and environmental fate. *Sci. Total Environ., 293,* 1-3, 117-127.

Thomas, K. V., McHugh, M., Hilton, M. & Waldock, M. (2003). Increased persistence of antifouling paint biocides when associated with paint particles. *Environ. Pollut., 123,* 1, 153-161.

U.S. Naval Institute (1981). Marine fouling and its prevention. Annapolis: Wood Hole Oceanographic Institute, U.S. Naval Institute, 1981, 165-205.

Van Loveren, H., Krajnc, E. I., Rombout, P. J. A., Blommaert, F. A. & Vos, J. G. (1990). Effects of ozone, hexachlorobenzene, and bis(tri-n-butyltin)oxide on natural killer activity in the rat lung. *Toxicol. Appl. Pharmacol., 102,* 21-33.

van Wezel, A. P. & van Vlaardingen, P. (2004). Environmental risk limits for antifouling substances. *Aquat. Toxicol., 66,* 4, 427-444.

Visser, T. (1993). *Infrared spectra of pesticides.* New York-Basel Hong Kong: Marcel Dekker, Inc., 425 p.

Vos, J. G., De Klerk, A., Krajnc, E. I., Kruizinga, W., Van Ommen, B. & Rozing, J. (1984). Toxicity of bis(tri-n-butyltin)oxide in the rat. II. Suppression of thymus-dependent immune responses and of parameters of nonspecific resistance after short-term exposure. *Toxicol. Appl. Pharmacol., 75,* 387-408.

Vos, J. G., De Klerk, A., Krajnc, E. I., Van Loveren, H. & Rozing, J. (1990). Immunotoxicity of bis(tri-n-butyltin)oxide in the rat: Effects on thymus-dependent-immunity and non-specific resistance following long-term exposure in young versus aged rats. *Toxicol. Appl. Pharmacol., 105,* 144-155.

Voulvoulis, N., Scrimshaw, M. D. & Lester, J. N. (2002a). Comparative environmental assessment of biocides used in antifouling paints. *Chemosphere, 47,* 7, 789-795.

Voulvoulis, N., Scrimshaw, M. D. & Lester, J. N. (2002b). Partitioning of selected antifouling biocides in the aquatic environment. *Mar. Environ. Res., 53,* 1, 1-16.

Will, F. & Krüger, E. (1999). Fungicide residues in strawberry processing. *J. Agric. Food Chem., 47,* 3, 858-861.

Wojdyla, A. T. (2003). Activity of some chemicals in the control of *Botrytis cinerea* on roses. *Commun. Agric. Appl. Biol. Sci., 68,* 4 Pt B, 711-715.

www.fluorideaction.org

Yamano, T. & Morita, S. (1993). Effects of pesticides on isolated rat hepatocytes, mitochondria, and microsomes. *Arch. Environ. Contam. Toxicol., 25,* 271-278.

Yebra, D. M., Kiil, S. & Dam-Johansen, K. (2004). Antifouling technology - Past, present and future steps towards efficient and environmentally friendly antifouling coatings. *Prog. Org. Coat., 50*, 2, 75-104.

In: Fungicides
Editors: P. De Costa and P. Bezerra

ISBN: 978-1-60692-631-4

Chapter V

EFFECT OF TOLYLFLUANID ON MICRONUCLEUS INDUCTION IN SHEEP PERIPHERAL BLOOD LYMPHOCYTES *IN VITRO*

***I. Šutiaková*[1,*], *N. Kovalkovičová*[2,†], *J. Legáth*[2], *V Šutiak*[2]**
[1]University of Prešov, Ul. 17. Novembra 1, 081 16 Prešov, Slovak Republic
[2]University of Veterinary Medicine, Komenského 73, 041 81 Košice, Slovak Republic

ABSTRACT

Micronucleus assay is a widely used test in evaluating the genotoxic consequences of exposures to environmental and occupational contaminants. In this study a fungicide tolylfluanid was investigated for its ability to induce micronuclei *in vitro* using sheep peripheral lymphocytes. Lymphocyte cultures from three donors were exposed to three different concentrations of fungicide (1×10^{-4}, 1×10^{-5} and 1×10^{-6} M/L) for 48 h. At the lowest concentration (1×10^{-6} M/L) the frequency of micronuclei was not significantly different (32.33 ± 3.51/1000 binucleated cells at this concentration versus 30.33±2.82/1000 binucleated cells in DMSO control, P = 0.44). Higher concentrations of fungicide (1×10^{-4} and 1×10^{-5} M/L) resulted in a significant dose dependent increase in the number of micronuclei in comparison with control (74.0 ± 13.0/1000 binucleated cells and 52.67 ± 10.12/1000 binucleated cells versus 30.33±2.82/1000 binucleated cells in DMSO control, P = 0.005 and 0.020, respectively, Anova test). Many of the treated cells also possessed multiple micronuclei. Tolylfluanid did not affect nuclear division index (NDI) at all treatment concentrations. Our results thus demonstrate a weak genotoxic effect of tolylfluanid in sheep peripheral lymphocytes *in vitro*.

Keywords: genotoxicity; micronucleus assay; fungicides; tolylfluanid; sheep peripheral lymphocytes

* E-mail: sutiakova@pobox.sk
† E-mail: kovalkovicova@uvm.sk

1. INTRODUCTION

Agronomic practices used in recent years have made the agrarian sector dependent heavily on pesticides. At the present, there are more than 1,000 chemicals classified as pesticides. Pesticides are designed to control target pests, either diseases or weeds. They have undoubtedly increased crop yields and reduced post-harvest losses, but at the same time they represent an important group of environmental pollutants to which man and animals are daily exposed, mainly as a consequence of their wide use in agriculture. Exposure to pesticides is likely to continue and possibly may increase in the near future, because of increased use and their persistence in the environment. Moreover, exposure to pesticides has been related to several diseases including several kinds of cancer, e.g. leukemia, bladder and pancreatic cancer. Cancer is a complex disease in which cells with altered gene expression, grow abnormally, invade other tissues and disrupt their normal function (Fenech, 2002; Norppa et al., 2006; El-Zein et al., 2006). To evaluate genetic damage induced by physical and chemical agents, various test systems have been described in bacteria, plants and in mammalian cells *in vivo* and *in vitro* (Kirkland et al., 2005; Jawich et al., 2006; Gadeva and Dimitrov, 2008). For many years cytogenetic alternations in cultured peripheral blood lymphocytes, such as chromosomal aberrations, sister chromatid exchanges, and micronuclei have been applied as biomarkers of genotoxic exposure and early effects of genotoxic carcinogens (Norppa, 2004). In this regard, particular attention is focused on chromosome aberrations because these are considered as an early warning signal for cancer development (Bonassi et al., 1995, 2000; Hagmar et al., 1998, 2004). The induction of sister chromatid exchanges has also been described as a rapid and sensitive end-point for clastogenicity tests and can be an indicator of persistent DNA damage (Cardoso et al., 2001). Micronuclei are defined as small, round, DNA-containing cytoplasmic bodies formed during cell division by loss of acentric chromatin fragments or whole chromosomes. The cytokinesis-blocked micronucleus assay is a simple and quick test extensively used for both *in vitro* and *in vivo* studies of the environmental genotoxicity. It is considered to be a suitable alternative to the chromosomal aberration assay, with the advantage that exposure to both clastogens and aneugens may be detected. In addition, this assay also allows the detection of effects on cell proliferation and cytotoxicity (Fenech, 2000, 2006). In addition to genotoxicity, stimulation of cellular proliferation may contribute to the carcinogenity of chemicals (Holland et al., 2002).

Pesticides are of great concern for their toxic effects and also for their potential as a long-term genetic hazard. The most problematic pesticides are fungicides since about 90 % of them used currently or formely have been determined to be carcinogenic in experimental animals (Saunders and Harper, 1994). The genotoxicity of many antifungal agents has been investigated *in vivo* and *in vitro*, including pyrimidine fungicides fenarimol (Paolini et al., 1996a,b; Aydemir and Bilaloglu, 2003; Poli et al., 2003; de Castro et al., 2005) and nuarimol (Tyrkiel et al., 1998); carbamate fungicides propamocarb (Aydemir and Bilaloglu, 2003) and thiophanate-methyl (Paolini et al., 1999; Fimognari et al., 1999); dithiocarbamate fungicides maneb (Steenland et al., 1997; Bertini et al., 2000; Osaba et al., 2002), zineb (Gerber et al., 2002; Osaba et al., 2002; Soloneski et al., 2001, 2002a,b, 2003), ferbam (Shanthi and Krishnamoorthy, 2002), thiram (Villani et al., 1998; Andrés et al., 1999), ziram (Crebelli et al., 1992; Franekić et al., 1994), mancozeb (Steenland et al., 1997; Shukla et al., 2004;

Calviello et al., 2005), tetrametylthiuramdisulfide (Rannug and Rannug, 1984), propineb (Rolandi et al., 1984) and zinc dimethyl (Zenzen et al., 2001). Furthermore the genotoxic potential of other fungicides was studied, e.g. benzimidazole fungicides carbendazim (McCarroll et al., 2002; Goumenou and Machera, 2003), thiabendazole (Watanabe-Akanuma et al., 2003, 2005; Vindas et al., 2004) and benomyl (McCarroll et al., 2002; Amer et al., 2003); phthalimide fungicides captan (Goumenou and Machera, 2003; Lebailly et al., 2003; Mouchet et al., 2006), folpet (Quest et al., 1993) and captafol (Rahden-Staron, 2002; Robbiano et al., 2004); aromatic fungicides chlorothalonil (Rosenkranz, 1999; Knopper et al., 2005), hexachlorobenzene (Canonero et al., 1997) and pentachlorophenol (Ateeq et al., 2002); organotin fungicides triphenyltin acetate, triphenyltin hydroxide (Oshiro et al., 1991; Chao et al., 1999) and bis(tri-n-butyltin)oxide – TBTO (Davis et al., 1987); acylamino acid fungicide metalaxyl (Hrelia et al., 1996a, Paolini et al., 1996c; Demsia et al., 2007); dinitrophenol fungicide dinocap (Çelik et al., 2004); oxazole fungicide vinclozolin (Hrelia et al., 1996b; Kevekordes et al., 1996; Lioi et al., 1998a,b; Wu et al., 2005; Zavala-Aguirre et al., 2007). Except of above mentioned fungicides the genotoxic activities have been studied in organomercury fungicide phenylmercury acetate (Lee et al., 1997; 1998); quinone fungicide dithianon (Paolini et al., 1997); dichlorophenyl dicarboximide fungicide procymidone (Hosokawa et al., 1993; Sapone et al., 2003); antibiotic fungicides cycloheximide (Basić-Zaninović et al., 1991), griseofulvin (Albertini et al., 1993) and aureofungin (Mujumdar et al., 1994); organophosphorus fungicides fosetyl (Quest et al., 1991) and pyrazophos (Yüzbaşioğluet et al., 2006); phenylsulphamide fungicide dichlofluanid (Heil et al., 1991); conazole fungicides imazalil (Vindas et al., 2004), hexaconazole (Yilmaz et al., 2008) and triadimefon (Kevekordes et al., 1996); amide fungicide prochloraz (Zelesco et al., 1990) and unclassified fungicides hexachloro (1,3) butadiene (Vamvakas et al., 1988) and o-phenylphenol (Suzuki et al., 1985; Eastmond, 1993; Balakrishnan and Eastmond, 2006; Brusick, 2005). Considering the contradictory results there is a need to allocate more investigations in order to evaluate the potential genotoxic effects of fungicides.

For this study tolylfluanid, 1,1-dichloro-N-[(dimethylamino)-sulfonyl]-1-fluoro-N-(4-methylphenyl) methanesulfenamide, was chosen because it was heavily used in agriculture by the year 2007 and represented one of the most frequently detected pesticides in vegetables and fruit (Nowacka, 2002). Tolylfluanid has a multi-site mode of action against phytophagous mites and fungal diseases caused by *Botrytis, Didymella, Drepanopeziza* in strawberries, raspberries, hops, apples, ribes, vine and tomatoes. It is very rapidly degradated in soil and water and because it is strongly absorbed by soil particules it has no potential to migrate into deeper soil layers (The Pesticide Manual, 2000; EPA, 2002).

However, it has recently been discovered that tolylfluanid can have an unexpected effect on drinking water. Specifically, the use of a certain plant protection product, Euparen M WG which contains tolylfluanid, leads to the formation of a metabolite of tolylfluanid, namely dimethylsulfamide, which is likely to be found in the soil, and in groundwater and surface water. By a standard drinking water preparation process (ozonisation) this metabolite is converted into a nitrosamine (NDMA) which is harmful to health. Therefore Slovakia and other Member States of the European Community have already suspended the outdoor use of products containing tolylfluanid (Commission Decision, 2007). But residues of this fungicide may be present in imported food-stuffs and pose the source of exposure.

In animals tolylfluanid is rapidly absorbed and hydrolysed within 48 h to dimethylamino sulfotoluidide (DMST) and then transformed to the main metabolite 4-(dimethylaminosulfonylamino) benzoic acid which can be further demethylated. There is no accumulation in organs and tissues (Abbink and Weber, 1988). Subchronic and chronic toxicity studies conducted in animals showed altered liver enzyme activities, fluoride and thyroid hormone levels, accompanied by an increased incidence of hyperplastic and neoplastic lesions of the thyroid (primarily adenomas) and damage of renal cortical tubules (PFPC Newsletter Special Issue, 1999). In sheep, tolylfluanid, administered orally, caused anorexia, weakness of the extremities and loose faeces (Hoffmann, 1983).

The data regarding tolylfluanid genotoxicity in animals are limited. In this study an attempt has been made to evaluate the ability of tolylfuanid to induce micronuclei in sheep peripheral lymphocyte cultures *in vitro*.

2. Materials and Methods

2.1. Chemicals

The Tested Pesticide

Tolylfluanid (Sigma-Aldrich, USA, refer to Figure 1 for details on chemical name, formula, molecular weight and CAS number of the tested fungicide) was dissolved in dimethylsulfoxide (DMSO) and freshly prepared before each experiment at concentrations of 1×10^{-4}, 1×10^{-5} and 1×10^{-6} M/L. The final concentration of DMSO in the cultures was 0.5 %. The tested substance was added at 24 h after culture initiation and left until the end of cultivation (48 h treatment time).

The Other Chemicals

Cytochalasin-B (Cyt-B, CAS No. 14930-96-2), mytomycin C (MMC, CAS No. 50-07-7) and dimethylsulfoxide (DMSO, CAS No. 67-68-5), penicillin G (benzylpenicillin sodium salt; CAS No. 200-710-2) were obtained from Sigma, USA. Streptomycin (streptomycin sulfate salt; CAS No. 3810-74-0) was obtained from Sigma-Aldrich, USA. Cyt-B was disolved in DMSO. MMC at a final concentration of 0.25 μg/mL was disolved in distilled water and served as positive control to ensure the validity of the assay. Chromosome medium serumfree Panserin 701 (CAS No. P0 -710701 M), and 7.5 % $NaHCO_3$ were obtained from PAN Systems GmbH, Biotechnologische Producte, Germany. Heparin (heparinum natrium) was obtained from Zentiva, a. s., Czech Republic.

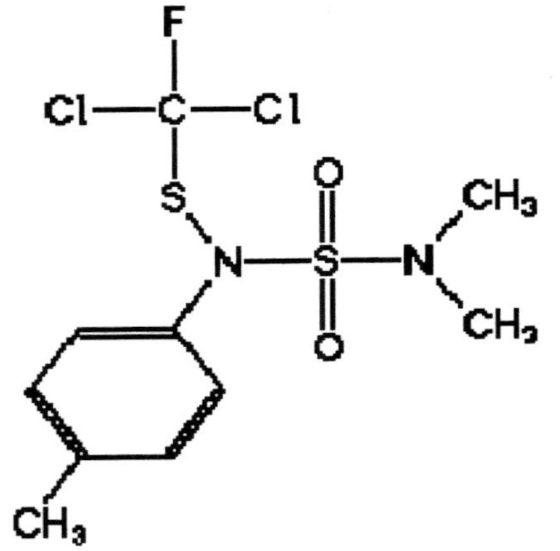

IUPAC name:
N-dichlorofluoromethylthio-*N'*,*N'*-dimethyl-*N*-*p*-tolylsulfamide
CAS name:
1,1-dichloro-*N*-[(dimethylamino)sulfonyl]-1-fluoro-*N*-(4-methylphenyl)methanesulfenamide
CAS registry No.:
[731-27-1]
Molecular formula:
$C_{10}H_{13}Cl_2FN_2O_2S_2$
Molecular Weight:
347.26
Purity:
99.7%

Figure 1. Tolylfluanid chemical data.

2.2. Lymphocyte Cultures

For the micronucleus assay, heparinised blood (100 IU/mL) from 3 clinically healthy donors (18-month-old female Merino sheep), obtained by *jugular vein* puncture, was used. Whole blood 0.4 mL was added to 7.0 mL chromosome medium supplemented with fetal calf serum, phytohemagglutinin-L, L-glutamine, penicillin G (100 IU/mL), streptomycin (100 μg/mL) and 7.5 % $NaHCO_3$.

2.3. Micronucleus Analysis

Lymphocyte cultures were divided into treated cultures, solvent and positive controls and incubated at 37 °C for 72 h. Cytokinesis was blocked by Cyt-B which was added 44 h after culture initiation to get a final concentration of 6 μg/mL. The cells were treated with hypotonic solution (0.035 M KCl) for 20 min at 37 °C and fixed with cold methanol:glacial acetic acid (3:1, v/v). The slides were air-dried and stained with 10 % Giemsa Romanowski in Sörensen phosphate buffer, pH 6.8, for 3–6 min. Using a Nicon microscope (CCD-100 camera system, Mitsubishi) the coded slides were scored blinded at magnifications of 400 x and 1000 x. Micronuclei were counted in 1000 binucleated cells per donor and per concentration and identified using well-known criteria (Countryman and Heddle, 1976; Surallés and Natarajan, 1997; Fenech, 2000; Gillian Clare et al., 2006).

2.4. Nuclear Division Index

Effects on the cellular proliferation rate were estimated by calculating nuclear division index (NDI). 500 lymphocytes per donor (total 1500 lymphocytes) were scored to evaluate the percentage of cells with 1–4 nuclei and NDI was calculated according to Eastmond and Tucker (1987) as

$$NDI = \frac{[M1 + (2M2 + 3M3 + 4M4)]}{N}$$

where M1 – M4 represent the number of cells with one to four nuclei, respectively, and N is the number of cells scored.

2.5. Statistical Analysis

The Sigma Stat program (Statistical software™, Jandel Scientific) was employed for statistical evaluation of the results. The mean frequency of micronuceated cells and the NDIs were calculated based on the results of three independent experiments, and the statistically significant differences between control and treatment values were determined using analysis of variance (ANOVA) followed by Tukey´s test at the 95 % confidence level.

3. Results

Table 1 shows the levels of micronuclei observed in sheep peripheral lymphocytes cultured in the presence of different concentrations of tolylfluanid. At the lowest concentration (1×10^{-6} M/L) the frequency of micronuclei was not significantly different ($P = 0.44$). Higher concentrations of tolylfluanid (1×10^{-4} and 1×10^{-5} M/L) resulted in significant dose dependent increase in the number of micronuclei ($P = 0.005$ and 0.02, respectively, ANOVA test). Many of the treated cells also possessed multiple micronuclei.

The NDI value in sheep peripheral lymphocytes after 48 h exposure to tolylfluanid was not significantly decreased compared with the negative control ($P > 0.05$; Table 2).

Table 1. Induction of micronuclei produced by tolylfluanid in sheep lymphocytes *in vitro*

Test substance	Treatment		Binucleated cells (BN) scored	Distribution of BN cell according to the No. of MN				Total No. of MN	MN/cell	Number of MN per 1000 BN			
	Period (h)			0	1	2	3			Mean	± SD	SEM	P
DMSO (negative control)	48		3000	2920	69	11	0	91/3000	0.030	30.33	2.82	1.20	-
MMC (positive control)	48	0.25 μg/mL	3000	2684	295	19	2	339/3000	0.113	113.00	8.72	5.03	***†
Tolylfluanid	48	1 x10^{-4} M/L	3000	2812	161	20	7	222/3000	0.074	74.00	13.00	7.51	**†
		1 x10^{-5} M/L	3000	2859	126	13	2	158/3000	0.053	52.67	10.12	5.84	*†
		1 x10^{-6} M/L	3000	2911	81	8	0	97/3000	0.032	32.33	3.51	2.03	ns

MN – micronucles; BN – binucleated cell; DMSO – dimethylsulphoxide; MMC – mitomycin C; SD – standard deviation; SEM – standard error mean.

*** Significatly different from the control P =< 0.001 (ANOVA).

** Significatly different from the control P = 0.005 (ANOVA).

* Significatly different from the control P = 0.020 (ANOVA).

† Significantly different from the control P < 0.05 (Tukey test, all pairwise multiple comparison procedures); ns – statistically non-significant difference; P = 0.44 (ANOVA).

Table 2. Nuclear division index (NDI) in sheep peripheral blood lymphocytes after 48 h exposure to tolylfluanid

Test substance	N/donor	NDI			Statistical values			
		A	B	C	Mean	± SD	SEM	P =
DMSO (negative control)	1500	1.20	1.09	1.01	1.101	0.09	0.05	-
MMC (positive control) 0.25 μg/mL	1500	1.08	1.05	1.07	1.065	0.02	0.01	0.55^{ns}
Tolylfluanid 1×10^{-4} M/L	1500	1.16	1.16	1.20	1.171	0.03	0.01	0.27^{ns}
1×10^{-5} M/L	1500	1.15	1.16	1.15	1.152	0.01	0.01	0.39^{ns}
1×10^{-6} M/L	1500	1.11	1.06	1.04	1.069	0.04	0.02	0.61^{ns}

ns – statistically non-significant differences (ANOVA); DMSO – dimethylsulphoxide; MMC – mitomycin C; N – total number of cells scored; A, B, C – donors; ± SD – standard deviation; SEM – standard error mean; P – statistical value.

4. Discussion

The agricultural chemicals marketed to increase food production may not only combat pests and weeds but also present toxic properties and cause genetic damage to the fauna and flora. Large amounts of these chemicals are released into the environment and many of them affect non-target organisms, being a potential hazard to human health. According to Garret et al. (1986) such genotoxic effects are of special concern due to the irreversible nature of the process. Genotoxicity is of interest as a pesticide health effect because most human and animal carcinogens are genotoxic, and genotoxicity may be a useful biomarker as an intermediate endpoint in carcinogenesis (Albertini et al., 2000; Hagmar et al., 2001).

In the past, risk assessment of pesticides was limited to the danger to human health, but currently ecological risks are also taken into account. In this regard, further studies are required in order to determine mechanism of action of pesticides, including how they interfere with metabolism, genetic damage they induce and their detoxification mechanisms in domestic and wildlife animals (Lioi et al., 1998a). About two-thirds to four-fifths of food animals are exposed to toxic substances (Bőhmer et al., 1991) that can be an important risk factors to human health (Cristaldi et al., 2004; Udroiu, 2007). Free living, grazing animals are among the animal groups immediately exposed to and most affected by the harmful influence of pesticides. We have used sheep as a model animal source of peripheral blood leukocytes because they are similar to wild ruminants and are a better indicator of environmental exposure than rodents, which are kept strictly under laboratory conditions.

The mutagenicity of tolylfluanid has not yet been firmly established. It was variably active in a variety of *in vitro* assays, e.g. weakly positive in the Ames test (Herbold, 1979) and positive in the forward mutation test in mouse lymphoma cells (Hoorn, 1985) and in the cytogenetic assay in human lymphocytes (Herbold, 1984a, 2000a). A weakly clastogenic effect of fungicide was observed in chromosomal aberration test in Chinese hamster V79 cells in the presence of S9 activation at 30 h incubation (Herbold, 1996). These studies indicated that tolylfluanid might have a clastogenic effect. On the other hand, there were several negative responses in the *vitro* studies, i.e. in uncheduled DNA synthesis test (Brendler-Schwaab, 1995), gene mutation test in Chinese hamster V79 cell line and ovary cells CHO-K1-BH_4 (Heidemann and Mietenburger, 1987; den Boer, 1987), in reverse mutation test in *Sacharomyces* (Hoorn, 1984) and *S. typhimurium* (Herbold, 1994).

No indications of mutagenic effects on germ cells were observed (Herbold, 1984b; Völkner, 1988a). Most of the *in vivo* tests with somatic cells were negative, i.e. micronucleus formation in mouse (Herbold, 1980) and Chinese hamster bone marrow (Herbold, 1983; 2000b), chromosomal aberration test in Chinese hamster and mouse bone marrow (Völkner, 1990; Herbold, 2004), test of sister chromatid exchanges in NMRI mice (Völkner, 1988b), DNA adduct formation test in Wistar rat lung, liver and thyroid (Calcagnotto et al., 1997). On the other hand, after subchronic oral exposure an induction of structural chromosomal aberrations and micronuclei by this fungicide in sheep lymphocytes was observed (Šutiaková et al., 2006). But in this study the pesticide formulation instead of purified active ingredient was used. All substances contained in this formulation (by-products of the active compound synthesis, adjuvants) that are kept secret by manufacturers might present risk for genetic stability in exposed organisms. Therefore in the present study the pure active ingredient was used to evaluate its genotoxicity by inducing micronuclei in mammalian testing system.

Formation of micronuclei and chromosome aberrations are two important cytogenetic endpoints considered to be biomarkers of early biological effects from exposure to mutagenic agents (Bonassi and Au, 2002; Gao and Zhan, 2007; Baumstark-Khan and Horneck, 2007). Over the past several years the cytokinesis-block micronucleus assay has evolved into a comprehensive method for measuring chromosome breakage, chromosome loss, non-disjuction, necrosis, apoptosis and cytostasis (Fenech, 2006, 2007). Micronuclei are thought to arise from both clastogenic (chromosome breakage) and aneugenic (chromosome lagging and spindle) effects, while structural chromosome aberrations are thought to arise from chromosome breakage and exchange. In this study tolylfluanid significantly increased micronucleus frequency at the higher concentrations tested only (1×10^{-4} and 1×10^{-5} M/L).

Cellular proliferation rate is a phenomenon that may be causally associated with the induction of chromosomal damage for a number of compounds which are non-DNA reactive and thus are treshold *in vitro* clastogens (Müller and Kasper, 2000). One of the parameter of cellular proliferation rate is nuclear division index which can be used for the evaluation of effect of chemicals on cell division (Eastmond and Tucker, 1987, 1989). In our study, nuclear division index was not significantly decreased in exposed lymphocytes in comparison with controls.

Here we report, for the first time to our knowledge, an induction of mitotic micronuclei by tolylfluanid in cultured sheep lymphocytes *in vitro*. We conclude that there is only a weak genotoxic effect of this fungicide in sheep peripheral lymphocytes *in vitro*.

Acknowledgments

This work was supported by VEGA Grant No. 1/0545/08 and the National Reference Laboratory for Pesticides University of Veterinary Medicine in Košice., Slovak Republic.

References

Abbink, J. & Weber, H. (1988). *Phenyl-UL-14C-tolylfluanid: investigation of the biokinetic behaviour in the rat* [online]. Institute of Metabolism Research, Bayer AG. Unpublished report No. 181081-9. Submitted to WHO by Bayer AG, Bayerwerk, FRG. Available from: URL: http://www.inchem.org/documents/ jmpr/jmpmono/ 2002pr13.htm

Albertini, S., Brunner, M. & Würgler, F. E. (1993). Analysis of the six additional chemicals for *in vitro* assays of the European Economic Communities' EEC aneuploidy programme using *Saccharomyces cerevisiae* D61.M and the *in vitro* porcine brain tubulin assembly assay. *Environ. Mol. Mutagen., 21,* 2, 180-192.

Albertini, R. J., Anderson, D., Douglas, G. R., Hagmar, L., Hemminki, K., Merlo, F., Natarajan, A. T., Norppa, H., Shuker, D. E. G., Tice, R., Waters, M. D. & Aitio, A. (2000). IPCS guidelines for the monitoring of genotoxic effects of carcinogens in humans. *Mutat. Res./Rev. Mutat. Res., 463,* 2, 111-172.

Amer, S. M., Donya, S. M. & Aly, F. A. (2003). Genotoxicity of benomyl and its residues in somatic and germ cells of mice fed on treated stored wheat grains. *Arch. Toxicol., 77,* 12, 712-721.

Andrés, J. A, Correa, N. S. & Rosas, S. B. (1999). The mutagenic potential of the fungicide thiram. *Rev. Argent. Microbiol., 31,* 2, 82-86.

Ateeq, B., Abul Farah, M., Niamat Ali, M. & Ahmad, W. (2002). Clastogenicity of pentachlorophenol, 2,4-D and butachlor evaluated by *Allium* root tip test. *Mutat. Res., 514,* 1-2, 105-113.

Aydemir, N. & Bilaloglu, R. (2003). The investigation of the genotoxic effects of fenarimol and propamocarb in mouse bone marrow *in vivo*. *Toxicol. Lett., 147,* 1, 73-78.

Balakrishnan, S. & Eastmond, D. A. (2006). Micronuclei and cell proliferation as early biological markers of ortho-phenylphenol-induced changes in the bladder of male F344 rats. *Food Chem. Toxicol., 44,* 8, 1340-1347.

Basić-Zaninović, T., Papes, D. & Franekić, J. (1991). Cycloheximide genotoxicity in *in vitro* and *in vivo* test systems. *Mutat. Res., 263,* 4, 203-210.

Baumstark-Khan, C. & Horneck, G. (2007). Results from the „technical workshop on genotoxicity biosensing“ on the micro-scale fluorometric assay of deoxyribonucleic acid unwinding. *Anal. Chimica Acta, 593,* 1, 75-81.

Bertini, S., Del Carratore, R., Giorgi, M., Bronzetti, G. & Della Croce, C. (2000). Genotoxic and mono-oxygenase system effects of the fungicide maneb. *Arch. Toxicol., 74,* 7, 415-420.

Böhmer, D., Ujházy, E., Tomo, I., Škorvaga, P. & Balonová, T. (1991). Experimental possibilities for detection of embryotoxicity risk of xenobiotics. *Agrochémia, 31,* 55-57.

Bonassi, S., Abbondandolo, A., Camurri, L., Dal Pra, L., De Ferrari, M. & Degrassi, F. (1995). Are chromosome aberrations in circulating lymphocytes predictive of future cancer onset in humans? Preliminary results of an Italian cohort study. *Cancer Genet. Cytogenet., 79,* 133-135.

Bonassi, S., Hagmar, L., Stromberg, U., Montagud, A. H., Tinnerberg, H. & Forni, A. (2000). Chromosomal aberrations in lymphocytes predict human cancer independently of exposure to carcinogens. European Study Group on Cytogenetic Biomarkers and Health. *Cancer Res., 60,* 1619-1625.

Bonassi, S. & Au, W. W. (2002). Biomarkers in molecular epidemiology studies for health risk prediction. *Mutat. Res./Rev. Mutat. Res., 511,* 1, 73-86.

Brendler-Schwaab, S. (1995). KUE 13183b - Test on unscheduled DNA synthesis in rat liver primary cell cultures *in vitro* [online]. Unpublished report No. 24436 31 October 1995 from Bayer AG, Institute of Toxicology, Wuppertal, Germany. Submitted to WHO by Bayer AG, Bayerwerk, Germany. Available from: URL: http://www.inchem.org/documents/jmpr/jmpmono/2002pr13.htm

Brusick, D. (2005). Analysis of genotoxicity and the carcinogenic mode of action for ortho-phenylphenol. *Environ. Mol. Mutagen., 45,* 5, 460-481.

Calcagnotto, A. M., Jeffrey, A. M. & Luo, F.-Q. (1997). ^{32}P-Postlabelling assay for detection of adduct formation by tolylfluanid (TF) in rat lung, thyroid and liver DNA [online]. Unpublished report No. R6933 25 August 1997 from American Health Foundation. Submitted to WHO by Bayer AG, Bayerwerk, Germany. Available from: URL: http://www.inchem.org/documents/jmpr/jmpmono/ 2002pr13.htm

Calviello, G., Piccioni, E., Boninsegna, A., Tedesco, B., Maggiano, N., Serini, S., Wolf, F. I. & Palozza, P. (2005). DNA damage and apoptosis induction by the pesticide Mancozeb in rat cells: involvement of the oxidative mechanism. *Toxicol. Appl. Pharmacol., 211,* 2, 87-96.

Canonero, R., Campart, G. B., Mattioli, F., Robbiano, L. & Martelli, A. (1997). Testing of p-dichlorobenzene and hexachlorobenzene for their ability to induce DNA damage and micronucleus formation in primary cultures of rat and human hepatocytes. *Mutagenesis, 12,* 1, 35-39.

Cardoso, R. S., Takahashi-Hyodo, S., Peitl, P. Jr, Ghilardi-Neto, T. & Sakamoto-Hojo, E. T. (2001). Evaluation of chromosomal aberrations, micronuclei, and sister chromatid exchanges in hospital workers chronically exposed to ionizing radiation. *Teratog. Carcinog. Mutagen., 21,* 6, 431-439.

Çelik, M., Ünal, F., Yüzbaşıoğlu, D., Ergün, M. A., Arslan, O. & Kasap, R. (2004). *In vitro* effect of karathane LC (dinocap) on human lymphocytes. *Mutagenesis, 20,* 2, 101-104.

Chao, J. S., Wei, L. Y., Huang, M. C., Liang, S. C. & Chen, H. H. (1999). Genotoxic effects of triphenyltin acetate and triphenyltin hydroxide on mammalian cells *in vitro* and *in vivo. Mutat. Res., 444,* 1, 167-174.

Commission Decision of 4 May 2007 laying down protective measures concerning uses of plant protection products containing tolylfluanid leading to the contamination of drinking water *(notified under document number C(2007) 1865)* (Text with EEA relevance), (2007/322/EC) [online]. Official Journal of the European Union, L 119/49, 9.5.2007. Available from: URL: http://eur-lex.europa.eu/LexUriServ/ LexUriServ.do?uri= OJ:L:2007:119:0049:0050:EN:PDF

Countryman, P. I. & Heddle, J. A. (1976). The production of MN from chromosome aberrations in irradiated cultures of human lymphocytes. *Mutat. Res.*, *41,* 321-332.

Crebelli, R., Zijno, A., Conti, L., Crochi, B., Leopardi, P., Marcon, F., Renzi, L. & Carere, A. (1992). Further *in vitro* and *in vivo* mutagenicity assays with thiram and ziram fungicides: Bacterial reversion assays and mouse micronucleus test. *Teratog. Carcinog. Mutagen., 12,* 3, 97-112.

Cristaldi, M., Ieradi, A. L., Udroiu, I. & Zilli, R. (2004). Comparative evaluation of background micronucleus frequencies in domestic mammals. *Mutat. Res., 559,* 1-2, 1-9.

Davis, A., Barale, R., Brun, G., Forster, R., Günther, T., Hautefeuille, H., van der Heijden, C. A., Knaap, A. G., Krowke, R. & Kuroki, T. (1987). Evaluation of the genetic and embryotoxic effects of bis(tri-n-butyltin)oxide (TBTO), a broad-spectrum pesticide, in multiple *in vivo* and *in vitro* short-term tests. *Mutat. Res., 188,* 2, 65-95.

de Castro, V. L., de Mello, M. A., Poli, P. & Zucchi, T. M. (2005). Prenatal and perinatal fenarimol-induced genotoxicity in leukocytes of *in vivo* treated rats. *Mutat. Res., 583,* 1, 95-104.

Demsia, G., Vlastos, D., Goumenou, M. & Matthopoulos, D. P. (2007). Assessment of the genotoxicity of imidacloprid and metalaxyl in cultured human lymphocytes and rat bone-marrow. *Mutat. Res., 634,* 1-2, 32-39.

den Boer, W. C. (1987). Mutagenicity test on KUE 13183b in the CHO/HGPRT forward mutation assay [online]. Unpublished report No. R4204 24 August 1987 from Hazleton Biotechnologies, Netherlands. Submitted to WHO by Bayer AG Bayerwerk. Available from: URL: http://www.inchem.org/documents/jmpr/ jmpmono/ 2002pr13.htm

Eastmond, D. A. & Tucker, J. D. (1987). Identification of inducing agents using cytokinesis-blocked human lymphocytes and an antikinetochore antibody. *Environ. Mol. Mutagen., 13,* 34-43.

Eastmond, D. A. & Tucker, J. D. (1989). Kinetochore localization in micronucleated cytokinesis-blocked Chinese hamster ovary cells: a new and rapid assay for identifying aneuploidy-inducing agents. *Mutat. Res., 224,* 4, 517-525.

Eastmond, D. A. (1993). Induction of micronuclei and aneuploidy by the quinone-forming agents benzene and o-phenylphenol. *Toxicol. Lett., 67,* 1-3, 105-118.

El-Zein, R. A., Schabath, M. B., Etzel, C. J., Lopez, M. S., Franklin, J. D. & Spitz, M. R. (2006). Cytokinesis - blocked micronucleus assay as a novel biomarker for lung cancer risk. *Cancer Res., 66*, 12, 6449-6456.

EPA (2002). Federal Register: Tolylfluanid [online]. Pesticide Tolerance, 67, 186, 60130-60142. Available from: URL: http://www.epa.gov/fedrgstr/EPA-PEST/ 2002/September/ Day-25/p24094.htm

Fenech, M. (2000). The *in vitro* micronucleus technique. *Mutat. Res., 445,* 81-95.

Fenech, M. (2002). Biomarkers of genetic damage for cancer epidemiology. *Toxicology, 181-182,* 411-416.

Fenech, M. (2006). Cytokinesis-block micronucleus assay evolves into a "cytome" assay of chromosomal instability, mitotic dysfunction and cell death. *Mutat. Res., 600,* 1-2, 58-66.

Fenech, M. (2007). Cytokinesis-block micronucleus cytome assay. *Nat. Protoc., 2,* 5, 1084-1104.

Fimognari, C., Nüsse, M. & Hrelia, P. (1999). Flow cytometric analysis of genetic damage, effect on cell cycle progression, and apoptosis by thiophanate-methyl in human lymphocytes. *Environ. Mol. Mutagen., 33,* 2, 173-176.

Franekić, J., Bratulić, N., Pavlica, M. & Papes, D. (1994). Genotoxicity of dithiocarbamates and their metabolites. *Mutat. Res., 325,* 2-3, 65-74.

Gadeva, P. & Dimitrov, B. (2008). Genotoxic effects of the pesticides rubigan, omite and rovral in root – meristem cells of *Crepis capillaris L. Mutat. Res., 652,* 191-197.

Gao, N. & Zhan, D.-S. (2007). Biocompatibility of self-made ceramic alloy evaluated by micronuclei experiments. *J. Clinic. Rehab. Tissue Engin. Res., 11,* 31, 6268-6270.

Garrett, N. E., Stack, H. F. & Waters, M. D. (1986). Evaluation of the genetic activity profiles of 65 pesticides. *Mutat. Res., 168,* 3, 301-326.

Gerber, G. B., Léonard, A. & Hantson, Ph. (2002). Carcinogenicity, mutagenicity and teratogenicity of manganese compounds. *Crit. Rev. Oncol. Hematol., 42,* 1, 25-34.

Gillian Clare, M., Lorenzon, G., Akhurst, L. C., Marzin, D., van Delf, J., Montero, R., Botta, A., Bertens, A., Cinelli, S., Thybaud, V. & Lorge, E. (2006). SFTG international collaborative study on *in vitro* micronucleus test II. Using human lymphocytes. *Mutat. Res., 607,* 1, 37-60.

Goumenou, M. & Machera, K. (2003). Genotoxic potency of the combination of carbendazim and captan formulations and their interaction, determined by the *in vivo* bone marrow micronucleus test. *Toxicol. Lett., 144,* 1, 148.

Hagmar, L., Bonassi, S., Stromberg, U., Brogger, A., Knudsen, L. E. & Norppa, H. (1998). Chromosomal aberrations in lymphocytes predict human cancer: a report from the European Study Group on Cytogenetic Biomarkers and Health (ESCH). *Cancer Res., 58,* 4117-4121.

Hagmar, L., Strömberg, U., Tinnerberg, H. & Mikoczy, Z. (2001). The usefulness of cytogenetic biomarkers as intermediate endpoints in carcinogenesis. *Int. J. Hyg. Environ. Health, 204,* 1, 43-47.

Hagmar, L., Strömberg, U., Bonassi, S., Hansteen, I.-L., Knudsen, L. E. & Lindholm, C. (2004). Impact of types of lymphocyte chromosomal aberrations on human cancer risk: results from Nordic and Italian cohorts. *Cancer Res., 64,* 2258-2263.

Heidemann, A. & Miltenburger, H. G. (1987). KUE 13183b, detection of gene mutations in somatic mammalian cells in culture: HGPRT-test with V79 cells [online]. Unpublished report No. R4103 8 May 1987 from Laboratory for Mutagenicity Testing, Technical University, Darmstadt, Germany. Submitted to WHO by Bayer AG, Bayerwerk, Germany. Available from: URL: http://www.inchem.org/documents/jmpr/jmpmono/2002pr13.htm

Heil, J., Reifferscheid, G., Hellmich, D., Hergenröder, M. & Zahn, R. K. (1991). Genotoxicity of the fungicide dichlofluanid in seven assays. *Environ. Mol. Mutagen., 17,* 1, 20-26.

Herbold, B. (1979). 13183b/*Salmonella*-microsome test for point mutagenic effects. Institute for Toxicology, Bayer AG [online]. Unpublished report No. 8265. Submitted to WHO by Bayer AG, Bayerwerk, FRG. Available from: URL: http://www.inchem.org/documents/jmpr/jmpmono/2002pr13.htm

Herbold, B. (1980). KUE 13183b (tolylfluanid) - Micronucleus-test on the mouse to evaluate for mutagenic effect [online]. Unpublished report No. 9149 13 May 1980 from Institute of Toxicology, Bayer AG. Submitted to WHO by Bayer AG, Bayerwerk, Germany. Available from: URL: http://www.inchem.org/ documents/jmpr/jmpmono/2002pr13.htm

Herbold, B. (1983). KUE 13183b (c.n. tolylfluanid/Euparen M/Preventol VP OC 3017) - Cytogenetic study of the Chinese hamster's bone marrow *in vivo* to evaluate for mutagenic effect [online]. Unpublished report No. 11792 10 May 1983 from Institute of Toxicology, Bayer AG. Submitted to WHO by Bayer AG, Bayerwerk, Germany. Available from: URL: http://www.inchem.org/documents/jmpr/jmpmono/ 2002pr13.htm

Herbold, B. (1984a). KUE 13183b/Cytogenetic study with human lymphocyte cultures *in vitro* to evaluate for harmful effect on chromosomes. Institute of Toxicology, Bayer AG [online]. Unpublished report No. 12836. Submitted to WHO by Bayer AG, Bayerwerk, FRG. Available from: URL: http://www.inchem.org/documents/jmpr/jmpmono/ 2002pr13.htm

Herbold, B. (1984b). KUE 13183b/Cytogenetic study of the spermatogonia of the Chinese hamster *in vivo* to evaluate for mutagenic effect. Institute of Toxicology, Bayer AG [online]. Unpublished report No. 12739. Submitted to WHO by Bayer AG, Bayerwerk, FRG. Available from: URL: http://www.inchem.org/ documents/jmpr/jmpmono/ 2002pr13.htm

Herbold, B. (1994). KUE 13183b - *Salmonella*/microsome test [online]. Unpublished report No. 22843 27 January 1994 from Institute of Toxicology, Bayer AG. Submitted to WHO by Bayer AG, Bayerwerk, FRG. Available from: URL: http://www.inchem.org/ documents/jmpr/jmpmono/2002pr13.htm

Herbold, B. (1996). KUE 13183b - *In vitro* mammalian chromosome aberration test with Chinese hamster V79 cells [online]. Unpublished report No. 24581 2 January 1996 from Institute of Toxicology, Bayer AG. Submitted to WHO by Bayer AG, Bayerwerk, Germany. Available from: URL: http://www.inchem.org/documents/jmpr/jmpmono/ 2002pr13.htm

Herbold, B. (2000a). KUE 13183b - First amendment to final report No. 12836 of 6 August 1984 - Cytogenetic investigations in human lymphocyte *in vitro* to test for clastogenic effects [online]. Unpublished report No. 12836A. 13 October 2000 from Institute of Toxicology, Bayer AG. Submitted to WHO by Bayer AG, Bayerwerk, FRG. Available from: URL: http://www.inchem.org/documents/jmpr/ jmpmono/2002pr13.htm

Herbold, B. (2000b). KUE 13183b - First amendment to final report No. 11792 of 10 May 1983 - Cytogenetic investigations in the bone marrow of Chinese hamsters *in vivo* to test for clastogenic effects [online]. Unpublished report No. 11792A 13 October 2000 from Institute of Toxicology, Bayer AG. Submitted to WHO by Bayer AG, Bayerwerk,

Germany. Available from: URL: http://www.inchem.org/documents/jmpr/jmpmono/2002pr13.htm

Herbold, B. (2004). KUE 13183B - *In vivo* bone marrow cytogeneic study using male mice. Bayer Health Care AG [online]. Unpublished report No. AT01134, 8 April 2004, Submitted to WHO by Bayer AG, Bayerwerk, Germany. In: Final addendum to the Draft Assessment Report (DAR) - public version - Initial risk assessment provided by the rapporteur Member State Finland for the existing active substance. Tolylfluanid of the second stage of the review programme referred to in Article 8(2) of Council Directive 91/414/EEC. February 2005. Available from: URL: http://www.inchem.org/documents/jmpr/jmpmono/2002pr13.htm

Hoffmann, K. (1983). KUE 13183b/Acute toxicity to the sheep after oral administration. Institute of Toxicology, Bayer AG [online]. Unpublished report No. 11975. Submitted to WHO by Bayer AG, Bayerwerk, FRG. Available from: URL: http://www.inchem.org/documents/jmpr/jmpmono/2002pr13.htm

Holland, N. T., Duramad, P., Rothman, N., Figgs, L. W., Blair, A., Hubbard, A. & Smith, M. T. (2002). Micronucleus frequency and proliferation in human lymphocytes after exposure to herbicide 2,4-dichlorophenoxyacetic acid *in vitro* and *in vivo*. *Mutat. Res., 521,* 1-2, 165-178.

Hoorn, A. J. W. (1984). Mutagenicity evaluation of KUE 13183b (c.n. tolylfluanid) in the reverse mutation induction assay with *Saccharomyces cerevisiae* strains S138 and S211*alpha* [online]. Unpublished report No. R3060 29 August 1984 from Litton Bionetics, Netherlands. Submitted to WHO by Bayer AG, Bayerwerk, Germany. Available from: URL: http://www.inchem.org/documents/jmpr/jmpmono/ 2002pr13.htm

Hoorn, A. J. W. (1985). KUE 13183b/Mutagenicity evaluation of KUE 13183b in the mouse lymphoma forward mutation assay. Litton Bionetics. The Netherlands [online]. Unpublished report No. 3192. Submitted to WHO by Bayer AG, Bayerwerk, FRG. Available from: URL: http://www.inchem.org/documents/jmpr/jmpmono/2002pr13.htm

Hosokawa, S., Murakami, M., Ineyama, M., Yamada, T., Koyama, Y., Okuno, Y., Yoshitake, A., Yamada, H. & Miyamoto, J. (1993). Effects of procymidone on reproductive organs and serum gonadotropins in male rats. *J. Toxicol. Sci., 18,* 2, 111-124.

Hrelia, P., Maffei, F., Fimognari, C., Vigagni, F. & Cantelli-Forti, G. (1996a). Cytogenetic effects of Metalaxyl on human and animal chromosomes. *Mutat. Res., 369,* 1-2, 81-86.

Hrelia, P., Fimognari, C., Maffei, F., Vigagni, F., Mesirca, R., Pozzetti, L., Paolini, M. & Cantelli Forti, G. (1996b). The genetic and non-genetic toxicity of the fungicide Vinclozolin. *Mutagenesis, 11,* 5, 445-453.

Jawich, D., Lteif, R., Pfohl-Leszkowicz, A. & Strehaiano, P. (2006). Effects of penconazole on two yeast strains: Growth kinetics and molecular studies. *Mol. Nutr. Food Res., 50,* 552-556.

Kevekordes, S., Gebel, T., Pav, K., Edenharder, R. & Dunkelberg, H. (1996). Genotoxicity of selected pesticides in the mouse bone-marrow micronucleus test and in the sister-chromatid exchange test with human lymphocytes *in vitro*. *Toxicol. Lett., 89,* 1, 35-42.

Kirkland, D., Aardema, M. Henderson, L. & Műller, L. (2005). Evaluation of the ability of a battery of three *in vitro* genotoxicity tests to discriminate rodent carcinogens and non-carcinogens. I. Sensitivity, specificity and relative predictivity. *Mutat. Res.,* 584, 1-256.

Knopper, L. D., Mineau, P., McNamee, J. P. & Lean, D. R. (2005). Use of comet and micronucleus assays to measure genotoxicity in meadow voles (*Microtus pennsylvanicus*) living in golf course ecosystems exposed to pesticides. *Ecotoxicology, 14,* 3, 323-335.

Lebailly, P., Devaux, A., Pottier, D., De Meo, M., Andre, V., Baldi, I., Severin, F., Bernaud, J., Durand, B., Henry-Amar, M. & Gauduchon, P. (2003). Urine mutagenicity and lymphocyte DNA damage in fruit growers occupationally exposed to the fungicide captan. *Occup. Environ. Medicine, 60,* 910-917.

Lee, C. H., Lin, R. H., Liu, S. H. & Lin-Shiau, S. Y. (1997). Distinct genotoxicity of phenylmercury acetate in human lymphocytes as compared with other mercury compounds. *Mutat. Res., 392,* 3, 269-276.

Lee, C. H., Lin, R. H., Liu, S. H. & Lin-Shiau, S. Y. (1998). Effects of germanium oxide and other chemical compounds on phenylmercury acetate-induced genotoxicity in cultured human lymphocytes. *Environ. Mol. Mutagen., 31,* 2, 157-162.

Lioi, M. B., Scarfi, M. R., Santoro, A., Barbieri, R., Zeni, O., Di Berardino, D. & Ursini, M. V. (1998a). Genotoxicity and oxidative stress induced by pesticide exposure in bovine lymphocytes cultures *in vitro*. *Mutat. Res., 403,* 13-20.

Lioi, M. B., Scarfi, M. R., Santoro, A., Barbieri, R., Zeni, O., Salvemini, F. & Di Berardino, D. & Ursini, M. V. (1998b). Cytogenetic damage and induction of pro-oxidant state in human lymphocytes exposed *in vitro* to glyphosate, vinclozolin, atrazine, and DPX-E9636. *Environ. Mol. Mutagen., 32,* 1, 39-46.

McCarroll, N. E., Protzel, A., Ioannou, Y., Frank Stack, H. F., Jackson, M. A., Waters, M. D. & Dearfield, K. L. (2002). A survey of EPA/OPP and open literature on selected pesticide chemicals. III. Mutagenicity and carcinogenicity of benomyl and carbendazim. *Mutat. Res., 512,* 1, 1-35.

Mouchet, F., Gauthier, L., Mailhes, C., Ferrier, V. & Devaux, A. (2006). Comparative evaluation of genotoxicity of captan in amphibian larvae (*Xenopus laevis* and *Pleurodeles waltl*) using the comet assay and the micronucleus test. *Environ. Toxicol., 21,* 3, 264-277.

Mujumdar, A. M., Shinde, S. L., Karekar, V. R., Joshi, S. S., Dhuley, J., Shanbhag, V. & Ghaskadbi, S. (1994). Genotoxicity assessment of the antifungal antibiotic aureofungin in *Salmonella typhimurium* and Swiss albino mice. *Mutat. Res., 321,* 1-2, 13-17.

Müller, L. & Kasper, P. (2000). Human biological relevance and the use of threshold-arguments in regulatory genotoxicity assessment: experience with pharmaceuticals. *Mutat. Res., 464,* 19-34.

Norppa, H. (2004). Cytogenetic biomarkers and genetic polymorphisms. *Toxicol. Lett., 149,* 1-3, 309-334.

Norppa, H., Bonassi, S., Hansteen, I. L., Hagmar, L., Strömberg, U., Rössner, P., Boffetta, P., Lindholm, C., Gundy, S., Lazutka, J., Cebulska-Wasilewska, A., Fabiánová, E., Srám, R. J., Knudsen, L. E., Barale, R. & Fucic, A. (2006). Chromosomal aberrations and SCEs as biomarkers of cancer risk. *Mutat. Res., 600,* 1-2, 37-45.

Nowacka, A. (2002). Residues of the most frequently applied fungicide in vegetables and fruit (1997 – 2001). *Progress-in-Plant-Protection, 42,* 1, 118-130.

Osaba, L., Rey, M. J., Aguirre, A., Alonso, A. & Graf, U. (2002). Evaluation of genotoxicity of captan, maneb and zineb in the wing spot test of *Drosophila melanogaster*: role of nitrosation. *Mutat. Res./Genetic Toxicol. and Environ. Mutagen., 518,* 1, 95-106.

Oshiro, Y., Piper, C. E., Balwierz, P. S. & Soelter, S. G. (1991). Chinese hamster ovary cell assays for mutation and chromosome damage: Data from non-carcinogens. *J. Appl. Toxicol., 11,* 3, 167-177.

Paolini, M., Mesirca, R., Pozzetti, L., Sapone, A. & Cantelli-Forti, G. (1996a) Molecular non-genetic biomarkers related to Fenarimol cocarcinogenesis: organ- and sex-specific CYP induction in rat. *Cancer Lett., 101,* 2, 171-178.

Paolini, M., Mesirca, R., Pozzetti, L., Maffei, F., Vigagni, F., Hrelia, P. & Cantelli-Forti, G. (1996b). Genetic and non-genetic biomarkers related to carcinogenesis in evaluating toxicological risk from Fenarimol. *Mutat. Res., 368,* 1, 27-39.

Paolini, M., Mesirca, R., Pozzetti, L., Sapone, A. & Cantelli-Forti, G. (1996c). Biomarkers of effect in evaluating metalaxyl cocarcinogenesis. Selective induction of murine CYP 3A isoform. *Mutat. Res., 361,* 2-3, 157-164.

Paolini, M., Mesirca, R., Pozzetti, L., Sapone, A. & Cantelli-Forti, G. (1997). Biomarkers of effect in evaluating dithianon cocarcinogenesis: selective induction and suppression of murine CYP3A isoform. *Cancer Lett., 113,* 1-2, 221-228.

Paolini, M., Pozzetti, L., Perocco, P., Mazzullo, M. & Cantelli-Forti, G. (1999). Molecular non-genetic biomarkers of effect related to methyl thiophanate cocarcinogenesis: organ- and sex-specific cytochrome P450 induction in the rat. *Cancer Lett., 135,* 2, 203-213.

PFPC Newsletter Special Issue: Hidden Sources of Fluoride – Pesticides, 1999, 1-8.

Poli, P., de Mello, M. A., Buschini, A., de Castro, V. L. S. S., Restivo, F. M., Rossi, C. & Zucchi, T. M. A. D. (2003). Evaluation of the genotoxicity induced by the fungicide fenarimol in mammalian and plant cells by use of the single-cell gel electrophoresis assay. *Mutat. Res./Genetic Toxicol. and Environ. Mutagen., 540,* 1, 57-66.

Quest, J. A., Hamernik, K. L., Engler, R., Burnam, W. L. & Fenner-Crisp, P. A. (1991). Evaluation of the carcinogenic potential of pesticides. 3. Aliette. *Regul. Toxicol. Pharmacol., 14,* 1, 3-11.

Quest, J. A., Fenner-Crisp, P. A., Burnam, W., Copley, M., Dearfield, K. L., Hamernik, K. L., Saunders, D. S., Whiting, R. J. & Engler, R. (1993). Evaluation of the carcinogenic potential of pesticides. 4. Chloroalkylthiodicarboximide compounds with fungicidal activity. *Regul. Toxicol. Pharmacol., 17,* 1, 19-34.

Rahden-Staroń, I. (2002). The inhibitory effect of the fungicides captan and captafol on eukaryotic topoisomerases *in vitro* and lack of recombinagenic activity in the wing spot test of *Drosophila melanogaster. Mutat. Res./Genetic Toxicol. Environ. Mutagen., 518,* 2, 205-213.

Rannug, A. & Rannug, U. (1984). Enzyme inhibition as a possible mechanism of the mutagenicity of dithiocarbamic acid derivatives in *Salmonella typhimurium. Chem. Biol. Interact., 49,* 3, 329-340.

Robbiano, L., Baroni, D., Carrozzino, R., Mereto, E. & Brambilla, G. (2004). DNA damage and micronuclei induced in rat and human kidney cells by six chemicals carcinogenic to the rat kidney. *Toxicology, 204,* 2-3, 187-195.

Rolandi, A., De Marinis, E. & De Caterina, M. (1984). Dithiocarbamate pesticides: activity of Propineb in the micronucleus test in mice. *Mutat. Res., 135,* 3, 193-197.

Rosenkranz, H. S. (1999). Chlorothalonil: lack of genotoxic potential. *Mutat. Res., 423,* 1-2, 183-186.

Sapone, A., Affatato, A., Canistro, D., Broccoli, M., Trespidi, S., Pozzetti, L., Biagi, G. L., Cantelli-Forti, G. & Paolini, M. (2003). Induction and suppression of cytochrome P450 isoenzymes and generation of oxygen radicals by procymidone in liver, kidney and lung of CD1 mice. *Mutat. Res., 527,* 1-2, 67-80.

Saunders, D. S. & Harper, C. (1994). *Pesticides. Principles and Methods of Toxicology.* New York, Raven Press, 386-415.

Shanthi, R. & Krishnamoorthy, M. (2002). Evaluation of the aneugenic potential of the fungicide Ferbam in mice. *Teratog. Carcinog. Mutagen., 22,* 6, 451-459.

Shukla, Y., Taneja, P., Arora, A. & Sinha, N. (2004). Mutagenic potential of Mancozeb in *Salmonella typhimurium. J. Environ. Pathol. Toxicol. Oncol., 23,* 4, 297-302.

Soloneski, S., González, M., Piaggio, E., Apezteguía, M., Reigosa. M. A. & Larramendy, M. L. (2001). Effect of the dithiocarbamate pesticide zineb and its commercial formulation azzurro. I. Genotoxic evaluation on cultured human lymphocytes exposed *in vitro. Mutagenesis, 16,* 6, 487-493.

Soloneski, S., Reigosa, M. A. & Larramendy, M. L. (2002a). Effect of dithiocarbamate pesticide zineb and its commercial formulation, azzurro. II. Micronucleus induction in immunophenotyped human lymphocytes. *Environ. Mol. Mutagenesis, 40,* 1, 57-62.

Soloneski, S., Gonzalez, M., Piaggio, E., Reigosa, M. A. & Larramendy, M. L. (2002b). Effect of dithiocarbamate pesticide zineb and its commercial formulation, azzurro. III. Genotoxic evaluation on Chinese hamster ovary (CHO) cells. *Mutat. Res., 514,* 1-2, 201-212.

Soloneski, S., Reigosa, M. A. & Larramendy, M. L. (2003). Vitamin E prevents ethylene bis(dithiocarbamate) pesticide zineb-induced sister chromatid exchange in Chinese hamster ovary cells. *Mutagenesis, 18,* 6, 505-510.

Steenland, K., Cedillo, L., Tucker, J., Hines, C., Sorensen, K., Deddens, J. & Cruz, V. (1997). Thyroid hormones and cytogenetic outcomes in backpack sprayers using ethylenebis (dithiocarbamate) (EBDC) fungicides in Mexico. *Environ. Health Perspect., 105,* 10, 1126-1130.

Surrallés, J. & Natarajan, A. T. (1997). Human lymphocytes micronucleus assay in Europe. An international survey. *Mutat. Res., 392,* 165-174.

Šutiaková, I., Kovalkovičová, N., Pistl, J., Novotný, J., Legáth, J., Kováč, G., Hlinčíková, S. & Šutiak, V. (2006). Chromosomal aberrations and frequency of micronuclei in sheep subchronically exposed to the fungicide Euparen Multi (tolylfluanid). *Ecotoxicol. Environ. Safety*, *64,* 3, 312-320.

Suzuki, H., Suzuki, N., Sasaki, M. & Hiraga, K. (1985). Orthophenylphenol mutagenicity in a human cell strain. *Mutat. Res., 156,* 1-2, 123-127.

The Pesticide Manual. 12th ed., Version 2.0, The British Crop Protection Council, 2000.

Tyrkiel, E., Wiadrowska, B. & Ludwicki, J. K. (1998). The effect of nuarimol on the mutagenic activity of n-nitrosodimethylamine and 2-acetylaminofluorene in mouse erythrocytes. *Rocz. Panstw. Zakl. Hig., 49,* 1, 55-66.

Udroiu, I. (2007). Cytogenetic assays applied to animal-derived food control. *Rev. vet., 18*, 1, 62-64.

Vamvakas, S., Kordowich, F. J., Dekant, W., Neudecker, T. & Henschler, D. (1988). Mutagenicity of hexachloro-1,3-butadiene and its S-conjugates in the Ames test -role of activation by the mercapturic acid pathway in its nephrocarcinogenicity. *Carcinogenesis, 9,* 6, 907-910.

Villani, P., Andreoli, C., Crebelli, R., Pacchierotti, F., Zijno, A. & Carere, A. (1998). Analysis of micronuclei and DNA single-strand breaks in mouse splenocytes and peripheral lymphocytes after oral administration of tetramethylthiuram disulfide (thiram). *Food. Chem. Toxicol., 36,* 155-164.

Vindas, R., Ortiz, F., Ramírez, V. & Cuenca, P. (2004). Genotoxicity of three pesticides used in Costa Rican banana plantations. *Rev. Biol. Trop., 52,* 3, 601-609.

Völkner, W. (1988a). Mouse germ-cell cytogenetic assay with KUE 13183b [online]. Unpublished report No. R4485 1 July 1988 from Cytotest Cell Research GmbH & Co. KG, Germany. Submitted to WHO by Bayer AG, Bayerwerk, Germany. Available from: URL: http://www.inchem.org/documents/jmpr/jmpmono/ 2002pr13.htm

Völkner, W. (1988b). Sister chromatid exchange assay in bone marrow cells of the mouse with KUE 13183b [online]. Unpublished report No. R4422 2 May 1988 from Cytotest Cell Research GmbH & Co. KG, Germany. Submitted to WHO by Bayer AG, Bayerwerk, Germany. Available from: URL: http://www.inchem.org/documents/ jmpr/jmpmono/2002pr13.htm

Völkner, W. (1990). Chromosome aberration assay in bone marrow cells of Chinese hamster with KUE 13183b [online]. Unpublished report No. R5153 20 September 1990 from Cytotest Cell Research GmbH & Co. KG, Germany. Submitted to WHO by Bayer AG, Bayerwerk, Germany. Available from: URL: http://www.inchem.org/documents/ jmpr/jmpmono/2002pr13.htm

Watanabe-Akanuma, M., Ohta, T. & Yamagata, H. (2003). Photomutagenicity of thiabendazole, a postharvest fungicide, in bacterial assays. *Environ. Mol. Mutagen., 41,* 2, 92-98.

Watanabe-Akanuma, M., Ohta, T. & Sasaki, Y. F. (2005). A novel genotoxic aspect of thiabendazole as a photomutagen in bacteria and cultured human cells. *Toxicol. Lett., 158,* 3, 213-219.

Wu, X. J., Lu, W. Q., Roos, P. H. & Mersch-Sundermann, V. (2005). Vinclozolin, a widely used fungicide, enhanced BaP-induced micronucleus formation in human derived hepatoma cells by increasing CYP1A1 expression. *Toxicol. Lett., 159,* 1, 83-88.

Yilmaz, S., Aksoy, H., Űnal, F., Çelik, M. & Yüzbaşioğlu, D. (2008). Genotoxic action of fungicide Conan 5FL (hexaconazole) on mammalian cells *in vivo* and *in vitro. Genetika, 44,* 3, 323-328.

Yüzbaşioğlu, D., Celik, M., Yilmaz, S., Unal, F. & Aksoy, H. (2006). Clastogenicity of the fungicide afugan in cultured human lymphocytes. *Mutat. Res., 604,* 1-2, 53-59.

Zavala-Aguirre, J. L, Torres-Bugarin, O. & Zamora-Perez, A. L. (2007). Aquatic ecotoxicology approaches in Western Mexico. *J. Environ. Sci. Health A Tox. Hazard Subst. Environ. Eng., 42*, 10, 1503-1511.

Zelesco, P. A., Barbieri, I. & Graves, J. A. (1990). Use of a cell hybrid test system to demonstrate that benomyl induces aneuploidy and polyploidy. *Mutat. Res., 242,* 4, 329-335.

Zenzen, V., Fauth, E., Zankl, H., Janzowski, C. & Eisenbrand, G. (2001). Mutagenic and cytotoxic effectiveness of zinc dimethyl and zinc diisononyldithiocarbamate in human lymphocyte cultures. *Mutat. Res./Genetic Toxicol. Environ. Mutagen., 497,* 1-2, 89-99.

In: Fungicides
Editors: P. De Costa and P. Bezerra
ISBN: 978-1-60692-631-4

Chapter VI

ANTIMICROBIAL TREATMENTS OF INDOOR MOLD AND BACTERIA

Marc Y. Menetrez*

U. S. Environmental Protection Agency, Office of Research and Development,
National Risk Management Research Laboratory,
Air Pollution Prevention and Control Division, Research Triangle Park, NC 27711, USA

ABSTRACT

Biological contaminants especially mold in buildings are known to act as sources of indoor air pollution, discomfort, asthma and pulmonary disease in building occupants. Sick buildings are evidence of extremely problematic indoor air quality (IAQ), often resulting from unacceptable concentrations of biological contaminants, particulates and odors, and extreme temperatures and humidity. Biological contaminants can cause allergic, toxic, or inflammatory responses in building occupants. The risk-management approach to limiting exposure has been to implement a reduction in indoor levels of biological contamination. Antimicrobial agents, called fungicides, sporicides or biocides have long been used to control, prevent, and remediate microbial growth. The antimicrobial efficacy of EPA-FIFRA registered chemicals and encapsulants, over the counter cleaners, and mechanical devices (such as UV irradiation) to reduce concentrations of mold and bacteria have only recently been investigated. Standard methods to test these control measures such as ASTM 6329-98, (2003) have recently been established, and now pertain to a wide set of applications.

* Phone 919-541-7981, fax 919-541-2157; Email menetrez.marc@epa.gov

AUTHOR SUMMARY

The following information on biological research is a conglomerate of old established knowledge, newly developed evaluations, qualitative comparisons of performance, and exact quantitative measurements. At times the non-heterogeneous nature of the evaluations can appear to be only loosely-bound and inconsistent in approach. However, the unique nature of science and the research which is constantly changing is specific for each area. Each area of work addressed below represents the best methodology at a point in time. Research to further develop the methods utilized will continue efforts toward standardized and comparable methods of evaluation.

ANTIMICROBIAL TREATMENTS AS CONTROL TECHNOLOGIES

The efficacy of antimicrobial treatments to eliminate or control biological growth in the indoor environment can easily be tested on nonporous surfaces. However, the testing of antimicrobial efficacy on porous surfaces, such as those found in the indoor environment [i.e., gypsum wallboard (GWB), heating, ventilating, and air-conditioning (HVAC) duct-liner insulation, and wood products] can be more complicated and prone to incorrect conclusions. Additionally, the capability to test antimicrobial efficacy has been advanced through the development of a static microbial test chamber (SMTC) constructed from acrylic sheeting (measures 32 x 39 x 51 cm) with shelves for samples and a saturated salt solution on the chamber bottom to control the equilibrium relative humidity (ERH) [1]. The SMTC was tested using ASTM 6329-98, *Standard Guide for Developing Methodology for Evaluating the Ability of Indoor Materials to Support Microbial Growth Using Static Environmental Chambers* (2003) [1]. This method was developed as part of on-going indoor air biocontaminant research. Multiple SMTCs were used to evaluate fungal growth on product coupons such as square sections of fiberglass duct-liner (FGDL) or GWB at various environmental conditions. The SMTC was developed to assess potential microbial growth on a variety of common building materials. Temperature and relative humidity (RH) are controlled to simulate the desired environmental conditions. Prior to chamber testing, materials can be treated by soaking to simulate a wetting event or treated with an antimicrobial to simulate mitigation practices [1].

(A) Antimicrobial Encapsulants

Research to control biological growth using three separate antimicrobial encapsulants which were spray-painted on contaminated (with *Aspergillus versicolor*) FGDL by method ASTM 6329-98 [1] has been performed in laboratory testing using visual inspection to estimate growth on coupons. The estimation of growth was made by optical inspection of the coupon surfaces. The numerical ranking of mold growth followed was;

0 = No Growth,

1 = minimal growth,
2 = growth covering 33.3% of coupon,
3 = growth covering 50% of coupon,
4 = growth covering 75% of coupon,
5 = growth covering the majority of the coupon with few bare spots remaining.

Triplicate sample coupons were processed for each of the 14 cleaning products and six GWB surface types. The results indicate differences in antimicrobial efficacy for the period of testing [2]. An encapsulant or coating is a covering that is applied to an object. The aim of applying coatings is to improve surface properties of a bulk material usually referred to as a substrate.

Three common HVAC (or HAC) antimicrobial encapsulants were evaluated for their use on FGDL in both laboratory and field application experiments. The antimicrobial encapsulants tested are manufactured for use in HVAC system components and on duct surfaces. Coating I was a polyacrylate copolymer containing 9% barium metaborate and 0.16% iodo-2-propynyl butylcarbamate; Coating II was an acrylic coating containing decabromodiphenyl oxide and antimony trioxide; and Coating III was an acrylic primer containing phosphoric acid compounds with a phosphated quaternary amine complex [diethanolamine n-coco alkyl derivatives; 2,2'-(coco ankylimino)bis-ethanol].

The results of the chamber experiments are shown in Tables 1 and 2, for sections of FGDL that were removed from the test house. Surface samples indicated that the population of A. versicolor on untreated FGDL increased by 3 logs (1,000 fold) by the end of the first month (see Table 1), and remained approximately level through the 3.5-month study.

Table 1 shows a slight variation (increase followed by a decrease) in *A. versicolor* population for Coatings I and III on FGDL, for the period of 3.5 months. This was in contrast to the increased populations observed in samples with Coating II. The increase in fungi population for Coating II was comparable to that observed in the untreated samples, as compared with successful limiting of growth accomplished by Coatings I and III.

Soiled FGDL experiments resulted in similar populations of *A. versicolor* for untreated and Coating II samples, as shown in Table 2. The results were again similar for Coatings I and III, in which variations in fungi populations were observed to increase in month 1, and then decrease. The results indicate that antimicrobials can remain effective with moderate dust loading.

Table 1. Growth of *A. versicolor* on the surface of FGDL maintained at 94% RH dynamic chamber

FGDL Sample	Biological growth (log CFUs/10 cm^2)			
	Start	Month 1	Month 2	Month 3.5
Untreated	0	3.8	4.40	4.2
Coating I	0	0.9	0.7	0.1
Coating II	0	2.9	3.1	3.3
Coating III	0	1.0	1.1	0

Table 2. Growth of *A. versicolor* on the surface of soiled FGDL maintained at 94% RH dynamic chamber

FGDL Sample	Biological Growth (log CFUs/10 cm^2)			
	Start	Month 1	Month 2	Month 3.5
Untreated	0	2.9	4.1	3.8
Coating I	0	1.5	1.6	1.0
Coating II	0	3.3	3.8	4.3
Coating III	0	1.5	0.8	0

Table 3. Change in log CFUs/10 cm^2 of *A. versicolor*

Treatment	Static chamber				Dynamic chamber
Not Soiled	70% RH	85% RH	90% RH	94% RH	94% RH
Untreated	BDL*	1.4	4.4	4.4	4.2
Coating I	BDL	BDL	BDL	< 1.0	<1.0
Coating II	< 1.0	1.9	3.4	4.3	3.3
Coating III	< 1.0	BDL	BDL	BDL	<1.0
Artificially Soiled					
Untreated	BDL	< 1.0	4.4	5.1	3.8
Coating I	< 1.0	< 1.0	BDL	< 1.0	1.0
Coating II	BDL	3.6	4.7	4.7	4.3
Coating III	< 1.0	BDL	BDL	BDL	<1.0

* BDL=Below Detection Limit.

A comparison of the results obtained with dynamic and static chamber testing is shown in Table 3. The additional static chamber testing was performed at 70, 85, 90, and 94% RH, for comparison with the 94% RH dynamic chamber testing. Table 3 indicates that static chamber results at 94% RH are in good agreement with dynamic chamber results at 94% RH. Studies also demonstrated that static chamber fungi growth decreases with decreasing RH. Both methods indicate greater effectiveness in controlling growth with Coatings I and III.

Laboratory SMTC experiments conducted at 21.7 °C (71 °F) and from 65% to saturated relative humidity showed differences in degrees of efficacy for three antimicrobial coatings. Two antimicrobial coatings limited fungal contamination for the duration of testing. The most effective coatings were Coatings I and III while Coating II was ineffective. Although all three antimicrobials are registered with the EPA, they were not equally effective, nor should they be expected to perform equally in field use [2].

Additional methods of testing antimicrobial efficacy are needed to be standardized to evaluate differences in products having or seeking EPA registration. The standard methods should cover treatment techniques pertaining to liquids, fumigants and irradiation. The following text addresses these research subjects and is the first step in the development of standard methods. Additionally, the series of experiments described in Menetrez et al. (2002), are adequate tests for viable mold [2]. However, in addition to viable mold, additional testing may be needed for viable bacteria (bacteria cells and spores), nonviable mold (mycotoxins) and bacteria (endotoxins), as well as viruses and some forms of allergens (e.g., dust mites), to determine whether the manufacturers' claims apply [2 - 4].

(B) Antimicrobial Cleaners

Mold contaminated building materials are often not entirely removed from problem buildings. These colonized porous materials frequently have surface cleaners applied in an attempt to alleviate the problem. The efficacy of antimicrobial cleaners to remove, eliminate or control mold growth on surfaces can easily be tested on non-porous surfaces. However, the testing of antimicrobial cleaner efficacy on porous surfaces, such as those found in the indoor environment such as GWB can be more complicated and prone to incorrect conclusions regarding residual organisms and microbial toxins [2, 3]. The mold *Stachybotrys chartarum* has been found to be associated with idiopathic pulmonary hemorrhage in infants and has been studied for toxin production and its occurrence in water damaged buildings [4]. Growth of *S. chartarum* on building materials such as gypsum wallboard has been frequently documented [5, 6]. Research to control *S. chartarum* growth using 13 separate antimicrobial cleaners on contaminated gypsum wallboard has been performed in laboratory testing. Laboratory SMTC experiments conducted at 21.1 °C, (70.0 °F) and 100% relative humidity showed differences in degrees of efficacy. Common brands of cleaning products were tested following directions printed on the product packaging and are listed in Table 4. A variety of gypsum wallboard surfaces were used to test these cleaning products at high relative humidity using a modification of ASTM 6329-98. Visual inspection for *S. chartarum* regrowth of the coupons within static chambers extended up to six months. Only those samples that exhibited heavy amounts of regrowth were stopped prior to six months. The estimation of regrowth was made by optical inspection of the coupon surfaces. The numerical ranking of mold growth followed was;

0 = No Growth,
1 = minimal growth,
2 = growth covering 33.3% of coupon,
3 = growth covering 50% of coupon,
4 = growth covering 75% of coupon,
5 = growth covering the majority of the coupon with few bare spots remaining.

Triplicate sample coupons were processed for each of the 14 cleaning products and six GWB surface types. Visual inspection for *S. chartarum* regrowth of the coupons within the static chambers occurred for six months or until it was judged to have extensive growth (a numerical ranking of 5). The results were numerically ranked from best (0 represented no growth) to worst (5 represented extensive growth) and are listed in Table 5a. Six varieties of surfaces were used to evaluate *S. chartarum* growth. The surfaces were constructed over standard GWB, they were:

Table 4. Cleaning products tested for removing *Stachybotrys chartarium* growth

Cleaning Product	Directions For Use	Concentration
Lysol (concentrated)	To disinfect/deodorize hard, non-porous surfaces, remove heavy soil first, then add 1.3 oz to one gallon water then apply with a sponge or mop wetting all surfaces thoroughly. Let stand 10 minutes, then wipe away excess.	189 mL H_2O 1.89 mL Lysol
Lysol All Purpose Cleaner Orange Breeze scent	For a cleaner, fresher household, dilute 2 oz. with a gallon of warm water. Good for everyday cleaning throughout the house. For your toughest household messes; use full strength and rinse thoroughly.	full strength
Lysol All Purpose Cleaner Orange Breeze scent	For a cleaner, fresher household, dilute 2 oz. with a gallon of warm water. Good for everyday cleaning throughout the house. For your toughest household messes; use full strength and rinse thoroughly.	250 mL H_2O 3.75 mL Lysol Orange Breeze
Lysol IC - Brand Quaternary Disinfectant Cleaner	Remove heavy soil deposits from surfaces, then thoroughly wet them with a solution of 1/2 oz of the concentrate per gallon of water. The solution can be applied with a cloth, mop, sponge or coarse spray or soaking. Let solution remain on surface for a minimum of 10 minutes. Allow to air dry.	378.5 mL H_2O 1.48 mL Lysol I.C.
Spray Nine Multi-Purpose Cleaner & Disinfectant	1. Spray on soiled surface. 2. Wipe immediately with a clean, damp sponge or cloth. 3. Repeat application making sure to wet all surfaces thoroughly. 4. Allow to stand for 3 minutes when treating for fungus. 5. Wipe off with a clean, damp sponge or cloth then rinse thoroughly.	full strength
Johnson Wax Professional Mildew Stain Remover with Bleach	Spray using full strokes, 6-8" from surface. Wait until stains disappear. Wipe with sponge. Rinse promptly.	full strength
Commercial Solutions Ultra Clorox Germicidal Bleach	Prewash surface, then mop or wipe with bleach solution. Allow solution to contact surface for at least 2 minutes. Rinse well and air dry. Dilute 2/3 cup bleach to 1 gallon water.	189 mL H_2O 7.89 mL bleach
SporKlenz	Remove any obvious debris or organic material from the surface to be sterilized. Dilute Spor-Klenz concentrate 100x (1 part Spor-Klenz to 99 parts purified water). Spray onto surfaces using a plastic spray bottle. Allow to remain on surface for 10 minutes. Let air dry or rinse with purified water.	175 mL H_2O 1.75 mL SporKlenz
Borax	Sprinkle borax into water and wipe with damp sponge.	473 mL of warm water 1 Tablespoon Borax

Pine Sol	For general disinfecting: Apply Original Pine-Sol Brand cleaner with a sponge or cloth full strength. Wet surfaces, let stand 5 minutes, then remove excess. For highly soiled areas, clean excess dirt first.	full strength
Tilex	Spray surface until thoroughly wet, let stand 5 minutes and rinse. Do not use on wood or painted surfaces. Avoid contact with aluminum, clothes, fabric, carpet or paper surfaces as they will discolor.	full strength
Fantastik Orange Action	Spray 6-8 inches from surface. After spraying, wipe with a dry paper towel or cloth.	full strength
Orange Glo Multipurpose Degreaser	Spray on soiled area and wipe clean. Rinse if necessary. For baked-on grease or thick soap film, wait several minutes before wiping.	full strength
Formula 409 Multipurpose Cleaner	Spray 6-8 inches from surface. General cleaning: Spray product straight onto soils and wipe clean with a dry paper towel or lint free cloth. Repeat for heavily soiled areas. Not recommended for use on soft vinyl, varnishes or aluminum.	full strength

1. Plain GWB, no paint.
2. Vinyl (100 percent vinyl) covered GWB.
3. GWB with vinyl coated wallpaper removed before cleaning and replaced.
4. GWB with vinyl coated wallpaper not removed before cleaning.
5. GWB with oil-based paint.
6. GWB with acrylic (latex) paint.

Table 5a. Comparison *Stachybotrys chartarium* growth for cleaners on six GWB surface types

	Surface Type*					
Mean growth ranked 0 to 5 for each surface type	**1**	**2**	**3**	**4**	**5**	**6**
Lysol All-Purpose Cleaner- Orange Breeze (full strength)	0.0	3.7	0.0	0.0	0.0	0.0
Borax	0.0	0.0	1.0	2.0	0.0	0.0
Orange Glo Multipurpose Degreaser	0.0	0.0	0.0	0.0	1.0	4.0
Fantastik Orange Action	0.0	3.3	2.3	0.7	0.3	2.3
Lysol IC - Brand Quaternary Disinfectant Cleaner	0.7	0.0	1.0	1.0	3.0	5.0
Formula 409 Multipurpose Cleaner	1.3	0.0	2.0	1.0	1.0	4.0
Lysol (concentrated)	3.0	0.0	1.0	3.0	0.0	1.7
Tilex	2.0	0.0	1.7	2.7	0.7	2.0
Spray Nine Multi-Purpose Cleaner & Disinfectant	2.7	0.0	1.0	3.0	1.0	1.7
SporKlenz	2.3	0.7	0.7	2.0	2.0	0.0
Pine Sol	2.0	0.0	0.3	2.0	0.7	0.7
Commercial Solutions Ultra Clorox Germicidal Bleach	5.0	0.0	1.0	3.3	1.7	0.7
Johnson Wax Professional Mildew Stain Remover with Bleach	3.7	0.0	1.0	2.3	1.7	1.3
Lysol All Purpose Cleaner Orange Breeze scent (diluted)	4.0	4.3	5.0	0.0	3.0	3.3

Table 5b. Comparison ranking of cleaners performance for six GWB surface types

	Surface Type*					
Cleaners ranked for each surface type	**1**	**2**	**3**	**4**	**5**	**6**
Lysol All-Purpose Cleaner- Orange Breeze (full strength)	1	13	1	1	1	1
Borax	1	1	5	7	1	1
Orange Glo Multipurpose Degreaser	1	1	1	1	7	12
Fantastik Orange Action	1	12	13	4	4	10
Lysol IC - Brand Quaternary Disinfectant Cleaner	5	1	5	5	13	14
Formula 409 Multipurpose Cleaner	6	1	12	5	7	12
Lysol (concentrated)	11	1	5	12	1	7
Tilex	7	1	11	11	5	9
Spray Nine Multi-Purpose Cleaner & Disinfectant	10	1	5	12	7	7
SporKlenz	9	11	4	7	12	1
Pine Sol	7	1	3	7	5	4
Commercial Solutions Ultra Clorox Germicidal Bleach	14	1	5	14	10	4
Johnson Wax Professional Mildew Stain Remover with Bleach	12	1	5	10	10	6
Lysol All Purpose Cleaner Orange Breeze scent (diluted)	13	14	14	1	13	11

* Surface Type.
1) Plain GWB, no paint.
2) Vinyl (100 percent vinyl) covered GWB.
3) GWB with vinyl coated wallpaper removed before cleaning and replacement.
4) GWB with vinyl coated wallpaper not removed before cleaning.
5) GWB with oil-based paint.
6) GWB with acrylic (latex) paint.

The object of this research was to test the antimicrobial efficacy of these cleaning and disinfectant products for removing and preventing, or restricting growth of *S. chartarum* growth on the six varieties of GWB surfaces listed above, and with variations in RH.

The mean results (of triplicate samples) of 14 cleaning products for the six types of GWB surfaces varied extensively (see Tables 5a and 5b). However, three cleaning products exhibited significantly better results than others. Lysol All-Purpose Cleaner-Orange Breeze (full strength) demonstrated results which ranked among the best in five of the six surfaces tested. Both Borax and Orange Glo Multipurpose Degreaser demonstrated results which ranked among the best in four of the six surfaces tested [6].

Eight other cleaning products ranked among the best in at least one surface test, they were: Formula 409, Lysol IC, Pine Sol, bleach, Spray Nine, Mildew Stain Remover with bleach SporKlenz, Tilex, Fantastik Orange Action, and Lysol All-Purpose Cleaner-Orange Breeze (diluted). Every product tested demonstrated to be among the best in at least one surface test [6].

The results of *S. chartarum* regrowth listed in Table 5a was sorted in a comparative ranking of antimicrobial efficacy performance. Those products listed Table 5a which best limited regrowth were given a ranking of 1, and those that demonstrated the most regrowth were given a ranking of 5. The 14 products tested are listed from 1 (best performance) to 14 (worst performance) in Table 5b. Numerous products received the same equivalent ranking in

Table 5b when their test results listed in Table 5a were equal. Table 5b illustrates the comparison of antimicrobial cleaning product performance [6].

The results indicate differences in antimicrobial efficacy for the six month period of testing by not allowing mold regrowth [6]. The preferred antimicrobial cleaner to choose is often dependent on the type of surface to be cleaned of *S. chartarum* contamination. For Plain GWB, no paint, the best cleaners were Borax, Lysol All-Purpose Cleaner-Orange Breeze (full strength), Orange Glo Multipurpose Degreaser, and Fantastik Orange Action [6].

For Vinyl (100 percent vinyl, removed, cleaned and replaced) covered GWB, the best cleaners were Formula 409, Lysol IC, Pine Sol, Borax, Lysol, Bleach, Spray Nine, Mildew Stain Remover with Bleach, Tilex, and Orange Glo Multipurpose Degreaser [6]. For GWB with vinyl coated wallpaper removed before cleaning and replaced, the best cleaners were Lysol All-Purpose Cleaner-Orange Breeze (full strength), and Orange Glo Multipurpose Degreaser [6]. For GWB with vinyl coated wallpaper not removed before cleaning, the best cleaners were Lysol All-Purpose Cleaner-Orange Breeze (full strength), and Orange Glo Multipurpose Degreaser, and Lysol All-Purpose Cleaner-Orange Breeze (diluted) [6]. For GWB with oil-based paint, the best cleaners were Lysol All-Purpose Cleaner-Orange Breeze (full strength), Lysol and Borax [6]. For GWB with acrylic (latex) paint, the best cleaners were Borax, Lysol All-Purpose Cleaner-Orange Breeze (full strength) and SporKlenz [6].

Lysol All-Purpose Cleaner-Orange Breeze (full strength) demonstrated results which ranked among the best in five of the six surfaces tested. Both Borax and Orange Glo Multipurpose Degreaser demonstrated results which ranked among the best in four of the six surfaces tested.

Every product tested demonstrated to be among the best in at least one surface test [6].

(C) Antimicrobial Paints

Employing antimicrobial paints can in some cases effectively prevent mold regrowth. The accepted recommendation in handling *S. chartarum* contaminated gypsum wallboard is removal and replacement. This practice is however, not always followed completely. Often mold contaminated building materials are not properly removed, some surface cleaning is performed and paint is applied in an attempt to alleviate the problem. The efficacy of antimicrobial paints to eliminate or control mold regrowth on surfaces can easily be tested on non-porous surfaces. However, the testing of antimicrobial efficacy on porous surfaces found in the indoor environment such as gypsum wallboard can be more complicated and prone to incorrect conclusions regarding residual organisms. Growth of *S. chartarum* on building materials such as gypsum drywall has been frequently documented. Research to control *S. chartarum* growth using seven separate antimicrobial paints and two commonly used paints on contaminated gypsum wallboard has been performed in laboratory testing. The nine paint products and manufacturers tested are listed in Tables 6a and b along with the product active ingredients.

Laboratory SMTC experiments conducted at 21.1 °C, (70.0 °F) and 100% relative humidity showed differences in degrees of efficacy. Manufacturers directions were followed and common gypsum wallboard was used as the base to test these products at high relative humidity. The results indicate differences in antimicrobial efficacy for the six month period of testing by not allowing mold regrowth. When the cost of replacing walls may prevent remediation, antimicrobial paint can lend a possible low-cost alternative [7]. Each coupon is visually assigned a numerical ranking of mold growth from 0 to 5 for the entire averaged coupon surface. Each paint result was the average of three coupons surfaces. Inspection for *S. chartarum* regrowth of the coupons within the static chambers extended up to six months. The estimation of regrowth was made by visual inspection of the coupon surfaces. Triplicate sample coupons were processed for each of the nine paint products and two cleaning techniques. The numerical ranking of mold growth followed was;

0 = No Growth,
1 = minimal growth, (growth covering less than 33.3% of sample)
2 = growth covering 33.3% of sample,
3 = growth covering 50% of sample,
4 = growth covering 75% of sample,
5 = growth covering the majority (greater than 75%) of the sample with few bare spots remaining.

Table 6a. Antimicrobial encapsulant paint products

Manufacturer	Antimicrobial Paint Products	Active Ingredients
Alistagen Corp. New York, NY 10016	Caliwel 1 Caliwel 2 with BNA (Bi-Neutralizing Agent)	18.7 % Hydrated Lime (calcium hydroxide)
PPG Industries Pittsburg, PA 15272	Portersept	10.0-20.0 % wt Titanium dioxide 1.0-10.0 % Propylene glycol 1.0-10.0 % Kaolin <1% Crystalline silica-quartz
Homax Products Inc. Bellingham, WA 98226	Mil-Kil Additive	40.0 % wt diiodomethyl p-tolyl sulfone added to acrylic/latex paint
Jomaps, Inc. Alpharetta, GA 63052	M-1 Additive	51.8 % Chlorothalonil 2, 4, 5, 6-Tetrachloroisophthalonitrile added to acrylic/latex paint
Masterchem Industries, Inc. Imperial, MO 63052	Kilz (interior/exterior water based)	Acrylic resin emulsion Titanium dioxide Calcium carbonate Ethylene glycol
Zinsser Company, Inc. Somerset, NJ 08873	Permawhite (satin, water based)	Limestone Titanium dioxide Ethylene glycol Mica Zinc oxide Magnesium aluminum silcate

Table 6b. Paint products

Manufacturer	Paint Products	Paint Type
The Valspar Corporation, Wheeling, Illinois 60090	American Tradition, Interior 100 % Acrylic	Acrylic/latex
The Valspar Corporation, Wheeling, Illinois 60090	Interior one coat Oil Semi-Gloss Enamel	Oil-based

Two techniques of preparing the GWB surfaces were used (cleaned with water only and cleaned with a bleach and water solution) to test these paint products at high relative humidity using a modification of ASTM 6329-98. The observed regrowth results were averaged for each of the seven antimicrobial paint products and the two standard paint products listed in Tables 7a and b. Results of regrowth of *S. chartarum* on GWB are listed in Table 7a. The test results of Table 7a list paint used on water cleaned GWB, and paint used on bleach and water cleaned GWB (the method recommended by most manufacturers) [7].

Results for the nine types of paint products on GWB surfaces varied. However, three antimicrobial encapsulant paint products exhibited no mold re-growth. Permawhite, M-1 Additive, and Porterscept demonstrated results which ranked among the best in tests (see Table 7a). Mil-Kil ranked among the best for water cleaned GWB (Table 7a), and near the best for bleach and water cleaned GWB (Table 7b). The remaining three antimicrobial encapsulant paints and two common paints did not perform as well. The Kilz performance was not even as good as the acrylic/latex or oil-based paint [7].

The results of *S. chartarum* regrowth listed in Table 7a was sorted in a comparative ranking of antimicrobial efficacy performance. The nine products tested are listed from 1 (best performance) to 9 (worst performance) in Table 7b. Numerous products received the same equivalent ranking in Table 7b when their test results listed in Table 7a were equal. Table 7b illustrates the comparison of antimicrobial paint product performance.

Table 7a. Growth ranking for cleaned and painted GWB

Paint products used on cleaned GWB	Mean *S. chartarum* growth ranking for water cleaned GWB	Mean *S. chartarum* growth ranking for bleach and water cleaned GWB
Permawhite	0	0
Portersept	0	0
Mil-Kil	0	0
M-1 Additive	0	0.3
Caliwell 1	4.0	1.7
Caliwell 2	4.0	0.7
Acrylic/Latex	4.0	4.0
Oil-Based	4.0	4.0
Kilz	5.0	5.0

Table 7b. Comparison ranking of cleaned and painted GWB

Paint products used on cleaned GWB	**Mean *S. chartarum* growth ranking for water cleaned GWB**	**Mean *S. chartarum* growth ranking for bleach and water cleaned GWB**
Permawhite	1	1
Portersept	1	1
Mil-Kil	1	1
M-1 Additive	1	4
Caliwell 1	5	6
Caliwell 2	5	5
Acrylic/Latex	5	7
Oil-Based	5	7
Kilz	9	9

Based on the study results the best antimicrobial encapsulant paints for dealing with *S. chartarum* contamination on GWB was Permawhite, M-1 Additive, and Porterscept. The results for Mil-Kil were close in comparison. Although two of these four products contain titanium-dioxide, they all contain unique formulations that make it difficult to draw conclusions regarding antimicrobial performance [7].

(D) Antimicrobial UVC Irradiation

Ultraviolet (UV) irradiation has been used for the disinfection of air streams for many years [8, 9]. The range of UV wavelengths found to be most effective was 220 to 300 nanometers (nm), and the peak effectiveness was determined to be 265 nm [10]. The production of UV light employs an electrical discharge through low-pressure mercury vapor enclosed in a quartz glass tube [10]. This technique produces a tube type bulb with a primary wavelength of 253.7 nm, and is within the "C" band of UV (UVC) [10]. The UVC or UV germicidal (UVGI) form of irradiation has been demonstrated to deactivate bacteria, fungi, viruses, and mycoplasmas [11- 15]. Ultraviolet irradiation has commonly been used in the indoor environment to eliminate or control infectious diseases in medical care facilities. HVAC system components such as duct-liners, cooling coils, drip-pans, interior insulation and areas subjected to high levels of moisture can create an environment which is prone to biological contamination. The movement of indoor air being dominated by HVAC system operation can carry biological contaminants which can expose large numbers of building occupants to bioaerosols. In addition, possible terrorist activities could release biological agents into ambient air, or directly into a building environment, or HVAC system may expose multitudes of individuals to dangerous pathogens.

A single UVC light-bulb was placed inside a galvanized steel square HVAC duct mock-up. The exposure chamber was maintained at room temperature which was 22 °C (71.6 °F). A method to determine the antimicrobial efficacy of UVC irradiation was developed and tested on the surface of agar plates with four species of vegetative bacteria, seven species of fungi and eight varieties of *Bacillus* bacteria spores. *B. anthracis* surrogates were used for their expected similar inactivation responses to UVC irradiation. The exposure time (from 5 to 900 seconds depending on the microorganism) was initiated when an internal guillotine was very quickly lifted allowing the UV light to travel down the duct to impact the plates. Only half of the inoculated agar plate was exposed to UV light by shading half of the plate. At the end of the exposure time, the guillotine was quickly lowered back into the duct mock-up. In all experiments, the plates were kept the same distance from the light (144.0 cm, or 56 in.). With distance and irradiance constant, time of exposure is the controlling variable. The percent kill and k value for each organism were calculated for various periods of exposure [16, 17].

For constant and uniform irradiance, the disinfection effect of UVC on a population of microorganisms can be expressed by the following set of equations [18]:

$$N_t/N_0 = \exp(- k \bullet \text{dose}) \tag{1}$$

Where:

N_t =	the number of microorganisms at any time t,
N_0 =	the number of microorganisms at start, before exposure begins,
N_t/N_0 =	the fraction of microorganisms surviving,
k =	a microorganism-dependent rate constant, $cm^2 / \mu W \bullet s$
dose =	the product of $E_{eff} \bullet \Delta t$, in $\mu W \bullet s / cm^2$ (measured irradiance • seconds of exposure),
W =	watts,
E_{eff} =	the effective irradiance received, in $\mu W \bullet s / cm^2$ (measured), and,
Δt =	exposure duration in seconds, s, between the start and time *t*.

The concentration-time product calculated in Equation 1 depicts the exponential decay of a population of viable organisms with constant exposure to UVC. Equation 1 can also indicate the ability of populations of microorganisms to withstand low to high doses of UVC irradiation [16, 17].

The plates were incubated until moderate growth was visible, then the colony forming units (CFUs) were counted. The percentage killed was obtained by the following Equation (2):

$$\% \text{ Kill} = 100 \times [1 - (C_E / C_{NE})] \tag{2}$$

where C_E is the number of colonies on the side of the plate exposed to UV (N_t) and C_{NE} is the number of colonies on the side of the plate not exposed to UV (N_0). Significant kill was achieved with increasing periods of exposure (up to a high kill rate of 81% for a 120 second exposure). Spores exposed to a similar dose of UV irradiation for an extended period (as would be found on surfaces such as cooling coil fins within an air-handler) would be expected to be relatively free of *Bacillus* bacteria. This research demonstrated that UVC lamp irradiation inactivated eight varieties of *Bacillus* bacteria spores to a reproducible degree with conditions of fixed dose. The k value and kill rate were calculated with above equations. The test organisms were deposited on the surface of an agar plate [16].

The eight varieties of *Bacillus* spores tested exhibited a level of resistence to UVGI irradiance that was similar. Each species had large variations in surviving populations, and no significant difference in resistance between species. The k values ranged from a high of 7.46e^{-05} cm^2 W-sec (for *B. s. orange*) to a low of 3.23e^{-05} cm^2 W-sec (for *B. megaterium*) [16].

The k value results showed variability for the three normally susceptible vegetative bacteria from 1.05 e^{-03} cm$^2\mu$W-sec to 3.60 e^{-05} cm$^2\mu$W-sec (with a range of relative standard deviation from 74 to 105%); yeast varied from 1.83 e^{-04} cm$^2\mu$W-sec to 1.73 e^{-05} cm$^2\mu$W-sec (with a range of relative standard deviations from 68 to 166%); and mold varied from 2.78 e^{-05} cm$^2\mu$W-sec to 7.39 e^{-06} cm$^2\mu$W-sec (with a range of relative standard deviation from 56 to 139%). Although highly variable the k values are both reproducible and similar for all varieties tested. *Deinococcus radiodurans* (bacteria), *Rhodotorula mucilaginosa* (yeast), and *Cladosporium cladosporioides* (mold) were the most difficult organisms to destroy in their groups. As anticipated, the four species of mold required a longer period of exposure to exhibit significant die-off than the vegetative bacteria. It is difficult to infer further UVC exposure effects between microorganisms as comparatively diverse as fungi and bacteria [17]. The ability to eliminate microorganism contaminants within commercial HVAC and residential HAC systems should contribute toward reducing occupant exposure and the opportunity for the spread of these organisms based on infectious diseases.

An example of the results of this work is listed in Figure 1 which depicts the percent kill as a function of the period (sec.) of UV. exposure. *D. radiodurans* (bacteria), *R. mucilaginosa* (yeast), and *C. cladosporioides* (mold) were the most difficult organisms to destroy: *G. candidum* and *C. albicans* of the yeast, *S. epidermidis*, *S. marcescens* and *P. fluorescens* of the bacteria, were the organisms which were most rapidly destroyed. Other than these specific microorganisms the four species of mold microorganisms required a longer period of exposure to exhibit significant die-off. It is difficult to infer further UV exposure effects between microorganisms as comparatively diverse as fungi and bacteria.

Heating, ventilating, and air-conditioning (HVAC) systems become colonized by microorganisms after a period of use, and distribute those organisms as well as those in the return air. Depending on the amount and type of microorganisms (bacteria, viruses and mold), the amount of dust and stationary film, cooling coil fouling may occur. It has been suggested that this fouling is responsible for a diminished coil capacity and increased energy consumption. Ultraviolet (UVC) irradiation is commonly used to eliminate or control microorganisms, and has recently been applied for indoor environments control and energy efficiency. ALTRU-V™ product line has two V-Smart software programs, to calculate the selection and application of UVC products and solutions for HVAC design and maintenance. UVC used to maintain HVAC equipment, and resulting in lower energy costs while providing cleaner air would greatly reduce occupant exposure and the opportunity for the spread of disease and allergic reactions. Effectively designing or retrofitting HVAC systems with ultraviolet products has formerly been performed without design criterion. The V-Smart software attempts to answer design questions such as how much UVC is required, what output performance can be expected.

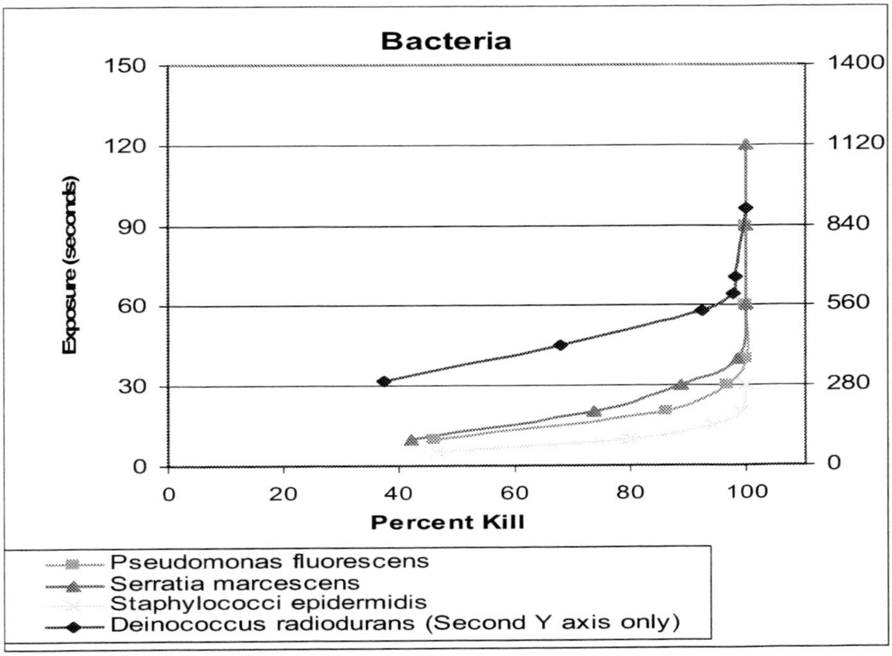

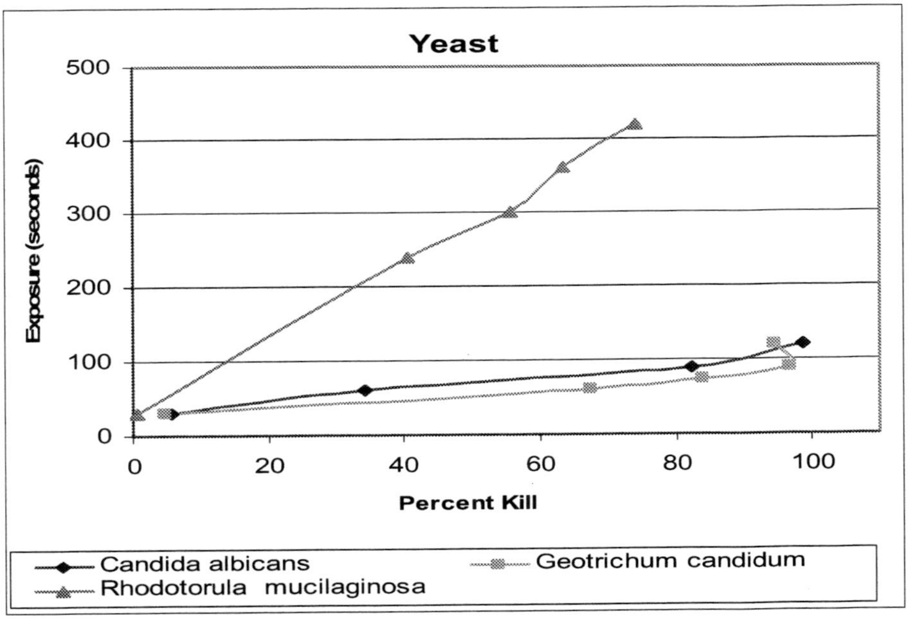

Figure 1. (Continued)

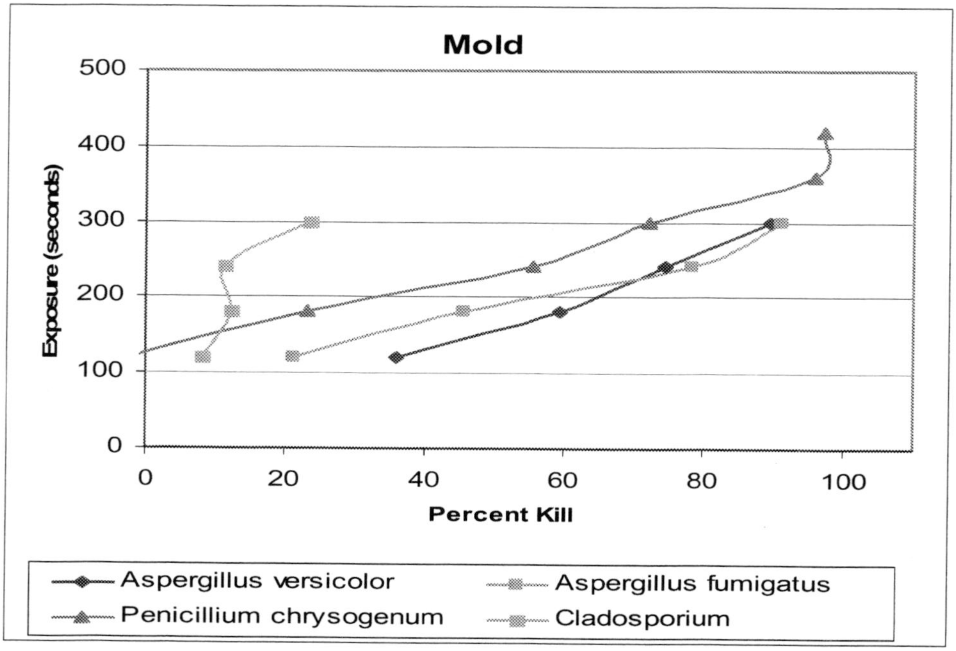

Figure 1. Comparison of percent kill by UV period of exposure.

(E) Ozone

Recent work evaluated the effects of exposing a variety of microorganisms (two bacteria and two fungi) to elevated gaseous ozone concentrations ranging from 100 – 1000 ppm [19]. In order to evaluate ozone under realistic "real world" conditions, the test organisms were inoculated onto the surfaces of building materials. The objective of this study was to evaluate the effects of exposing a variety of microorganisms to elevated gaseous ozone concentrations. Both porous and non-porous building materials were used to represent actual indoor surfaces, and controlled chamber exposures were conducted to maintain consistent exposure concentrations.

Both gypsum wallboard (porous) and glass slide (non-porous) building materials were employed as the test surfaces in a series of experiments. Four separate microorganisms and two levels of relative humidity (RH) were tested. The four organisms selected for testing in this study were: *Rhodotorula mucilaginosa*, *Penicillium brevicompactum*, *Bacillus atrophaeus*, and *Staphylococcus epidermidis*. Two fungi organisms [*R. mucilaginosa* (vegetative yeast cells) and *P. brevicompactum* (mold spores)], and two bacteria organisms [*B. atrophaeus* (gram-positive bacterial spores), and *S. epidermidis* (vegetative bacterium)] were used.

The ozone efficacy results varied for the organisms inoculated on the surface of glass slides and gypsum wallboard coupons. Exposures on the glass slides at low RH had no observed effect on the concentration of *B. atrophaeus* and *R. mucilaginosa*, while the *S. epidermidis* and *P. brevicompactum* both decreased at least 4 logs at the maximum exposure.

The high RH exposures on both glass slides and gypsum wallboard affected all of the organisms. However, the *R. mucilaginosa* were inactivated by 4 logs. On the gypsum wallboard at low RH, none of the organisms exposed were inactivated by as much as 2 logs. The organisms exposed to high concentrations of gaseous ozone were more readily killed on glass slides than on gypsum wallboard. Additionally, increasing RH was found to increase the biocidal capability of high levels of ozone [19].

The overall results of this study indicate that, even at relatively high concentrations of ozone, it is difficult to get significant inactivation (damage to genetic material causing non-viability) of organisms on surfaces. In agreement with earlier experiments conducted at low ozone concentrations, the organisms exposed to high concentrations of gaseous ozone were more readily killed on glass slides than on gypsum wallboard. Increasing RH increases the biocidal capability of high levels of ozone [19]. However, unlike the application of previously discussed antimicrobial treatments such as cleaners, paints or UV irradiation, gaseous ozone is not a realistic alternative for remediating biological contamination.

Although the specific results vary according to each of the four test organisms and the test surfaces, the overall results of this study indicate that, even at relatively high concentrations of ozone, it is difficult to get significant inactivation of organisms on surfaces. Maintaining consistently high concentrations of 1000 ppm of ozone gas could be difficult throughout the volume of air contained in a building remediation application due to unwanted reactions with building materials. Achieving a significant reduction of biocontamination concentrations on surfaces, as well as inside porous materials, wall cavities and voids within a building would be very difficult [19]. In addition to the difficulty in achieving these elevated concentrations, and the inadequate ability of gas phase ozone to reduce concentrations of microorganisms, the high risk to human health of exposure makes this treatment technique both ineffective and hazardous.

SUMMARY

The significant technical findings of the research discussed within this report are summarized and listed below. The discussions of the technical findings are only meant to summarize the referenced publications and not to restate technical results from those publications. The findings listed below summarize the evaluation of antimicrobial treatments as control technologies (Antimicrobial Encapsulants, Antimicrobial Cleaners, Antimicrobial Paints, Antimicrobial UVC Irradiation, and Ozone).

The results of antimicrobial product testing are not meant to endorse the incomplete removal of mold contaminated building materials. However, it is recognized that complete removal may not always be possible and solutions to control mold regrowth may contribute to reduced occupant exposure. Current recommendations of removal and replacement of porous building materials should be followed. It was not the intension of this discussion to endorse any product. Reporting on the performance of these products under the stated conditions was and remains the only purpose.

Technical Findings. Evaluation of Antimicrobial Treatments as Control Technologies

Finding that significant variation in antimicrobial efficacy of encapsulents to limit or eliminate biological growth indicates a need for widespread product testing and for the development of an efficacy testing protocol [2, 3, 7].

Lysol All-Purpose Cleaner-Orange Breeze (full strength) demonstrated results which ranked among the best in five of the six surfaces tested. Both Borax and Orange Glo Multipurpose Degreaser demonstrated results which ranked among the best in four of the six surfaces tested [3].

In instances (when mold damage is not substantial), cleaning surfaces and then painting with Permawhite, M-1 Additive, Porterscept, or Mil-Kil can offer a practical alternative to removing building materials [7].

UVC irradiation has the ability to eliminate microorganism contaminants within commercial HVAC and residential HAC systems and contribute toward reducing occupant exposure to microorganisms and the opportunity for the spread of these organisms as well as infectious diseases [8, 16, 17].

Maintaining high concentrations of ozone gas necessary for significant reduction of biocontamination concentrations on surfaces, as well as inside porous materials, wall cavities and voids within a building would be very difficult and impractical [19].

The findings listed above cover a broad expanse of research related to detecting and controlling mold contamination. Additional work is needed to further reduce human exposure to biological contaminants.

References

[1] ASTM 6329-98, (2003) *Standard Guide for Developing Methodology for Evaluating the Ability of Indoor Materials to Support Microbial Growth Using Static Environmental Chambers*.

[2] Menetrez, M. Y., and Foarde, K. K., Testing Antimicrobial Efficacy on Porous Materials, Indoor Built Environment: *The Journal of the International Society of the Built Environment,* October, 2002;11:202-207.

[3] Menetrez, M. Y., Foarde, K. K., Webber, T. D., Dean, T. R., and Betancourt, D. A., Testing Antimicrobial Cleaner Efficacy On Gypsum Wallboard Contaminated with *Stachybotrys chartarum, Journal of Environmental Science and Pollution Research,* March 2007, espr 2007.03.397.

[4] Dearborn D. G., Iwona Y, Sorenson W. G., Miller M. J.: Overview of investigations into pulmonary hemorrhage among infants in Cleveland, Ohio: *Environmental Health Perspectives*, 107 (Suppl. 3), June 1999, p 495-499.

[5] Vesper S. J., Dearborn D. G., Yike I., Allan T., Sobolewski J., Hinkley S.F., Jarvis B.B., Haugland R. A.: Evaluation of Stachybotrys chartarum in house of an infant with

pulmonary hemorrhage: quantitative assessment before, during, and after remediation: *Journal of Urban Health,* 77 (1), Mar 2000, pp 68-85.

[6] Vesper S. J., Vesper M. J.: Stachylysin may be a cause of hemorrhaging in humans exposed to Stachybotrys chartarum: *Infection and Immunity,* 70 (4), April 2002, pp 2065-2069.

[7] Menetrez, M. Y., Foarde, K. K., Webber, T. D., Dean, T. R., and Betancourt, D. A., Testing Antimicrobial Paint Efficacy On Gypsum Wallboard Contaminated with *Stachybotrys chartarum, The Journal of Occupational and Environmental Hygiene, 5*: 1-4, Feb. 2008.

[8] Shechmeister, I.L. (1991) Sterilization by ultraviolet radiation. In *Disinfection, Sterilization, and Preservation.* S.S. Block, Ed. Phildelphia: Lea & Febiger, 553-565.

[9] Cole, E.C. and Foarde, K.K. (1999) Chapter 16. Biocides and Antimicrobial Agents. Bioaerosols: Assessment and Control. J. Macher, ed. *American Conference of Governmental Industrial Hygienists,* Cincinnati, OH.

[10] VanOsdell, D., and Foarde, K.K. (2002) *Defining the Effectiveness of UV Lamps Installed in Circulating Air Ductwork,* ARTI-21CR/610-40030-01.

[11] Morey, P.R. (1988) Microorganisms in Buildings and HVAC Systems. A Summary of Environmental Studies. Proceedings of IAQ'88 - Engineering Solutions to Indoor Air Problems. Atlanta, GA. April 11-13. *American Society of Heating, Refrigerating and Air-Conditioning Engineers*: Atlanta, GA, 10-25.

[12] Lidwell, O.M. (1994) Ultraviolet radiation and the control of airborne contamination in the operating room, *J. of Hosp. Inf.,* 28, 245-248.

[13] Calvo, M.A., Agut, M., Calvo, R.M. and Larrondo, J. (1999) Effect of ultraviolet light irradiation and nitrosoguanidine on viability of 46 strains of Arthinium and their antibiotic production, *Microbios,* 98, 179-187.

[14] Slieman, T.A., and Nicholson, W.L. (2000) Artificial and Solar UV Radiation Induces Strand Breaks and Cyclobutane Pyrimidine Dimers in Bacillus subtilus Spore DNA, *Applied and Environmental Microbiology,* 66(1), 199-205.

[15] Peccia, J., Werth, H.M., Miller, S. and Hernandez, M. (2001) Effects of Relative Humidity on the Ultraviolet Induced Inactivation of Airborne Bacteria, *Aerosol Science and Technology,* 35, 728-740.

[16] Menetrez, M. Y., Foarde, K. K., Webber, T. D., Dean, T. R., and Betancourt, D. A., Efficacy of UV Irradiation on Eight Species of Bacillus, *Journal of Environmental Engineering and Science,* Volume 5, Number 4, July 2006, 329-334.

[17] Menetrez, M. Y., Foarde, K. K., Webber, T. D., Dean, T. R., and Betancourt, D. A., Testing The Effectiveness of UV Irradiation on Vegetative Bacteria and Fungi Surface Contamination, *Journal of Environmental Microbiology,* 2008.

[18] Phillips Lighting Division (1992) Disinfection by UV-radiation. *Booklet* 3222 C34; 00671.

[19] Menetrez, M. Y., Foarde, K. K., Webber, T. D., Dean, T. R., and Betancourt, D. A., An Evaluation of the Antimicrobial Effects of Gas-Phase Ozone, *The Journal of Ozone: Science and Engineering,* 2008.

In: Fungicides
Editors: P. De Costa and P. Bezerra

ISBN: 978-1-60692-631-4

Chapter VII

Determination of Fungicide Residues in Environmental Samples

Graciela M. Escandar
Instituto de Química Rosario (CONICET-UNR), Facultad de Ciencias Bioquímicas y Farmacéuticas, Universidad Nacional de Rosario,
Suipacha 531 (S2002LRK) Rosario, Argentina

Abstract

The current state of analytical methods devoted to the determination of common fungicide residues is reviewed, based on the concern of worldwide government agencies about their potential risk for human health. The review covers relevant analytical methods applied to samples of environmental interest, highlighting the analysis of natural waters and foodstuff for human consumption.

Introduction

This chapter discusses developments in methods devoted to the fungicide analysis in environmental samples the last fifteen years. Coverage is limited to the most significant papers in the field. Techniques and methods that best demonstrates the evolution of fungicide analysis are highlighted.

Fungicides are a type of pesticides that control fungal illnesses by specifically inhibiting or killing the fungus causing the disease. They are applied with the purpose of controlling a disease during the development of a crop, increasing its productivity, and improving the storage life and quality of harvested plants and crop. Because of that, the general population is exposed to fungicides and their possible toxic effects. Fungicides vary extremely in their potential for causing adverse effects in humans [1] and, fortunately, most of the newly developed chemicals have a low degree of toxicity to mammals [2]. However, because of concern about the possibilities of chronic health problems and environmental effects, many of those compounds that were commonly used in the past are now under review, since several studies determined that they could be carcinogenic [3]. In certain cases, it is the fungicide derivatives which are toxic. For instance, ethylenethiourea, derived from decomposition of dithiocarbamate fungicides in environment, has been suspected of causing teratogenic, carcinogenic, immunotoxic, and mutagenic effects [4]. World official agencies have shown a particular interest in monitoring and regulating the usage of pesticide residues in environmental samples [5]. These agencies report documents describing the method validation and analytical quality control requirements to support the validity of the data used for checking conformity to maximum residue limits (MRLs) and assessment of consumer exposure to pesticides [6, 7].

European and UK drinking water regulations require that potable water contains less than 0.1 μg L^{-1} of an individual pesticide (herbicide, insecticide or fungicide), and less than 0.5 μg L^{-1} of total pesticides [8], while they allow a maximum of 0.05 mg kg^{-1} of any pesticide in agricultural foodstuff [9]. According to these values, it is evident that sensitive analytical methods, providing very low limits of detection (LODs) and quantification (LOQs) are needed.

The large number of reviews and some books devoted to the analysis of priority pesticides in the evaluated period is an indication of the concern on this topic [10-39]. Since pesticides (herbicides, insecticides and fungicides) can have similar chemical structures, most methods employed for their determination focus the attention in their chemical properties rather than in their functions. Therefore, it is very common to fing methods devoted to the determination of several pesticides, regardless their specific activity.

The above cited reviews indicate that the most commonly employed analytical techniques are chromatographic ones, from the more simple methods to tandem-liquid or gas chromatography-mass spectrometric techniques (LC-MS and GC-MS respectively).

Different approaches directed to the improvement of the isolation, pre-concentration and cleanup of pesticide residue extracts from various environmental matrices have also been reviewed [15,18,19,37, 40-54].

This chapter has been organized by first discussing the most used separative methods, followed by the remaining employed methodologies, classified according to the nature of the instrumental signal which is measured.

SEPARATIVE METHODS

Chromatography

Although chromatographic techniques, such as supercritical-fluid [55-58], conventional and high-performance thin-layer [59-65] and ion chromatographies [66, 67], have been applied to analysis of pesticides, most of the analyses have been developed using gas chromatography and HPLC (high-performance liquid chromatography), which are described below.

Gas Chromatography

Capillary gas chromatography has been the CG technique selected for the analysis of pesticide residues in environment samples. Several methods using conventional detectors (i.e. electron-capture, nitrogen-phosphorus-selective or flame photometric detectors) were reported for fungicide determination in natural waters [68-76] and other environmental or natural matrices such as soils, wines, vegetables, fruits, medicinal herbs, rice fields, rice, black tea malt, spent grains, beer and plants (ginseng) [68,76–99]. In general, these methods are able to determine a limited number of fungicides, but the involved methodologies are fast and show very good sensitivity. Other specific detectors were also applied. Campillo et al. developed a method based on solid-phase microextraction followed by GC with microwave-induced plasma atomic emission detection for determining captan and other pesticides in honey [100]. Quantification was carried out by monitoring the chlorine, bromine and sulphur emission lines and the detection limits ranged from 0.02 to 10 ng g^{-1}. Captan was determined, by a similar procedure, in herbal and tea infusions [101].

Khummueng et al. reported the use of two-dimensional gas chromatography (GC×GC) with nitrogen-phosphorus detection for the quantitation of the fungicides chlorothalonil, iprodione, myclobutanil, penconazole, procymidone, propiconazole, tebuconazole and vinclozolin in vegetable samples [102].

In several cases, confirmation of the analysed compounds was performed by gas chromatography-mass spectrometry [84,89,90,91,96,102].

Gas Chromatography-Mass Spectroscopy

GC-MS is a common separation technique for thermally stable fungicide residue analysis, because of its sensitivity and selectivity, and the easy identification of compounds from the mass spectra. The residues are identified in screening analyses by means of the mass spectral libraries containing reference mass spectra and retention times of active ingredients and also of their metabolites.

Table 1 presents the different fungicides analyzed in water and foodstuff samples by using CG-MS in the reviewed period. In addition, features of the employed chromatographic techniques and the evaluated concentration levels are indicated.

The information in this table was organized by first giving the analyses carried out in water samples (including river, lake, sea, tap, mineral and waste waters) and then those performed in a large variety of environmental samples. Within each of these major groups, in turn, the citation is set in chronological order. This setup has the purpose of showing the evolution of strategies and employed instrumental.

As can be appreciated, fungicides are in most cases simultaneously determined with pesticides by using this analytical multiresidue method: samples with one hundred or more residues were analyzed [136,153,155,163,171].

Table 1. Gas chromatography-mass spectroscopic methods for fungicide determination in environmental samples

Fungicides	Matrix[a]	Method	Concentration Levels[b]	Ref.
captan, chlorothalonil, procymidone[c]	water	GC-MS (SIM)	LODs 0.14 μg L^{-1} (captan), 0.003 μg L^{-1} (chlorothalonil), 0.012 μg L^{-1} (procymidone)	103
ethylenethiourea (environmental metabolite of ethylenebis dithiocarbamate fungicides)	water	GC-CI-MS	0.05-50 μg L^{-1}	104
metalaxyl, triadimenol, tebuconazole[c,d]	water	SPE-GC-MS and SPE-GC-MS-MS	LODs 1-40 ng L^{-1}	105
dicloran, chlorothalonil, vinclozolin, dichlofluanid, captan, folpet, captafol	water	SPME-GC-MS	LODs 1-60 ng L^{-1}	106
captan, chloroneb, chlorothalonil, ediphenfos, etridiazole, fenarimol, flutolanil, iprobenfos, iprodione, isoprothiolane, mepronil, pencycuron, phthalide, probenazole, procymidone, quintozene, tolclofos-methyl, tricyclazole	water	SPE-GC-MS	LODs 0.01-0.1 μg L^{-1}	107
metalaxyl, folpet, vinclozolin[c,e]	water	SPE-GC-MS-MS	LODs < 48 ng L^{-1}, LOQs 160 ng L^{-1}	108
chlorothalonil, cyproconazole, difenoconazole, folpet, imazalil, imibenconazole, propiconazole, tebuconazole, triadimenol, triflumizole[c]	water	headspace SPME-GC-MS	< 5 μg L^{-1}	109
chlorothalonil, dichlofluanid, vinclozolin[c]	water	SPME-GC-MC (SIM)	LODs 1-56 ng L^{-1}	110
procymidone[c]	water	SPME-GC-ITD-MS-MS	LOD 0.003 μg L^{-1}	111
polycarbamate	water	TPI-GC-MS	0.3 μg L^{-1}	112
captan, etridiazole, propiconazole[c]	water	SBSE-TD-GC-MS	LODs 0.2-20 ng L^{-1}	113
captan, etridiazole, flusilazole, iprodione, oxadixyl,	water	SPE-GC-MS	0.1 μg L^{-1}	114

penconazole, propiconazole, tebuconazole, vinclozolin[c]				
procymidone[c]	water	SPE-isotope dilution-GC-MS	< 1 μg L^{-1}	115
iprodione, tebuconazole, triadimefon[c]	rain water	SPME-GC-ITD-MS-MS	LODs 5-500 ng L^{-1}	116
chlorothalonil, dichlofluanid[c]	water	SME-GC-MS	LOD 10 ng L^{-1}, LOQ 30 ng L^{-1} (chlorothalonil), LOD 32 ng L^{-1}, LOQ 97 ng L^{-1} (dichlofluanid)	117
diphenylamine, cyprodinil, thiabendazole, imazalil[c]	water	SPME-GC-TOF-MS	0.1-1 μg L^{-1}	118
fenpropimorphic acid (metabolite of fenpropimorph)	soil	GC-MS	LODs 1 μg kg^{-1}	119
N-n-alkyl-dimethylmorpholines	sediment	GC-MS	5-100 ng mL^{-1}	120
captan, thiabendazole, procymidone[c]	carrot	LP-GC-MS	LODs 8 ng g^{-1} (captan) 16 ng g^{-1} (thiabendazole) 0.2 ng g^{-1} (procymidone)	121
vinclozolin, iprodione, procymidone	white wines	SBSE-TD-GC-MS	LOQs 0.5 μg L^{-1} (vinclozolin and procymidone), 5 μg L^{-1} (iprodione)	122
cyprodinil, fludioxonil	white wines	SPME-GC-MS	LODs 0.1 μg L^{-1} (cyprodinil), 0.2 μg L^{-1} (fludioxonil)	123
metalaxyl	soil	GC-EII-MS	1-10 ng L^{-1}	124
pyrimethanil, kresoxim-methyl	grapes, strawberries, tomatoes, ketchup	HS-SPME-GC-MS	LODs 1.8-2.0 ng g^{-1} (pyrimethanil), 2.8-3.1 ng g^{-1} (kresoxim-methyl)	125
bitertanol, captan, tolclofos-methyl, vinclozolin, folpet, thiabendazole, imazalil, metalaxyl, difenoconazole, quintozene, tebuconazole, penconazole, propiconazole, pyrimethanil, fludioxonil, tecnazene, iprodione, myclobutanil, tolylfluanid[c]	fruits and vegetables	SPE-GC-MS	LOQs 0.01 mg kg^{-1}	126

Table 1. Continued

Fungicides	Matrix[a]	Method	Concentration Levels[b]	Ref.
captan, chlorothalonil, dichlofluanid, folpet, imazalil, metalaxil, o-phenylphenol, thiabendazole[c]	fruits and vegetables	DSPE-GC-MS	250 ng g^{-1}	127
procymidone, thiabendazole, captan[c]	fruits	GC×GC-TOF-MS	0.01 mg kg^{-1}	128
vinclozolin, dicloran	soil	SPME-UE-GC-MS	LODs 2-13 ng g^{-1}	129
captan, procymidone, thiabendazole[c]	cereal based foods	GC-TOF-MS	LOQs ≤ 0.01 mg kg^{-1}	130
pyrimethanil, kresoxim-methyl	soil, humic materials	HS-SPME-GC-MS	LODs 0.001 μg g^{-1} (pyrimethanil), 0.004 μg g^{-1} (kresoxim-methyl)	131
benalaxyl, cyprodinil, flusilazole, oxadixyl, thiabendazole[c]	fruits and vegetables	GC-MS (SIM)	at ng g^{-1} levels	132
procymidone, vinclozolin[c,g]	wine	MMLLE-GC-MS	LODs 0.03-0.4 μg L^{-1} LOQs 0.3-3.5 μg L^{-1}	133
quintozene[c]	fruit	GC-ICP-MS	at ng g^{-1} levels	134
procymidone[c]	marine sediments	SSLE-GC-MS-MS	LOD 1μg L^{-1}	135
procymidone[c]	marine sediments	MAE-GC-MS-MS	1μg L^{-1}	136
chlorothalonil, chlorpyrifos, cyproconazole, nuarimol, procymidone[c]	soil, juice, honey	GC-MS	LODs 1 ppb, LOQs 10 ppb	137
captan, cyproconazole, difenoconazole, epoxiconazole, etaconazole, etridiazole, fenbuconazole, fludioxonil, folpet, hexaconazole, imazalil, iprodione, myclobutanil, nuarimol, penconazole, prochloraz, propiconazole, quinoxyfen, quintozene, tebuconazole, tecnazene, tolylfluanid, triadimenol, triflumizole, triticonazole,	fruits and vegetables	GC-MS	≤ 50 ng g^{-1}	138

vinclozolin[c]				
benalaxyl, captan, cyproconazole, fludioxinil, hexaconazole, iprodione, kresoxim-methyl, metalaxyl, myclobutanil, oxadixyl, penconazole, procymidone, propiconazole, quintozene, tebuconazole, tetraconazole, triadimenol triflumizol, vinclozolin[c]	vegetables	GC-QqQ-MS	LODs 0.02-0.57 μg kg^{-1}	139
fenarimol, iprodione, metalaxyl, procymidone, quintozene[c]	sediment	GC-MS	2-10 μg kg^{-1}	140
captan, chlorothalonil, folpet, imazalil, metalaxyl, thiabendazole, vinclozolin[c]	vegetables, fruits	GC-MS (SIM)	10-100 ng g^{-1}	141
benalaxyl, chlorothalonil, cyproconazole, nuarimol, procymidone, triadimefon[c]	juice	SPE-GC-MS (SIM)	LODs 0.1-4.6 μg L^{-1}	142
imazalil, isoprothiolane [c]	food waste compost	PLE-GC-MS	0.02-0.04 μg g^{-1}	143
captan, cyprodinil, kresoxim-methyl, methidathion, myclobutanil, penconazole, tebuconazole[c]	apple	GC-MS	0.01 mg kg^{-1}	144
captan, kresoxim-methyl myclobutanil, penconazole, tebuconazole[c,f]	apple and baby food	SPE-GC-MS (SIM)	LOQs < 5 μg kg^{-1}	145
captan, cyprodinil, folpet, imazalil, tebuconazole, thiabendazole, tolylfluanid, procymidone, vinclozolin[c]	fruit-based baby food	GC-MS	10 ng g^{-1}	146
flusilazole, imibenconazole, propiconazole[c]	vegetables, fruits, and green tea	SBSE-TD-RTL-GC-MS	LODs 5 μg kg^{-1}	147
captan, kresoxim-methyl, myclobutanol, penconazole, tebuconazole[c]	apple	GC-MS	0.005 mg kg^{-1}	148
captan, folpet	khaki and cauliflower	SPE-GC-MS	LODs 0.01 mg kg^{-1}	149

Table 1. Continued

Fungicides	Matrix[a]	Method	Concentration Levels[b]	Ref.
bitertanol, cyproconazole, difenoconazole, fenarimol, flusilazole, flutolanil, imibenconazole, myclobutanil, propiconazole, tebuconazole[c]	green tea, water	dual SBSE-TD-LTM-GC-MS	LODs <10 ng L^{-1}	150
folpet[c]	washing waters of olive	SPE-GC-MS-MS	at ng L^{-1} levels	151
chlorothalonil, metalaxil, penconazole, procymidone, tetraconazole, triadimefon, triadimenol, triflumizole, vinclozolin[c]	vegetables	GC-MS-MS	LODs <3.2 μg kg^{-1}, LOQs 9.6 μg kg^{-1}	152
benalaxyl, cyfluthrin, difenoconazole, fludioxonil, hexaconazole, iprodione, oxadixyl, penconazole, propiconazole, tebuconazole, vinclozolin[c]	avocado	PLE-LP-GC-MS-MS	LOQs 0.04-8.33 μg kg^{-1}	153
captan, chlorothalonil, flusilazole, folpet, imazalil, metalaxyl, oxadixyl, procymidone, pyrimethanil, tebuconazole, thiabendazole, triadimefon, vinclozolin[c]	tomato	LP-GC-MS-MS	LODs 0.1-0.4 μg kg^{-1}	154
azaconazole, benaxalil, bromuconazole, cyproconazole, diclobutrazol, dicloran, difenoconazole, dimethomorph, diniconazole, fenbuconazole, fenpropimorph, fludioxonil, fluquinconazole, flusilazole, folpet, hexaconazole, myclobutanil, propiconazole, tebuconazole, vinclozolin[c]	spinach, soybean and orange	SFE-GC-MS	0.05 μg g^{-1}	155
carbendazim, thiabendazole, bitertanol, epoxiconazole, flusilazole, imazalil, prochloraz, propiconazole,	apple	UPLC-MS-MS	LODs 0.5-8 μg kg^{-1}	156

tebuconazole, thiabendazole[c]				
bitertanol, captafol, captan, chlorothalonil dichlofluanid, folpet, imazalil, iprodione, myclobutanil, oxadixyl, procymidone, pyrifenox, pyrimethanil, triadimefon, triadimenol, vinclozolin[c]	apple juice	LVI-PTV-GC-MS (SIM)		157
chlorothalonil, cyprodinil, folpet, penconazole, procymidone[c]	fruit and vegetable	SBSE-TD-RTL-GC-MS	1-50 μg kg^{-1}	158
folpet[c]	olive oil	GC-MS-MS	LOD 5 μg kg^{-1}, LOQ 10 μg kg^{-1}	159
benalaxyl, metalaxyl, procymidone[c]	soils	SFE-GC-MS-MS	0.1-3.7 μg kg^{-1}	160
prochloraz, tebuconazole	mushroom	GC-MS	LOQs 0.01 mg kg^{-1}	161
o-phenylphenol	beer	GC-MS	0.1 μg L^{-1}	162
chlorobenzilate, chlorothalonil, dichlofluanid, iprodione, propiconazole, quintozene, uniconazole, vinclozolin[c]	unpolished rice	GPC-SPE-GC-MS (SIM)	LODs 1-20 ng g^{-1}	163
cyprodinil, dimethomorph, fludioxonil, iprodione, myclobutanil, pyrimethanil, quinoxyfen, vinclozolin[c]	lemon, raisins, wheat flour, cucumber	DSPE-GC-MS-MS	0.005, 0.01, 0.02, 0.2 mg kg^{-1}	164
folpet[c]	olives	GC-MS-MS	LOD 5 μg kg^{-1}	165
procymidone, iprodione, captan, tolylfluanid[c]	herbal crude drugs	SPE-GC-MS	LODs 0.003-0.006 mg kg^{-1}	166
vinchlozolin, triadifemon, procymidone, hexaconazole, myclobutanil, krezoxim-methyl, propiconazole, tebuconazole[c,f]	wheat grain, peach, lettuce	SPE-GC-MS	LOQs 0.005-0.01 mg kg^{-1}	167
chlorophenols	industrial efluents	SPME-GC-MS	lowest level 0.5 ng mL^{-1}	168
cyproconazole, difenoconazole, flusilazole, imazalil, myclobutanil, penconazole, prochloraz, propiconazole, tebuconazole, triadimefon, triadimenol	honeybee	SPE-GC-MS (SIM)	LODs 0.001-0.005 μg per bee	169

Table 1. Continued

Fungicides	Matrix[a]	Method	Concentration Levels[b]	Ref.
captan, captafol, folpet	air	LVI-CI-GC-MS	LODs 2.5 μg L^{-1} (captan, folpet), 5.0 μg L^{-1} (captafol)	170
bitertanol, captafol, captan, chlorobenzilate, cyproconazole, dichlofluanid, difenoconazole, flusilazole, flutolanil, imibenconazole, iprodione, myclobutanil, tebuconazole, triadimenol, tricyclazole[c]	potato, cabbage, carrot, apple, orange, cucumber, rice	GPC-DSPE-GC-MS	0.1 mg kg^{-1}	171
chlorothalonil and degradate products	soil, sediment	SPE-GC-MS	LODs 1-5 μg kg^{-1}	172

[a] Water samples include natural and/or waste waters. [b] They are given as LODs, LOQs or evaluated concentrations. [c] Other pesticides and/or organic pollutants are included in the analysis. [d] Nitrogen - phosphorus detection (NPD) was also applied. [e] NDP and electron-capture detection (ECD) were also applied, [f] ECD was also applied. [g] Flame-ionization detection (FID) was also applied. CI chemical ionization. DSPE dispersive solid-phase extraction. EII electron-impact ionization. GPC gel permeation chromatography. HS headspace. ITD ion trap. ICP inductively coupled plasma. LP low-pressure. LTM low thermal mass. LVI large-volume injection. MAE microwave-assisted extraction. MMLLE microporous membrane liquid-liquid extraction. PLE pressurized liquid extraction. PTV programmed-temperature vaporization. QqQ triple quadrupole. RTL retention time locked. SBSE stir bar sorptive extraction. SFE supercritical fluid extraction. SIM selected-ion monitoring. SPE solid-phase extraction. SPME solid-phase micro extraction. SSLE sequential superheated liquid extraction. TD thermal desorption. TOF time of flight. TPI temperature-programmable inlet. UE ultrasonic extraction.

High Performance Liquid Chromatography

In the 1990s, HPLC with UV-spectrophotometric detection, including single wavelength and diode array detection, was one of the most used methods for the determination of fungicides in water [173-188] and other natural samples [189-193]. Nowadays, this simple and fast method is still being applied for the determination of widely used fungicides in water, milk, soil, fruits, vegetables and food [194-213].

With the purpose of increasing selectivity, many of LC methods are combined with modern extraction techniques such as molecularly imprinted solid-phase extraction [212]. Molecularly imprinted polymers were also prepared for the SPE of tebuconazole in biological and environmental samples (cabbage, pannage, shrimp, orange juice and tap water) [214].

The native fluorescence emission of benzimidazole fungicides was used for their detection in water samples [215-217], food [218] and soil [219], at part per billion levels after chromatographic separation. A thiabendazole-imprinted column was used for the HPLC-fluorescence determination of this fungicide in orange, lemon, grape and strawberry extracts at low concentration levels and in less than 15 min, without any need for a clean-up step in the analytical protocol [200]. Thiabendazole was determined in orange juice by HPLC with fluorescence detection [221], reaching detection and quantitation limits of 0.15 and 0.50 μg kg^{-1}, respectively. The confirmation of thianbendazole residues on positive samples was performed by gas chromatography with mass spectrometric detection using selected ion monitoring.

HPLC with fluorescence detection was also used for the determination of ortho-phenylphenol, diphenyl and diphenylamine in apples and oranges [222].

HPLC with post-column photolysis and fluorimetric, conductometric or electrochemical detection was evaluated for determination of more than 100 pesticides, including chlorothalonil, etridiazole and fenarimol, in groundwater samples [223].

The fungicides thiram [224], folpet, captan and captafol [225] were quantified in river water by HPLC with electrochemical detection.

Circular dichroism (CD) detectors were used when enantiomeric resolution of chiral fungicides was required [201,211,226].

HPLC-Mass Spectroscopy

Since the beginning of the present century, LC-MS has been gaining popularity as the major analytical method for pesticides, including fungicides. Fungicides are in most cases polar compounds of low volatility and in certain cases of thermal lability, facts that make LC-MS the technique of choice. Although GC-MS and LC-MS are complementary techniques, there is a clear trend to increase the number of LC-MS applicantions in pesticide residue analysis.

The on-line coupling of LC-MS is more difficult to accomplish than the GC-MS coupling. However, the problem has been overcome thanks to the development of a number of LC-MS interfaces, such as particle-beam, thermospray and atmospheric pressure chemical ionization interfaces, and continuous-flow fast-atom bombardment and electrospray. On the other hand, the coupling of LC with tandem mass spectrometry detection (MS-MS), which provides greater discrimination from matrix interferences, has notably improved the method performance and justifies why it is becoming popular for pesticide residue analysis.

Soler and Picó [39] have reported a review with a large number and variety of pesticides, including fungicides, which can be determined in food, using LC-MS-MS. The work includes the merits of the different mass analyzers, the improvements brought about by tandem MS and the most recent instrument designs.

Table 2 shows the references reviewed which apply LC-MS methods. The information was organized as in Table 1.

Because of the high separation and detecting power of the LC-MS method, fungicides shown in Table 2 were in many cases selected from usually large lists of determined pesticide residues.

HPLC and LC-ESI-MS using monolithic columns, which consist of continuous beds with macro and mesopores, were used to analyze pesticides, including the fungicides carbendazim, hexaconazole, tebuconazole and triadimefon [227]. Their advantages were evaluated and compared with those obtained using conventional packed columns.

Table 2. Liquid chromatography-mass spectroscopic methods for fungicide determination in environmental samples

Fungicide	Matrix[a]	Method	Concentration Levels[b]	Ref.
tebuconazole, triadimefon, fenpropimorph, tridemorph, benomyl, carbendazim[c]	water	LC-TS-MS	LODs 10-100 ng L^{-1}	228
pentachlorophenol and other acidic pesticides	water	LC-ESI-MS	LODs 2-25 ng L^{-1}	229
carbendazim, prochloraz, propiconazole[c]	water	SPE-LC-ESI-MS	LODs 2-4 ng L^{-1}	230
carbendazim, prochloraz, triadimenol, flusilazole, hexaconazole, tebuconazole, penconazole, propiconazole, triadimenol, fenpropimorph[c]	water	SPE-LC-APCI-MS and LLE-LC-APCI-MS	LOQs 0.02-0.1 μg L^{-1} (TCI), LOQs 0.004-0.02 μg L^{-1} (SIM)	231
carbendazim, prochloraz[c]	water	SPE-LC-ESI-MS	LODs 0.05-1.5 ng L^{-1}	232
oxine-copper, iprodione, thiram[c]	water	LC-ESI-MS	LODs 0.7-2.1 pg mL^{-1}	233
tricyclazole[c]	water	LC-PB-MS	0.1 μg mL^{-1}	234
carbendazim[c]	water	SPE-LC-ESI-MS-MS	25 ng L^{-1}	235
manzeb, maneb, zineb	water	LC-ESI-MS	0.05-2 μg mL^{-1}	236
carbendazim[c]	water	SPE-LC-MS-MS	25 ng L^{-1}	237
benzothiazoles	water	SPE-LC-ESI-MS	LOQs 20-200 ng L^{-1}	238
flusilazol, chlorthalonil[c,d]	water	LC-APCI-MS	LODs 7 ng L^{-1} (flusilazol), 15 ng L^{-1} (chlorthalonil)	239
carbendazim, imazalil[c]	water	SPE-LC-QqQ-MS-MS and SPE-LC-Q-TOF-MS-MS	0.37 μg L^{-1} (carbendazim), 0.22 μg L^{-1} (imazalil)	240
benomyl, carpropamid, thiram, oxine-copper, tricyclazole[c]	water	SFE-LC-TOF-MS	LODs 0.0034-3.3 μg L^{-1}	241
carbendazim, imazalil[c]	water	SPE-LC-ESI-MS-MS	LOQ 25 ng L^{-1}	242
azoxystrobin[c]	water	SPE-LC-ESI-MS^n	LOQ 16.7 μg L^{-1}	243

flubendazole, propiconazole, ketoconazole, miconazole, rabeprazole, itraconazole[c]	water	SPE-LC-ESI-MS-MS	10 ng L^{-1}	244
manzeb, maned, zineb, thiram, ziram	water	SPE-LC-APCI-MS-MS	LOQ 0.11 μg L^{-1}	4
imazalil, thiabendazole[c]	water	UPLC-TOF-MS	μg L^{-1} levels	245
ethylenethiourea (environmental metabolite of ethylenebis dithiocarbamate fungicides)	crops	PB-LC-MS	LOD 5 ng g^{-1}	246
carbendazim[c]	aquatic and sediment samples	LC-ISP-MS and LC-TS-MS	LODs 30 pg (ISP), 900 pg (TS)	247
carbendazim, imazalil, thiophanate-methyl, thiabendazole, benomyl	orange	LC-ESI-MS and LC-APCI-MS	LODs <0.03 mg kg^{-1}	248
carbendazim, thiabendazole	apple juice	SPE-LC-ESI-MS	10-70 μg L^{-1} (carbendazim), 2-130 μg L^{-1} (thiabendazole)	249
imidacloprid, metalaxyl, myclobutanil, thiabendazole	strawberry, orange, potato, pear, melon	DSPE-LC-APCI-MS	LODs < 0.05 mg kg^{-1}	250
carbendazim, imazalil, kresoxim-methyl, myclobutanil, penconazole, propiconazole, tebuconazole, thiabendazole[c]	grape, kiwi, lemon, peach, nectarine, spinach, strawberry	LC-ESI-MS-MS	0.01 and 0.8 mg kg^{-1}	251
carbendazim, thiabendazole, iprodione[c]	fruit juices	DSPE-LC-MS-MS	LODs < 0.2 ng g^{-1}	252
imazalil, iprodione, triflumizole[c]	fruits, vegetables, rice	SFE-LC-ESI-MS	LODs 0.04-148 ng g^{-1}	253
thiabendazole[c]	cow's milk	LC-ESI-MS-MS	< 1 μg L^{-1}	254
carbendazim, thiabendazole, imazalil, propiconazole, prochloraz, epoxiconazole, flusilazole, tebuconazole, bitertanol[c]	apple, apricot	LC-ESI-MS-MS	LODs 0.1-3 μg kg^{-1}	255

Table 2. Continued

Fungicide	Matrix[a]	Method	Concentration Levels[b]	Ref.
dichloran, flutriafol, o-phenylphenol, prochloraz, tolclofos-methyl	cherry, lemon, orange, peach	SPE-LC-IT-MS and SPE-LC-IT-MS-MS	LOQs 0.002–0.01 μg g^{-1} (LC-MS) and 0.0005-0.01 μg g^{-1} (LC-MS-MS)	256
carbendazim, fenpropimorph, imazalil[c]	crops	LC-ESI-MS-MS	0.01mg kg^{-1}	257
fenhexamid	caneberry, blueberry, pomegranate	LC-MS-MS	LOD 0.009 μg g^{-1} LOQ 0.020 μg g^{-1}	258
carbendazim, imazalil, thiabendazole, thiophanate-methyl[c]	fruit and vegetables	LC-MS-MS	0.01-0.5 mg kg^{-1}	259
cyprodinil, fenpropimorph, imazalil, metalaxyl, spiroxamine, tebuconazole, thiabendazole[c]	tomato, lemon, wheat flour, raisins, cucumber	ECHO-LC-APCI-MS-MS, ECHO-LC-ESI-MS-MS	0.01-0.1 mg kg^{-1}	260
carbendazim, cyprodinil, fenpropimorph, imazalil, metalaxyl, kresoxim-methyl, spiroxamine, thiabendazole, tolylfluanid, triadimefon[c]	apple, lettuce, orange	LC-ESI-MS-MS	0.01-0.1 mg kg^{-1}	261
carbendazim, cymoxanil, cyprodinil, prochloraz, thiabendazole, tridemorph[c]	green bean, cucumber, pepper, tomato, eggplant, watermelon, melon, zucchini	LC-ESI-MS-MS	LOQs <1 ng g^{-1}	262
carbendazim, cymoxanil, cyproconazole, difenoconazole, fluquinconazole, imazalil, metalaxyl, oxadixyl, prochloraz, tebuconazole, thiabendazole[c]	fruits, vegetables	LC-ESI-MS-MS	LOQ 0.01 mg kg^{-1}	263
o-phenylphenol, diphenyl, thiabendazole, imazalil	citrus fruits	LC-APPI-MS	LODs 0.01 μg g^{-1}, 0.05 μg g^{-1} (diphenyl)	264
tridemorph, carbendazim, thiabendazole, imazalil, propiconazole, bitertanol	banana, orange	LC-ESI-MS-MS	LOQ 0.05 mg kg^{-1}	265
carbendazim, thiabendazole,	pepper, lettuce,	LC-ESI-MS-MS	LODs $\leq$ 0.01 mg kg^{-1}	266

triflumizole[c]	aubergine			
carbendazim, imazalil, pyrimethanil, thiabendazole, thiophanate-methyl[c]	apple, avocado, carrot, lettuce, orange, potato, wheat	LC-ESI-MS-MS	0.02, 0.04, 0.20 mg kg^{-1}	267
carbendazim, imazalil, thiabendazole[c]	orange	LC-APCI-MS^3	LOQs 0.001-0.3 mg kg^{-1}	268
iprodione, procymidone[c]	apple, grape	LC-TOFMS	2 μg g^{-1}	269
carbendazim, thiabendazole[c]	apple-based infant foods	LC-ESI-MS-MS	LODs ≤ 0.2 μg kg^{-1}	270
imazalil, prochloraz, degradation products	citrus fruits	LC-TOF-MS, LC-ITD-MS-MS	1 mg kg^{-1}	271
propiconazole, fenbuconazole, cyproconazole, difenoconazole, tebuconazole, hexaconazole, bromuconazole, epoxiconazole, tetraconazole, triticonazole, triadimefon, triadimenol, myclobutanil	apple, peach, flour, water	SPE-LC-ESI-MS-MS	25-50 μg L^{-1} (food commodities), 0.50 μg L^{-1} (water)	272
fludioxonil, famoxadone	fruits, vegetables	LC-ESI-MS-MS	0.002 mg kg^{-1} (fludioxonil), 0.010 mg kg^{-1} (famoxadone)	273
carbendazim, thiophanate-methyl	tomato skin	LC-ESI-MS TOF and LC-ESI-IT-MS^2	0.2-1.8 μg g^{-1}	274
bitertanol, cyproconazole, epoxiconazole, flusilazole, hexaconazole, imazalil, myclobutanil, penconazole, prochloraz, propiconazole, tebuconazole, triadimefon, triadimenol	wine	LC-ESI-MS-MS	LOQs 0.25-7.5 ng mL^{-1}	275
carbendazim, pentachloro phenol, prochloraz, propanil, propiconazole[c]	bovine milk	SPE-LC-MS-MS	LOQs 0.008-1.4 μg L^{-1}	276
carbendazim, cyprodinil, dimethomorph, imazalil, oxadixyl, thiabendazole, triflumizole[c]	tomato, lemon, raisin, avocado	SPE-LC-ESI-QqQ-MS-MS	0.01-0.1 mg kg^{-1}	277

Table 2. Continued

Fungicide	Matrix[a]	Method	Concentration Levels[b]	Ref.
2,4-dichlorophenol, 2,4,5-trichlorophenol, pentachlorophenol[c]	cereals	PLE-LC-ESI-MS	LODs 0.003-0.013 μg g^{-1}	278
fenhexamid, pyrimethanil, tolylfluanid, kresoxim methyl	strawberry	LC-ESI-MS	0.03-0.66 mg kg^{-1}	279
benomyl, carbendazim, imazalil, metalaxyl, thiabendazol[c]	fruits, vegetables	LC-ESI-MS-MS	LODs 0.002-0.007 mg kg^{-1}	280
carbendazim, thiabendazol, oxadixyl, imazalil[c]	fruits	UPLC-ESI-MS-MS	0.01 mg kg^{-1}	281
cymoxanil, cyprodinil, carbendazim, fludioxonil, imazalil, thiabendazole, triadimefon, triadimenol[c]	cereal-based baby foods, orange, potato	UPLC-ESI-MS-MS	0.01 mg kg^{-1}	282
carbendazim, difenoconazole, fenpropimorph, flutolanil, imazalil, prochloraz, tebuconazole, thiabendazole	orange, red wine, red grape, raisin, wheat flour	DSPE-LC-MS-MS	0.01-0.1 mg kg^{-1}	164
dichlofluanid, diniconazole, epoxiconazole, fenarimol, imazalil, iprodione, kresoxim-methyl, myclobutanil, prochloraz, procymidone, pyrimethanil, thiabendazole, thiophanate-methyl, triadimefon, triadimenol[c]	apple, banana, grape, lettuce, orange, tomato	DSPE-LC-ESI-MS	LODs 1-30 μg kg^{-1} LOQs 4-100 μg kg^{-1}	283
carbendazim, thiabendazole, imazalil, prochloraz, iprodione and metabolites	fruit juices	SFE-LC-ESI-TOF-MS	LODs 0.08-0.45 μg L^{-1}	284
benomyl, ethirimol, imazalil, oxycarboxim, thiabendazol[c]	leaf	LC-ESI-IT-MS	LODs 1.5-218 μg kg^{-1} LOQs 4.8-725 μg kg^{-1}	285
azaconazole, bitertanol, bromuconazole, carbendazim, carpropamid, cyproconazole, cyprodinil, dichlofluanid, difenoconazole,	soya grain	LC-ESI-MS-MS	LODs 0.1-0.25 ng L^{-1}	286

dimethomorph, diniconazole, dodemorph, epoxiconazole, fenbuconazole, fenpropimorph, fluquinconazole, flusilazole, imazalil, kresoxim-methyl, metalaxyl, metconazole, myclobutanil,nuarimol, oxadixyl, penconazole, prochloraz, propiconazole, spiroxamine, tebuconazole, tetraconazole, thiabendazole, triadimefon, triadimenol, tricyclazole, triflumizole, triticonazole, zoxamide[c]				
trifloxystrobin and metabolites	soil	ASE-LC-MS-MS	LOQs 2.5 ng g^{-1}	287

[a] Water samples include natural and/or waste waters. [b] They are given as LODs, LOQs or evaluated concentrations. [c] Other pesticides and/or organic pollutants are included in the analysis. [d] Also determined by diode array detector. ASE accelerated solvent extraction. APCI atmospheric pressure chemical ionization, APPI atmospheric pressure photoionization. DSPE dispersive solid-phase extraction. ESI electrospray interface. ISP ionspray. IT ion trap. PB particle beam. PLE pressurized liquid extraction. SIM selected ion monitoring mode. QqQ triple quadrupole. Q-TOF quadrupole time of flight combination. SPE solid-phase extraction. TCI total ion current. TS thermospray. UPLC ultra-performance liquid chromatography.

GC-MS–LC-MS

Multiresidue methods combinig gas and liquid chromatography have been and continue to be a strategy profusely applied for monitoring purposes [288-295]. A fast method for the determination of residues of more than 200 pesticides (including more than thirty fungicides) in fruits and vegetables using gas and liquid chromatographies with mass spectrometric detection was developed by Lehotay et al. [296, 297].

Determination of multiclass pesticides, including 13 fungicides in vegetable samples was carried out using pressurized liquid extraction followed by LC-MS-MS (which allows for the analysis of more polar compounds) and GC-MS-MS, for the analysis of apolar and semipolar pesticides [298].

Determination of residues of 446 pesticides (including fungicides such as flusilazole, imazalil, propiconazole, tetraconazole and vinclozolin) in apples, oranges, grapes, cabbage, tomatoes and celery was performed using GC-MS and LC-MS-MS [299]. The same research group carried out the determination of 660 and 405 pesticide residues in tissues (beef, mutton, pork, chicken, and rabbit) and grains (maize, wheat, oat, rice and barley), respectively, also using CG-MS and LC-MS-MS methods [300, 301]. Recently, Pihlström et al. have presented a multiresidue method for the determination of 309 pesticides, including numerous fungicides, in fruit and vegetables, using both gas and liquid chromatography with tandem mass spectrometry [302].

Capillary Electrophoresis

Capillary electrophoresis (CE) is a suitable tool for determining fungicide in environmental matrices, because of its simplicity and high separation efficiency. Menzinger et al. [5], Picó et al. [303] and Hernández Borges et al. [304] have discussed the application of this method to the determination of agrochemical residues.

The determination of the fungicide ferbam (ferric dimethyldithiocarbamate) was carried out in wheat samples using UV detection [305].

A CE method was developed for the determination of ziram and zineb in wheat samples, using direct UV absorbance detection [306], with detection limits of 0.57 $\mu g\ mL^{-1}$ and 0.68 $\mu g\ mL^{-1}$, respectively.

CE with UV detection was applied to the simultaneous determination of thiabendazole, prochloraz and procymidone in real grape samples [307]. SPE was used for the isolation and preconcentration of the fungicides, providing limits of detection lower than the maximum residue limits.

Carbendazim and thiabendazole were analyzed by CE-diode array detection in lemon [308]. The limits of detection obtained for thiabendazole and carbendazim were 2.3 and 2.0 $\mu g\ mL^{-1}$ respectively.

A CE-electrospray mass spectrometry method for determining procymidone and thiabendazole in apples, grapes, oranges, pears, strawberries and tomatoes was described [309]. Fungicide residues were preconcentrated by both SPE and injection of large sample volumes into the capillary by a stacking technique. The frequent presence of both fungicides in real fruit and vegetables was demonstrated.

A method based on SPE and micellar electrokinetic chromatography (MEKC) was developed for the simultaneous determination of post-harvest fungicides (carbendazim, imazalil, methylthiophanate, o-phenylphenol, prochloraz, procymidone, thiabendazole and triadimefon) in grape, lettuce, orange and tomato [310]. The reproducibility and repeatability of the combination of SPE pre-treatment and MEKC were good for all the fungicides, except for imazalil and o-phenylphenol in oranges, due to some matrix compounds interfering with the separation.

A synthesized polyaniline was evaluated as a sorbent for SPE of carbendazim, chlorothalonil and a variety of polar pesticides from tap and river water samples [311]. The determination of these pesticides was carried out using cyclodextrin-modified MEKC equipped with diode array detection. The detection limits were in the range of 0.01-0.5 $\mu g\ L^{-1}$ using 350 mL water samples.

Validamycin A, a main component of the antibiotic validamycin complex, which is used to control sheath blight disease of rice plants, was determined by CE with indirect UV detection [312].

The quantitative determination of six pesticides in peaches and nectarines, including the fungicides procymidone, pyrimethanil and thiabendazole, was performed by CE-ESI-MS-MS [313]. The samples were preconcentrated by SPE using C_{18} silica gel. Under optimized CE-MS-MS conditions, the minimum detectable levels for the six pesticides in spiked peach samples were between 0.01 $mg\ kg^{-1}$ for pirimicarb and 0.05 $mg\ kg^{-1}$ for procymidone, which constitutes a severalfold increase in sensitivity compared to CE-MS and to conventional CE-

UV. The authors also indicated that the pesticides most often detected in real samples were thiabendazole and procymidone.

The separation and on-line concentration of carbendazim, 2-aminobenzimidazole, thiabendazole and other pesticides by CE with formic acid-ammonium formate (a volatile migration buffer applicable to MS detection) were investigated [314].

A test mixture of five pesticides and metabolites (including thiabendazole and carbendazim) was investigated by MECK with an ultraviolet diode array detector [315]. These compounds were separated in less than10 min. The method was applied to the analysis of the pesticides in cultivated vegetables such as cucumbers, which were extracted with a liquid-liquid extraction procedure.

The fungicides carbendazim, thiabendazole, imazalil, procymidone, triadimefon, and prochloraz were determined by CE with absorbance UV detection [316]. Limits of detection were improved by increasing the optical path length through a proper connection of the column to a capillary detection cell of 180 μm optical path length.

Pyrimethanil, nuarimol, procymidone, cyprodinil and the insecticide pirimicarb were determined in wine by MEKC with UV detection using the on-line preconcentration strategy called reversed electrode polarity stacking mode (REPSM) [317]. The combination of the off-line SPME and on-line REPSM preconcentration strategies allowed obtaining limits of detection between 17.6 and 32.3 $\mu g\ L^{-1}$.

A scheme to elucidate the degradation behavior of both enantiomers of the fungicide imazalil in soil using cyclodextrin-modified capillary zone electrophoresis was presented by Chu et al. [318].

SPECTROSCOPIC METHODS

Spectrophotometry

A colorimetric method for the determination of captafol (a fungicide belonging to the sulfanilamide group) based on its reaction with a dithiocarbamate was applied to residues in grains and apples [319].

Several spectrophotometric methods for the determination of dithiocarbamate fungicides have been reported in the evaluated period. Second-derivative UV-spectrophotometry was used to determine thiram in water [321] and also in apples, lettuce, potatoes, brussels sprouts and cabbages [321]. Ziram was spectrophotometrically determined up to a level of 1 $\mu g\ mL^{-1}$ in samples of potato, cabbage and wheat, by using a thiocyanate and rhodamine 6G method [322]. Zineb was quantified in the range 0.12-0.87 $\mu g\ mL^{-1}$ by the ethylene blue method in polluted water, vegetables and fruits [323]. A spectrophotometric method for the determination of zineb, ziram and thiram in a concentration range between 0.02 and 0.32 $\mu g\ mL^{-1}$ was applied to samples of water, vegetables and grains [324]. Ziram, zineb and ferbam in foodstuffs were determined through the convertion of ziram and zineb into a zinc–phenylfluorone complex and ferbam into an iron-phenylfluorone complex [325]. Ferbam was also spectrophotometrically determined in the range 0.5-20 $\mu g\ mL^{-1}$ in wheat grains by converting the fungicide into iron(II)-bathophenanthroline complex [326].

A spectrophotometric determination of some pesticides (including thiram) in river water samples after preconcentration with *Saccharomyces cerevisiae* immobilized on sepiolite was developed [327]. The calibration curve was linear up to 20 μg mL^{-1}, and the limit of detection for thiram was 0.161 μg mL^{-1}.

Ferbam [328], ziram and zineb [329] were determined in fog-water by either spectrophotometry or flame-atomic absorption spectrometry (flame-AAS). The spectrophotometric determinations are based on complex formation between certain reagents and the metal ions Fe(III) or Zn(II), which are contained in these fungicides. Alternatively, either the zinc or iron content are directly analyzed using flame-AAS. The detection limits for the spectrophotometric detection were 62, 20 and 21 μg L^{-1} for ferbam, ziram and zineb, respectively, and 1, 145 and 144 μg L^{-1} for the flame-AAS detection.

Sharma et al. determined ziram in wheat grains by using fourth derivative spectrophotometry [330]. The procedure was based on converting the fungicide into its copper(II) dimethyldithiocarbamate complex, which was then dissolved in Triton X-100. Beer's law was obeyed over the concentration range 0.5-30 μg mL^{-1} in the final solution.

Luminescence

Due to the high sensitivity of the photoluminescence signals based on fluorescence and phosphorescence, and the additional advantage of these methods in avoiding the use of large volumes of organic solvents, they have been widely applied to the determination of fungicide residues.

Fletcher et al. reviewed the literature in the field of molecular fluorescence, phosphorescence and chemiluminescence spectrometries, as applied to different analytes, including several fungicides [331].

Determination of thiabendazole residues in tap, natural, waste, residual and sea-water samples was performed by solid-phase (Sephadex G-15 gel) spectrofluorimetry [332].

Fuberidazole was fluorimetrically determined in irrigation water at low (10-100 ng mL^{-1}) levels [333]. 1-Naphthylacetic acid was quantified in natural waters by solid-phase (Sephadex QAE A-25 anion-exchanger) spectrofluorimetry [334], and limits of detection and quantification of 0.09 and 0.3 ng mL^{-1}, respectively, were obtained.

Phosphorescence emission was used for the determination of the fungicide morestan (quinomethionate) in different water samples [335]. The method is based on solid-phase room temperature phosphorescence using a device which consists of a disposable polyester sheet with a circular micro zone formed by poly-(vinyl chloride) and tributyl phosphate as a plasticizer. Morestan is fixed in the sensing zone of the sensor and its phosphorescence emission is directly measured. The concentration range is linear in the range 1-200 ng mL^{-1}, with a detection limit of 0.28 ng mL^{-1}.

Different approaches have been and are still being used by analysts for the enhancement of the already notable sensitivity of molecular emission measurements. One of these approaches is the use of organized media, since microscopically organized chemical assemblies frequently modify the physicochemical properties of analytes, which can be exploited for analytical purposes. Among the compounds used for obtaining microheterogeneous media, cyclodextrins and surfactants (above their critical micelle concentration) have been applied in fungicide analysis [336]. Thiabendazole was determined by micellar (sodium dodecylsulfate)-stabilized room-temperature phosphorimetry in canned pineapple samples, using thallium (I) as heavy metal to promote the intersystem crossing [337]. Room-temperature phosphorescence determination of thiabendazole through the formation of the thiabendazole/β-cyclodextrin/triton X-100 ternary complex was carried out in tap water, lake water and pineapples [338] with a detection limit of 2.1 ng mL^{-1}. Thiabendazole has also been determined by room-temperature phosphorescence without a protective medium, but only with the presence of high concentrations of heavy atom perturbers [339], and by nylon-induced phosphorimetry [340].

The applicability of heavy-atom induced room-temperature phosphorescence to determine pesticides in real samples was also demonstrated through the quantification of the fungicide fuberidazole [341].

The fluorescence enhancement of carbendazim due to a 1:1 guest-host inclusion complex formation with cucurbit[6]uril has been reported [342].

Luminescence detection coupled to flow-injection systems is a frequent approach used by analysts in the determination of fungicides in environmental samples. A micellar enhanced flow-injection fluorimetric method was developed for the determination of carbendazim in natural water samples [343]. The use of cetyltrimethylammonium bromide as micellar medium provided an 11.6-fold enhancement of sensitivity comparing with that found in the absence of micelles, reaching a limit of detection of 2.5 μg L^{-1} for carbendazim.

A stopped-flow fluorimetric sequential-injection method was developed for the simultaneous determination of carbaryl, fuberidazole, thiabendazole and warfarin in micellar media [344].

The determination of fuberidazole and thiabendazole in a sequential-injection system with a fluorimetric detector was also performed [345].

Flow-injection systems combined with solid-surface fluorescence or phosphorescence detection have been a useful means of pre-concentrating the sample, preserving the sampling frequency. A continuous-flow online solid-phase fluorescence-based system (optosensor) was proposed for the simultaneous determination of benomyl and carbendazim [346]. The continuous-flow system is based on the online preconcentration and resolution of the pesticides on a solid sensing zone, followed by the sequential measurement of their native fluorescence, and subsequent desorption of these analytes from the flow-through cell filled with C_{18} silica gel. The same authors developed fluorescence-based optosensors for the determination of benomyl and thiabendazole [347], o-phenylphenol and thiabendazole [348], fuberidazole, carbaryl and benomyl [349] and carbendazim, carbofuran, and benomyl [350] in water samples.

A novel flow-though optosensor formed by powder nylon was employed for the determination of thiabendazole in water samples of different origins [351].

A single flow-through optosensor spectrofluorimetric system, using C_{18} silicagel as an active sorbent, was proposed for the resolution of mixtures of α-naphthol, o-phenylphenol and thiabendazole, at μg L^{-1} levels, in environmental waters using a partial least-squares (PLS) multivariate calibration approach [352].

Luminescence spectroscopy, as other spectroscopic techniques, is prone to be affected by spectral interferences. The lack of selectivity is generated by spectral overlapping among the investigated compounds and/or by the emission from the matrix itself. Resolution of overlapping fluorescence or phosphorescence profiles can be achieved using derivative spectroscopy or multivariate calibration. The simultaneous determination of carbaryl and thiabendazole in different types of water samples was also performed by using three-dimensional derivative variable-angle and synchronous room-temperature phosphorescence spectroscopy in the presence of sulfite as the O_2 scavenger, and an external heavy atom salt [353]. Limits of detection ranged between 1.4 ng mL^{-1} for TBZ and 1.7 ng mL^{-1} for CBL.

Application of PLS multivariate calibration for the determination of mixtures of carbaryl and thiabendazole in waters by solid phase (Whatman No. 4 filter-paper) spectrophosphorimetry was developed [354]. A PLS multivariate calibration model was developed and applied to the spectral data to quantify the fungicides. The calibration graphs were linear between 0.5-4 mg L^{-1} and 0.16-1.2 mg L^{-1} for carbaryl and thiabendazole, respectively. A similar phosphorescent procedure was used for the same authors for the determination of thiabendazole in potatoes, green beans, lettuce and different types of water [355]. The most serious interference in this univariate method was produced by carbaryl and warfarin.

Trace determination of carbendazim, fuberidazole and thiabendazole in water was performed by application of multivariate calibration to cross-sections of three-dimensional excitation-emission fluorescence matrices [356].

De Armas et al. performed the simultaneous determination of fluorophores with overlapped spectra, including the fungicides fuberidazole and thiabendazole, by sequential-injection analysis coupled to variable angle scanning fluorescence spectrometry and algorithms based on linear regression [357].

Ternary mixtures of carbendazim, fuberidazole and thiabendazole were resolved by using fluorescence spectroscopy and PLS [358].

The multivariate net analyte signal (NAS)-based method HLA (hybrid linear analysis), a modification of the original hybrid linear analysis (HLA) method, was used to determine carbendazim, fuberidazole and thiabendazole in water samples [359].

The application of the generalised rank annihilation method (GRAM) and the trilinear decomposition (TLD) method to the resolution and quantitation of fluorescence excitation-emission matrices of a ternary mixture of carbendazim, fuberidazole and thiabendazole in water samples has been described [360]. These fungicides were also quantified by multivariate curve resolution-orthogonal projection approach (MCR-OPA), multivariate curve resolution-alternating least squares (MCR-ALS) [361] and parallel factor analysis (PARAFAC) [362] of three-dimensional excitation-emission fluorescence matrices.

The simultaneous determination of carbendazim and thiabendazole in water samples was achieved by using a chemometric second-order algorithm: PLS with residual bilinearization (PLS/RBL) [363]. The chemometric study was performed using fluorescence excitation-emission matrices obtained after the extraction of the analytes over a C_{18}-membrane surface. The work demonstrates the power of PLS/RBL for predicting the concentration of analytes in the presence of both inner-filter effects and unsuspected species.

Chemiluminescence and electrogenerated chemiluminescence methods based on the tris(2,2'-bipyridine) ruthenium(II) chemiluminescence reaction were carried out and compared for the analysis of morpholine fungicides [364].

Fourier Transform Infrared Spectrometry

A flow injection Fourier transform infrared spectrometry (FT-IR) procedure was developed for the determination of ziram and thiram in soils [365]. Absorbance measurements, in the wavenumber range of 1600-1460 cm^{-1} for ziram and 1400-1315 cm^{-1} for thiram were carried out, and the peak areas as a function of time were interpolated in external calibration lines prepared from standard solutions of ziram and thiram in chloroform. Absolute detection limits of 400 μg for ziram and 785 μg for thiram were obtained.

The potential of FT-IR to be used in screening and determination of selected pyrethroid and organochlorine pesticides in fresh water was analyzed by Columé et al. [366]. A representative compound of each main group (dichlofuanid, the fungicide captan and fenpropathrin) was selected and their direct simultaneous determination in fresh water was investigated. Using a PLS calibration, it could be shown that all three analytes could be quantified in fresh water in a concentration range from 1.2 to 4.8 μg L^{-1}.

A general strategy for the determination of six pesticides (including the fungicides iprodione, procymidone and tricyclazole) in agrochemicals by FT near infrared (FT-NIR) spectroscopy was developed by Moros et al. [367]. The methodology is based on extraction of the active principles with acetonitrile, and direct determination by transmission measurements, using glass vials as measurement cells, and univariate calibration at selected wavenumbers depending on the pesticide to be analyzed. FT-NIR provided limit of detection values ranging from 0.004 to 0.17 mg g^{-1}, and offered a 10 times faster methodology than chromatography, as well as an environmentally friendly alternative which reduces the reagent consumption.

The surface variability of powder-free nitrile rubber gloves was investigated for analysis of captan .contamination [368], using attenuated total reflection Fourier transform infrared (ATR-FT-IR) spectrophotometry. ATR-FT-IR proved to be a useful analytical tool for measuring glove variability, detecting surface humidity effects, and choosing selective wavelengths for analysis of nonvolatile surface contaminants.

Atomic Spectroscopy

Atomic absorption spectroscopy (AAS) is applied for the determination of fungicides containing metal ions, such as dithiocarbamates.

Indirect determination of ziram by atomic absorption spectrometry at levels 3.2-8.0 μM was proposed [369]. The method was based on the formation of the dithiocarbamate-Cu(II) complex, which was extracted into isobutyl methyl ketone in a flow-injection system and determined by AAS.

By combination of an HPLC and an atomic absorption method, the fungicides zineb, maneb, and mancozeb could be distinguished, in formulated products, by comparing the total Zn and Mn contents [370].

A flow-injection system for the online pre-concentration of metal dithiocarbamate fungicides by sorption on a C60 fullerene column was developed [371]. The fungicides are directly retained on the sorbent column, eluted from it, and fed into a flame atomic-absorption spectrometer. The method was applied to the resolution of synthetic mixtures, as well as to the speciation/determination of ziram, maneb and febam in spiked grain samples, all with acceptable recoveries.

The determination of copper in powdered chocolate samples by slurry-sampling flame atomic-absorption spectrometry was carried out by dos Santos et al. [372]. The determination of copper in chocolate is important because copper compounds are extensively used as fungicides in the farming of cocoa. The method allowed determination of copper in chocolate with a detection limit of 0.4 $\mu g\ g^{-1}$.

The indirect determination of zineb and ferbam in water, tomato and wheat grain by flame atomic absorption spectrometry was carried out [373]. Metals liberated upon decomposition of the fungicides were determined, and fungicide content was calculated by using the stoichiometric relationship between the metal and the corresponding fungicide. The fungicides were determined with relative standard deviations and relative errors which were less than 5%.

As was indicated in Table 1, Pröfrock et al. reported a method for the determination of pesticides (including quintozene) based on the simultaneous element-specific determination of P, S, Cl, Br, and I by GC hyphenated with octopole reaction cell-inductively coupled plasma mass spectrometry (ICP-MS) [134].

Copper concentrations were measured in Australian vineyard soils using inductively coupled plasma atomic emission spectrometry (ICP-AES) [374]. This work was performed to assess the extent of copper accumulation resulting from the use of Cu-based fungicides and to indicate the likely risks to long-term soil fertility.

Finally, some applications of atomic spectrometry to the fungicide analysis in environmental samples are included in the review of Butler et al. [375].

Other Spectroscopic Methods

Franko appraised the achievements related to the application of thermal lens spectrometry (TLS) in food analysis and environmental research [376]. All the applications are associated with the use of an appropriate analytical procedure providing sufficient selectivity, which cannot be achieved by TLS itself. Although the work does not specifically analyze fungicides, the study can be extended to this type of pesticides. The main advantages of novel analytical methods include improved sensitivity and selectivity, simplicity, minimized need for sample preparation and handling, as well as reduced time of analysis.

Flow-injection electrospray ionization-tandem mass spectrometry was developed for the determination of thiabendazole, imazalil, and o-phenylphenol in citrus fruit [377]. The method involves the combined use of stable isotopically labeled internal standards and a multiple reaction monitoring technique. The average recoveries for the fungicides at the tolerance levels (thiabendazole and o-phenylphenol, 10 mg kg^{-1}; imazalil, 5 mg kg^{-1}) ranged from 77 to 101%.

Advanced spectroscopic and microscopic methods were used to elucidate the Cu contamination, as a result of fungicide application, in a contaminated calcareous soil [378]. Microscopically focused synchrotron-based XRF (μ-SXRF) was used to map the elemental distribution in the soils. Bulk and microscopically focused X-absorption near edge structure (XANES) and extended X-ray absorption fine structure (EXAFS) spectra indicated that the Cu in the soil was predominantly Cu adsorbed on soil organic matter. Results provided information on the molecular coordination of Cu in a contaminated soil, which is critical for understanding the long-term fate and best management practices for Cu in the environment.

Electrochemical Methods

In the earliest 90's, thiram was voltammetrically determined (LOD = 0.3 μg L^{-1}) in both powder formulations and water, following the adsorptive accumulation on a rotating-gold-disc electrode [379].

An electrochemical study based on direct current and differential pulse polarography and coulometry for folpet, captan, captafol and their hydrolysis products was carried out [380]. The electrochemical behaviour of the assayed fungicides was interpreted according to the polarographic and coulometric data and with the aid of other techniques such as FT-IR, nuclear magnetic resonance (NMR) spectroscopy and GC-MS, which were used to identify the products obtained in the coulometry assays. Also, different polarographic procedures were proposed for the determination of the fungicides, reporting that it is not possible to perform simultaneous polarographic quantification of the three compounds. The polarographic signals of these compounds in their mixture show a high overlapping and, therefore, chemometric methods such as PLS calibration and artificial neuronal netwoks were utilized for the simultaneous determination of these compounds in river samples [381].

Determination of organic pollutants, including the fungicides carbendazim and o-chlorophenol, in a range 1×10^{-4} to 1.5 mg mL^{-1} in a flow stream was developed using a wall-jet electrode system and square-wave stripping principles [382].

The voltammetric behaviour of fenbendazole, albendazole, thiabendazole and mebendazole at a glassy carbon electrode was studied, and their determination was carried out by flow injection with amperometric detection [383]. LODs in the 0.01-0.1 μM concentration range were achieved. As an application, fenbendazole was determined in spiked food samples at the 30 and 180 μg g^{-1} concentration levels, which correspond to the lower and upper concentrations for fenbendazole administration to treated poultry.

Cyclic voltammetric studies of the herbicide isoproturon and the fungicide carbendazim in soil and water samples using polypyrrole modified glassy carbon electrodes were carried out [384]. The LOD for carbendazim was 5 ng mL^{-1}. The same authors investigated the redox behaviour of two herbicides, isoproturon and methyl parathion, and of the fungicide carbendazim, using heteropolyacid montmorillonite clay-modified glassy carbon electrodes in the presence and absence of the surfactant cetyltrimethylammonium bromide [385]. The presence of the surfactant enhanced the peak current, and hence stripping voltammetric determination procedures for all the three pesticides were developed. The applicability of the method was verified in soil and water samples.

An electroanalytical procedure was proposed for the determination of triflumizole in formulated, soil and natural water samples using differential pulse polarography [386]. Limits of detection and quantification were obtained as 0.72 and 2.39 μmol L^{-1}, respectively.

IMMUNOANALYTICAL METHODS

During the evaluated period, immunoanalytical techniques for environmental monitoring and determination of fungicide residues and other pesticides were reviewed [387-389] Metalaxyl was determined in wine samples by using an enzyme-linked immunosorbent assay (ELISA) with microtitre plates coated with a polyclonal antibody [390]. The limit of detection for metalaxyl was 0.5 ppb and the pesticides alachlor, furalxyl and metalachlor exhibited 90% cross-reactivity.

The fungicide benadaxyl was determined in water and wine through an ELISA [391]. A derivative of benalaxyl was synthesized, linked to bovine serum albumin, and the immunogen was used to immunize three mice and one chicken, which responded by producing specific antibodies to benalaxyl with negligible cross-reactivity to various structuraly related pesticides. LODs of 0.35 μg L^{-1} (with mouse antibodies) and 0.20 μg L^{-1} (with chicken antibody) were obtained. The suitability of the ELISA for benalaxyl quantification in wine was also studied in the working range 2-50 μg L^{-1}.

An ELISA for thiabendazole was developed to the analysis of orange, grapefruit, banana, apple and pear juices [392]. The immunoassay was based on a monoclonal antibody derived from a hapten functionalized at the nitrogen atom in the 1-position of the thiabendazole structure. The immunoassay was able to accurately determine thiabendazole in a range of 1 to 20 ng mL^{-1} depending on the studied juice.

Three diagnostic immunoassays, i.e., ELISA, fluorescence polarization, and time-resolved fluorescence, were developed with regard to quantification of azoxystrobin, up to 400 pg mL^{-1}, in grape extract and natural water samples [393]. While the three formats were comparable in terms of performance, the fluorescence polarization assay was the least labor-intensive and required the lowest time to be performed.

A monoclonal antibody-based indirect competitive ELISA was developed for the analysis of gossypol, a polyphenol derived from the cotton plant and which has fungicidal effect, in cottonseed meals [394]. The LOD for gossypol was 0.024 μg mL^{-1}.

An optical biosensor consisting of a glutathione-S-transferase(GST)-immobilized gel film was developed to detect captan up to 2 μg mL^{-1} in contaminated water [395]. The sensing scheme was based on the decrease of yellow product produced from substrates, 1-chloro-2,4-dinitrobenzene and glutathione, due to the inhibition of GST reaction by captan. Absorbance of the product as the output of enzyme reaction was detected and the light was guided through the optical fibers.

Recently, a paper describing the synthesis of functionalized haptens of kresoxim-methyl, the production of monoclonal antibodies, and the development of enzyme-linked immunosorbent assays was reported [396].

CONCLUSION

Figure 1 illustrates the distribution of the employed fungicide methods, abstrated from the earliest '90s to the present. More than 70 % of research works are devoted to gas and liquid chromatographic resolutions, including both conventional and mass spectrometry detection. In the last years, a noticeable growth of chromatography coupled to mass spectrometry is registered. The success of both CG and LC coupled to mass spectroscopy can be attributed to the fact that multiresidue determination can be carried out in a relatively easy way. Although the number of works using gas chromatography is similar to those applying liquid chromatography, the current tendency towards the use of more polar fungicides, which present lower persistence and toxicity than the apolar ones, suggests that LC methods will increase in the future.

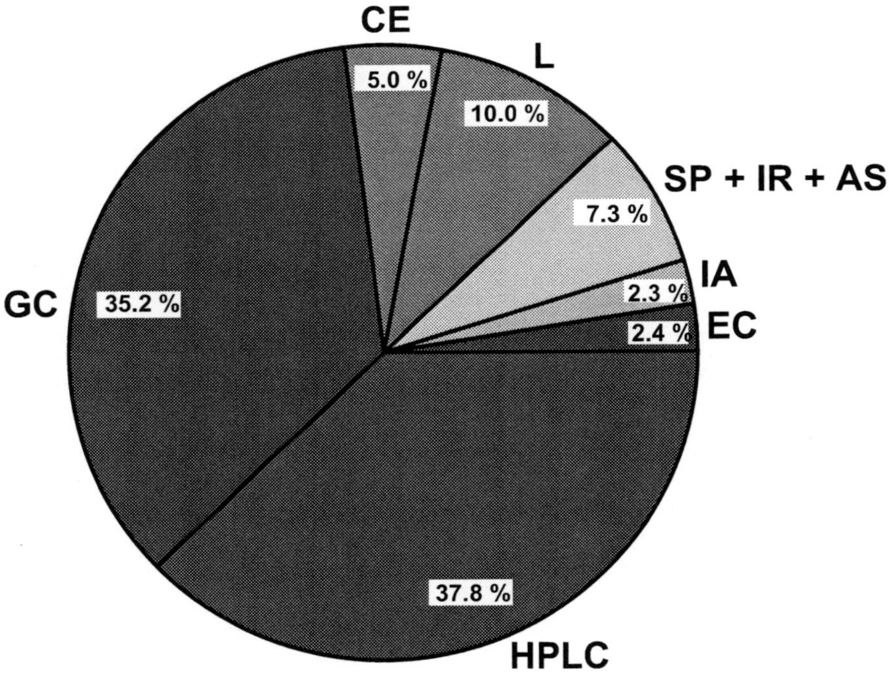

Figure 1. Distribution of the relevant methods employed for fungicide determination in environmental samples in the last fifteen years. AS atomic spectroscopy. CE capillary electrophoresis. EC electrochemical methods. GC gas chromatography. HPLC high-performance chromatography. IA immunoanalytical methods. IR infrared methods. L luminescence. SP spectrophotometry.

On the other hand, CE has also a high separation eficiency, with the advantage that very small consumption of toxic solvents is involved. However, because of the small sample volumes injected, its sensitivity is inadequate for residue determinations, and must be enhanced by using approaches to trace enrichment or improving detection systems.

Among the spectroscopic methods, which comprise about 17 % of the total, the most used for fungicide determination are those based on either fluorescence or phosphorescence detection. This fact can be ascribed to the high sensitivity of these methods. Furthermore, their coupling to modern multivariate methods with their concomitant contribution to selectivity, has produced a significant increase in the use of these techniques in complex matrices.

In addition to sensitivity and selectivity, other important properties are required by environmental sample analysis. The necessity to enhance the control of ecological contamination induces the development of faster methods, with simplification of sample preparation procedures and increasing the sample throughput by automation. Finally, efforts should also be focused on reducing the consumption of toxic solvents as this is essential for environmental safety.

ACKNOWLEGMENTS

The author gratefully acknowledge the Universidad Nacional de Rosario, the Agencia Nacional de Promoción Científica y Tecnológica (Project PAE No 22204) and the Consejo Nacional de Investigaciones Científicas y Técnicas for financially supporting this work.

REFERENCES

[1] Fong, W. G. Pesticide Residues in Foods. Methods, Techniques and Regulations; Wiley: New York, NY, 1999; pp 205-225.

[2] Peters, H. A.; Gocmen, A.; Cripps. D. J. *Arch. Neurol.* 1992, *39*, 744-749.

[3] Smith, R. A.; Christenson, W. R.; Bartels, M. J.; Arnol, L. L.; St. John, M. K.; Cano, M.; Garland, E. M.; Lake, S. G.; Wahle, B. S.; MacNett, D. A.; Cohen, S. M. *Toxicol. Appl. Pharmacol.* 1998, *150*, 402-413.

[4] Hayama, T.; Yada, K.; Onimaru, S.; Yoshida, H; Todoroki, K.; Nohta, H.; Yamaguchi, M. *J. Chromatogr.* A 2007, *1141*, 251-258.

[5] Menzinger, F.; Schnitt Kopplin, Ph.; Freitag, D.; Kettrup, A. *J. Chromatogr. A* 2000, *891*, 45-67.

[6] European Comission, document SANCO/2007/3131, *Method Validation and Quality Control Procedures for Pesticide Residues Analysis in Food and Feed*, 31 October 2007.

[7] Website of the United State Environmental Protection Agency (U.S. EPA): www.epa.gov/pesticides/

[8] European Directive 80/778/EEC, European Commission, Brussels, 1980.

[9] European Directive 93/57/EEC and 93/58/EEC, European Commission, Brussels, 1993.

[10] Aaron, J. J.; Tran-Minh, C.; Colliss, J. S.; Smart, N. A. *Anal. Proc.* 1993, *2*, 72-77.

[11] MacCarthy, P.; Klusman, R. W.; Cowling, S. W.; Rice, J. A. *Anal. Chem.* 1993, *65*, 244R-292R.

[12] Barceló, D. *J. Chromatogr.* 1993, *643*, 117-143.

[13] Singh, R. P.; Chiba, M. *J. Chromatogr.* 1993, *643*, 249-260.

[14] Honing, M.; Barceló, D.; van Baar B. L. M., Brinkman U. A. Th., *Techn. Instrum. Anal. Chem.* 1995, *17*, 535-562.

[15] Tekel, J.; Hatrik, S. *J. Chromatogr. A* 1996, *754*, 397-410.

[16] van Zoonen, P. (Ed.) *Analytical Methods for Pesticide Residues in Foodstuffs. General Inspectorate for Health Protection*, sixth ed., Ministry of Public Health, Welfare and Sports, The Netherlands, 1996.

[17] Hatrik, S.; Tekel, J. *J. Chromatogr. A* 1996, *733*, 217-233.

[18] Liska, I.; Slobodnik, J. *J. Chromatogr. A.* 1996, *733*, 235-258.

[19] Balinova, A. *J. Chromatogr. A* 1996, *754*, 125-135.

[20] Biziuk, M.; Przyjazny, A.; Czerwinski, J.; Wiergowski, M. *J. Chromatogr. A* 1996, *754*, 103-123.

[21] Jain, C. K.; Ali, I. *Int. J. Environ. Anal. Chem.* 1997, *68*, 83-101.

[22] Fernåndez Alba, A. R.; Agüera, A.; Contreras, M.; Peñuela, G.; Ferrer, I., Barceló, D. *J. Chromatogr. A* 1998, *823*, 35-47.

[23] Coly, A., Aaron, J. J. *Talanta* 1998, *46*, 815-843.

[24] Aaron, J. J.; Coly, A. *Analusis* 2000, *28*, 699-709.

[25] Van der Hoff, G. R.; van Zoonen, P. *J. Chromatogr. A* 1999, *843*, 301-322.

[26] Vessella, J.; Acobas, F.; Benanou, D.; Guinamant, J. L. *Spectra Anal.* 2001, *220*, 32-36.

[27] Dunec, A. F.; Cheregi, M.; Calatayud, J. M.; Mateo,-JVG; Enein, H. Y. A. *Crit. Rev. Anal. Chem.* 2003, *33*, 57-68.

[28] Lee, P. W.; Aizawa, H.; Barefoot, A. C.; Murphy, J. J. (Eds.) *Handbook of Residue Analytical Methods for Agrochemicals*, Wiley: New York, NY, 2003, Vol. 2.

[29] Sharma, V. K.; Aulakh, J. S.; Malik, A. K. *J. Environ. Monitor.* 2003, *5*, 717-723.

[30] Tadeo, J. L.; Sánchez Brunete, C.; Albero, B.; González, L. *Crit. Rev. Anal. Chem.* 2004, *34*, 121-131.

[31] Andreu, V.; Picó, Y. *Trends Anal. Chem.* 2004, *23*, 772-789.

[32] Picó, Y.; Blasco, C.; Font, G. *Mass Spectrom. Rev.* 2004, *23*, 45-85.

[33] Koester, C. J. *Anal. Chem.* 2005, *77*, 3737-3754.

[34] Picó, Y.; Font, G; Ruiz, M. J.; Fernández, M. *Mass Spectrom. Rev.* 2006, *25*, 917-960.

[35] Kuster, M.; López de Alda, M.; Barceló, D. *Mass Spectrom. Rev.* 2006, *25*, 900-916.

[36] Sancho, J. V.; Pozo, O. J.; Ibañez, M.; Hernández, F. *Anal. Bioanal. Chem.* 2006, *386*, 987-997.

[37] Richardson, S. D. *Anal. Chem.* 2006, *78*, 4021-4046.

[38] Lambropoulou, D. A.; Albanis, T. A. *Anal. Bioanal. Chem.* 2007, *389*, 1663-1683.

[39] Soler, C.; Picó, Y. *Trends Anal. Chem.* 2007, *26* 103-115.

[40] Schuelein, J.; Martens, D.; Spitzauer, P.; Kettrup, A. *Fresenius' J. Anal. Chem.* 1995, *352*, 565-571.

[41] Barceló, D.; Hennion, M. C. *Anal. Chim. Acta* 1995, *318*, 1-41.

[42] Eisert, R.; Levsen, K. *J. Chromatogr. A* 1996, *733*, 143-157.

[43] Hatrík, S.; Tekel, J. *J. Chromatogr. A* 1996, *733*, 217-233.
[44] Bruzzoniti, M. C.; Sarzanini, C.; Mentasti, E. *J. Chromatogr. A* 2000, *902*, 289-309.
[45] Taguchi, S.; Sun, H. F.; Hata, N.; Kasahara, I. *Bunseki Kagaku* 2000, *49*, 941-952.
[46] Alpendurada, M. F. *J. Chromatogr. A* 2000, *889*, 3-14.
[47] Lipinski, J. *Fresenius' J. Anal. Chem.* 2000, *367*, 445-449.
[48] Lipinski, J. *Fresenius' J. Anal. Chem.* 2001, *369*, 57-62.
[49] Pihlström, T.; Isaac, G.; Waldebäck, M.; Österdahl, B. G.; Markides, K. E. *Analyst*, 2002, *127*, 554-559.
[50] Smith, R. M. *J. Chromatogr. A* 2002, *975*, 31-46.
[51] Kataoka, H. *Anal. Bioanal. Chem.* 2002, *373*, 31-45.
[52] Richardson, S. D. *Anal. Chem.* 2004, *76*, 3337-3364.
[53] Aulakh, J. S.; Malik, A.; Kaur, V.; Schmitt Kopplin, P. *Crit. Rev. Anal. Chem.* 2005, *35*, 71-85.
[54] Raynie, D. E. *Anal. Chem.* 2006, *78*, 3997-4003.
[55] Sandra, P.; Kot, A.; Medvedovici, A.; David, F. *J. Chromatogr. A* 1995, *703*, 467-478.
[56] Toribio, L.; del Nozal, M. J.; Bernal, J. L.; Jiménez, J. J.; Serna, M. L. *J. Chromatogr. A* 1998, *823*, 163-170.
[57] Bernal, J. L.; Jiménez, J. J. ; Rivera, J. M.; Toribio, L.; del Nozal, M. J. *J. Chromatogr. A* 1996, *754*, 145-157.
[58] Henry, M. C.; Yonker, C. R. *Anal. Chem.* 2006, *78*, 3909-3915.
[59] Wassmuth Wagner, I.; Jork, H. *J. Planar Chromatogr. Mod. TLC* 1989, *2*, 297-303.
[60] Burger, K.; Koehler, J.; Jork, H., *J. Planar Chromatogr. Mod. TLC* 1990, *3*, 504-510.
[61] de la Vigne, U.; Janchen, D. E.; Weber, W. H. *J. Chromatogr.* 1991, *553*, 489-496.
[62] Balinova, A. *Anal. Chim. Acta* 1995, *311*, 423-427.
[63] Tuzimski, T.; Bartosiewicz, A. *Chromatographia* 2003, *58*, 781-788.
[64] Tuzimski, T.; Soczewiński, E. *Chromatographia* 2004, *59*, 121-128.
[65] Tuzimski, T. *J. Planar Chromatogr. Mod. TLC* 2005, *105*, 349-357.
[66] Kubáň, P.; Flowers, H. *J. Agric. Food Chem.* 2001, *49*, 2848-2852.
[67] Kubáň, P.; Flowers, H. *Anal. Chim.* Acta 2001, *437*, 115-122.
[68] Xiao, Y.; Fan, D.; Chen, H. *J. Assoc. Off. Anal. Chem.* 1990, *73*, 761-763.
[69] Suzuki, T.; Yaguchi, K.; Ohnishi, K.; Yamagishi, T. *J. Chromatogr. A* 1994, *662*, 139-146.
[70] de la Colina, C.; Peña, A.; Mingorance, M. D.; Sánchez Rasero, F. *J. Chromatogr. A* 1996, *733*, 275-281.
[71] Oubiña, A.; Martínez, E.; Gascón, J.; Barceló, D.; De Alleluia, I. B. *Int. J. Environ. Anal. Chem.* 1998, *70*, 75-91. Gil García, M. D.; Martínez Galera, M.; Pablos Espada, M. C.; Garrido Frenich, A.; Martínez Vidal, J. L. *J. AOAC Int.* 2000, *83*, 1068-1075.
[73] Zanella, R.; Marozzin Mistura, C.; Kurz, M. H. S.; Primel, E. G.; Ferreira Goncalves, F. *Anal. Lett.* 2003, *36*, 1393-1400.
[74] Luthje, K.; Hyotylainen, T.; Riekkola, M. L. *Anal. Bioanal. Chem.* 2004, *378*, 1991-1998.
[75] Pan, H. J.; Ho, W. H. *Anal. Chim. Acta* 2004, *527*, 61-67.
[76] Liu, Y.; Zhao, E. C.; Zhou, Z. Q. *Anal. Lett.* 2006, *39*, 2333-2344.
[77] Perz, R. C.; van Lishaut, H.; Schwack, W. *J. Agric. Food Chem.* 2000, *48*, 792-796.

[78] Jiménez, J. J.; Bernal, J. L.; del Nozal, M. J.; Toribio, L.; Arias, E. *J. Chromatogr. A* 2001, *919*, 147-156.

[79] Lee, W.; Wong, S. *Analyst* 1995, *120*, 2475-2478.

[80] Nerin, C.; Batlle, R.; Cacho, J. *J. Chromatogr. A* 1998, *795*, 117-124.

[81] Menkissoglu Spiroudi, U.; Fotopoulou, A. *Int. J. Environ. Anal. Chem.* 2004, *84*, 15-27.

[82] Boulaid, M.; Aguilera, A.; Camacho, F.; Soussi, M.; Valverde, A. *J. Agric. Food Chem.* 2005, *53*, 4054-4058.

[83] Tang, F.; Yue, Y. D.; Hua, R.; Ge, S. M.; Tang, J. *J. AOAC Int.* 2005, *88*, 720-728.

[84] Fenoll, J.; Hellin, P.; Marin, C.; Martínez, C. M.; Flores, P. *J. Agric. Food Chem.* 2005, *53*, 7661-7666.

[85] Yi, X.; Lu, Y. *Chemosphere* 2006, *65*, 639-643.

[86] Karthika, C.; Sachin, P. J. *J. Zhejiang Univ. Sci.* 2008, *9*, 160-164.

[87] Bempelou, E. D.; Konstantinos S. Liapis, K. S. *Int. J. Environ. Anal. Chem.* 2006, *86*, 63- 68.

[88] D'Aquino, S.; Schirra, M.; Palma, A.; Tedde, M.; Angioni, A.; Garau, A.; Cabras, P. *J. Agric. Food Chem.* 2007, *55*, 825-831.

[89] Vela, N.; Pérez, G.; Navarro, G.; Navarro, S. *J. AOAC Int.* 2007, *90*, 544-549.

[90] Navarro, S.; Pérez, G.; Vela, N.; Mena, L.; Navarro, G. *J. Agric. Food Chem.* 2005, *53*, 8572-8579.

[91] Aguilera, A.; Rodríguez, M.; Brotons, M.; Boulaid, M.; Valverde, A. *J. Agric. Food Chem.* 2005, *53*, 9374-9382.

[92] Tang, F.; Yue, Y. D.; Hua, R. M.; Cao, H. Q. *J. AOAC Int.* 2006, *89*, 498-502.

[93] Georgiou, P. P.; Liapis, K. S.; Miliadis, G. E. ; Siskos, P. A. *Int. J. Environ. Anal. Chem.* 2006, *86*, 69-76.

[94] Janska, M.; Lehotay, S. J.; Mastovska, K.; Hajslova, J.; Alon, T.; Amirav, A. *J. Sep. Sci.* 2006, *29*, 66-80.

[95] Zhu, X. L.; Qi, X. Y; Yue, J. N.; Lei, W. J. *Fenxi Huaxue* 2007, *35*, 259-262.

[96] Fenoll, J.; Hellin, P.; Martínez, C. M.; Flores, P. *J. AOAC Int.* 2007, *90*, 263-270.

[97] Kende, A.; Vrabecz, A.; Angyal, V.; Rikker, T.; Eke, Z.; Torkos, K. *Chromatographia* 2006, *63*, 181-187.

[98] Anagnostopoulos, C.; Miliadis, G. E.; Aplada Sarlis, P.; Ziogas, B. N. *Int. J. Environ. Anal. Chem.* 2006, *86*, 77-82.

[99] Park, Y. S.; El-Aty, A. M. A.; Choi, J. H; Cho, S. K.; Shin, D. H.; Shim, J. H. *Biomed. Chromatogr.* 2007, *21*, 29-39.

[100] Campillo, N.; Penalver, R.; Aguinaga, N.; Hernández Córdoba, M. *Anal. Chim. Acta* 2006, *562*, 9-15.

[101] Campillo, N.; Penalver, R.; Hernández Córdoba, M. *Talanta* 2007, *71*, 1417-1423.

[102] Khummueng, W.; Trenerry, C.; Rose, G.; Marriott, P. J. *J. Chromatogr. A* 2006, *1131*, 203-214.

[103] Kadokami, K; Morimoto, M.; Haraguchi, K.; Koga, M.; Shinohara, R. *Anal. Sci.* 1991, *7*, 247-252.

[104] Meiring, H. D.; de Jong, A. P. J. M. *J. Chromatogr. A* 1994, *683*, 157-165.

[105] Garrido Frenich, A.; Martínez Vidal, J. L.; Pablos Espada, M. C.; Gil García, M. D.; Arrebola, F. J. *Chromatographia* 2000, *52*, 614-620.

[106] Lambropoulou, D. A.; Konstantinou, I. K.; Albanis, T. A. *J. Chromatogr. A* 2000, *893*, 143-156.

[107] Tanabe, A.; Mitobe, H.; Kawata, K.; Sakai, M.; Yasuhara, A. *J. AOAC Int.* 2000, *83*, 61-77.

[108] Garrido Frenich, A; Pablos Espada, M. D. C.; Martínez Vidal, J. L.; Molina, L. *J. AOAC Int.* 2001, *84*, 1751-1762.

[109] Sakamoto, M.; Tsutsumi, T. *J. Chromatogr. A* 2004, *1028*, 63-74.

[110] Albanis, T. A.; Hela, D. G.; Lambropoulou, D. A.; Sakkas Vasilios, A. *Int. J. Environ. Anal. Chem.* 2004, *84*, 1079-1092.

[111] Gonçalves, C.; Alpendurada, M. F. *J. Chromatogr. A* 2004, *1026*, 239-250.

[112] Kawamoto, T.; Yano, M.; Makihata, N. *J. Chromatogr. A* 2005, *1074*, 155-161.

[113] Nakamura, S.; Daishima, S. *Anal. Bioanal. Chem.* 2005, *382*, 99-107.

[114] Leandro, C. C.; Bishop, D. A.; Fussell, R. J.; Smith, F. D.; Keely, B. J. *J. Agric. Food Chem.* 2006, *54*, 645-649.

[115] Planas, C.; Puig, A.; Rivera, J.; Caixach, J. *J. Chromatogr. A* 2006, *1131*, 242-252.

[116] Scheyer, .A; Morville, S.; Mirabel, P.; Millet, M. *Anal. Bioanal. Chem.* 2006, *384*, 475-487.

[117] Beceiro González, E.; Concha Graña, E.; Guimaraes, A.; Gonçalves, C.; Muniategui Lorenzo, S.; Alpendurada, M. F. *J. Chromatogr. A* 2007, *1141*, 165-173.

[118] Hernández, F.; Portoles, T.; Pitarch, E.; López, F. J. *Anal. Chem.* 2007, *79*, 9494-9504.

[119] Dieckmann, H.; Kreuzig, R.; Baḥadir, M. *Fresenius' J. Anal. Chem.* 1996, *355*, 183-186.

[120] Klöppel, H.; Jürling, H. *Fresenius' J. Anal. Chem.* 1997, *357*, 353-355.

[121] Mastovska, K.; Lehotay, S. J.; Hajslova, J. *J. Chromatogr. A* 2001, *926*, 291-308.

[122] Sandra, P.; Tienpont, B.; Vercammen, J.; Tredoux, A.; Sandra, T.; Davis, F. *J. Chromatogr. A* 2001, *928*, 117-126.

[123] Rial Otero, R.; Yagüe Ruiz, C.; Cancho Grande, B.; Simal Gándara, J. *J. Chromatogr. A* 2002, *942*, 41-52.

[124] Buser H. R.; Müller, M. D.; Poiger, T.; Balmer, M. E. *Environ. Sci. Technol.* 2002, *36*, 221-226.

[125] Navalón, A.; Prieto, A.; Araujo, L.; Vilchez, J. L., *J. Chromatogr. A* 2002, *975*, 355-360.

[126] Stajnbaher, D.; Zupancic Kralj, L. *J. Chromatogr. A* 2003, *1015*, 185-198.

[127] Anastassiades, M.; Lehotay, S.J.; Stajhbaher, D.; Schenck, F. J. *J. AOAC Int.* 2003, *86*, 412-431.

[128] Zrostlikova, J.; Hajslova, J.; Cajka, T. *J. Chromatogr. A* 2003, *1019*, 173-186.

[129] Lambropoulou, D. A.; Albanis, T. A. *Anal. Chim. Acta* 2004, *514*, 125-130.

[130] Cajka, T.; Hajslova, J. *J. Chromatogr. A* 2004, *1058*, 251-261.

[131] Navalón, A.; Prieto, A.; Araujo, L.; Vilchez, J. L. *Anal.Bioanal. Chem.* 2004, *379*, 1100-1105.

[132] Mercer, G. E.; Hurlbut, J. A. *J. AOAC. Int.* 2004, *87*, 1224-1236.

[133] Hyotylainen, T.; Luthje, K.; Rautiainen Rama, M.; Riekkola, M. L. *J. Chromatogr.A* 2004, *1056*, 267-271.

[134] Pröfrock, D.; Leonhard, P.; Wilbur, S.; Prange, A. *J. Anal. At. Spectrom.* 2004, *19*, 623-631.

[135] Morales Muñoz, S.; Luque García, J. L.; Ramos, M. J.; Fernández Alba, A.; Luque de Castro, M. D. *Anal. Chim. Acta* 2005, *552*, 50-59.

[136] Morales Muñoz, S.; Luque García, J. L.; Ramos, M. J; Martínez Bueno, M. J.; Luque de Castro, M. D. *Chromatographia* 2005, *62*, 69-74.

[137] Sánchez Brunete, C.; Albero, B.; Martín, G.; Tadeo, J. L. *Anal. Sci.* 2005, *21*, 1291-1296.

[138] Mercer, G. E. *J. AOAC Int.* 2005, *88*, 1452-1462.

[139] Garrido Frenich, A.; González Rodríguez, M. J.; Arrebola Liebanas, F. J.; Martínez Vidal, J. L. *Anal. Chem.* 2005, *77*, 4640-4648.

[140] Kawata, K.; Asada, T.; Oikawa, K.; Tanabe, A. *J. AOAC. Int.* 2005, *88*, 1440-1451.

[141] Mastovska, K.; Lehotay, S. J.; Anastassiades, M. *Anal. Chem.* 2005, *77*, 8129-8137.

[142] Albero, B.; Sánchez Brunete, C.; Tadeo, J. L. *Talanta* 2005, *66*, 917-924.

[143] Kawata, K; Asada, T.; Oikawa, K. *J. Chromatogr. A* 2005, *1090*, 10-15.

[144] Kirchner, M.; Matisova, E.; Hrouzkova, S.; de Zeeuw, J. *J. Chromatogr. A* 2005, *1090*, 126-132.

[145] Hercegova, A.; Domotorova, M.; Matisova, E.; Kirchner, M.; Otrekal, R.; Stefuca, .V *J. Chromatogr. A* 2005, *1084*, 46-53.

[146] Cajka, T.; Mastovska, K.; Lehotay, S. J.; Hajslova, J. *J. Sep. Sci* 2005, *28*, 1048-1060.

[147] Ochiai, N.; Sasamoto, K.; Kanda, H.; Yamagami, T.; David, F.; Tienpont, B.; Sandra, P. *J. Sep. Sci.* 2005, *28*, 1083-1092.

[148] Kirchner, M.; Matisova, E.; Otrekal, R.; Hercegova, A.; de Zeeuw, J. *J. Chromatogr. A* 2005, *1084*, 63-70.

[149] Barreda, M.; López, F. J.; Villarrova, M.; Beltran, J.; García-Baudín, J. M.; Hernández, F. *J. AOAC Int.* 2006, *89*, 1080-1087.

[150] Ochiai, N.; Sasamoto, K.; Kanda, H.; Nakamura, S. *J. Chromatogr. A* 2006, *1130*, 83-90.

[151] Guardia Rubio, M.; Ruiz Medina, A.; Molina Díaz, A.; Fernández de Córdova, M. L. *J. Sep. Sci.* 2006, *29*, 1578-1586.

[152] Martínez Vidal, J. L.; Arrebola Liebanas, F. J.; González Rodríguez, M. J.; Garrido Frenich, A.; Fernández Moreno, J. L. *Rapid Commun. Mass Spectrom.* 2006, *20*, 365-375.

[153] Fernández Moreno, J. L.; Arrebola Liebanas, F. J.; Garrido Frenich, A.; Martínez Vidal, J. L. *J. Chromatogr. A* 2006, *1111*, 97-105.

[154] Walorczyk, S.; Gnusowski, B. *J. Chromatogr. A* 2006, *1128*, 236-243.

[155] Ono, Y.; Yamagami, T.; Nishina, T.; Tobino, T. *Anal. Sci.* 2006, *22*, 1473-1476.

[156] Kovalczuk, T.; Jech, M.; Poustka, J.; Hajšlová, J. *Anal. Chim. Acta* 2006, *577*, 8-17.

[157] Wang, J. H.; Zhang, Y. B.; Wang, X. L. *J. Sep. Sci.* 2006, *29*, 2330-2337.

[158] Kende, A.; Csizmazia, Z.; Rikker, T.; Angyal, V.; Torkos, K. *Microchem. J.* 2006, *84*, 63-69.

[159] Guardia Rubio, M.; Fernández de Córdova, M. L.; Ayora Cañada, M. J.; Ruiz Medina, A. *J. Chromatogr. A* 2006, *1108*, 231-239.

[160] Gonçalves, C.; Carvalho, J. J.; Azenha, M. A.; Alpendurada, M. F. *J. Chromatogr. A* 2006, *1110*, 6-14.

[161] Kastanias, A.; Chrysayi Tokousbalides, M.; Coward, S.; Philippoussis, A.; Diamantopoulou, P. *Bull. Environ. Contam. Toxicol.* 2006, *77*, 149-154.

[162] Coelhan, M.; Bromig, K. H.; Glas, K.; Roberts, A. L. *J. Agric. Food Chem.* 2006, *54*, 5731-5735.

[163] Zhang, W. G.; Chu, X. G.; Cai, H. X.; An, J.; Li, C. J. *Rapid Commun. Mass Spectrom.* 2006, *20*, 609-617.

[164] Payá, P.; Anastassiades , M.; Mack, D.; Sigalova, I.; Tasdelen, B.; Oliva, J.; Barba, A.; *Anal. Bioanal. Chem.* 2007, *389*, 1697-1714.

[165] Guardia Rubio, M.; Marchal López, R. M.; Ayora Cañada, M. J.; Ruiz Medina, A. *J. Chromatogr. A* 2007, *1145*, 195-203.

[166] Oh, C. H., *Bull. Environ. Contam. Toxicol.* 2007, *78*, 314-318.

[167] Balinova, A.; Mladenova, R.; Shtereva, D. *J. Chromatogr. A* 2007, *1150*, 136-144.

[168] Pino, V.; Ayala, J. H.; González, V.; Afonso, A. M. *Int. J. Environ. Anal. Chem.* 2007, *87*, 159-175.

[169] Charlton, A. J. A.; Jones, A. *J. Chromatogr. A* 2007, *1141*, 117-122.

[170] Bailey, R.; Belzer, W. *J. Agric. Food Chem.* 2007, *55*, 1150-1155.

[171] Liu, L. B.; Hashi, Y.; Qin, Y. P.; Zhou, H. X.; Lin, J. M. *J. Chromatogr. B* 2007, *845*, 61-68.

[172] Hladik, M. L.; Kuivila, K. M. *J. Agric. Food Chem.* 2008, *56*, 2310-2314.

[173] Hogendoorn, E. A.; Van Zoonen, P.; Brinkman, U. A. T. *Chromatographia* 1991, *31*, 285-292.

[174] Di Corcia, A; Marchetti, M. *Environ. Sci. Technol.* 1992, *26*, 66-74.

[175] Yamada, N.; Tomita, B.; Chaya, K.; Murakami, N. *Jpn. J. Toxicol. Environ. Health* 1992, *38*, 188-191.

[176] Brinkman, U. A. T.; Van Hout, P. J. M.; Macrae, R. *Chromatogr. Anal.* 1994, *31*, 9-11.

[177] de la Colina, C.; Baez, M. E.; Pena, A.; Romero, E.; Dios, G.; Sánchez Rasero, F. *Sci. Total Environ.* 1994, *153*, 1-6.

[178] Nouri, B.; Fouillet, B.; Toussaint, G.; Chambon, P.; Chambon, R. *Analyst* 1995, *120*, 1133-1136.

[179] Papantoni, M. ; Mathiasson, L.; Nilsson, U. *J. Agric. Food Chem.* 1995, *43*, 157-164.

[180] Dupas, S.; Guenu, S.; Pichon, V.; Montiel, A.; Welte, B.; Hennion, M. C. *Int. J. Environ. Anal. Chem.* 1996, *65*, 53-68.

[181] Guenu, S.; Hennion, M. C. *J. Chromatogr. A* 1996, *737*, 15-24.

[182] Aguilar, C.; Borrull, F.; Marce, R. M. *Chromatographia* 1996, *43*, 592-598.

[183] Martínez Vidal, J. L.; Parrilla, P.; Martínez Galera, M.; Garrido Grenich, A. *Analyst* 1996, *121*, 1367-1372.

[184] Martínez Galera, M.; Martínez Vidal, J. L.; Garrido Frenich, A.; Gil García, M. D. *J. Chromatogr. A* 1997, *778*, 139-149.

[185] Parrilla, P.; Martínez Galera, M.; Garrido Frenich, A.; Martínez Vidal, J. L. *J. Liq. Chromatogr. Relat. Technol.* 1997, *20*, 425-442.

[186] Weissmahr, K. W.; Houghton, C. L.; Sedlak, D. L. *Anal. Chem.* 1998, *70*, 4800-4804.
[187] Martínez Galera, M.; Garrido Frenich, A.; Martínez Vidal, J. L. *J. Liq. Chromatogr. Relat. Technol.* 2000, *23*, 1187-1202.
[188] Garrido Frenich, A.; Martínez Galera, M.; Gil García, M. D.; Martínez Vidal, J. L.; Catasus, M.; Marti, L.; Mederos, M. V. *J. Liq. Chromatogr. Relat. Technol.* 2001, *24*, 651-668.
[189] Di Muccio, A.; Camoni, I.; Ventriglia, M.; Attard Barbini, D.; Mauro, M.; Pelosi, P.; Generali, T.; Ausili, A.; Girolimetti, S. *J. Chromatogr. A* 1995, *697,* 145-152.
[190] Santos, T. C. R.; Rocha, J. C.; Barceló, D. Int. *J. Environ. Anal. Chem.* 1998, *70*, 19-28.
[191] Kontou, S.; Tsipi, D.; Oreopoulou, V.; Tzia, C. *J. Agric. Food Chem.* 2001, *49*, 1090-1097.
[192] Di Muccio, A.; Girolimetti, S.; Attard Barbini, D.; Pelosi, P.; Generali, T.; Vergori, L.; De Merulis, G.; Leonelli, A.; Stefanelli, P. *J. Chromatogr. A* 1999, *833*, 61-65.
[193] Falqui Cao, C.; Wang, Z.; Urruty, L.; Pommier, J. J.; Montury, M. *J. Agric. Food Chem.* 2001, *49*, 5092-5097.
[194] Young, M. S.; Phillips, D. J.; Iraneta, P. C.; Krol, J. *J. AOAC Int.* 2001, *84*, 556-561.
[195] Msagati, T. A. M.; Muzi Nindi, M. *J. Sep. Sci.* 2001, *24*, 606-614.
[196] Sandahl, M.; Mathiasson, L; Jönsson, J. A. *J. Chromatogr. A* 2002, *975*, 211-217.
[197] van Hoof, F.; van Wiele, P.; Acobas, F.; Guinmant, J.L.; Bruchet, A.; Scmitz, I.; Bobeldijk, I.; Sacher, F.; Ventura, F.; Boleda, R. *J. AOAC Int.* 2002, *85*, 375-383.
[198] Hutta, M.; Rybar, I.; Chalanyova, M. A. D. *J. Chromatogr. A* 2002, *959*, 143-152.
[199] Millán, S.; Sanpedro, M.; Unceta, N.; Goicolea, M.; Rodríguez, E.; Barrio, R. *J. Chromatogr. A* 2003, *995*, 135-142.
[200] Aulakh, J. S.; Malik, A. K.; Mahajan, R. K. *Talanta* 2005, *66*, 266-270.
[201] Guo, Y. N.; Jiang, Z. S.; Zhang, M.; Feng, L. J.; Zhao, J. Y.; Li, J. C. *Fenxi Huaxue* 2005, *33*, 395-397.
[202] Liu, D. H.; Wang, P.; Zhou, W. F.; Gu, X.; Chen, Z. S.; Zhou, Z. Q. *Anal. Chim. Acta* 2006, *555*, 210-216.
[203] Dimou, A. D.; Sakellarides, T. M.; Vosniakos, F. K.; Giannoulis, N.; Leneti, E.; Albanis, T. *Int. J. Environ. Anal. Chem.* 2006, *86*, 119-130.
[204] Zhou, Q.; Xiao, J.; Ding, Y. *Anal. Chim. Acta* 2007, *602*, 223-228.
[205] Veneziano, A.; Vacca, G.; Arana, S.; De Simone, F.; Rastrelli, L. *Food Chem. Sep.* 2004, *87*, 383-386.
[206] Singh, S. B.; Foster, G. D.; Khan, S. U. *J. Agric. Food Chem.* 2004, *52*, 105-109.
[207] Prousalis, K. P.; Polygenis, D. A.; Syrokou, A.; Lamari, F. N.; Tsegenidis, T. O. *Anal. Bioanal. Chem.* 2004, *379*, 458-463.
[208] Maity, A.; Mukherjee, I. *J. AOAC Int.* 2004, *87*, 157-161.
[209] Topuz, S.; Özhan, G.; Alpertunga, B. *Food Control* 2005, *16,* 87-92.
[210] Qu, T. L.; Meng, Z. L.; Li, J. Q. *Fenxi Huaxue* 2006, *34*, 1023-1026.
[211] Wang, P; Liu, D. H.; Wang, Y. H.; Shan, W. L.; Jiang, S. R.; Zhou, Z. Q. *Fenxi Huaxue* 2006, *34*, 1524-1528.
[212] Baggiani, C.; Baravalle, P.; Giraudi, G.; Tozzi, C. *J. Chromatogr. A* 2007, *1141*, 158-164.

[213] D'Archivio, A. A; Fanelli, M.; Mazzeo, P.; Ruggieri, F. *Talanta* 2007, *71*, 25-30.
[214] Hu, M. L.; Jiang, M.; Wang, P.; Mei, S. R.; Lin, Y. F.; Hu, X. Z.; Shi, Y.; Lu, B.; Dai, K. *Anal. Bioanal. Chem.* 2007, *387*, 1007-1016.
[215] Halko, R.; Padrón Sanz, C.; Sosa Ferrera, Z.; Santana Rodríguez, J. J. *Chromatographia* 2004, *60*, 151-156.
[216] López Monzón, A.; Vega Moreno, D.; Torres Padrón, M. E.; Sosa Ferrera, Z.; Santana Rodríguez, J. J. *Anal. Bioanal. Chem.* 2007, *387*, 1957-1963.
[217] Moral, A.; Sicilia, M. D.; Rubio, S.; Pérez Bendito, D. *Anal. Chim. Acta* 2006, *569*, 132-138.
[218] Pawlowski, T. M.; Poole, C. F. *J. Agric. Food Chem.* 1998, *46*, 3124-3132.
[219] Halko, R.; Sanz, C. P.; Ferrera, Z. S.; Rodriguez, J. J. S. *J. AOAC Int.* 2006, *89*, 1403-1409.
[220] Turiel, E.; Tadeo, J. L.; Cormack, P. A. G.; Martin Esteban, A. *Analyst* 2005, *130*, 1601-1607.
[221] Albero, B.; Sánchez Brunete, C.; Tadeo, J. L. *J. AOAC Int.* 2004, *87*, 664-670.
[222] Saad, B.; Haniff, N. H.; Saleh, M. I.; Hashim, N. H.; Abu, A.; Ali, N. *Food Chem.* 2004, *84,* 313-317.
[223] Miles, C. J. *J. Chromatogr.* 1992, *592*, 283-290.
[224] Ubeda, M. R.; Sevilla Escribano, M. T.; Hernández Hernández, L. *Microchem. J.* 1990, *41*, 22-28.
[225] Carabias Martínez, R.; Rodríguez Gonzalo, E.; García Jimenez, M. G.; García Pinto, C.; Pérez Pavón, J. L.; Hernández Mendez, J. *J. Chromatogr. A* 1996, *754*, 85-96.
[226] Wang, P.; Jiang, S. R.; Liu, D. H.; Zhang, H. J.; Zhou, Z. Q. *J. Agric. Food Chem.* 2006, *54*, 1577-1583.
[227] Wang, J. F.; Xu, Y. J.; Liu, S. G.; Jiang, S. R.; Pan, C.P. *J. Sep. Sci.* 2007, *30*, 3-7.
[228] Volmer, D.; Levsen, K; Wuensch, G. *J. Chromatogr. A* 1994, *660*, 231-248.
[229] Crescenzi, C.; Di Corcia, A.; Marchese, S.; Samperi, R. *Anal. Chem.* 1995, *67*, 1968-1975.
[230] Crescenzi, C.; Di Corcia, A.; Guerriero, E.; Samperi, R. *Environ. Sci. Technol.* 1997, *31*, 479-488.
[231] Jeannot, R.; Sauvard, E. *Ital. J. Food Sci.* 2000, *12*, 219-231.
[232] Di Corcia, A.; Nazzari, M.; Rao, R.; Samperi, R.; Sebastiani, E. *J. Chromatogr. A* 2000, *878*, 87-98.
[233] Takino, M.; Daishima, S.; Yamaguchi, K.; Nakahara, T. *Bunseki Kagaku* 2001, *50*, 309-317.
[234] Miles, C. J.; Doerge, D. R.; Bajic, S. *Micromass Technical Note*, 2001, *202*, 4.
[235] Hernández, F.; Sancho, J. V.; Pozo, O.; Lara, A; Pitarch, E. *J. Chromatogr. A* 2001, *939*, 1-11.
[236] Hanada, Y.; Tanizaki, T.; Koga, M.; Shiraishi, H.; Soma, M. *Anal. Sci.* 2002, *18*, 441-444.
[237] Sancho, J. V.; Pozo, O. J.; Hernández, F. *Analyst* 2004, *129*, 38-44.
[238] Kloepfer, A; Jekel, M; Reemtsma, T. *J. Chromatogr. A* 2004, *1058*, 81-88.
[239] Irace Guigand, S.; Aaron, J. J.; Scribe, P.; Barceló, D. *Chemosphere* 2004, *55*, 973-981.

[240] Hernández, F.; Pozo, O. J.; Sancho, J. V.; López, F. J.; Marin, J. M.; Ibañez, M. *Trends Anal. Chem.* 2005, *24*, 596-612.

[241] Sasaki, H.; Yonekubo, J.; Hayakawa, K. *Anal. Sci.* 2006, *22*, 835-840.

[242] Marin, J. M,; Sancho, J. V.; Pozo, O. J.; López, F. J.; Hernández, F. *J. Chromatogr. A* 2006, *1133*, 204-214.

[243] Polati, S.; Bottaro, M.; Frascarolo, P.; Gosetti, F.; Gianotti, V.; Gennaro, M. C. *Anal. Chim. Acta* 2006, *579*, 146-151.

[244] de Streene, J. C.; Mortier, K. A.; Lambert, W. E. *J. Chromatogr. A* 2006, *1123*, 71-81.

[245] Ibáñez, M.; Sancho, J. V.; McMillan, D.; Rao, R.; Hernández, F. *Trends Anal. Chem.* 2008, *27*, 481-489

[246] Doerge, D. R. Miles, C. J. *Anal. Chem.* 1991, *63*, 1999-2001.

[247] Honing, M.; Riu, J.; Barceló, D.; van-Baar, B. L. M.; Brinkman, U. A. T. *J. Chromatogr. A* 1996, *733*, 283-294.

[248] Fernández, M.; Rodríquez, R.; Picó, Y.; Manes, J. *J. Chromatogr. A* 2001, *912*, 301-310.

[249] Young, M. S.; Early, M. F.; Mallet, C. R.; Krol, J. *J. AOAC Int.* 2001, *84*, 1608-1613.

[250] Pous, X.; Ruiz, M. J.; Picó, Y.; Font, G. *Fresenius' J. Anal. Chem.* 2001, *371*, 182-189.

[251] Taylor, M. J.; Hunter, K.; Hunter, K. B.; Lindsay, D.; Le Bouhellec, S. *J. Chromatogr. A* 2002, *982*, 225-236.

[252] Perret, D.; Gentili, A.; Marchese, S.; Sergi, M.; D'Ascenzo, G. *J. AOAC Int.* 2002, *85* , 724-730.

[253] Kaihara, A.; Yoshii, K.; Tsumara, Y.; Ishimitsu, S.; Tonogai,Y. *J. Health Sci.* 2002, *48*, 173-178.

[254] de Ruyck, H.; Daeseleire, E.; de Ridder, H.; van Renterghem, R. *J. Chromatogr. A* 2002, *976*, 181-194.

[255] Zrostlikova, J.; Hajslova, J.; Kovalczuk, T.; Stepan, R.; Poustka, J. *J. AOAC. Int.* 2003, *86*, 612-622.

[256] Blasco, C.; Font, G.; Manes, J.; Picó, Y. *Anal. Chem.* 2003, *75*, 3606-3615.

[257] Klein, J.; Alder, L. *J. AOAC Int.* 2003, *86*, 1015-1037.

[258] Hengel, M.; Hung, B.; Engebretson, J.; Shibamoto, T. *J. Agric. Food Chem.* 2003, *51*, 6635-6639.

[259] Jansson, C.; Pihlströem, T.; Östedahl, B. G.; Markides, K. E. *J. Chromatogr. A* 2004, *1023*, 93-104.

[260] Alder, L.; Luederitz, S.; Lindtner, K.; Stan, H. J. *J. Chromatogr. A* 2004, *1058*, 67-79.

[261] Hetherton, C. L.; Sykes, M. D.; Fussell, R. J.; Goodall, D. M. *Rapid Commun. Mass Spectrom.* 2004, *18*, 2443-2450.

[262] Garrido Frenich, A.; Martínez Vidal, J. L.; López López, T.; Cortés Aguado, S.; Martínez Salvador, I. *J. Chromatogr. A* 2004, *1048*, 199-206.

[263] Ortelli, D.; Edder, P.; Corvi, C. *Anal. Chim. Acta* 2004, *520*, 33-45.

[264] Yoshioka, N.; Akiyama, Y.; Teranishi, K. *J. Chromatogr. A* 2004, *1022*, 145-150.

[265] Zamora, T.; Pozo, O. J.; López, F. J.; Hernández, F. *J. Chromatogr. A* 2004, *1045*, 137-143.

[266] Agüera, A.; López, S.; Fernández Alba, A. R.; Contreras, M.; Crespo, J.; Piedra, L. *J. Chromatogr. A* 2004, *1045*, 125-135.

[267] Granby, K.; Andersen, J. H.; Christensen, H. B. *Anal. Chim. Acta* 2004, *520*, 165-176.

[268] Blasco, C.; Font, G.; Picó, Y. *J. Chromatogr. A* 2004, *1043*, 231-238.

[269] García Reyes, J. F.; Ferrer, I.; Thurman, E. M.; Molina Díaz, A.; Fernández Alba, A. R. *Rapid Commun. Mass Spectrom.* 2005, *19*, 2780-2788.

[270] Wang, J.; Cheung, W.; Grant, D. *J. Agric. Food Chem.* 2005, *53*, 528-537.

[271] Thurman, E. M.; Ferrer, I.; Zweigenbaum, J.; García Reyes, J. F.; Woodman, M.; Fernández Alba, A. R. *J. Chromatogr. A* 2005, *1082*, 71-80.

[272] Schermerhorn, P. G.; Golden, P. E.; Krynitsky, A. J.; Leimkuehler, W. M. *J. AOAC Int.* 2005, *88*, 1491-1502.

[273] Sannino, A.; Bandini, M., *J. AOAC Int.* 2005, *88*, 1822-1826.

[274] Thurman, E. M.; Ferrer, I.; Fernández Alba, A. R. *J. Chromatogr. A* 2005, *1067*, 127-134.

[275] Troesken, E. R.; Bittner, N.; Voelkel, W. *J. Chromatogr. A* 2005, *1083*, 113-119.

[276] Bogialli, S.; Curini, R.; Di Corcia, A.; Lagana, A.; Stabile, A.; Sturchio, E. *J. Chromatogr. A* 2006, *1102*, 1-10.

[277] Hernández, F.; Pozo, O. J.; Sancho, J. V.; Bijlsma, L.; Barreda, M.; Pitarch, E. *J. Chromatogr. A* 2006, *1109*, 242-252.

[278] Carabias Martínez, R.; Rodríguez Gonzalo, E.; Revilla Ruiz, P. *J. Chromatogr. A* 2006, *1137*, 207-215.

[279] Rabolle, M.; Spliid, N. H.; Kristensen, K.; Kudsk, P. *J. Agric. Food Chem.* 2006, *54*, 900-908.

[280] Botitsi, H.; Economou, A.; Tsipi, D. *Anal. Bioanal. Chem.* 2007, *389*, 1685-1695.

[281] Pozo, O. J.; Barreda, M.; Sancho, J. V.; Hernández, F.; Lliberia, J. Ll.; Cortés, B.; Bagó, B. *Anal. Bioanal. Chem.* 2007, *389*, 1765-1771.

[282] Leandro, C. C.; Hancock, P.; Fussell, R. J.; Keely, B. J. *J. Chromatogr. A* 2007, *1144*, 161-169.

[283] Wang, S. L.; Xu, Y. J.; Pan, C. P.; Jiang, S. R.; Liu, F. M. *Anal. Bioanal. Chem.* 2007, *387*, 673-685.

[284] Gilbert López, B.; García Reyes, J. F.; Mezcua, M.; Molina Díaz, A.; Fernández Alba, A. R. *J. Agric. Food Chem.* 2007, *55*, 10548-10556.

[285] Lesueur, C.; Gartner, M.; Mentler, A.; Fuerhacker, M. *Int. J. Environ. Anal. Chem.* 2007, *87*, 1013-1032.

[286] Pizzutti, I. R.; de Kok, A.; Zanella, R.; Adaime, M. B.; Hiemstra, M.; Wickert, C.; Prestes, O. D. *J. Chromatogr. A* 2007, *1142*, 123-136.

[287] Chen, J.; Loo, B.; Ray, C. *J. Agric. Food Chem.* 2008, *56*, 1829-1837.

[288] Brennecke, R. *Fresenius' J. Anal. Chem.* 1991, *339*, 399-401.

[289] Simal Gandara, J.; Paseiro Losada, P.; González Rodríguez, V.; Romero Rodríguez, A. *J. Agric. Food Chem.* 1993, *41*, 674-677.

[290] Rietveld, R.; Quirijns, J. *J. Chromatogr. A* 1994, *683*, 151-1553.

[291] Salau, J. S.; Alonso, R.; Batllo, G.; Barceló, D. *Anal. Chim. Acta.* 1994, *293*, 109-117.

[292] de Almeida Azevedo, D.; Lacorte, S.; Vinhas, T.; Viana, P.; Barceló, D. *J. Chromatogr. A* 2000, *879*, 13-26.

[293] Geerdink, R. B.; Niessen, W. M. A.; Brinkman, U. A. T. *J. Chromatogr. A* 2002, *970*, 65-93.

[294] Brito, N. M.; Navickiene, S.; Polese, L.; Jardim, E. F. G.; Abakerli, R. B.; Ribeiro, M. L. *J. Chromatogr. A* 2002, *957*, 201-209.
[295] Lehotay, S. J.; Mastovska, K.; Lightfield, A. R. *J. AOAC Int.* 2005, *88*, 615-629.
[296] Lehotay, S. J.; de Kok, A.; Hiemstra, M.; van Bodegraven, P. *J. AOAC Int.* 2005, *88*, 595-614.
[297] Lehotay, S. J. *J. AOAC Int.* 2007, *90*, 485-520.
[298] Garrido Frenich, A.; Martínez Salvador, I.; Martínez Vidal, J. L.; López López, T. *Anal. Bioanal. Chem.* 2005, *383*, 1106-1118.
[299] Pang, G. F.; Fan, C. L.; Liu, Y. M.; Cao, Y. Z.; Zhang, J. J.; Li, X. M.; Li, Z. Y.; Wu, Y. P.; Guo, T. T. *J. AOAC Int.* 2006, *89*, 740-771.
[300] Pang, G. F.; Cao, Y. Z.; Zhang, J. J.; Fan, C. L.; Liu, Y. M.; Jia, G. Q.; Li, Z. Y; Shi, Y. Q.; Wu, Y. P.; Guo, T. T.; Li, X. M. *J. Chromatogr. A* 2006, *1125*, 1-30.
[301] Pang, G. F.; Liu, Y. M.; Fan, C. L.; Zhang, J. J.; Cao, Y. Z.; Li, X. M.; Li, Z. Y.; Wu, Y. P.; Guo, T. T. *Anal. Bioanal. Chem.* 2006, *384*, 1366-1408.
[302] Pihlström, T.; Blomkvist, G.; Friman, P.; Pagard, U.; Österdahl, B. G. *Anal. Bioanal. Chem.* 2007, *389*, 773-1789.
[303] Picó, Y.; Rodríguez, R.; Manes, J. *Trends Anal. Chem.* 2003, *22*, 133-151.
[304] Hernández Borges, J.; Frias García, S.; Cifuentes, A.; Rodríguez Delgado, M. A. *J. Sep. Sci.* 2004, *27*, 947-963.
[305] Malik, A. K.; Seidel, B. S.; Faubel, W. *J. Chromatogr. A* 1999, *857*, 365-368.
[306] Malik, A. K.; Faubel, W. *Talanta* 2000, *52,* 341-346.
[307] Rodríguez, R.; Boyer, I.; Font, G.; Picó, Y. *Analyst* 2001, *126*, 2134-2138.
[308] Kaltsonoudis, C. K.; Lamari, F. N.; Prousalis, K. P.; Karamanos, N. K.; Tsegenidis, T. *Chromatographia* 2003, *57*, 181-184.
[309] Rodríguez, R.; Picó, Y.; Font, G.; Mañes, J. *J. Chromatogr. A* 2002, *949*, 359-366.
[310] Rodríguez, R.; Picó, Y.; Font, G.; Mañes, J. *J. Chromatogr. A* 2001, *924*, 387-396.
[311] Bagheri, H.; Saraji, M.; Barceló, D. *Chromatographia* 2004, *59*, 283-289.
[312] He, J.; Chen, S. W.; Ruan, L. F.; Cao, L. L.; Yao, J.; Yu, Z. N. *J. Agric. Food Chem.* 2003, *51*, 7523-7527.
[313] Juan García, A.; Font, G.; Picó, Y. *Electrophoresis* 2005, *26*, 1550-1561.
[314] Takeda, S.; Fukushi, K.; Chayama, K.; Nakayama, Y.; Tanaka, Y.; Wakida, S. I. *J. Chromatogr. A* 2004, *1051*, 297-301.
[315] Segura Carretero, A.; Cruces Blanco, C.; Cortacero Ramírez, S.; Carrasco Pancorbo, A.; Fernández Gutiérrez, A. *J. Agric. Food Chem.* 2004, *52*, 5791-5795.
[316] Galhiane, M. S.; Rissato, S. R.; Apon, B. M. *J. Liq. Chromatogr. Relat. Technol.* 2005, *28*, 2349-2359.
[317] Molina Mayo, C.; Hernández Borges, J.; Borges Miquel, T. M.; Rodríguez Delgado, M. A. *J. Chromatogr. A* 2007, *1150,* 348-355.
[318] Chu, B. L.; Guo, B. Y.; Peng, Z. L.; Wang, Z. H.; Guo, G. S.; Lin J. M. *J. Sep. Sci.* 2007, *30*, 923-929.
[319] Verma, B. C.; Sharma, D. K.; Thakur, H. K.; Rao, B. G.; Sharma, N. K. *Analyst* 1991, *116*, 867-870.
[320] Schwack, W.; Nyanzi, S. *Z. Lebensm. Unters. Forsch.* 1994, *198*, 3-7.
[321] Nyanzi, S.; Karg, J.; Schwack, W. *Dtsch. Lebensm. Rundsch.* 1994, *90*, 239-242.

[322] Mathew, L.; Rao, T. P.; Iyer, C. S. P.; Damodaran, A. D. *Talanta* 1995, *42*, 41-43.
[323] Das, J. V.; Gupta, V. K. *Chem. Anal. (Warsaw)* 1995, *40*, 85-92.
[324] Kesari, R.; Gupta, V. K. *Talanta* 1998, *45*, 1097-1102.
[325] Malik, A. K.; Kapoor, J.; Rao, A. L. J. *J. Environ. Monitor.* 2000, *2*, 367-371.
[326] Malik, A. K. *J. Environ. Monitor.* 2000, *2*, 151-153.
[327] Tunceli, A.; Bag, H.; Turker, A. R. *Fresenius' J. Anal. Chem.* 2001, *371*, 1134-1138.
[328] Agarwal, S.; Aggarwal, S. G.; Singh, P. *Talanta* 2003, *61*, 871-877.
[329] Agarwal, S.; Aggarwal, S. G. *Talanta* 2005, *65*, 104-110.
[330] Sharma, V. K.; Aulakh, J. S.; Bansal, S.; Malik, A. K.; Mahajan, R. K. *Int. J. Environ. Anal. Chem.* 2004, *84*, 1105-1110.
[331] Fletcher, K. A.; Fakayode, S. O.; Lowry, M.; Tucker, S. A.; Neal, S. L.; Kimaru, I. W.; McCarroll, M. E.; Patonay, G.; Oldham, P. B.; Rusin, O.; Strongin, R. M.; Warner, I. M. *Anal. Chem.* 2006, *78*, 4047-4068.
[332] Capitán, F.; Alonso, E.; Avidad, R.; Capitán Vallvey, L. F.; Vilchez, J. L. *Anal. Chem.* 1993, *65*, 1336-1339.
[333] García Sánchez, F.; Aguilar Gallardo, A. *Microchem. J.* 1994, *50*, 161-168.
[334] Navalón, A.; Blanc, R.; Vilchez, J. L. *Mikrochim. Acta* 1997, *126*, 33-38.
[335] Capitán Vallvey; L. F.; Fernández Ramos, M. D.; Avidad, R.; Deheidel, M. K. A. *Anal. Chim. Acta* 2001, *440*, 131-141.
[336] Maggio, R.; Piccirilli, G. N.; Escandar, G. M. *Appl. Spectrosc.* 2005, *59*, 873-880.
[337] Segura Carretero, A.; Cruces Blanco, C.; Estrada Fernández, R.; Fernández Gutiérrez, A. *Fresenius' J. Anal. Chem.* 1998, *360*, 605-608.
[338] Tang, B.; Wang, X.; Wang, G. L.; Wang, Y.; Chen, Z. Z. *Analyst* 2005, *130*, 1038-1045.
[339] Segura Carretero, A.; Cruces Blanco, C.; Cañabate Díaz, B.; Fernández Sánchez, J. F.; Fernández Gutiérrez, A. *Anal. Chim. Acta* 2000, *417*, 19-30.
[340] Correa, R. A.; Escandar, G. M. *Anal. Chim. Acta* 2006, *571*, 58–65.
[341] Salinas, A.; Fernández Sánchez, J. F.; Segura Carreteto, A.; Fernández Gutiérrez, A. *Int. J. Environ. Anal. Chem.* 2005, *85*, 443-449.
[342] Saleh, N.; Al Rawashdeh, N. A. F. *J. Fluoresc.* 2006, *16*, 487-493.
[343] Sancenón, J.; de la Guardia, M. *Anal. Chim. Acta* 1994, *287*, 49-57.
[344] de Armas, G.; Miro, M.; Estela, J. M.; Cerda, V. *Luminescence* 2002, *17*, 259-260.
[345] de Armas, G.; Becerra, E.; Cladera, A.; Estela, J. M.; Cerda, V. *Anal. Chim. Acta* 2001, *427*, 83-92.
[346] García Reyes, J. F.; Ortega Barrales, P.; Molina Díaz, A. *Anal. Chim. Acta* 2003, *493*, 35-45.
[347] García Reyes, J. F.; Ortega Barrales, P.; Molina Díaz, A. *Agric. Food Chem.* 2004, *52*, 2197-2202.
[348] García Reyes, J. F.; Llorent Martínez, E. J.; Ortega Barrales, P.; Molina Díaz, A. *Anal. Bioanal. Chem.* 2004, *378*, 429-437.
[349] García Reyes, J. F.; Llorent Martínez, E. J.; Ortega Barrales, P.; Molina Díaz, A. *Talanta* 2004, *64*, 742-749.
[350] Llorent Martínez, E. J.; García Reyes, J. F.; Ortega Barrales, P.; Molina Díaz, A. *J. AOAC Int.* 2005, *88*, 860-865.

[351] Piccirilli, G. N.; Escandar, G. M. *Anal. Chim. Acta* 2007, *601*,196-203.
[352] Domínguez Vidal, A.; Ortega Barrales, P.; Molina Díaz, A. *J. Fluoresc.* 2007, *17*, 271-277.
[353] Cañabate Díaz, B.; Segura Carretero, A.; Cruces Blanco, C.; Fernández Gutiérrez, A. *Appl. Spectrosc.* 2003, *57*, 1585-1591.
[354] Capitán Vallvey, L. F.; Deheidel, M. K. A.; de Orbe, I.; Avidad, R. *Analyst* 1999, *124*, 49-53.
[355] Capitán Vallvey, L. F.; Deheidel, M. K.; Avidad, R. *Mikrochim. Acta* 1999, *130*, 273-279.
[356] Picón Zamora, D.; Martínez Galera, M.; Garrido Frenich, A.; Martínez Vidal, J. L. *Analyst* 2000, *125*, 1167-1174.
[357] de Armas, G.; Miro, M.; Estela, J. M.; Cerda, V. *Anal. Chim. Acta* 2002, *471*, 173-186.
[358] Martínez Galera, M.; Picón Zamora, D.; Martínez Vidal, J. L.; Garrido Frenich, A. *Anal. Lett.* 2002, *35*, 921-941.
[359] Martínez Galera, M.; Picón Zamora, D.; Martínez Vidal, J. L.; Garrido Frenich, A.; Espinosa Mansilla, A.; Muñoz de la Peña, A.; Salina López, F. *Talanta* 2003, *59*, 1107-1116.
[360] Garrido Frenich, A.; Picón Zamora, D.; Martínez Galera, M.; Martínez Vidal, J. L. *Anal. Bioanal .Chem.* 2003, *375*, 974-980.
[361] Garrido Frenich, A.; Picón Zamora, D.; Martínez Vidal, J. L.; Martínez Galera, M. *Anal.Chim. Acta* 2001, *449*, 143-155.
[362] Rodríguez Cuesta, M. J.; Boque, R.; Rius, F. X.; Picón Zamora, D.; Martínez Galera, M.; Garrido Frenich, A. *Anal. Chim. Acta* 2003, *491*, 47-56.
[363] Piccirilli, G. N.; Escandar, G. M. *Analyst* 2006, *131*, 1012-1020.
[364] González, J. M.; Greenway, G. M.; McCreedy, T.; Qijun, S. *Analyst* 2000, *125*, 765-769.
[365] Cassella, A. R.; Cassella, R. J.; Garrigues, S.; Santelli, R. E.; de Campos, R. C.; de la Guardia, M. *Analyst* 2000, *125*, 1829-1833.
[366] Columé, A.; Diewok, J.; Lendl. B. *Int. J. Environ. Anal. Chem.* 2004, *84*, 835-844.
[367] Moros, J.; Armenta, S.; Garrigues, S.; de la Guardia, M. *Anal. Chim. Acta* 2006, *579*, 17-24.
[368] Phalen, R. N.; Que Hee, S. S. *Appl. Spectrosc.* 2007, *61*, 204-211.
[369] Jiménez de Blas, O.; Pereda de Paz, J. L.; Hernández Méndez, J. *J. Anal. At. Spectrom.* 1990, *5*, 693-696.
[370] Lo, C. C.; Ho, M. H.; Hung, M. D. *J. Agric. Food Chem.* 1996, *44*, 2720-2723.
[371] Baena, J. R.; Galego, M.; Valcarcel, M. *Analyst* 2000, *125*, 1495-1499.
[372] dos Santos, W. N. L.; da Silva, E. G. P.; Fernandes, M. S.; Araujo, R. G. O.; Costa, A. C. S.; Vale, M. G. R.; Ferreira, S. L. C. *Anal. Bioanal. Chem.* 2005, *382*, 1099-1102.
[373] Turker, A. R.; Sezer, B. *Turk. J. Pharm. Sci.* 2005, *2*, 35-42.
[374] Wightwick, A. M.; Mollah, M. R.; Partington, D. L.; Allinson, G. *J. Agric. Food Chem.* 2008, *56,* 2457-2464.
[375] Butler, O. T.; Cook, J. M.; Harrington, C. F.; Hill S. J.; Rieuwerts, J.; Miles, D. L. *J. Anal. At. Spectrom.* 2008, *23*, 249-286.
[376] Franko, M. *Talanta* 2001, *54*, 1-13.

[377] Ito, Y.; Goto, T.; Oka, H.; Matsumoto, H.; Miyazaki, Y.; Takahashi, N.; Nakazawa, H. *J. Agric. Food Chem.* 2003, *51*, 861-866.

[378] Strawn, D. G.; Baker, L. L. *Environ. Sci. Technol.* 2008, *42*, 37-42.

[379] Sevilla, M. T.; Rodríguez Procopio, J.; Pinilla, J. M.; Hernández, L. *Electroanalysis (NY)* 1990, *2*, 475-479.

[380] Carabias Martínez, R.; Rodríguez Gonzalo, E.; García Jiménez, M. G.; Hernández Méndez, J. *J. Electroanal. Chem.* 1998, *456*, 193-202.

[381] Guiberteau Cabanillas, A.; Galeano Díaz, T; Mora Diez, N.; Salinas, F.; Ortiz Burguillos, J. M.; Viré, J. C. *Comput. Chem.* 2001, *25*, 459-473.

[382] Manisankar, P.; Selvanathan, G.; Viswanathan, S.; Gurumallesh Prabu, H. *Electroanalysis (NY)* 2002, *14*, 1722-1727.

[383] Guzmán Vázquez de Prada, A.; Mena, M. L.; Reviejo, A. J.; Pingarrón, J. M. *Anal. Lett.* 2004, *37*, 65-79.

[384] Manisankar, P.; Selvanathan, G.; Vedhi, C. *Int. J. Environ. Anal. Chem.* 2005, *85*, 409-422.

[385] Manisankar, P.; Selvanathan, G.; Vedhi, C. *Talanta* 2006, *68*, 686-692.

[386] Inam, R.; Gulerman, E. Z.; Sarigul, T. *Anal. Chim. Acta* 2006, *579*, 117-123.

[387] Montiel, A. *Analusis* 1991, *19*, 134-137.

[388] Schobel, U.; Barzen, C.; Gauglitz, G. *Fresenius' J. Anal. Chem.* 2000, *366*, 646-658.

[389] Lee, N. A.; Kennedy, I. R. *J. AOAC Int.* 2001, *84*, 1393-1406.

[390] Bushway, R. J.; Thome, E. Jr. *Food Agric. Immunol.* 1998, *10*, 23-28.

[391] Giraudi, G.; Rosso, I.; Baggiani, C.; Giovannoli, C.; Vanni, A.; Grassi, G. *Anal. Chim Acta* 1999, *392*, 85-94.

[392] Abad, A.; Manclus, J. J.; Moreno, M. J.; Montoya, A. *J. AOAC Int.* 2001, *84*, 156-161.

[393] Furzer, G. S.; Veldhuis, L.; Hall, J. C. *J. Agric. Food Chem.* 2006, *54*, 688-693.

[394] Wang, X.; Chen, F.; Wan, P. J.; Huang, G. *J. Agric. Food Chem.* 2004, *52*, 7793-7797.

[395] Choi, J. W.; Kim, Y. K.; Song, S. Y.; Lee, I. H.; Lee, W. H. *Biosens. Bioelectron.* 2003, *18*, 1461.

[396] Mercader, J. V.; Suárez Pantaleón, C.; Agulló, C.; Abad Somovilla, A.; Abad Fuentes, A. *J. Agric. Food Chem.* 2008, *56*, 1545-1552.

In: Fungicides
Editors: P. De Costa and P. Bezerra

ISBN: 978-1-60692-631-4

Chapter VIII

GLOBAL ADAPTIVE RESPONSE AND RESISTANCE TO AGRICULTURAL FUNGICIDES: LESSONS FROM YEAST AND PHYTOPATHOGENIC FUNGI

Tânia R. Cabrito, Miguel C. Teixeira, Isabel Sá-Correia

IBB – Institute for Biotechnology and Bioengineering, Centre for Biological and Chemical Engineering, Instituto Superior Técnico, 1049-001, Lisboa, Portugal

ABSTRACT

Agricultural fungicides are widely used in crop protection. However, they are potential pollutants and their accumulation in the environment can cause severe health problems. Moreover, its efficacy against a broad spectrum of phytopathogenic fungi is compromised by the emergence of multiresistant strains. Multiple drug resistance is in most cases due to the action of membrane transporters that, presumably, catalyze the extrusion of unrelated chemical compounds. The biological role and expression regulation of a number of these transporters conferring fungicide resistance in *Saccharomyces cerevisiae* and in other fungi are reviewed in this chapter.

Genome-wide analysis tools have been increasingly used to provide new insights into the mechanisms underlying organism-environment interactions. This new field of Environmental Toxigenomics may provide a better understanding of the toxicological effects of each potential environmental toxicant and on how cells are able to acquire resistance to these chemical stresses. It may also allow the identification of early and sensitive biomarkers of the toxicological response. Post-genomic experimental approaches have been applied with success to the yeast *S. cerevisiae*, a widely accepted eukaryotic model system. The knowledge gathered so far on the mechanisms underlying the toxicity of, and resistance to, agricultural fungicides in *S. cerevisiae* and in filamentous fungi based on these approaches and on more detailed analyses, is reviewed here. Emphasis is given to the systemic benzimidazole benomyl and the dithiocarbamate mancozeb.

ABBREVIATIONS

ABC ATP Binding Cassete
AH Aromatic Hydrocarbons
AP AnilinoPyrimidines
CAA Carboxylic Acid Amides
DMI DeMethylation Inhibitors
MBC Methyl Benzimidazole Carbamates
MBI Melanin Biosynthesis Inhibitors
MDR MultiDrug Resistance
MFS Major Facilitator Superfamily
PA PhenylAmides
PDR Pleiotropic Drug Resistance
PP PhenylPyrroles
QoI Quinone outside Inhibitors
QiI Quinone inside Inhibitors.

1. INTRODUCTION

Agricultural fungicides are pesticides that control fungal proliferation by specifically inhibiting or killing phytopathogenic fungi. Over 8000 species of fungi are known to cause disease in plants, often having a significant economic impact on crop yield (Adams, 1997). Thus, managing diseases is an essential component in crop production. Fungicides for plant protection are used not only with the intent of controlling fungal diseases, but also to increase crop productivity and quality (McGrath, 2004). Fungicides can be deposited in the surface of plants and attack non-specific targets in the fungal spore as it germinates or target very specific sites, such as single receptors or enzymes. Many specific fungicides are systemic in their action (they enter the plant and are transported in the xylem and phloem) while non-specific compounds tend to have a low systemic predisposition (Adams, 1997).

Although the use of fungicides is an unavoidable practice in current agriculture, given the need for higher food supplies world-wide, its usage may have negative outcomes. One of the major problems concerning the use of fungicides is the toxic effect that they can have in public health. For instance, DuPont's Benlate, which contains the benzimidazole-fungicide benomyl as the active principle and has been widely used in vine-growing in the USA since the 1970's, was taken off the U.S. market in 2001, being classified by the U.S. Environmental Protection Agency as a possible carcinogen (http://heritage.dupont.com/floater/fl_benlate/floater.shtml; http://www.apsnet.org/online/feature/fungi/). An association between environmental exposure to benomyl and anophthalmia has been suggested. Benomyl has also been identified as a potential teratogenic, having negative effects in rat embryonic development (Hewitt *et al.*, 2005). Its mode of action is believed to be related to its ability to inhibit the polymerization of brain tubulin, inhibiting neuronal cell differentiation at concentrations likely to be achieved during the development of fetal abnormalities in rats in vivo (McLean *et al.*, 1998). This fungicide affects many parameters of differentiation, including optic development even at levels below those that could be considered embryotoxic (Hewitt *et al.*, 2005).

Another commonly used fungicide is mancozeb, a mixture of manganese- and zinc-ethylene-bis-dithiocarbamate (Mn:Zn, 9:1), that is efficient against a broad spectrum of fungi (Ballantyne, 2004). This compound displays low acute toxicity, but acts as a pro-oxidant and exerts chronic adverse health effects, being associated to carcinogenesis and development of Parkinson's disease (Belpoggi *et al.*, 2002; Calviello *et al.*, 2006; Zhou *et al.*, 2004). Both mancozeb and maneb, another dithiocarbamate fungicide, are equipotent neurotoxicants and a recent study on the mechanisms of neural damage associated with mancozeb exposure has determined the role that generated reactive oxygen species (ROS) play in toxicity. Mancozeb exposure was associated with mitochondrial uncoupling in mesencephalic rat cells, a phenomenon known to increase free radical production (Domico *et al.*, 2007). DNA damage and apoptosis induction by mancozeb in rat fibroblasts was also observed, being possibly related to an oxidative mechanism (Calviello *et al.*, 2006). Other studies also relate the use of this fungicide with the presence in some wines of high levels of Mn and Zn, two essential micronutrients that are toxic at high concentrations (Calhelha *et al.*, 2006; La Pera *et al.*, 2008). The use of fungicides should be controlled due to its toxicological effects in humans and in other naturally occurring beneficial organisms, which is the case of some yeast genera used in food technologies, such as the genus *Saccharomyces*.

Table 1. Main classes of agricultural fungicides according to their mode of action, target site, and chemical group. Known cases of resistance are also indicated

Family name	Mode of action	Examples of fungicides	Examples of known resistant fungal phytopathogens
PhenylAmides (PA)	Biosynthesis of nucleic acid	benalaxyl, furalaxyl, metalaxyl, metalaxyl-M	
Hydroxypyrimidines		bupirimate, dimethirimol, ethirimol	*Erysiphe graminis f.sp. hordei, Sphaerotheca fuliginea*
Heteroaromatics		hymexazole, octhilinone	
Carboxylic acids		oxolinic acid	
Methyl Benzimidazole Carbamates (MBC)	Mitosis	benomyl, carbendazim, thiabendazole, thiophanate, thiophanate-methyl	*Alternaria alternata, Botrytis cinerea, Cladosporium fulvum*
Phenylcarbamates		diethofencarb	*Botrytis cinerea, Neurospora crassa, Verticillium fungicola*
Benzamides		zoxamide	

Table 1 (Continued)

Family name	Mode of action	Examples of fungicides	Examples of known resistant fungal phytopathogens
Phenylureas		pencycuron	*Rhizoctonia solani*
Pyrimidinamines	Respiration	diflumetorim	
Carboxamides		benodanil, flutolanil, mepronil, fenfuram, thifluzamide, furametpyr, penthiopyrad	*Aspergillus nidulans, Coprinus cinereus, Ustilago nuda*
Quinone outside Inhibitors (QoI)		azoxystrobin, enestrobin, picoxystrobin, pyraclostrobin, kresoxim-methyl, trifloxystrobin, dimoxystrobin, metominostrobin	*Alternaria alternata, Botrytis cinerea, Mycosphaerella graminicola*
Quinone inside Inhibitors (QiI)		cyazofamid, amisulbrom	*Saccharomyces cerevisiae*
AnilinoPyrimidines (AP)	Biosynthesis of amino acids and proteins	cyprodinil, mepanipyrim, pyrimethanil	*Botrytis cinerea*
Quinolines	Signal transduction	quinoxyfen	*Erysiphe graminis f. sp. hordei*
PhenylPyrroles (PP)		fenpiclonil, fludioxonil	*Alternaria brassicicola, Botryotinia fuckeliana*
Dicarboximides		chlozolinate, iprodione, procymidone, vinclozolin	*Alternaria alternate, Botrytis cinerea, Neurospora crassa*
Phosphorothiolates	Biosynthesis of lipids	edifenphos, iprobenfos (IBP), pyrazophos	*Bipolaris oryzae, Pyricularia oryzae*
Dithiolanes		isoprothiolane	
Aromatic Hydrocarbons (AH)		biphenyl, chloroneb, dicloran, quintozene (PCNB), tecnazene (TCNB), tolclofos-methyl	*Botrytis cinerea, Rhizoctonia solani, Sclerotium rolfsii*
Heteroaromatics		etridiazole	

Carbamates		iodocarb, propamocarb, prothiocarb, dimethomorph, flumorph	
Carboxylic Acid Amides (CAA)			
DeMethylation Inhibitors (DMI)	Biosynthesis of sterols	imazalil, oxpoconazole, pefurazoate, prochloraz, triflumizole, azaconazole, bitertanol, bromuconazole, cyproconazole, difenoconazole, diniconazole, epoxiconazole, etaconazole, fenbuconazole, fluquinconazole, flusilazole, flutriafol, hexaconazole, imibenconazole, ipconazole, metconazole, myclobutanil, penconazole, propiconazole, prothioconazole, simeconazole, tebuconazole, tetraconazole, triadimefon, triadimenol, triticonazole	*Aspergillus nidulans,, Botrytis cinerea, Mycosphaerella graminicola*
Amines		aldimorph, dodemorph, fenpropimorph, tridemorph, fenpropidin, piperalin, spiroxamine	*Erysiphe graminis f. sp. tritici, Erysiphe graminis f. sp. hordei, Nectria haematococca*
Hydroxyanilides		fenhexamid	*Botrytis cinerea*
Polyoxins	Biosynthesis of glucan	polyoxin	*Cochliobolus heterostrophus, Alternaria alternata, Alternaria kikuchiana*

Table 1 (Continued)

Family name	Mode of action	Examples of fungicides	Examples of known resistant fungal phytopathogens
Melanin Biosynthesis Inhibitors (MBI)	Biosynthesis of melanin	fthalide, pyroquilon, tricyclazole, carpropamid, diclocymet, fenoxanil	*Magnaporthe grisea*
Iorganic	Multiple sites / Not known	copper, sulphur	
Quinones		dithianon	
Dithiocarbamates		ferbam, mancozeb, maneb, metiram, propineb, thiram, zineb, ziram	*Botrytis cinerea, Helminthosporium halodes*
Phthalimides		captan, captafol, folpet	*Botrytis cinerea*
Chloronitriles		chlorothalonil	*Botrytis cinerea*
Phenylsulfamides		dichlofluanid, tolylfluanid	*Botrytis cinerea*
Aliphatic nitrogens		dodine, guazatine, iminoctadine	*Venturia inaequalis,, Penicillium digitatum, Penicillium italicum*
Triazines		anilazine	

Adapted from Compendium of Pesticide Common Names (http://www.alanwood.net/pesticides/), Crop Protection Compendium (http://www.cabi.org/AllOtherProducts.asp?SubjectArea=&PID=106) and APSnet - American Phytopathological Society (http://www.apsnet.org/online/feature/fungi/).

A second problem concerning the wide use of fungicides is the emergence of fungicide resistant phytopathogenic fungi strains, with severe agro-economical consequences. Cases of resistance (http://www.apsnet.org/online/feature/fungi/) have been described for many of the most widely used fungicide families, such as DMI (DeMethylation Inhibitors), QoI (Quinone outside Inhibitors), Dithiocarbamates and MBC (Methyl Benzimidazole Carbamates). For example, the first case of benzimidazole fungicides resistance was registered in 1969, just one year after their introduction. The reason for the rapid development of resistance was related with the fact that these fungicides are single site inhibitors of fungal microtubule assembly during mitosis (Smith, 1988). In Table 1 current knowledge on the main agricultural fungicide families and their mode of action, as well as examples of fungal phytopathogens that have developed resistance to specific fungicides are sumarized.

In this chapter, the knowledge gathered based on genome-wide approaches and on more detailed studies on the response and resistance to agricultural fungicides in the eukaryotic model *Saccharomyces cerevisiae* and in phytopathogenic fungi is reviewed, focusing the fungicides benomyl and mancozeb. The role of multidrug resistance transporters and of the regulatory networks that control their expression in fungicide resistance is highlighted.

2. Toxicological Assessment of Agricultural Fungicides and Underlying Mechanisms

Toxicological assessment of pesticides, including fungicides, has been based essentially on bioassays using mammals to detect either acute or mid-term toxic effects, while the ecotoxicological impact of these xenobiotic compounds has been mainly tested on birds, insects, aquatic organisms and soil microorganisms (Landis & Yu, 1999; Papaefthimiou *et al.*, 2004; Tomlin, 1997). Although these toxicity tests have been used for years and have a wide acceptance for fungicide regulation, there is an international demand for the development and validation of simpler and more rapid screening methods and for minimizing animal utilization and pain. Hence, in vitro protocols mostly based on the use of animal cell lines and cytotoxicity assays based on the use of eukaryotic microbes as test systems are currently in use or under validation for alternative toxicity testing (http://ecvamsis.jrc.it/invittox/static/index.html). Short-term toxicity assays based on the determination of the deleterious effects of xenobiotics on the biological function of bacteria, fungi, algae, and protozoa or on the activity of enzymes, are also being developed and used increasingly. These assays are simple, rapid, and cost-effective, require small sample volumes, and can be miniaturized (Papaefthimiou *et al.*, 2004). Among them are the growth inhibitory assays based on the measurement of changes in microbial cell concentration, through culture turbidity, to estimate the impact of toxic compounds on microbial growth kinetics and energetics.

Although these tests are current practice for pesticide toxicity assessment they provide little evidence on the molecular basis of the exerted toxicity. Moreover, it has become increasingly evident that many pesticides exert long-term toxicological effects occurring upon chronic exposure, those effects being hard to predict based on classical toxicological assays. Some detailed studies have been carried out in different model systems to assess fungicide toxicity at a molecular basis.

The single cell eukaryotic model *S. cerevisiae* is non-pathogenic, easy to manipulate genetically, well characterized, and exhibits fast and inexpensive growth. The paradigm of research using *S. cerevisiae* has changed following the publication of the genome sequence more than a decade ago (Goffeau *et al.*, 1996), and a large amount of biological information has been gathered over several years of post-genomic research facilitated by easy access to public databases (SGD, Saccharomyces Genome Database – www.yeastgenome.com; and YEASTRACT - http://www.yeastract.com, among others). Research on *S. cerevisiae* pioneered the development of several post-genomic experimental approaches and computational tools. Large-scale biological material has also been produced, including a collection of mutants in which each yeast gene was individually deleted, facilitating studies in yeast. This collection (EUROSCARF – http://web.uni-frankfurt.de/fb15/mikro/euroscarf) (Kelly *et al.*, 2001) allows quick, easy and high-throughput search for genes involved in the resistance or susceptibility to any given environmental stressor. Genome-wide expression analyses in yeast have been successfully used to assess the cellular and molecular changes imposed by different types of stress, in particular by xenobiotic compounds of agricultural interest, such as the herbicide sulfometuron methyl (Jia *et al.*, 2000), the dithiocarbamate fungicides thiuram, zineb and maneb (Kitagawa *et al.*, 2003), the benzimidazole fungicide benomyl (Lucau-Danila *et al.*, 2005), the pesticide lindane (Parveen *et al.*, 2003), and the herbicide 2,4-D (Teixeira *et al.*, 2005; Teixeira *et al.*, 2006a; Teixeira *et al.*, 2007). Even though many cytotoxic compounds used in agriculture may act in their target organisms via physiological mechanisms that do not exist in yeast, many of the basic mechanisms underlying resistance and adaptation to chemical and environmental stresses are apparently conserved among phylogenetically distant organisms (Adams, 1997; Landis & Yu, 1999). Therefore, the characterization of mechanisms of toxicity of fungicides in yeast cells has contributed and is expected to continue to contribute to the understanding of these mechanisms in more complex and less easily accessible eukaryotes, such as in phytopathogenic fungi.

3. Mechanisms of Resistance to Agricultural Fungicides Identified in Yeast and in Phytopathogenic Fungi through Gene-by-gene Analysis

3.1. The Multidrug Resistance (MDR) Phenomenon

Fungicide resistance, defined as the inherited ability of a fungus to survive and reproduce following exposure to a dose of fungicides normally lethal to the wild type, is a physiological characteristic that has the potential to cause large economic losses and environmental damages. The widespread use of fungicides has led to a growing number of resistant fungi that possess multiple-resistance to various classes of fungicides. Fungi may become resistant to fungicides through several mechanisms, including fungicide enzymatic inactivation, post-transcriptional or translational changes at the fungicide site of action, which leads to a decreased affinity to the toxic compound, overproduction of the target enzyme, synthesis of a substitute enzyme, which functions as a decoy, protecting the true target enzyme, bypass of the blocked site by the operation of alternative pathways and, most significantly, decrease fungicide accumulation resulting from decrease uptake or increase efflux of the toxic compound (Adams, 1997; Fluit *et al.*, 2001).

Phytopathogenic fungi that develop resistance to one fungicide may become simultaneously resistant to other fungicides that have a similar chemical structure and/or mode of action, which is known as "cross-resistance". For example, pathogenic strains that acquired resistance to the benzimidazole fungicide benomyl are usually also resistant to carbendazim, thiophanate-methyl or thiabendazole, other benzimidazole fungicides (Adams, 1997).

When resistance is due to the action of rather unspecific processes fungi may develop simultaneous resistance to structurally and functionally unrelated compounds, a phenomenon known as multidrug resistance (MDR). MDR can be mediated by various mechanisms. In a recent study aiming at providing a chemical genomic portrait of yeast, more than 500 genes were found to be required for MDR (Hillenmeyer *et al.*, 2008). These genes are highly enriched for Gene Ontology functions such as endosome transport, vacuolar degradation and transcription (Hillenmeyer *et al.*, 2008). However, in most cases, MDR is due to the action of active membrane transporters that are presumed to catalyze the extrusion of unrelated chemical compounds (fungicides, herbicides, antibiotics, etc.). The expression of genes encoding these pleiotropic efflux pumps was also shown to confer resistance to a number of unrelated chemical compounds in the referred chemical genomic assay (Hillenmeyer *et al.*, 2008). The emergence of the MDR phenomenon is implicated in the failure of many therapeutic actions, in the control of microorganisms responsible for food-poisoning and food-spoilage and in the eradication of plant pathogens and weeds. For instance, in agriculture, MDR has great economic impact: the extensive use of fungicides to provide crop protection has led to the emergence of resistant strains of many fungal pathogens, thus rendering such compounds useless (Sá-Correia & Tenreiro, 2002; Sá-Correia *et al.*, 2009). A classical example is the common occurrence of strains of *Botrytis cinerea* that have become resistant to various unrelated fungicides (*e.g.* benzimidazole and dicarboximide fungicides) (Adams, 1997).

3.2. Drug Efflux Pumps

3.2.1. The Drug Efflux Pumps

Multidrug efflux pumps found in the plasma membrane of all living cells are thought to recognize a wide variety of structurally and functionally unrelated chemicals and to actively extrude them from the cytoplasm to the outer medium, providing protection from these compounds (Jungwirth & Kuchler, 2006; Sá-Correia & Tenreiro, 2002; Sá-Correia *et al.*, 2009). However, the molecular mechanisms behind the apparent promiscuity of these multidrug efflux pumps remain elusive and a topic of debate (Jungwirth & Kuchler, 2006; Sá-Correia & Tenreiro, 2002; Sá-Correia *et al,* 2009). Several MDR transporters have been identified and thoroughly studied in different organisms, particularly those belonging to the ABC (ATP-Binding Cassette) superfamily (Jungwirth & Kuchler, 2006). A less well characterized family of transporters, the proton-motive-force-dependent multidrug transport systems, belonging to the Major Facilitator Superfamily (MFS), has received increasing attention in bacteria and yeast (Sá-Correia & Tenreiro, 2002; Sá-Correia *et al.*, 2009).

3.2.2. Resistance to Agricultural Fungicides Mediated by ABC Drug Efflux Pumps

ABC proteins can be found in the cells of all organisms, using the free energy of ATP hydrolysis to drive substrate transport across cell membranes (Bolhuis *et al.*, 1997). These proteins mediate diverse cellular transport processes, such as the excretion (over the plasma membrane or into a vacuole) of potentially toxic compounds, lipid translocation or the excretion of the yeast mating factor. They can also work as ion channels or display antigen activity (Martinoia *et al.*, 2002). ABC proteins constitute one of the largest protein superfamilies, with more than 3000 members operating from bacteria to man (Jungwirth & Kuchler, 2006). Quite remarkably, most members of the ABC protein family share a similar molecular architecture and domain organization (Jungwirth & Kuchler, 2006). The genome of the baker's yeast *Saccharomyces cerevisiae* harbours 30 distinct genes encoding ABC transporters, several of which carry out membrane translocation of hundreds of structurally and functionally unrelated xenobiotic compounds, mediating cellular detoxification and conferring pleiotropic drug resistance (PDR). These are generally referred to as ABC drug efflux pumps. Much of our understanding of ABC-driven multidrug resistance in fungi comes from studies in the yeast model (Jungwirth & Kuchler, 2006; Balzi & Goffeau, 1995). In fact, many ABC transporters from filamentous fungi involved in fungicide resistance were characterized based on previous results on their yeast homologues (Del Sorbo *et al.*, 1997; Del Sorbo *et al.*,2000; Nakaune *et al.*, 1998; Urban *et al.*, 1999). Yeast cells lacking endogenous ABC pumps, which are hypersensitive to many antifungal drugs, have been successfully used as host systems for heterologous expression of ABC transporters from fungal phytopathogens (de Waard *et al.*, 2006). The first fungal ABC transporter encoding gene characterized was *S. cerevisiae PDR5* (Balzi *et al.*, 1994). This ABC transporter has been implicated in resistance to more than 100 compounds, including several agricultural fungicides, like DMIs (namely, triflumizole and bitertanol), imidazoles (*e.g.* imazalil), anilinopyrimidines, benzimidazoles, dithiocarbamates, and many others (Del Sorbo *et al.*, 1997; Hnatova *et al.*, 2003; Kolaczkowski *et al.*, 1998). The transcription factors Pdr1p and Pdr3p were also demonstrated to be stress response factors (Fardeau *et al.*, 2007). Mutants containing disrupted chromosomal copies of the *PDR1* and *PDR3* genes or of the *PDR5* gene alone were found to be hypersensitive to QoI fungides (*e.g.* kresoxim-methyl and azoxystrobin) (Hnatova *et al.*, 2003).

Several ABC transporter encoding genes from the filamentous fungi model *Aspergillus nidulans*, a potential phytopathogenic fungus whose genome sequence was published in December 2005 (Galagan *et al.*, 2005), have been described. Expression of the genes *atrA*, *atrB*, *atrC* and *atrD* is up-regulated by numerous natural and synthetic toxic compounds, including DMI fungicides. The expression of the *A. nidulans* gene *atrB* in a *S. cerevisiae* strain devoid of a number of ABC transporters led to increased resistance towards the antibiotic cyclohexamide and to other drugs, suggesting a MDR role for this ABC transporter (de Waard *et al.*, 2006). In fact, functional expression of *atrB* was shown to complement imazalil hypersensitivity associated with *PDR5* deficiency in *S. cerevisiae* (Del Sorbo *et al.*, 1997). Through functional analysis in *A. nidulans*, the involvement of this same gene in protection against representative compounds from various classes of fungicides (*e.g.* the benzimidazole fungicide carbendazim, the phenylpyrrole fungicide fludioxonil and the QoI fungicide kresoxim-methyl) was also demonstrated (Andrade *et al.*, 2000a; Andrade *et al.*, 2000b; de Waard *et al.*, 2006). More recently, another ABC transporter encoding gene, *atrG*, was also shown to mediate resistance to DMI fungicides in *A. nidulans* (de Waard *et al.*, 2006).

Several ABC transporter encoding genes from the phytopathogenic fungus *Botrytis cinerea*, that affects many plant species, have already been identified. *BcatrB* encodes a protein with homology to ABC transporters from other fungi (Del Sorbo *et al.*, 2000), such as *PDR5* and *SNQ2* from *S. cerevisiae* and *AtrA* and *AtrB* from *A. nidulans*. Increased transcript levels from *BcatrB* were observed after a short period of exposure to phenylpyrrole, anilinopyrimidine and dicarboximide fungicides. In addition, *ΔBcatrB* deletion mutant is more sensitive to the phenylpyrrole fungicides fenpiclonil and fludioxonil, while *BcatrB* overexpression leads to decreased sensitivity to those fungicides. The expression of the ABC transporter *BcatrD* is also up-regulated by treatment with DMI, dicarboximide and benzimidazole fungicides. Moreover, deletion of the ABC transporter encoding gene *BcatrK* (also known as *BMR1*) leads to increased sensitivity to phosphorothiolate fungicides (*e.g.* iprobenfos) (de Waard *et al.*, 2006).

MDR was also described in the phytopathogenic fungus *Penicillium digitatum*, isolated from the surface of lemons (Nakaune *et al.*, 1998; Nakaune *et al.*, 2002). A homology search indicated that *PMR1* from this plant pathogen is significantly similar to several ABC-MDR transporters (47.7% and 38.8% identity with *S. cerevisiae PDR5* and *SNQ2*, respectively (Balzi *et al.*, 1994; Bissinger & Kuchler, 1994; Hirata *et al.*, 1994; Servos *et al.*, 1993) and 46.5% identity with *A. nidulans AtrA* (Del Sorbo *et al.*, 1997)). *PMR1* was demonstrated to be involved in resistance to DMI fungicides (Nakaune *et al.*, 1998). *PMR5*, another ABC transporter encoding gene from *P. digitatum*, shows 37% identity to *PMR1* from *P. digitatum,* 71% identity to *AtrB* from *A. nidulans*, and 65% identity to *BcatrB* from *B. cinerea* (Nakaune *et al.*, 2002). Disruption mutant for this gene displayed increased sensitivity to the benzimidazole fungicides, thiabendazole and benomyl and to the quinine fungicide, dithianon, among other compounds (Nakaune *et al.*, 2002). Transcription of both *PMR1* and *PMR5* was strongly induced in response to several toxicants, including DMIs that specifically induced *PMR1*, and dithianon, that specifically induced *PMR5* transcription. These ABC transporters may have complementary roles in multidrug resistance, each exhibiting different substrate-specificities (Nakaune *et al.*, 2002).

Four ABC MDR transporter encoding genes (*MgAtr1*, *MgAtr2*, *MgAtr4* and *MgAtr5*) have also been identified in the wheat pathogen *Mycosphaerella graminicola.* Their heterologous expression in a *S. cerevisiae* strain devoid of multiple ABC transporters showed that the expression of the first three genes leads to decreased yeast sensitivity to DMI fungicides (*e.g.* cyproconazole, propiconazole, tebuconazole). The role of *MgAtr1* in resistance to the fungicide cyproconazole was confirmed in *M. graminicola* laboratory isolates (de Waard *et al.*, 2006; Schuller *et al.*, 2007).

Rice blast fungus *Magnaporthe grisea* is the most devastating rice phytopathogenic fungus (Dean *et al.*, 2005). The *M. grisea ABC1* transporter encoding gene was identified in a mutagenesis screen for mutants exhibiting decreased pathogenicity. This ABC transporter is similar to yeast ABC MDR transporters, and its transcription is inducible by drugs (Urban *et al.*, 1999). Another ABC transporter from this plant pathogen, *ABC2,* shows a high level of homology with previously described ABC transporters such as, *BcatrK* and *BcatrD* from *B. cinerea* (64% and 35%) (Hayashi *et al.*, 2001; Nakajima *et al.*, 2001), *ABC2* from *Venturia inaequalis* (61%), *MgAtr5* from *M. graminicola* (38%) (Stergiopoulos *et al.*, 2002), *PMR5* from *P. digitatum* (38%) (Nakaune *et al.*, 2002) and *SNQ2* from *S. cerevisiae* (36%) (Servos *et al.*, 1993). *ABC2* is up-regulated after treatment with DMI fungicides and *Δabc2* deletion mutant derived from *M. grisea* is more sensitive than the parental strain to three DMI fungicides (bitertanol, myclobutanil, and tebuconazole) (Lee *et al.*, 2005).

Recently, a putative ATP-binding cassette (ABC) transporter gene (*BgABC1*) was isolated from the biotrophic pathogenic fungus *Blumeria graminis f. sp. tritici*, a fungus that causes powdery mildew on grasses, including cereals. Analysis of *BgABC1* trasncription using real-time PCR indicated that gene expression increases significantly when growing in wheat seedlings treated with the DMI fungicide triadimefon, suggesting that *BgABC1* can be involved in the protection of *Blumeria graminis* against fungicide toxicity (Hu *et al.*, 2008).

The obtained knowledge on drug transporters can be used to develop compounds that specifically inhibit these proteins, which can be used as new fungicides or fungicide coadjutants. This kind of compounds, known as ABC transporter blockers or modulators of ABC transporters, is already being developed in medical research, especially for use in chemotherapy. Concerning plant pathogens, it was recently demonstrated that a combinations of DMI or QoI fungicides with a hydroxyflavone derivative compound reverted the fungicide resistant phenotype of the wheat pathogen *Pyrenophora tritici-repentis* isolates (Reimann & Deising, 2005).

3.2.3. Resistance to Agricultural Fungicide Mediated by Drug-H$^+$ Antiporters

The major facilitator superfamily (MFS) is a very large and ancient protein superfamily found throughout nature, from bacteria to higher eukaryotes, whose biological function is energised by the electrochemical gradient across membranes. Diverse substrates show affinity to these transporters in a proton motive force dependent mechanism of symport, antiport or uniport. Some of the MFS transporters are involved in drug resistance, acting presumably as drug-H$^+$ antiporters (Paulsen *et al.*, 1996). Current understanding of the biological function and regulation of the MFS proteins involved in MDR is at an earlier stage compared with that of ABC transporters (Sá-Correia *et al.*, 2009). Although a large number of these MFS-MDR membrane transporters has been identified in bacteria and fungi, their contribution to drug tolerance is scarcely understood. The MFS-MDR transporters often share overlapping drug specificity with ABC drug efflux pumps, which may explain in part why the involvement of MFS transporters in multidrug resistance has been obscured by their better-publicized ABC relatives. The MFS-MDR include 22 proteins in *S. cerevisiae* (Sá-Correia *et al.*, 2009). The majority of these proteins were completely unknown before the release of the yeast genome sequence in 1996 (Goffeau *et al.*, 1996). Throughout the past 12 years some efforts have been carried out to characterize these transporters and several of them have been implicated in yeast resistance to agricultural fungicides (Sá-Correia & Tenreiro, 2002; Sá-Correia *et al.*, 2009). This is the case of *FLR1*, which confers resistance to mancozeb (Teixeira *et al.*, 2008) and benomyl (Brôco *et al.*, 1999).

In the phypathogenic fungi *B. cinerea,* the overexpression of the MFS transporter encoding gene *Bcmfs1* leads to decreased sensitivity to natural plant toxins and to structurally unrelated fungicides, such as DMI fungicides. The deletion of *Bcmfs1* gene in *ΔBcatrD* background further increased the sensitivity of this strain towards DMI fungicides (Hayashi *et al.*, 2002). The results indicate that *Bcmfs1* is an MFS-MDR transporter involved in protection against natural toxins and fungicides and has a substrate specificity that overlaps with the ABC transporter *BcatrD*. *Bcmfs1* may also be involved in protection of *B. cinerea* against plant defense compounds during the pathogenic phase of growth on host plants and against fungitoxic antimicrobial metabolites during its saprophytic phase of growth (Hayashi *et al.*, 2002).

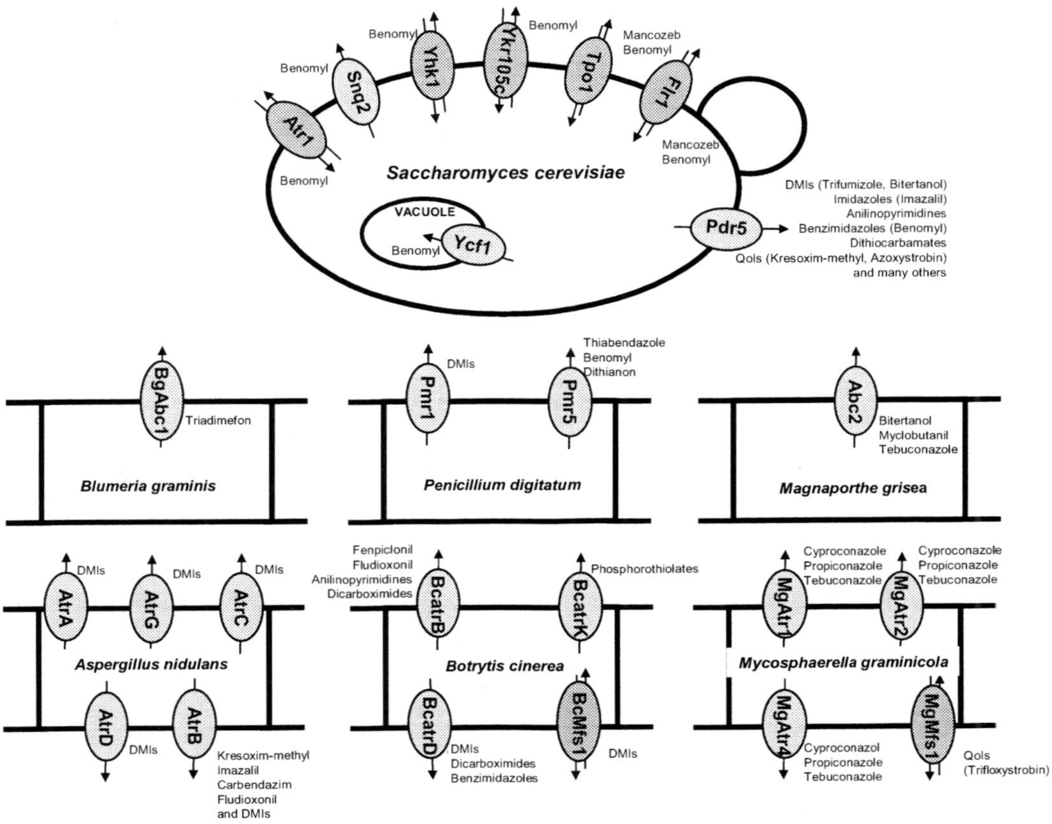

Figure 1. *S. cerevisiae* and phytopathogenic fungi ABC efflux pumps (blue) and MFS-MDR transporters (pink) described in the literature as being involved in cell response to agricultural fungicide induced stress.

MgMfs1 from *M. graminicola* was also implicated in mycotoxin secretion and multidrug resistance. Heterologous expression of *MgMfs1* in a hypersensitive *S. cerevisiae* strain resulted in a strong decrease in sensitivity to a broad range of unrelated synthetic and natural toxic compounds, including QoI fungicides. The sensitivity of the *Δmfs1* disruption mutant of *M. graminicola* to several of these fungicides and to the mycotoxin cercosporin is higher compared with the parental strain (Roohparvar *et al.*, 2007). More recently, it was suggested that overexpression of this gene in QoI-resistant field isolates may be a potential mechanism of QoI resistance under field conditions (Roohparvar *et al.*, 2008).

3.3. Transcriptional Regulation Networks Controlling Fungicide Resistance

ABC and MFS transporters involved in MDR in yeast are under tight regulation by the so-called PDR (Pleiotropic Drug Resistance) network. The binuclear $Zn(II)_2Cys_6$ zinc finger transcription factors Pdr1p and Pdr3p are the two master regulators of this network (Fardeau *et al.*, 2007; Jungwirth *et al.*, 2000). *PDR1* and *PDR3* display some functional redundancy, regulating shared target genes and binding to the same DNA motifs, the so called PDREs (pleiotropic drug response elements). Gain- or loss-of-function mutated forms of these proteins confer resistance or sensitivity to several unrelated drugs, through constitutive modifications to the expression of ABC drug efflux pumps (*e.g.* Pdr5p or Snq2p) or MFS-MDR drug-H^+ antiporters (*e.g.* Flr1p or Tpo1p) (Schuller *et al.*, 2007). Yrr1p and Pdr8p, two other $Zn(II)_2Cys_6$, as well as the basic-leucine zipper transcription factor Yap1p, are also involved in the regulation of the PDR network (Jungwirth *et al.*, 2000). Other transcription factors with specific roles in cell physiology or in metabolism related stress responses are also involved in regulation of MDR transporter encoding genes. These include Rpn4p, the regulator of genes encoding proteosome sub-units, and Hsf1p, involved in heat shock and other stress responses (Hahn *et al.*, 2006; Owsianik *et al.*, 2002).

The up-regulation of Flr1p in response to mancozeb or to benomyl induced stress is fully dependent on Yap1p expression and partially dependent on Pdr3p expression (Brôco *et al.*, 1999; Teixeira *et al.*, 2008; Tenreiro *et al.*, 2001). Under mancozeb induced stress conditions, the regulation of this gene was proved to be also dependent on Yrr1p and Rpn4p expression for maximal activation (Teixeira *et al.*, 2008). A qualitative model for the cross-talk between these regulators under mancozeb stress was recently proposed (Teixeira *et al.*, 2008) (Fig.2).

The transcriptional cascades leading to the PDR phenotype in wild-type cells are largely unknown. Fardeau *et al.* (2007) showed that within a few minutes of drug sensing yeast elicits an effective PDR response, involving tens of PDR genes. This early response is highly dependent on Pdr1p. The activity of this transcription factor in early drug response is apparently not drug-specific, since two chemically unrelated drugs, benomyl and fluphenazine, elicit identical, Pdr1p-dependent, early responses (Fardeau *et al.*, 2007).

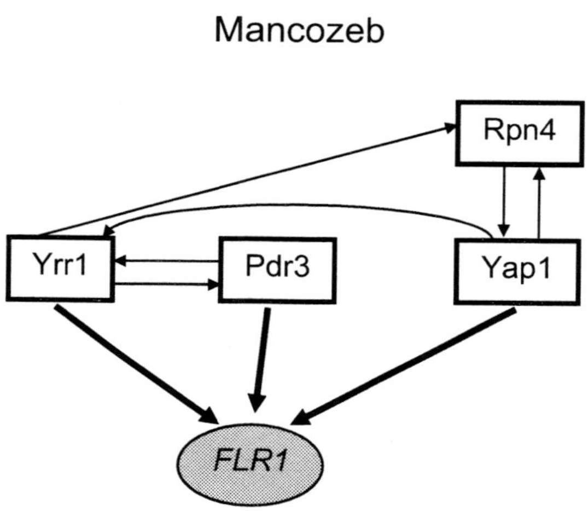

Figure 2. Transcription regulatory network controlling the up-regulation of the drug-H^+ antiporter encoding gene *FLR1* induced upon yeast exposure to mancozeb, as postulated by Teixeira *et al.* (2008).

M. grisea ABC efflux pumps encoding genes *ABC2* and *ABC1* contain an upstream coding region with conserved Pdr3p/Pdr1p-binding sites. These binding sites also occur in the promoter regions of ABC efflux pumps encoding genes from other pathogenic fungi, such as *MgAtr1* and *MgAtr5* from *M. graminicola*. Hence, in filamentous fungi some ABC transporter encoding genes may be regulated by transcription factors containing zinc-finger motifs similar to those previously implicated in the regulation of *S. cerevisiae* ABC transporter encoding genes, such as *PDR5* and *SNQ2* (Lee *et al.*, 2005).

4. Mechanisms of Toxicity of, and Resistance to, Agricultural Fungicides Identified through Genome-wide Approaches

4.1. Toxicogenomic Approaches

Genomic information and tools are beginning to be used to increase our understanding of how organisms of all types interact with the environment. The study of the expression of all genes at the genome (DNA), transcriptome (RNA), proteome (proteins) and metabolome (metabolites) level, in response to exposure to a toxicant, is known as toxicogenomics (Olden, 2006; Simmons & Portier, 2002) (Fig. 3). This new interdisciplinary area combines these genome-wide technologies with more traditional tools of pathology and toxicology to study the biological response to environmental toxicants. This systems biology approach offers a tool of unprecedented power to directly monitor the earlier stages of the toxicological response (Olden, 2006; Schwartz *et al.*, 2004; Simmons & Portier, 2002). Such alterations of global gene expression that can be monitored by microarrays or expression proteomics, for instance, occur almost immediately after exposure, whereas the clinical manifestation of toxicity might take several days or even years to develop. The assessment of these gene expression changes could potentially provide an earlier and more sensitive biomarker of a toxic response than traditional toxicological methods. There is increasing evidence that chemicals with similar toxicological properties produce a characteristic gene expression "fingerprint", also known as "signature profile" (Schwartz *et al.*, 2004; Simmons & Portier, 2002; Teixeira *et al.*, 2007). Hence, toxicogenomics has the potential to identify genes that are affected by chemical compounds inducing similar toxicological effects at the early stage of the toxicological response and to establish parallelisms between different organisms (Teixeira *et al.*, 2007).

The use of such global approaches applied to the yeast *S. cerevisiae* led to a number of new insights into the mechanisms of toxicity of, and resistance to, agricultural fungicides, particularly in the cases of benomyl and mancozeb.

4.2. Global Response to Benomyl in Yeast

Resistance to benzimidazoles developed rapidly in the late 1960's and early 1970's and has been detected in several fungal species. In most cases, fungal resistance to this type of fungicides correlates with point mutations in the β-tubulin gene, leading to the alteration of the amino acid sequence at the benzimidazole-binding site (Adams, 1997).

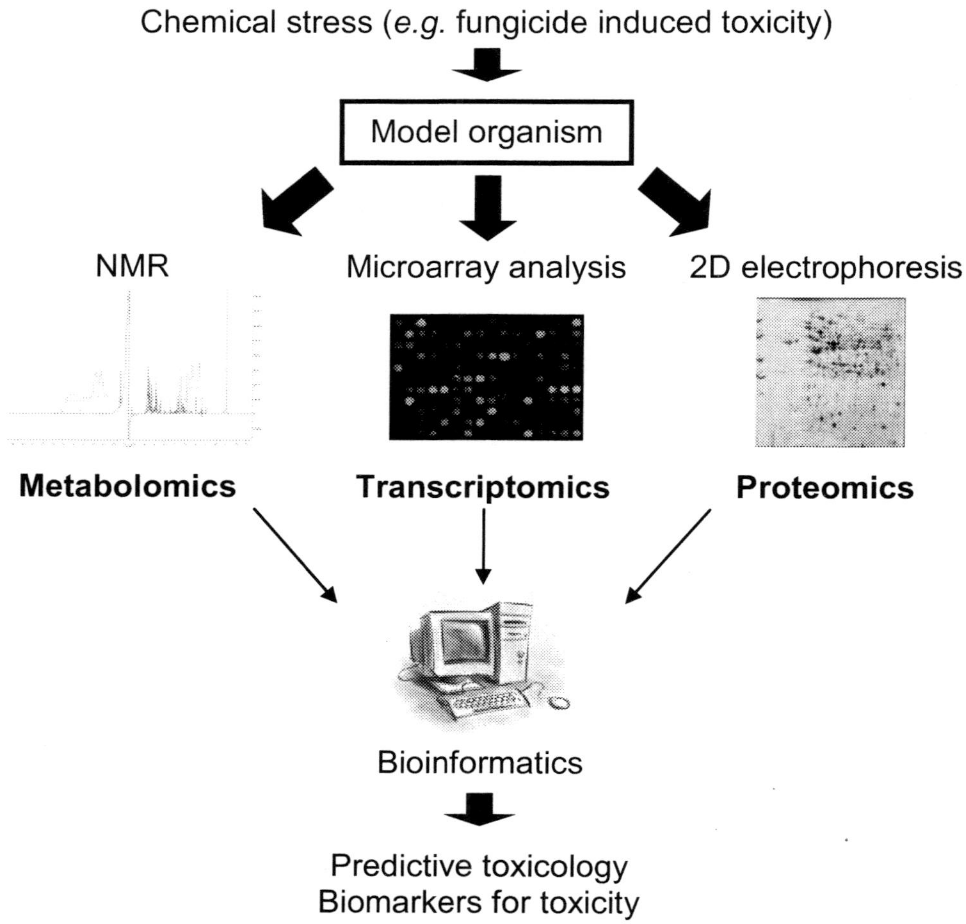

Figure 3. Toxicogenomic approach overview.

Through DNA microarrays, both the early and late response of yeast to benomyl induced stress was characterized (Lucau-Danila *et al.*, 2005). The obtained results show that cells exposed to this fungicide exhibit a transient transcriptional response that somehow mimics the known oxidative stress response, mainly dependent on the transcription activator Yap1p. As revealed by the use of the YEASTRACT database (Teixeira *et al.*, 2006b), 74% of genes that were found to be up-regulated under benomyl stress (Lucau-Danila *et al.*, 2005) are controlled by this transcription factor, suggesting a pro-oxidant effect in yeast. The early up-regulated genes by benomyl encode proteins mainly related to membrane functions, such as plasma membrane organization proteins and active MDR transporters of the ABC (*e.g. PDR5*) and the MF (*e.g. FLR1* and *TPO1*) Superfamilies. The late activated genes in response to benomyl include: several genes encoding protein folding chaperones, most of them containing an Yap1p biding site; most of the genes coding for redox-controlling enzymes (*e.g. GSH* and *TRX1*) and several transcription factors encoding genes previously involved in MDR regulation (*e.g. YRR1* and *CIN5*) (Lucau-Danila *et al.*, 2005). It is also interesting to point out that over 30% of the up-regulated genes are known targets of the general stress responsive transcription factors Msn2p/Msn4p or of the multidrug resistance regulators Pdr1p/Pdr3p.

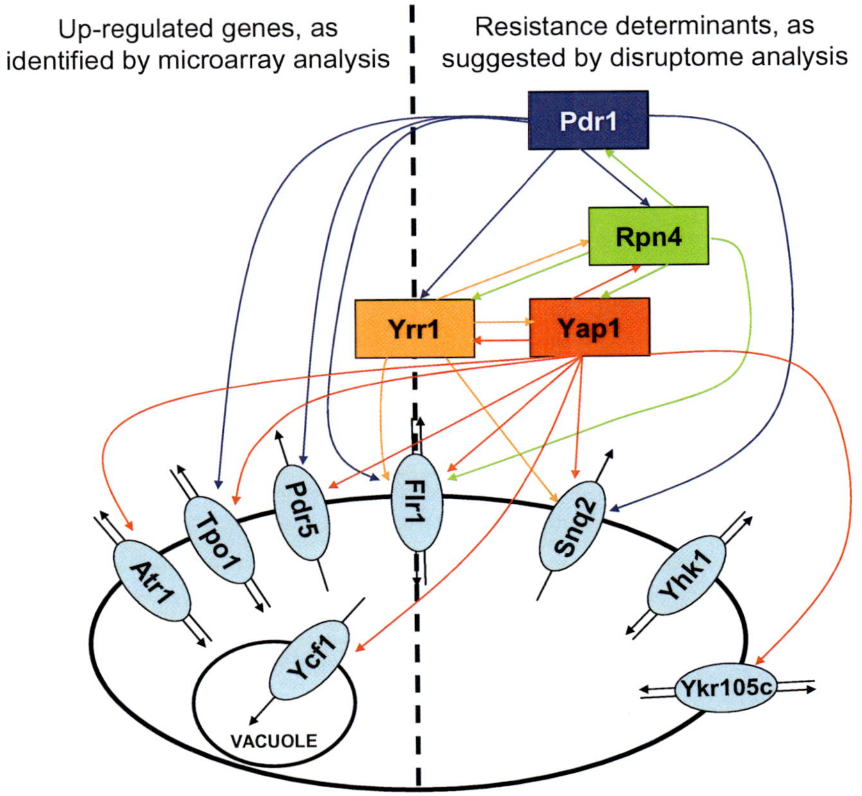

Figure 4. Suggested model for the activation of MDR transporters encoding genes involved in yeast adaptive response and resistance to benomyl. Pdr1, Rpn4, Yrr1 and Yap1 are transcription activators; Atr1, Tpo1, Flr1, Yhk1 and Ykr105c are MFS-MDR transporters; and Pdr5, Snq2 and Ycf1 are ABC efflux pumps. Adapted from the results obtained by Hillenmeyer *et al.* (2008) and Lucau-Danila *et al.* (2005), analysed in this work using the YEASTRACT database (Teixeira *et al.*, 2006b).

The susceptibility of a collection of yeast mutants in which each non-essential yeast gene was individually deleted, the so-called disruptome, towards benomyl stress was also recently tested (Hillenmeyer *et al.*, 2008). The authors of this study emphasized the fact that all eight chaperonin-containing t-complex genes, *TCP1*, *CCT2*, *CCT3*, *CCT4*, *CCT5*, *CCT6*, *CCT7*, and *YJL009w*, which are essential and conserved between yeast and human, confer resistance to benomyl. Further analysis revealed that several genes encoding MDR transporters also confer resistance to this benzimidazole. For instance, MFS-MDR transporters encoding genes, *FLR1*, *YKR105c* and *YHK8*, and the ABC drug efflux pump encoding gene *SNQ2* were identified as determinants of resistance to benomyl in this study. Besides, many transcription factors from the PDR network, such as Pdr1p, Yap1p, Yrr1p, Rpn4p and Msn2p, were also detected. These results are consistent with DNA microarrays data, since most of the referred transcription factors regulate a large number of the benomyl-induced up-regulated genes.

These two genome-wide approaches are highly complementary. As displayed in Fig. 4, the genes which are up-regulated in response to benomyl induced stress (revealed by microarray analysis) are not necessarily those individually required for benomyl resistance (revealed by the disruptome analysis). It is interesting to point out what seems to be the central role of Flr1p, the single MDR transporter being simultaneously benomyl-induced and a benomyl-resistance determinant.

4.3. Global Response to Mancozeb in Yeast

In spite of its toxicity, mancozeb is one of the most widely used agricultural fungicides (Maroni *et al.*, 2000), mainly due to the fact that it has maintained its efficacy against several phytopathogenic fungi. Its exact mode of action is not yet known; however, it has been proposed to act by inhibiting enzyme activity, being its high reactivity related to metal-chelating ability and high affinity for –SH group containing proteins (Allain & Krari, 1991; Vaccari *et al.*, 1999).

The early global response to mancozeb using the eukaryotic model *Saccharomyces cerevisiae* was recently analysed by expression proteomics using two-dimensional electrophoresis (2-DE) (Santos *et al.*, 2009). According to these results, the target genes (*e.g. TSA1, TSA2, SOD1, SOD2, AHP1, GRE2, GRX1, CYS3, PRE3, PRE6, PRE8, PRE9, EFT1, RPS5, TIF11, HSP31, HSP26, HSP104, HSP60, HSP70*-family) and the main transcription activators (e.g. Yap1p, Msn2p/Msn4p, Met4p, Hsf1p, Aft1p, Pdr1p, Skn7p, Rpn4p, Gcn4p) of the complex mancozeb-induced expression changes are related with yeast response to stress, in particular to oxidative stress, protein translation initiation and protein folding, disassembling of protein aggregates and degradation of damaged proteins (Santos *et al.*, 2009). In a recent screening of the susceptibility of the yeast disruptome towards mancozeb induced stress, genes encoding most of the referred transcription factors were found to be determinants of yeast resistance to this fungicide (Dias *et al.*, unpublished results). These proteins/genes may be useful as early and sensitive biomarkers of the toxicological response to mancozeb and the regulatory networks behind the yeast response to this toxicant have emerged from the expression proteomics study. These indications may be particularly relevant to mancozeb response in humans as 70% of the gene functions identified as having an altered expression under stress induced by this fungicide in yeast have human homologues (Santos *et al.*, 2009). Corroborating previous results, the MFS-MDR transporter, Flr1p, and also its homologue Tpo1p, were found to be determinants of yeast resistance to mancozeb (Dias *et al.*, unpublished results). Also, the transcriptional regulators Yap1, Rpn4 and Yrr1p were found to be required for yeast tolerance to mancozeb. These transcription factors, besides being among the major expression regulators underlying the observed proteome-wide changes occurring under mancozeb stress, were found to play a role in *FLR1* transcriptional regulation (Teixeira *et al.*, 2008) (Fig. 2).

Maneb, thiram and zineb are other dithiocarbamate fungicides commonly used in agriculture. Gene expression profiles, resulting from *S. cerevisiae* exposure to these three fungicides and other chemicals, were obtained by DNA microarrays (Kitagawa *et al.*, 2003). In this study, thirty genes, including *FLR1,* exhibited an increased expression, over 2 fold, when exposed to each of the three fungicides. Classification of the up-regulated genes by gene function (which may be used to understand fungicide toxicity) and hierarchical clustering (which may have application in predicting chemical structures that cause environmental toxicity) was performed. The obtained results suggest that DNA microarray technology has potential for predicting chemical structures that causes major environmental toxicity (Kitagawa *et al.*, 2003).

5. FINAL REMARKS AND FUTURE PERSPECTIVES

Toxicogenomic approaches applied to agricultural fungicide toxicity may accelerate our understanding of the underlying molecular mechanisms. However, genome-wide studies aiming at the establishment of a gene expression fingerprint for each fungicide family and its association to known toxic effects are needed in order to reach the goal of predictive toxicogenomics

In recent years, a boost of new insights into the role of multidrug ABC transporters from phytopathogenic fungi in fungicide resistance was registered. Nonetheless, the role and regulation of MDR transporters in fungicide resistance has been focused on a relatively small number of fungicide families and more work is still required to fully characterize the resistance mechanisms. Moreover, the involvement of MFS-MDR transporters on the widespread multifungicide resistance phenomenon is poorly understood.

In recent years, genome sequences of a number of the most common phytopathogenic fungi was made available (Dean *et al.*, 2005; Galagan *et al.*, 2005), rendering easier the elucidation of the adaptive responses to agricultural fungicides in their target organisms. Through global analysis, using microarrays, expression proteomics and metabolomics, more genes/proteins/metabolites with an important role in the cell response to a specific fungicide can be revealed. However, the application of this approach to phytopathogenic fungi is still relatively new and unexplored. Meyer *et al.* (2007) reported the first transcriptome-wide analysis of the adaptative response of *Aspergillus niger* to the antifungal drugs caspofungin and fenpropimorph. *A. niger* causes a disease called black mold on certain fruits and vegetables (Samson *et al.*, 2002). In this study, many important genes were identified as being up-regulated by caspofungin induced stress, mainly genes predicted to function in cell wall assembly and remodelling, cytoskeletal organization, signalling and oxidative stress response. These results are consistent with those previously obtained in *S. cerevisiae* (Meyer *et al.*, 2007). The application of such genome-wide approaches to the elucidation of the mechanisms of toxicity of, and resistance to, agricultural fungicides in their target organisms is expected to shed a lot more light into this fascinating area of applied research. It is also expected that the wealth of knowledge gathered on this subject using yeast as an experimental model system will continue to guide and facilitate many of these studies on phytopathogenic fungi and higher eukaryotes, with implications in Agriculture, Environmental Protection and Human Health.

6. References

Adams, D. J. (1997). Drug and pesticide resistance in fungi. In J. D. Hayes & C. R. Wolf (Eds.), *Molecular genetics of drug resistance* (1st ed., pp. 31-80). Amsterdam: Harwood Academic Publishers.

Allain, P. & Krari, N. (1991). Diethyldithiocarbamate, copper and neurological disorders. *Life Sci, 48(3)*, 291-299.

Andrade, A. C., Del Sorbo, G., Van Nistelrooy, J. G., & de Waard, M. A. (2000a). The ABC transporter AtrB from Aspergillus nidulans mediates resistance to all major classes of fungicides and some natural toxic compounds. *Microbiology, 146 (Pt 8)*, 1987-1997.

Andrade, A. C., Van Nistelrooy, J. G., Peery, R. B., Skatrud, P. L., & de Waard, M. A. (2000b). The role of ABC transporters from Aspergillus nidulans in protection against cytotoxic agents and in antibiotic production. *Mol Gen Genet, 263*(6), 966-977.

Ballantyne, B. (2004). Toxicology of fungicides. In T. C. Marrs & B. Ballantyne (Eds.), *Pesticide Toxicology and International Regulation* (1st ed., pp 191-303). John Wiley and Sons.

Balzi, E., & Goffeau, A. (1995). Yeast multidrug resistance: the PDR network. *J Bioenerg Biomembr, 27*(1), 71-76.

Balzi, E., Wang, M., Leterme, S., Van Dyck, L., & Goffeau, A. (1994). PDR5, a novel yeast multidrug resistance conferring transporter controlled by the transcription regulator PDR1. *J Biol Chem, 269*(3), 2206-2214.

Belpoggi, F., Soffritti, M., Guarino, M., Lambertini, L., Cevolani, D., & Maltoni, C. (2002). Results of long-term experimental studies on the carcinogenicity of ethylene-bis-dithiocarbamate (Mancozeb) in rats. *Ann N Y Acad Sci, 982*, 123-136.

Bissinger, P. H., & Kuchler, K. (1994). Molecular cloning and expression of the Saccharomyces cerevisiae STS1 gene product. A yeast ABC transporter conferring mycotoxin resistance. *J Biol Chem, 269*(6), 4180-4186.

Bolhuis, H., van Veen, H. W., Poolman, B., Driessen, A. J., & Konings, W. N. (1997). Mechanisms of multidrug transporters. *FEMS Microbiol Rev, 21*(1), 55-84.

Brôco, N., Tenreiro, S., Viegas, C. A. & Sá-Correia, I. (1999). FLR1 gene (ORF YBR008c) is required for benomyl and methotrexate resistance in Saccharomyces cerevisiae and its benomyl-induced expression is dependent on pdr3 transcriptional regulator. *Yeast, 15(15)*, 1595-1608.

Calhelha, R. C., Andrade, J. V., Ferreira, I. C., & Estevinho, L. M. (2006). Toxicity effects of fungicide residues on the wine-producing process. *Food Microbiol, 23*(4), 393-398.

Calviello, G., Piccioni, E., Boninsegna, A., Tedesco, B., Maggiano, N., Serini, S., *et al.* (2006). DNA damage and apoptosis induction by the pesticide Mancozeb in rat cells: involvement of the oxidative mechanism. *Toxicol Appl Pharmacol, 211*(2), 87-96.

de Waard, M. A., Andrade, A. C., Hayashi, K., Schoonbeek, H. J., Stergiopoulos, I., & Zwiers, L. H. (2006). Impact of fungal drug transporters on fungicide sensitivity, multidrug resistance and virulence. *Pest Manag Sci, 62*(3), 195-207.

Dean, R. A., Talbot, N. J., Ebbole, D. J., Farman, M. L., Mitchell, T. K., Orbach, M. J., *et al.* (2005). The genome sequence of the rice blast fungus Magnaporthe grisea. *Nature, 434*(7036), 980-986.

Del Sorbo, G., Andrade, A. C., Van Nistelrooy, J. G., Van Kan, J. A., Balzi, E., & de Waard, M. A. (1997). Multidrug resistance in Aspergillus nidulans involves novel ATP-binding cassette transporters. *Mol Gen Genet, 254*(4), 417-426.

Del Sorbo, G., Schoonbeek, H., & de Waard, M. A. (2000). Fungal transporters involved in efflux of natural toxic compounds and fungicides. *Fungal Genet Biol, 30*(1), 1-15.

Domico, L. M., Cooper, K. R., Bernard, L. P., Zeevalk, G. D. (2007). Reactive oxygen species generation by the ethylene-bis-dithiocarbamate (EBDC) fungicide mancozeb and its contribution to neuronal toxicity in mesencephalic cells. *Neurotoxicol, 28(6)*, 1079-1091.

Fardeau, V., Lelandais, G., Oldfield, A., Salin, H., Lemoine, S., Garcia, M., *et al.* (2007). The central role of PDR1 in the foundation of yeast drug resistance. *J Biol Chem, 282*(7), 5063-5074.

Fluit, A. C., Visser, M. R., & Schmitz, F. J. (2001). Molecular detection of antimicrobial resistance. *Clin Microbiol Rev, 14*(4), 836-871, table of contents.

Galagan, J. E., Calvo, S. E., Cuomo, C., Ma, L.-J., Wortman, J. R., Batzoglou, S., *et al.* (2005). Sequencing of Aspergillus nidulans and comparative analysis with A. fumigatus and A. oryzae. *Nature, 438*(7071), 1105-1115.

Goffeau, A., Barrell, B. G., Bussey, H., Davis, R. W., Dujon, B., Feldmann, H., *et al.* (1996). Life with 6000 genes. *Science, 274(5287)*, 563-567.

Hahn, J. S., Neef, D. W. & Thiele, D. J. (2006) A stress regulatory network for co-ordinated activation of proteasome expression mediated by yeast heat shock transcription factor. *Mol Microbiol, 60(1),* 240-251.

Hayashi, K., Schoonbeek, H. J. & de Waard, M. A. (2002) Bcmfs1, a novel major facilitator superfamily transporter from Botrytis cinerea, provides tolerance towards the natural toxic compounds camptothecin and cercosporin and towards fungicides. *Appl Environ Microbiol, 68(10),* 4996-5004.

Hayashi, K., Schoonbeek, H. J., Sugiura, H. & de Waard, M. A. (2001). Multidrug resistance in *Botrytis cinerea* associated with decreased accumulation of the azole fungicide oxpoconazole and increased transcription of the ABC transporter gene BcatrD. *Pestic Biochem Physiol, 70*, 168-179.

Hewitt, M. J., Mutch, P., & Pratten, M. K. (2005). Potential teratogenic effects of benomyl in rat embryos cultured in vitro. *Reprod Toxicol, 20*(2), 271-280.

Hillenmeyer, M. E., Fung, E., Wildenhain, J., Pierce, S. E., Hoon, S., Lee, W., *et al.* (2008). The chemical genomic portrait of yeast: uncovering a phenotype for all genes. *Science, 320*(5874), 362-365.

Hirata, D., Yano, K., Miyahara, K., & Miyakawa, T. (1994). Saccharomyces cerevisiae YDR1, which encodes a member of the ATP-binding cassette (ABC) superfamily, is required for multidrug resistance. *Curr Genet, 26*(4), 285-294.

Hnatova, M., Gbelska, Y., Obernauerova, M., Subikova, V., & Subik, J. (2003). Cross-resistance to strobilurin fungicides in mitochondrial and nuclear mutants of Saccharomyces cerevisiae. *Folia Microbiol (Praha), 48*(4), 496-500.

Hu, W., Yan, L., & Ma, Z. (2008). Cloning and Expression Analysis of a Putative ABC Transporter Gene BgABC1 from the Biotrophic Pathogenic Fungus Blumeria graminis f. sp. tritici. *J Phytopathol, 156*(2), 120-124.

Jia, M. H., Larossa, R. A., Lee, J. M., Rafalski, A., Derose, E., Gonye, G., *et al.* (2000). Global expression profiling of yeast treated with an inhibitor of amino acid biosynthesis, sulfometuron methyl. *Physiol Genomics, 3*(2), 83-92.

Jungwirth, H., & Kuchler, K. (2006). Yeast ABC transporters-- a tale of sex, stress, drugs and aging. *FEBS Lett, 580*(4), 1131-1138.

Jungwirth, H., Wendler, F., Platzer, B., Bergler, H., & Hogenauer, G. (2000). Diazaborine resistance in yeast involves the efflux pumps Ycf1p and Flr1p and is enhanced by a gain-of-function allele of gene YAP1. *Eur J Biochem, 267*(15), 4809-4816.

Kelly, D. E., Lamb, D. C., & Kelly, L. (2001). Genome-wide generation of yeast deletion strains. *Comp Funct Genom, 2*, 236-242.

Kitagawa, E., Momose, Y., & Iwahashi, H. (2003). Correlation of the structures of agricultural fungicides to gene expression in Saccharomyces cerevisiae upon exposure to toxic doses. *Environ Sci Technol, 37*(12), 2788-2793.

Kolaczkowski, M., Kolaczowska, A., Luczynski, J., Witek, S., & Goffeau, A. (1998). In vivo characterization of the drug resistance profile of the major ABC transporters and other components of the yeast pleiotropic drug resistance network. *Microb Drug Resist, 4*(3), 143-158.

La Pera, L., Dugo, G., Rando, R., Di Bella, G., Maisano, R., & Salvo, F. (2008). Statistical study of the influence of fungicide treatments (mancozeb, zoxamide and copper oxychloride) on heavy metal concentrations in Sicilian red wine. *Food Addit Contam, 25*(3), 302-313.

Landis, W. G., & Yu, M. H. (1999). Introduction to Environmental Toxicology: Impacts of chemicals upon ecological systems (3rd ed.). Boca Raton, FL: Lewis Publishers.

Lee, Y.-J., Yamamoto, K., Hamamoto, H., Nakaune, R., & Hibi, T. (2005). A novel ABC transporter gene ABC2 involved in multidrug susceptibility but not pathogenicity in rice blast fungus, Magnaporthe grisea. *Pesticide Biochemistry and Physiology, 81*(1), 13-23.

Lucau-Danila, A., Lelandais, G., Kozovska, Z., Tanty, V., Delaveau, T., Devaux, F., *et al.* (2005). Early expression of yeast genes affected by chemical stress. *Mol Cell Biol, 25*(5), 1860-1868.

Maroni, M., Colosio, C., Ferioli, A., & Fait, A. (2000). Biological Monitoring of Pesticide Exposure: a review. Introduction. *Toxicology, 143*(1), 1-118.

Martinoia, E., Klein, M., Geisler, M., Bovet, L., Forestier, C., Kolukisaoglu, U., *et al.* (2002). Multifunctionality of plant ABC transporters--more than just detoxifiers. *Planta, 214*(3), 345-355.

McGrath, M. T. (2004). What are Fungicides?, *The Plant Health Instructor*: The American Phytopathological Society.

McLean, W. G., Holme, A. D., Janneh, O., Southgate, A., Howard, C. V., & Reed, M. G. (1998). The effect of benomyl on neurite outgrowth in mouse NB2A and human SH-SY5Y neuroblastoma cells in vitro. *Neurotoxicology, 19*(4-5), 629-632.

Meyer, V., Damveld, R. A., Arentshorst, M., Stahl, U., van den Hondel, C. A., & Ram, A. F. (2007). Survival in the presence of antifungals: genome-wide expression profiling of Aspergillus niger in response to sublethal concentrations of caspofungin and fenpropimorph. *J Biol Chem, 282*(45), 32935-32948.

Nakajima, M., Suzuki, J., Hosaka, T., Hibi, T., & Akutsu, K. (2001). Functional analysis of an ATP-Binding Cassette transporter gene in Botrytis cinerea by gene disruption. *Journal of General Plant Pathology, 67*(3), 212-214.

Nakaune, R., Hamamoto, H., Imada, J., Akutsu, K., & Hibi, T. (2002). A novel ABC transporter gene, PMR5, is involved in multidrug resistance in the phytopathogenic fungus Penicillium digitatum. *Mol Genet Genomics, 267*(2), 179-185.

Nakaune, R., Adachi, K., Nawata, O., Tomiyama, M., Akutsu, K., & Hibi, T.(1998). A novel ATP-Binding Cassette transporter involved in multidrug resistance in the phytopathogenic fungus Penicillium digitatum. *Appl Environ Microbiol, 64*(10), 3983–3988.

Olden, K. (2006). Toxicogenomics--a new systems toxicology approach to understanding of gene-environment interactions. *Ann N Y Acad Sci, 1076*, 703-706.

Owsianik, G., Balzi, l. L. & Ghislain, M. (2002) Control of 26S proteasome expression by transcription factors regulating multidrug resistance in Saccharomyces cerevisiae. *Mol Microbiol, 43(5)*,1295-308.

Papaefthimiou, C., Cabral M. de, G., Mixailidou, C., Viegas, C. A., Sá-Correia, I., & Theophilidis, G. (2004). Comparison of two screening bioassays, based on the frog sciatic nerve and yeast cells, for the assessment of herbicide toxicity. *Environ Toxicol Chem, 23*(5), 1211-1218.

Parveen, M., Momose, Y., Kitagawa, E., Kurita, S., Kodama, O., & Iwahashi, H. (2003). Bioassay of pesticide Lindane using yeast-DNA microarrays technology. *Chem-Bio Informatics Journal, 3*(1), 12-29.

Paulsen, I. T., Skurray, R. A., Tam, R., Saier, M. H., Jr., Turner, R. J., Weiner, J. H., *et al.* (1996). The SMR family: a novel family of multidrug efflux proteins involved with the efflux of lipophilic drugs. *Mol Microbiol, 19*(6), 1167-1175.

Reimann, S., & Deising, H. B. (2005). Inhibition of efflux transporter-mediated fungicide resistance in Pyrenophora tritici-repentis by a derivative of 4'-hydroxyflavone and enhancement of fungicide activity. *Appl Environ Microbiol, 71*(6), 3269-3275.

Roohparvar, R., de Waard, M. A., Kema, G. H., & Zwiers, L. H. (2007). MgMfs1, a major facilitator superfamily transporter from the fungal wheat pathogen *Mycosphaerella graminicola*, is a strong protectant against natural toxic compounds and fungicides. *Fungal Genet Biol, 44*(5), 378-388.

Roohparvar, R., Mehrabi, R., Van Nistelrooy, J. G., Zwiers, L. H., & de Waard, M. A. (2008). The drug transporter MgMfs1 can modulate sensitivity of field strains of the fungal wheat pathogen Mycosphaerella graminicola to the strobilurin fungicide trifloxystrobin. *Pest Manag Sci, 64*(7), 685-693.

Sá-Correia, I., dos Santos, S. C., Teixeira, M. C., Cabrito, T. R., & Mira, N. P. (2009). Drug:H(+) antiporters in chemical stress response in yeast. *TRENDS in Microbio,* 17(1):22-31.

Sá-Correia, I., & Tenreiro, S. (2002). The multidrug resistance transporters of the major facilitator superfamily, 6 years after disclosure of *Saccharomyces cerevisiae* genome sequence. *J Biotechnol, 98*(2-3), 215-226.

Santos, P. M., Simões. T., Sá-Correia, I. (2009). Insights into yeast adaptive response to the agricultural fungicide mancozeb: A toxicoproteomics approach. *Proteomics,* 9(3):657-670.

Samson, R. A., Houbraken, J., Summerbell, R. C., Flannigan, B., & Miller, J. D. (2002). Common and important species of fungi and actinomycetes in indoor environments. In B. Flannigan, R. A. Samson & J. D. Miller (Eds.), *Microogranisms in Home and Indoor Work Environments: Diversity, Health Impacts, Investigation and Control* (1st ed., pp. 287-292). New York: CRC Press.

Schuller, C., Mamnun, Y. M., Wolfger, H., Rockwell, N., Thorner, J., & Kuchler, K. (2007). Membrane-active compounds activate the transcription factors Pdr1 and Pdr3 connecting pleiotropic drug resistance and membrane lipid homeostasis in Saccharomyces cerevisiae. *Mol Biol Cell, 18*(12), 4932-4944.

Schwartz, D. A., Freedman, J. H., & Linney, E. A. (2004). Environmental genomics: a key to understanding biology, pathophysiology and disease. *Hum. Mol. Genet., 13*(suppl_2), R217-224.

Servos, J., Haase, E., & Brendel, M. (1993). Gene SNQ2 of Saccharomyces cerevisiae, which confers resistance to 4-nitroquinoline-N-oxide and other chemicals, encodes a 169 kDa protein homologous to ATP-dependent permeases. *Mol Gen Genet, 236*(2-3), 214-218.

Simmons, P. T., & Portier, C. J. (2002). Toxicogenomics: the new frontier in risk analysis. *Carcinogenesis, 23*(6), 903-905.

Smith, C. M. (1988). History of benzimidazole use and resistance. In C. J. Delp (Ed.). *Fungicide Resistance in North America* (1st ed., pp. 23-24). St. Paul, MN: The American Phytopathological Society.

Stergiopoulos, I., Gielkens, M. M., Goodall, S. D., Venema, K., & de Waard, M. A. (2002). Molecular cloning and characterisation of three new ATP-binding cassette transporter genes from the wheat pathogen Mycosphaerella graminicola. *Gene, 289*(1-2), 141-149.

Teixeira, M. C., Dias, P. J., Simoes, T., & Sa-Correia, I. (2008). Yeast adaptation to mancozeb involves the up-regulation of *FLR1* under the coordinate control of Yap1, Rpn4, Pdr3, and Yrr1. *Biochem Biophys Res Commun, 367*(2), 249-255.

Teixeira, M. C., Duque, P., & Sa-Correia, I. (2007). Environmental genomics: mechanistic insights into toxicity of and resistance to the herbicide 2,4-D. *Trends Biotechnol, 25*(8), 363-370.

Teixeira, M. C., Fernandes, A. R., Mira, N. P., Becker, J. D., & Sá-Correia, I. (2006a). Early transcriptional response of *Saccharomyces cerevisiae* to stress imposed by the herbicide 2,4-dichlorophenoxyacetic acid. *FEMS Yeast Res, 6*(2), 230-248.

Teixeira, M. C., Monteiro, P., Jain, P., Tenreiro, S., Fernandes, A. R., Mira, N. P., *et al.* (2006b). The YEASTRACT database: a tool for the analysis of transcription regulatory associations in *Saccharomyces cerevisiae. Nucleic Acids Res, 34*(Database issue), D446-451.

Teixeira, M. C., Santos, P. M., Fernandes, A. R., & Sá-Correia, I. (2005). A proteome analysis of the yeast response to the herbicide 2,4-dichlorophenoxyacetic acid. *Proteomics, 5*(7), 1889-1901.

Tenreiro S., Fernandes, A. R. & Sá-Correia, I. (2001) Transcriptional activation of FLR1 gene during Saccharomyces cerevisiae adaptation to growth with benomyl: role of Yap1 and Pdr3p. *Bioch Biophys Res Commun, 280,* 216-222.

Tomlin, C. D. S., Ed. (1997). The pesticide manual (11th ed.). London: British Crop Protection Council.

Urban, M., Bhargava, T., & Hamer, J. E. (1999). An ATP-driven efflux pump is a novel pathogenicity factor in rice blast disease. *EMBO J, 18*(3), 512-521.

Vaccari, A., Saba, P., Mocci, I., Ruiu, S. (1999) Dithiocarbamate pesticides affect glutamate transport in brain synaptic vesicles. *J Pharmacol Exp Ther, 288(1)*, 1-5.

Zhou, Y., Shie, F. S., Piccardo, P., Montine, T. J., & Zhang, J. (2004). Proteasomal inhibition induced by manganese ethylene-bis-dithiocarbamate: relevance to Parkinson's disease. *Neurosci, 128*(2), 281-291.

In: Fungicides
Editors: P. De Costa and P. Bezerra

ISBN: 978-1-60692-631-4

Chapter IX

FUNGICIDE RESIDUE ANALYSIS IN ENVIRONMENTAL, BIOLOGICAL AND FOOD SAMPLES: A REVIEW

***Lidia M. Ravelo-Pérez*[1], *Javier Hernández-Borges*[2], *and Miguel Ángel Rodríguez-Delgado*[1,*]**

[1]Departamento de Química Analítica, Nutrición y Bromatología, Facultad de Química, Universidad de La Laguna (ULL), Avda. Astrofísico Francisco Sánchez s/nº, 38206 La Laguna, Tenerife, Islas Canarias, Spain

[2]Departamento de Protección Vegetal, Instituto Canario de Investigaciones Agrarias (ICIA), Apdo. 60, 38200, La Laguna, Tenerife, Islas Canarias, Spain

ABSTRACT

Fungicides are a group of chemicals used in agriculture to control plant diseases caused by fungal attack (fungi are the number one cause of crop loss worldwide). As a result of their widespread use and their relative persistence, fungicide residues present in waters, food, etc., can reach the consumer and may therefore represent a risk for human health. Moreover, animals can accumulate some of these substances from contaminated feed and water and also from indoor fungicide practices. All these aspects have originated the need to develop analytical methodologies that allow the determination of these compounds below their established maximum residue limits (according to current legislation) in the different countries especially in environmental and food samples. The present chapter attempts to show the current situation of the analysis of fungicide residues in environmental, biological and food samples, describing the analytical methods used for their determination.

* Corresponding author. Tel: +34 922 318046; Fax: +34 922 318003; Email: mrguez@ull.es

Abbreviations

BSTFA	*N*-(*tert*butyldimethylsilyl)-*N*-methyltrifluoroacetamide
APCI	Atmospheric pressure chemical ionization
ASE	Accelerated solvent extraction
CD	Cyclodextrin
CE	Capillary electrophoresis
CI	Chemical ionization
CX/PDMS	Carboxen/polydimethylsiloxane
CW/DVB	Carbowax/divinylbenzene
CW/TPR	Cabowax/templated resin
CZE	Capillary zone electrophoresis
DAD	Diode array detection
ECD	Electron capture detection
EI	Electron impact ionization
ESI	Electrospray ionization
ETU	Ethylenethiourea
EU	European Union
FAO	Food and Agricultural Organization
FD	Fluorescence detection
FPD	Flame photometric detection
GC	Gas chromatography
HCB	Hexachlorobenzene
HCH	Hexachlorocyclohexane
HLB	Hydrophilic-lypophilic balance
HPLC	High-performance liquid chromatography
HR	High resolution
LLE	Liquid-liquid extraction
LOD	Limit of detection
LOQ	Limit of quantification
LPME	Liquid-phase microextraction
MAE	Microwave-assisted extraction
MASE	Membrane-assisted solvent extraction
MEKC	Micellar electrokinetic chromatography
MIP	Molecularly imprinted polymers
MRL	Maximum residue limit
MS	Mass spectrometry
MSPD	Matrix solid-phase dispersion
MWCNTs	Multiwalled-carbon nanotubes
NPD	Nitrogen-phosphorus detection
PA	Polyacrylate
PDA	Photodiode array detection
PDMS	Polydimethylsiloxane
PDMS/DVB	Polydimethylsilane/divinylbenzene

PLE	Pressurized-liquid extraction
REPSM	Reversed-electrode polarity stacking mode
SAESC	Sonication-assisted extraction in small columns
SBSE	Stir bar sorptive extraction
SDE	Steam distillation extraction
SDME	Single-drop microextraction
SLE	Solid-liquid extraction
SPE	Solid-phase extraction
SPME	Solid-phase microextraction
TD-cGC	Thermal desorption capillary-gas chromatograpy
TTCA	2-thiazolidinethione-4-carboxylic acid
UAE	Ultrasound-assisted extraction
UN	United Nations
UPLC	Ultra performance liquid chromatography
UV	Ultraviolet
WHO	World Health Organization

1. INTRODUCTION

Pesticides comprise a large number of substances that belong to many different chemical classes. They are applied to crops at various stages of cultivation (preemergence, postemergence, etc.) to provide protection against pests and to prevent/reduce agricultural losses and thus improve the production yield [1]. They are also applied during post-harvest storage in order to preserve/improve crop quality in terms of cosmetic appeal, often important to buyers. Pesticides can also improve the nutritional value of food and sometimes its safety. They are essential in the modern stage of agricultural practices but, due to their biocide activity and potential risk for the consumer, the control of pesticide residues especially in food and water is a growing source of concern for the general population.

Fungi are one of several causative agents of crop diseases that can reduce the yield and quality of food crops [2]. They sometimes produce toxic compounds that can make the final product unfit to eat: The fungal pathogens that cause crop diseases adapt quickly to their new environmental/resistant situations. As a result, although plant breeders can sometimes incorporate resistance to a specific disease, this resistance often breaks down [3]. A fungicide is a particular type of pesticide that controls fungal disease by specifically inhibiting or killing the target fungus. They are extremely important in three ways: they reduce production yield losses, they improve the quality and appearance of harvested products and they make some crops much safer to eat by reducing the natural toxins that fungi can produce. Ragsdale *et al.* [4] wrote a detailed report on the benefits of fungicides in agriculture, citing many examples in which their use is essential for food safety.

After their application, fungicides are gradually dispersed like other pesticides. Their dispersion rate depends on several factors including the species cultivated, the chemical formulation and application method [5, 6], climatic conditions (especially rainfall and temperature), physical causes (mainly volatilization), and chemical degradation, in which sunlight plays an important part [7, 8]. As a result, fungicides are distributed into the environment, and due to their relative persistence, they can contaminate to a variable extent water, soil and agricultural products. In addition, animals can accumulate such substances from contaminated feed and water and also from indoor fungicide practices. Moreover, the indications of the correct use of the fungicides (adequate application, following the security guidelines for their application, applying the correct doses and respecting the indicated "security times") are not always followed and, if there is not an appropriate control, these compounds can finally reach the consumer and may therefore represent a risk for human health.

The adverse effects of fungicides on both human health and the environment are a matter of public concern. Thus, because of possible health effects, there is an increasing need to monitor fungicides in environmental, biological and food samples. In order to ensure the safety of food for consumers and regulate international trade, the Food and Agricultural Organization (FAO) and the World Health Organization (WHO) of the United Nations (UN) have set up the Joint FAO/WHO Codex Alimentarius commission which has established universal maximum residue limits (MRLs) for pesticides in foodstuff. Moreover, each country sets its own MRLs or even authorizes the use of certain pesticides which are forbidden or not used in other countries.

Great efforts are exerted to develop sensitive methods with low limits of quantification (LOQs) to determine residual level of fungicides. Among the various methods of analysis, chromatographic methods [gas chromatography (GC) and high performance liquid chromatography (HPLC)] have the advantages of robustness, sensitivity and selectivity and therefore they are the most frequently used for this purpose. Generally, GC has been used with class-selective detectors such as the electron capture (ECD), flame photometric (FPD), nitrogen-phosphorus (NPD) or mass spectrometry (MS) detectors [9, 10], and HPLC has been used with ultraviolet (UV), diode-array (DAD), fluorescence (FD) or MS detection [11, 12]. All of these detectors are subject to interferences from the matrix. To lessen these effects, extensive clean-up and extraction procedures have been used, e.g. liquid-liquid extraction (LLE), solid-liquid extraction (SLE), solid-phase extraction (SPE), solid-phase microextraction (SPME), single-drop microextraction (SDME), ultrasound-assisted extraction (UAE), sonication-assisted extraction in small columns (SAESC), steam distillation extraction (SDE), microwave-assisted extraction (MAE), accelerated solvent extraction (ASE), pressurized liquid extraction (PLE), molecularly imprinted polymers-solid-phase extraction (MIP-SPE), stir-bar sorptive extraction (SBSE), matrix solid-phase dispersion (MSPD) and liquid-phase microextraction (LPME).

The use of GC and HPLC as separation methods implies a high cost of the instrumentation and chemicals as well as lengthy analysis time. In this sense, a good alternative that highly reduces this daily cost is capillary electrophoresis (CE) which is increasingly being used in the analysis of fungicides due to its simplicity, high separation efficiency, speed of analysis and low consumption of sample and reagents [13]. The main disadvantage of the CE is its low sensitivity when compared to GC or HPLC, although the development of preconcentration procedures before the CE separation has allowed the feasible quantification of fungicides at very low levels [14].

The present chapter attempts to be a critical and updated revision of the current methods of analysis of fungicide residues in different types of samples, concentrating basically on environmental, biological and food samples. The different detectors as well as the sample pretreatments used in combination with the analytical methods for their analysis in these samples will also be discussed.

2. ANALYTICAL METHODS OF FUNGICIDE RESIDUES

Nowadays, the development of an analytical methodology for pesticide determination should be able enough to allow the determination of such pesticides below the MRL established for that compound. In general MRLs in foods are between 0.01 and 10 mg/kg, depending on the pesticide and the commodity. Concerning water samples the limits are even lower. The European Union (EU), for example, has established that pesticide levels should not reach 0.1 μg/L for individual compounds and 0.5 μg/L as a total content [15].

Methods used to analyze fungicides and their residues below their MRLs are similar to those used for other pesticides. In most cases they are not analyzed alone, but together with other groups of pesticides, GC being the classical method, and GC coupled to MS (GC-MS) the preferred technique for multiresidual analysis and for confirmation purposes, besides the traditional detectors [16]. MS is in general the most desired detection system, especially when working with highly complex samples like the biological ones [17]. MS provides information about the molecular weight of the compounds of interest and provides unequivocal structural information via fragmentation patterns that can be obtained with MS^n procedures. GC coupled to tandem mass spectrometry (GC-MS/MS) has also become an alternative for routine fungicide monitoring, on account of the low cost and relative simplicity of commercial bench-top ion traps [18-20]. As an example, Wittke *et al.* [20] determined 3,5-dichloroaniline (metabolite of the fungicides vinclozolin, procymidone, iprodione and chlozolinate) and 3,4-dichloroaniline (metabolite of some herbicides) in human urine by GC-MS/MS, GC-MS and GC-ECD. SDE and LLE were used as preconcentration techniques: Results showed that in contrast to the MS mode, the baseline noise and interferences are almost eliminated in the MS/MS mode. In addition, 3,4-dichloroaniline was not detectable in the MS mode (3,4-dichloroaniline was detectable in MS/MS mode and ECD). Moreover, referring to the signal-to-noise ratio, in the MS/MS mode more than ten orders of magnitude better sensitivity were achieved. By the analysis of identical native urine and spiked urine samples with the GC-ECD and GC-MS/MS methods, a good correspondence of the results of these independent techniques was achieved. Although different ionization techniques have been interfaced with GC, the most commonly used have been electron impact ionization (EI) and chemical ionization (CI) [12]. A recent example of the application of GC-CI/MS in fungicide analysis is the work of Bailey and Belzer [21] who developed a combination of a SPE procedure with GC-CI/MS to the analysis of three fungicides (captan, captafol and folpet) from organic extracts of air samples.

Among the classical detectors used in GC, ECD, FPD and NPD are the most employed for the analysis of fungicides in environmental, biological and food samples. As an example, Navarro *et al.* [22] separated and determined a group of eight fungicides (captan, carboxin, fludioxonil, flutolanil, folpet, pyrimethanil, quintozene and tebuconazole) in fruits and vegetables by GC with ECD, NPD and MS detection, using MSPD as previous preconcentration step. Results showed that similar recoveries, LOQs and linearity were obtained for GC-NPD and GC-ECD, but the chromatograms obtained by GC-MS clearly demonstrated a better selectivity compared to that by GC-ECD or GC-NPD. Vrizas *et al.* [23] used GC with FPD for the analysis of a group of five dithiocarbamate fungicides (maneb, zineb, mancozeb, thiram and ziram) in dry tobacco leaves and peaches using MAE as extraction procedure.

In spite of the numerous advantages that GC shows for the analysis of fungicide residues (such as high sensitivity and selectivity for the detection of these compounds as well as a high robustness), many fungicides are not volatile enough or are thermally unstable to be analyzed by this methodology, although these aspects may be solved in some occasions by introducing a suitable derivatization step -in some cases large and tedious- prior to the GC injection. HPLC, like GC, is a very robust technique which has proven to be a good approach in fungicide residue analysis. Moreover, HPLC is very effective in separating non-volatile and thermally labile compounds. Most HPLC-based methods use common UV, DAD or FD detectors. The literature concerning the analysis of fungicide residues in different matrices (environmental, biological and food samples) using HPLC with some of these classical detectors is extensive. As an example, Liu *et al.* [24] used HPLC-UV for the purpose to determine benalaxyl in soils and waters, using UAE and SPE as preconcentration techniques. HPLC-DAD was applied by Carlucci *et al.* [25] with the aim to analyze the fungicides iprodione and vinclozolin in human urine, being SPE the previous preconcentration step. An example of the application of HPLC-FD in fungicide analysis is the work of Saad *et al.* [26] who developed a method in combination with a SPE procedure for the determination of three fungicides (*o*-phenylphenol, diphenyl and diphenylamine) in apples and oranges. FD provides in general a higher sensitivity (and selectivity) but it is specific for compounds with native fluorescence (which are not many) or compounds that can easily be transformed into fluorescent and stable derivatives. The first is the case of fungicides like thiabendazole, benomyl, carbendazim or fuberidazole (benzimidazole fungicides) [27] and the second of fungicides like thiram, nabam, maneb, mancozeb or propineb (alkylenebis(dithiocarbamate) fungicides), especially those with amino groups, for which dansyl chloride, *o*-phthalaldehyde (OPA) or fluorescamine are frequently used as derivatizing agents [28].

However, like in any separation method, the preferred detection system is MS (HPLC-MS). Thus, HPLC-MS or HPLC-MS/MS have become a powerful tool for fungicide residue analysis in a variety of complex matrices, because of its already known advantages: high selectivity and sensitivity, substantial reduction of sample treatment steps compared with other more conventional techniques, e.g. GC-MS, HPLC-UV or HPLC-FD, and reliable quantification and confirmation at the low concentrations required [29-32]. Trösken *et al.* [33] have described a HPLC-MS/MS method for the determination of 13 fungicides (penconazole, myclobutanil, cyproconazole, triadimefon, triadimenol, imazalil, tebuconazole, hexaconazole, fusilazole, epoxiconazole, bitertanol, propiconazole and prochloraz) in wine. Centrifugation was the only sample preparation step used to eliminate particles, such as crystals of tartar and yeast of very young wine. The interfaces most commonly used in HPLC for the analysis of fungicides are electrospray ionization (ESI) and atmospheric pressure chemical ionization (APCI). Compared to traditional detectors, these interfaces in combination with MS instruments have increased the sensitivity of HPLC by several orders of magnitude and thus, have helped make HPLC-MS routine. As an example, Sagratini *et al.* [34] have used SPME-HPLC with ESI/MS and ESI/MS/MS detection to the determination of carbamates and phenylurea pesticide residues (i.e. four insecticides, three herbicides and the fungicide diethofencarb) in fruit juices, achieving limits of detection (LODs) in the range 0.001-0.01 mg/kg. Other example of the use of these interfaces in fungicide analysis is the work of Blasco *et al.* [35] who developed a combination of a MSPD procedure with HPLC-ESI/MS and HPLC-APCI/MS for the analysis of the fungicides dazomet, disulfiram, and thiram and the metabolites ethylenthiourea and propylenthiourea in fruits, vegetables and cereals (avocados, cherries, lemons, nuts, oats, oranges, rice and tomatoes). Moreover, a comparison of APCI and ESI interfaces was also carried out, finding that APCI achieved better sensitivity. In addition, APCI was more robust and gave reproducible spectra of the studied compounds without adduct formation.

Although GC and HPLC are the typical analytical separation methods to determine fungicide residues, these techniques have several disadvantages (such as high cost of the instrumentation and chemicals as well as large analysis time). Side by side with the classical techniques for detecting fungicide residues (GC or HPLC) an increasing number of methods involve the use of CE [13, 36-39]. CE joints separation of compounds with GC-like resolution, and the capability of HPLC to determine thermally labile or non-volatile compounds. It shows great potential in the analysis of fungicides in environmental, biological and food samples, because of its features, such as higher separation efficiency, shorter analysis time, simplicity with regards to instrumentation and very less consumption of expensive reagents and solvents [13, 36]. One of the major limitations of CE compared to other techniques like GC or HPLC is its low sensitivity in terms of solute concentration, which is caused by the short optical path-length of the capillary used as detection cell and also by the small volumes that can be introduced into the capillary (normally a few nanoliters). To overcome this problem, several off-line and on-line preconcentration strategies have been developed with success [37-42], enabling pesticide determination well below their MRLs in different matrices.

From the various different CE modes, capillary zone electrophoresis (CZE) and micellar electrokinetic chromatography (MEKC) have the higher number of applications in environmental and food science fields [36-38]. In addition, the works most recently published concerning the application of CE in fungicide analysis imply the use of classical detection (UV and DAD). As an example of its use and application to fungicide analysis, Kaltsonoudis *et al.* [43] have investigated a CZE-UV method for the determination of two fungicides (carbendazim and thiabendazole) in lemons while Molina and Silva [44] used a LLE-MEKC-UV method for the multiresidue analysis of eight fungicides (carbendazim, metalaxyl, captan, procymidone, folpet, captafol, vinclozolin and iprodione) in fruit juices.

MS detection is also compatible with CE. Presently, the coupling of CE to MS and tandem mass spectrometry (MS/MS) is one of the most powerful techniques of choice for identification of fungicide residues because the acquisition of mass information facilitates the identification and characterization of the analytes and overcomes a large number of interfering substances. Among the ionization techniques, ESI (which is a soft ionization technique) is often considered the most suitable technique for on-line coupling of CE with MS [45-48]. As an example, Rodríguez *et al.* [49] developed a method based on SPE-CE-ESI-MS to determine two fungicides (procymidone and thiabendazole) in fruits and vegetables (apples, grapes, oranges, pears, strawberries and tomatoes), achieving LOQs in the range 0.005-0.05 mg/kg. This is also the case of the work by Hernández-Borges *et al.* [14] who developed a SPME-CE-ESI-MS procedure for the determination of three fungicides (pyrifenox, cyprodinil, pyrimethanil) together with other two pesticides in grape and orange juice.

Therefore, the determination of fungicide residues is usually accomplished by chromatographic or electrophoretic techniques (GC, HPLC or CE). The complexity of the environmental, biological and food samples as well as unsuitable LODs, especially in CE, make it necessary to use an appropriate extraction or preconcentration procedure to their chromatographic or electrophoretic determination. Several extraction approaches (mainly classical solvent extraction followed by either SPE or SPME) have been employed for this purpose. Regarding the extraction of fungicides with organic solvents, the most employed techniques are LLE or SLE either assisted by ultrasounds (UAE) or microwaves (MAE), or developed with pressurized liquids (PLE). Other methods very used for the extraction and enrichment of fungicides from matrices of different characteristics prior to their analysis by GC, HPLC or CE procedures are SPE [50-54], SPME [55-59], ASE [60], SDME [61], SBSE [62-66], MSPD [67], MIP-SPE [68] and LPME [69]. Some of these techniques in combination with GC, HPLC or CE methods for the determination of fungicides in environmental, biological and food samples will be commented in the next sections.

3. Analysis of Fungicide Residues in Environmental Samples

Because of the indiscriminate use of fungicides for different applications, important environmental problems are emerging, which represent a serious risk to plant, animal and human health. Fungicides are applied directly to the soil or they are sprayed over crop fields and hence they are released into the environment [70]. Many of them readily penetrate plants through the roots and leaves (systemic fungicides) and can contaminate soils and surface water directly as spray drift or run-off, and also via drainage through the soils of treated agricultural land.

Air can be contaminated by fungicides which may also be transferred into the atmosphere by vaporization or spray drift once they are applied. In confined atmospheres (e.g. greenhouses, stockrooms, etc.), which are especially important for human safety, the contamination of the air becomes intensive during and after application of the fungicides increasing the potential risk exposure of workers. In fact, the inhalation exposure to fungicides in greenhouses is considered as more critical than outdoors, because greenhouse walls restrict their rapid distribution and dilution via air-flow. Although concern has risen about possible health risk upon re-entry in greenhouses after the application of fungicides, investigations on airborne residues are still limited [71].

An overview of several papers published in recent years concerning the analysis of fungicide residues in environmental samples is presented in Table 1. Due to the very low levels at which these compounds are usually present in the environment and the complexity of the environmental matrices, most of the methods used for the identification and determination of fungicides in this type of samples include an appropriate preconcentration step followed by a chromatographic (in most cases) or electrophoretic analysis. Sample preparation is usually the most important and time-consuming part of the overall analysis and it limits overall performance of the method.

Table 1. Some examples of the analysis of fungicide residues in environmental samples

Fungicide	Matrix	Analytical method and detection system	Sample pretreatment	Observations	Ref.
Waters					
Fluquinconazole, bromuconazole, dimethomorphe, tetraconazole, tebuconazole, pyridabene, prosulfocarb, hexaconazole	Waste, surface and ground waters	HPLC-MS/MS	SPE (on Strata C_{18})	Simultaneous determination with other type of pesticides. LODs: 0.4-12.3 ng/L Recoveries: 93-118%	[129]
Iprobenfos	Milli-Q, tap and river waters	GC-MS	SPE (on MWCNTs)	Simultaneous determination with other type of pesticides. LOD: 0.01 µg/L Recoveries: 93-104%	[75]
Chlorothalonil, hexaconazole, penconazole, procymidone, tetraconazole, vinclozolin	Farm water	GC-ECD	Hollow-fiber-LPME (toluene)	LODs: 0.004–0.025 µg/L Recoveries: 91-98%	[69]

Table 1. Continued

Fungicide	Matrix	Analytical method and detection system	Sample pretreatment	Observations	Ref.
Metalaxyl, diethofencarb, myclobutanil, tebuconazole	Tap, ground, rain and reservoir waters	HPLC-UV	SPE (on MWCNTs)	Simultaneous determination with other type of pesticides. LODs: 3.0-6.9 ng/L Recoveries: 79-109%	[130]
Carbendazim, metalaxyl, pyrimethanil, procymidone, nuarimol, azoxystrobin, fenarimol, benalaxyl, penconazole	Mineral, stagnant, and tap waters	MEKC-UV	SPE (on Oasis HLB)	Simultaneous determination with other type of pesticides. LODs: 0.558-0.064 µg/L Recoveries: 57-112%	[51]
Carbendazim, chlorothalonil	Tap and river waters	CD-MEKC-DAD	SPE (on polyaniline)	Simultaneous determination with other type of pesticides. LODs: 0.01-0.5 µg/L Recoveries: 59-95%	[74]
Chlorothalonil, triadimefon, hexaconazole, diniconazole	Tap and river waters	GC-µECD	SDME (xylene)	LODs: 0.006–0.01 µg/L Recoveries: 80-102%	[61]
Soils					
Cymoxanil	Drinking water and soil	HPLC-UV	SPE (on Strata X and Strata $C_{18}E$ for water and soil samples, respectively)	LODs: 0.025 mg/L for water samples and 0.025 mg/kg for soil samples Recovery (%): 85%	[131]
Carbendazim, imidacloprid, cymoxanil, cyprodinil	Agricultural waters and soils	HPLC-ESI-MS	SPE (on Oasis HLB)	Simultaneous determination with other type of pesticides. LODs: 0.010-0.025 µg/L for water samples and 0.5-2.5 µg/kg for soil samples Recoveries: 76-99%	[53]

				for water samples and 70-85% for soil samples	
Cyprodinil, fludioxonil, metalaxyl, penconazole, pyrimethanil, procymidone, tebuconazole, vinclozolin	Vineyard soil	GC-MS	UAE and LLE (ethyl acetate)	LODs: 2.0-20 μg/kg Recoveries: 14-124%	[132]
Imazalil enantiomers	Soil	CD-CZE-UV	UAE (methanol)	LODs: 0.24-0.26 μg/mL Recoveries: 81-83% Study of the degradation of imazalil in soil	[85]
Chlorothalonil, procymidone, hexaconazole, tebuconazole, triadimefon, triadimenol, pyrifenox, cyproconazole	Greenhouse soil	GC-NPD and GC-MS	UAE and LLE (dichloromethane)	Simultaneous determination with other type of pesticides. LODs: 0.3-6.2 μg/kg (GC-NPD) and 1.3-9.3 μg/kg (GC-MS) Recoveries: 75-87% (GC-NPD)	[83]
Epoxiconazole	Soil	HPLC-DAD	SPE (on silica gel)	Simultaneous determination with other type of pesticides. LODs: 0.007-0.018 mg/kg Recoveries: 74-85%	[133]
Triadimefon, myclobutanil, cyproconazole, procymidone, tolclofos-methyl, pyrazophos, nuarimol, fenarimol, benalaxyl, ofurace, oxadixyl, dichlofluanid, quintozene, chlorothalonil	Soil	GC-ECD and GC-NPD	SAESC (ethyl acetate)	LODs: 2.0-10 μg/kg Recoveries: 87-111% (GC-ECD) and 89-106% (GC-NPD) Study of the influence of the residue residence time on fungicide recoveries	[86]

Table 1. Continued

Fungicide	Matrix	Analytical method and detection system	Sample pretreatment	Observations	Ref.
Imazalil, isoprothiolane	Compost	GC-MS	PLE (acetonitrile)	Simultaneous determination with other type of pesticides. LODs: 0.03 μg/g Recoveries: 81-100%	[134]
Air samples					
Propineb and its metabolites: ETU and propylenethiourea	Air	GC-MS (propineb) HPLC-UV (metabolites)	SPE (on silica gel)	LODs: 0.8-1.0 ng/m^3 (propineb) and 40-49 ng/m^3 (metabolites) Recoveries: 86-89% (propineb) and 98-100% (metabolites)	[52]
Folpet, procymidone, quintozene, chlorothalonil, penconazole	Greenhouse air	GC-MS	SPME (on PDMS fiber)	Simultaneous determination with other type of pesticides. LODs: 0.03-77 μg/m^3 Study of the concentration of procymidone in the greenhouse air after application of the pesticide	[55]

Concerning water samples, MRLs established by the current legislations are very low (see section 2). Thus, to achieve these limits, a suitable extraction or preconcentration procedure is necessary. The technique most widely used for isolation and preconcentration of fungicides from water samples (the most intensively analyzed samples have been tap, mineral and ground waters) is SPE, which has a number of well-documented advantages, such as high recovery values, low cost and the consumption of relatively low volumes of organic solvents [72]. SPE of pesticides from water samples is generally performed by passing between 0.1 and 1 L of sample (pH is frequently adjusted) through the sorbent supported in a column, cartridge or disk format. An example of the application of SPE as previous preconcentration step in fungicide analysis is the work of Ravelo-Pérez *et al.* [51] who developed a combination of a SPE procedure with MEKC-UV for the analysis of a group of twelve pesticides (i.e., nine fungicides (carbendazim, metalaxyl, pyrimethanil, procymidone, nuarimol, azoxystrobin, fenarimol, benalaxyl and penconazole), two insecticides (pirimicarb and tebufenozide) and one acaricide (tetradifon)) in mineral, tap and stagnant waters. In this work, the sensitivity is enhanced by combining MEKC-UV analysis with off-line (i.e., SPE on Oasis HLB as stationary phase) and on-line (i.e. reversed-electrode polarity stacking mode (REPSM)) preconcentration techniques [38]. On-line preconcentration procedures, also named as stacking or sweeping techniques, have helped to considerably improve the LODs achieved by CE. Figure 1 shows the influence of the composition of the sample in the on-line preconcentration of these twelve analytes. From the figure it is clear that for this specific case, the mixture 1:3 (v:v) water:100 mM sodium tetraborate at pH 8.5 (Figure 7A) provided a good sensitivity improvement. In this case, after appropriate optimization of the injection time LODs between 33.6 and 216 μg/L were achieved, which are well below the LODs frequently achieved in CE without an on-line preconcentration procedure (which are in the mg/L level). SPE cartridges allowed an ulterior preconcentration of the pesticides from water samples down to 927 ng/L.

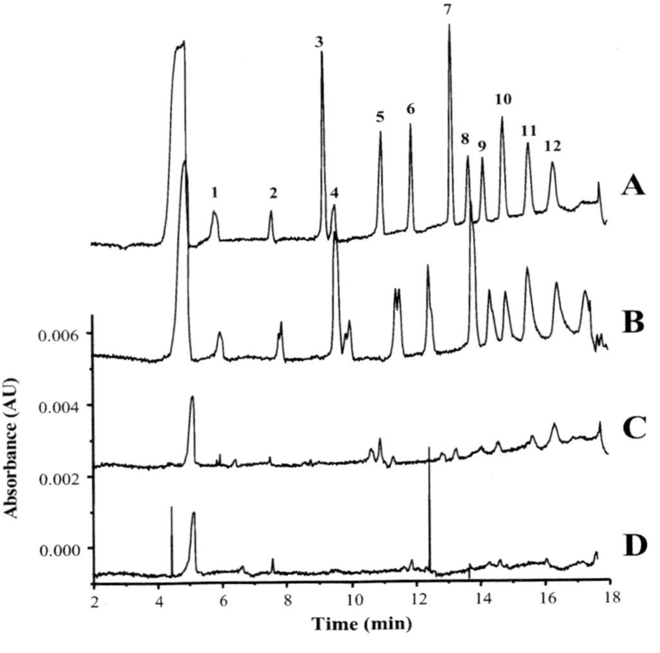

Figure 1. REPSM-MEKC-UV electropherograms showing the effect of the dissolution used for sample preparation. Injection: 11 s at 20 psi. A) Sample in 1:3 (v:v) water:100 mM sodium tetraborate at pH 8.5. B) Sample in 1:1 (v:v) water:100 mM sodium tetraborate at pH 8.5. C) Sample in 3:1 (v:v) water:100 mM sodium tetraborate at pH 8.5 D) Sample in Milli-Q water. Separation electrolyte: 100 mM sodium tetraborate, 30 mM SDS, pH 8.5 and 6% 1-propanol. Total length of the capillary 57 cm (50 cm effective length). Voltage, +22 kV. Temperature, 25ºC. UV detection at 210 nm. Peak identification: (1) carbendazim, (2) pirimicarb, (3) metalaxyl, (4) pyrimethanil, (5) procymidone, (6) nuarimol, (7) azoxystrobin, (8) tebufenozide, (9) fenarimol, (10) benalaxyl, (11) penconazole, and (12) tetradifon. Sample: 5 mg/L of each pesticide except for (2) pirimicarb, (3) methalaxyl (10 mg/L), and (9) fenarimol (2.5 mg/L). Reprinted from [51] with permission from Wiley-VCH.

Oasis HLB, C_{18} and Strata X are the extraction sorbents more used in SPE for the preconcentration of fungicides. D`Archivio *et al.* [73] investigated the retention ability of five commercially available SPE cartridges based on different kinds of sorbents (C_{18} bonded silica, graphitized carbon black, Lichrolut EN, Oasis HLB and Strata X) for the preconcentration of a group of 5 fungicides (metalaxyl, dicloran, iprodione, procymidone and vinclozolin) together with other 11 pesticides in groundwater samples. Finally, these analytes were determined by HPLC-DAD. Oasis HLB and Strata X provided the best results in the preconcentration of the samples, yielding average recoveries higher than 70%, except for phenmedipham that rapidly degrades in groundwater. LODs of the target pesticides provided by the SPE-HPLC-DAD procedure were between 0.003 and 0.040 μg/L. Recently, other extraction sorbents (such as polyaniline and MWCNTs) have also been employed in some cases. Bagheri *et al.* [74] developed a cyclodextrin (CD)-MEKC-DAD method to analyze carbendazim and chlorothalonil (together with other types of pesticides) in tap and river water. In this article, polyaniline was used and evaluated as a sorbent for SPE of these pesticides, finding that in comparison with C_{18}, polyaniline shows higher recoveries especially for very polar compounds. Wang *et al.* [75] studied the use of multiwalled-carbon nanotubes (MWCNTs) as SPE sorbent for the simultaneous extraction of twelve pesticides (the fungicide iprobenfos and other eleven pesticides) in Milli-Q, tap and river waters and their later separation and quantification by GC-MS. Recoveries achieved with spiked water samples were in the range of 82.0–103.7%.

SPME has also become popular for the analysis of fungicides in water samples [76-78]. As an example, Lambropoulou *et al.* [76] have used SPME for the extraction of seven fungicides (dicloran, chlorothalonil, vinclozolin, dichlofluanid, captan, folpet and captafol) from river, lake, sea and ground waters and their later determination by GC-ECD and GC-MS. In this case, four types of fibers were compared: polyacrilate (PA), polydimethylsiloxane (PDMS), carbowax/divinylbenzene (CW/DVB) and polydimethylsiloxane/divinylbenzene (PDMS/DVB). PDMS stationary phase provided the best results and LODs achieved for the whole procedure ranged between 1.0 and 60 ng/L. However, the coated fiber is expensive and in some cases sample carry-over problems do exist. Therefore, other preconcentration techniques based also on microextraction have also been employed, such as LPME [69, 79] or SDME [61] with good results. Concerning the first of them, since 1990, only ten compounds from three fungicide families (dicarboximide, benzimidazole and triazole fungicides) have been determined, using LPME for different aqueous matrices, including ground, surface, deionized, farm and tap waters [69, 80-82].

The concentrations of fungicides present in soil are generally much higher than those present in water. Moreover, the complexity of the sample matrices and the analytical difficulties involved in bringing the analytes into solution are also greater in soils. Therefore, extraction and preconcentration procedure play an important role in this type of environmental samples.

The extraction of fungicides from soil samples requires the use of organic solvents, which compete in the release of the analytes retained owing to high activity of the matrix. Conventionally, the most frequently used methods for the extraction of fungicides from soils including agitation, sonication and soxhlet [12, 83, 84], with subsequent clean-up of the extracts, in some cases, before chromatographic or electrophoretic determination. An example of the application of UAE in fungicide analysis is the work of Chu *et al.* [85] who studied the degradation of imazalil enantiomers in soil using UAE in combination with CD-CZE-UV method. Methanol was used as extraction solvent and the separation buffer was 50 mM NaH_2PO_4, 5 mM $NH_4H_2PO_4$ and 5 mM β-CD (pH 3.0). The recovery for (-)- and (+)-imazalil was 81 and 83%, respectively. However, as it is well known, a number of disadvantages were observed with these extraction methods: they are laborious, involve large volumes of toxic solvents under aggressive shaking and/or temperature conditions and require long extraction times. These drawbacks may be overcome by using other extraction techniques, such as SPE, SAESC and SPME. Sánchez-Brunete *et al.* [86], for example, developed a rapid method for the determination of 14 fungicides (triadimefon, myclobutanil, cyproconazole, procymidone, tolclofos-methyl, pyrazophos, nuarimol, fenarimol, benalaxyl, ofurace, oxadixyl, dichlofluanid, quintozene and chlorothalonil) in soil, based on the ultrasound assisted extraction of soil samples with low volumes of organic solvents (SAESC) and their later separation and quantification by GC-ECD and GC-NPD. Ethyl acetate, acetone and methanol were employed as extraction solvent, being ethyl acetate the one that provided the best recoveries. LODs of the fungicides studied varied from 2.0 to 10 μg/kg.

Regarding the use of SPME, Lambropoulou and Albanis [87] evaluated a SPME procedure (with PA as stationary phase) coupled to ultrasonic extraction for extracting trace amounts of two fungicides (vinclozolin and dicloran) in soil samples. The combination of SPME with GC-MS allowed the determination of these fungicides down to 13 ng/g in soil samples, with recoveries higher than 91%.

For air sampling and analysis, methods of preconcentration as adsorption onto solid sorbents are becoming more widely used because of their advantages in the selection of the appropriate sorbent for a given group of fungicides in air. Usual sampling consists of collecting high volumes of contaminated air that are filtered through an adapted solid-phase material and washed out with organic solvents. In a further processing step, analytes have to be desorbed and/or concentrated before being chromatographied (CE has still not been applied for the analysis of fungicides in air samples). SPE and mainly SPME are the preconcentration methods more used. A relatively recent example of the application of SPME in fungicide analysis is the work of Ferrari *et al.* [55] who developed a combination of a SPME procedure with GC-MS for the analysis of eleven pesticides (the fungicides folpet, procymidone, quintozene, chlorothalonil and penconazole and other six pesticides) in the greenhouse air after pesticide application. After testing different SPME fibers (PDMS, PDMS/DVB, PA and carboxen/polydimethylsiloxane (CX/PDMS)), they found that PDMS stationary phase provided the best results. LODs achieved for the whole procedure ranged between 0.03 and 77 $\mu g/m^3$.

4. ANALYSIS OF FUNGICIDE RESIDUES IN BIOLOGICAL SAMPLES

Despite the obvious benefits of fungicides, their potential impact on the environment and public health is substantial. Fungicides vary in their persistence. Some are non-persistent (e.g. bisdithiocarbamates, like maneb, mancozeb, ziram, etc.; phthalimides, like captan or folpet; chlorophenyls, such as dicloran; chloronitriles, such as chlorothalonil; acylalalines, like metalaxyl and dicarboximides, such as vinclozolin, procymidone, chlozolinate or iprodione) and control only the pathogen on contact and shortly after being applied. By nature, most non-persistent fungicides decompose within several weeks with exposure to sunlight and water. In addition, these fungicides tend not to bioaccumulate; they are typically metabolized and excreted from the body in a few days. However, persistent fungicides (mainly organochlorine fungicides, such as hexachlorobenzene (HCB), forbidden in Europe) are effective for a longer time and tend to bioaccumulate in humans and other animals and thus biomagnify up to 70 000 times in the food chain [88-90].

Due to the heavy agricultural use of fungicides and their movement into the environment, humans are continually exposed to many of these compounds via the food chain and also through residential use [17]. Regarding agricultural workers, exposure is different according to jobs. Thus, applicators could show the highest levels of fungicide excretion, whereas growing, post-harvesting and maintenance workers could show lower levels of exposure. Moreover, higher levels of fungicide excretion could be observed in greenhouses compared to open field workers [91].

The growing toxicological concern over fungicides has prompted studies on analytical techniques for their better monitoring in biological samples, such as human body fluids (e.g. whole blood, plasma, urine or serum) or human tissues and animal fluids or tissues. Biological monitoring is becoming an increasingly important element of field studies designed to assess the risk from occupational fungicide exposure for preventive purposes. Biological monitoring of exposure to fungicides is aimed at estimating at effective internal dose according to the fate of the fungicide in the body. This monitoring can be divided into four areas [92]: direct measurement of unchanged fungicides in biological media, determination of their metabolites in urine or blood, quantification of biological effects related to the internal dose, and measurement of active chemicals interaction with a the target or non-target molecules.

A summary of the relatively recent analysis of fungicide residues in biological samples is showed in Table 2. Due to the lower concentration levels and the only small sample amounts available, analytical procedures for the determination of fungicides or their metabolites in these biological samples have to be more powerful than those for food or workplace monitoring. In addition, biological samples such as blood, plasma, serum, urine and tissues are complicated multi-component mixtures. Therefore, suitable extraction, clean-up or specific isolation procedures for a target compound is necessary prior to their detection by various methods. LLE, SPE and SPME are being used as extraction techniques in the field of analytical toxicology [93]. Moreover, GC and HPLC are widely used for analyses of fungicides in biological samples (CE has not yet been applied with this purpose).

Table 2. Some examples of the analysis of fungicide residues in biological samples

Fungicide	Matrix	Analytical method and detection system	Sample pretreatment	Observations	Ref.
Human urine					
Iprodione, vinclozolin	Human urine	HPLC-DAD	SPE (on C_{18})	LODs: 10 ng/mL Recoveries: 89-96%	[25]
ETU	Human urine	GC-MS	LLE (dichloromethane) and derivatization (with anhydrous acetonitrile, BSTFA and tertbutyldimethyi-lsilyl chloride)	LOD: 0.6 μg/L Recoveries: >90%	[94]
3,4-dichloroaniline (metabolite of vinclozolin, procymidone, iprodione and chlozolinate)	Human urine	GC-ECD, GC-MS and GC-MS/MS	SDE (cyclohexane), LLE (with sulphuric acid) and derivatization (with heptafluorobutyric anhydride)	Simultaneous determination with other type of pesticides. LODs: 0.05 μg/L (GC-ECD), 0.5 μg/L (GC-MS) and 0.03 μg/L (GC-MS/MS) Recoveries: 79-117% (GC-MS/MS)	[20]
TTCA	Human urine	GC-MS	LLE (diethyl ether) and derivatization (with diazoethane/ toluene)	LOD: 0.7 μg/L Recoveries: 86-98%	[95]
Human blood					
HCB	Human serum and urine	GC-ECD	SPME (on PDMS fiber)	Simultaneous determination with other type of pesticides. LODs: 2 ng/mL Recoveries: 80-127%	[96]

Table 2. Continued

Fungicide	Matrix	Analytical method and detection system	Sample pretreatment	Observations	Ref.
HCB	Human serum	GC-ECD and GC-MS	Acid digestion	LOD: 0.2 ng/mL Study of the association of HCB and individuals urinary porphyrins	[135]
Chlorothalonil, dicloran, metalaxyl, phthalimide, tetrahydrophthalimide	Human serum and plasma	GC-HR-MS	SPE (Oasis column with a mixed polarity phase)	Simultaneous determination with other type of pesticides. LODs: 1.0-20 pg/g Recoveries: 14-91%	[97]
HCB	Human serum	GC-MS	LLE (n-hexane/diethyl ether)	Simultaneous determination with other type of pesticides. LODs: 0.01 ng/mL Study of the relations with consumption of dietary components	[136]
HCB	Human serum	GC-ECD	LLE (hexane)	Simultaneous determination with other type of pesticides. -	[137]
Other biological samples					
Fenarimol	Human blood, liver, kidney and gastric content	HPLC-DAD/MS	SPE (on Bond Elut Certify® LRC columns)	LODs: 20-60 ng/g -	[138]

HCB	Human adipose tissue	GC-ECD	LLE (hexane)	Simultaneous determination with other type of pesticides. -	[139]
Phthalimide, phthalamic acid (metabolites of folpet)	Rat plasm	HPLC-UV/DAD	SPE (on Oasis HLB)	LODs: 5.0-10 ng/mL Recoveries: 76-90%	[140]
HCB	Hamster liver and fat	GC-MS	-	Simultaneous determination with other type of pesticides. LODs: 0.001 mg/kg Recoveries: 90-110%	[141]
Metalaxyl enantiomers: (-)-(R)-metalaxyl and (+)-(S)-metalaxyl	Rabbit plasma, liver and kidney	HPLC-DAD and GC-MS	LLE (ethyl acetate)	LODs: 0.01 µg/mL Recoveries: 82-87%	[142]
HCB	Edible tissues from marine species	GC-MS	Cold-extraction with petroleum ether/acetone; liquid-liquid partition with n-hexane and SPE on C_{18}.	Simultaneous determination with other type of pesticides. LODs: 0.1-0.5 ng/g Recoveries: 80-110%	[143]

Regarding urine samples, an obvious advantage of biological monitoring in urine is its ease of availability. In addition, the analysis is not usually limited by the volume of sample available. Therefore, less sensitive instrument could be used by compensating for the decreased instrument sensitivity with increased sample. The analysis of urine is further enhanced because the concentrations of fungicides or their metabolites are higher in urine than in blood, due to their relatively rapid metabolism and excretion. However, an increase in the sample size is generally accompanied by an increase in background noise of the sample.

SPE (C_{18} is the most common sorbent packing material), SPME (PDMS is the fiber coating more used) and LLE (with dichloromethane, ethyl acetate, hexane or diethyl ether as common extraction solvents) are the common preconcentration methods for extracting fungicides of this type of biological samples. A work of Carlucci *et al.* [25] is an example of the application of SPE (on C_{18} cartridges) for the extraction of two fungicides (vinclozolin and iprodione) from human urine of greenhouse operators. Their later separation and quantification were carried out by HPLC-DAD and recoveries obtained were in the range of 89-96%. Two metabolites of alkylene bisdithiocarbamate fungicides (i.e. ethylenethiourea (ETU) and 2-thiazolidinethione-4-carboxylic acid (TTCA)) have also been measured in urine. Fustinoni *et al.* [94] reported the determination of ETU in human urine by GC-MS using LLE (with dichloromethane) as previous preconcentration step. The recoveries achieved were higher than 90%. In this work, they also studied the urinary ETU excretion in 13 vineyard workers (pre- and post-exposure samples) and in 14 controls, finding ETU levels in all samples (<1.6 μg/kg of creatinine). Weiss *et al.* [95] described the determination of TTCA in human urine by LLE (with diethyl ether)-GC-MS, yielding average recoveries higher than 89%. In addition, they analyzed urine samples from people occupationally exposed and the results were compared with the levels of TTCA excreted in urine by 50 control persons without known exposure to dithiocarbamates. The results showed that persons occupationally exposed to these fungicides excrete higher levels of TTCA in urine than the general population, finding a highly significant difference between the exposed and unexposed collective.

Regarding blood samples or its products (i.e. plasma and serum), the major disadvantages of blood measurements are the venipuncture required to obtain the sample and the low toxicant concentrations. Unfortunately, the invasive nature of venipuncture sampling limits researchers´ ability to get high participation rates in large-scale studies. In addition, when samples can be obtained, the amount of blood available to perform the analysis is often limited; therefore, ultrasensitive analytical techniques may be required. For non-persistent fungicides, analysis of blood is further complicated by the inherently low toxicant concentrations that are generally present in blood (ng/L) when compared with urinary metabolite concentrations (μg/L) [17].

HCB is a persistent organochlorine fungicide which is most commonly measured as the intact fungicide and/or its metabolite in whole blood, serum or plasma. Typically, serum or plasma is extracted using LLE, SPE or SPME, and the extract is mainly analyzed using GC-ECD or GC-MS. As an example, López *et al.* [96] determined organochlorine and organophosphorus pesticides (HCB among them) in human serum and urine by SPME-GC-ECD/FPD. In this case, four types of fibers were compared: PA, PDMS, CX/PDMS and CW/DVB. PDMS stationary phase provided the best results and LODs achieved for the whole procedure ranged between 1.0 and 10 ng/mL for serum samples and between 0.1 and 0.4 ng/mL in urine samples. Organochlorine pesticides (HCB among them) were analyzed by GC-ECD, whereas organophosphorus pesticides by GC-FPD. Figure 2 shows the chromatograms obtained when applying the SPME-GC-ECD/FPD procedures to serum samples spiked at 50 and 10 ng/mL for organochlorine and organophosphorus pesticides, respectively.

Other fungicides (non-persistent) such as chlorothalonil, dicloran, tetrahydrophthalimide, phtalimide and metalaxyl have also been analyzed in human serum and plasma. Barr *et al.* [97] developed a SPE (on Oasis column with a mixed polarity phase)-GC-high resolution (HR)-MS procedure to the simultaneous determination of these fungicides with other type of pesticides in serum and plasma. LODs achieved were in the range of 1.0-20 pg/g. In addition, the method developed was employed to measure plasma pesticide concentrations in females living in an urban area, finding detectable concentrations of many widely used residential pesticides in the plasma of the urban females.

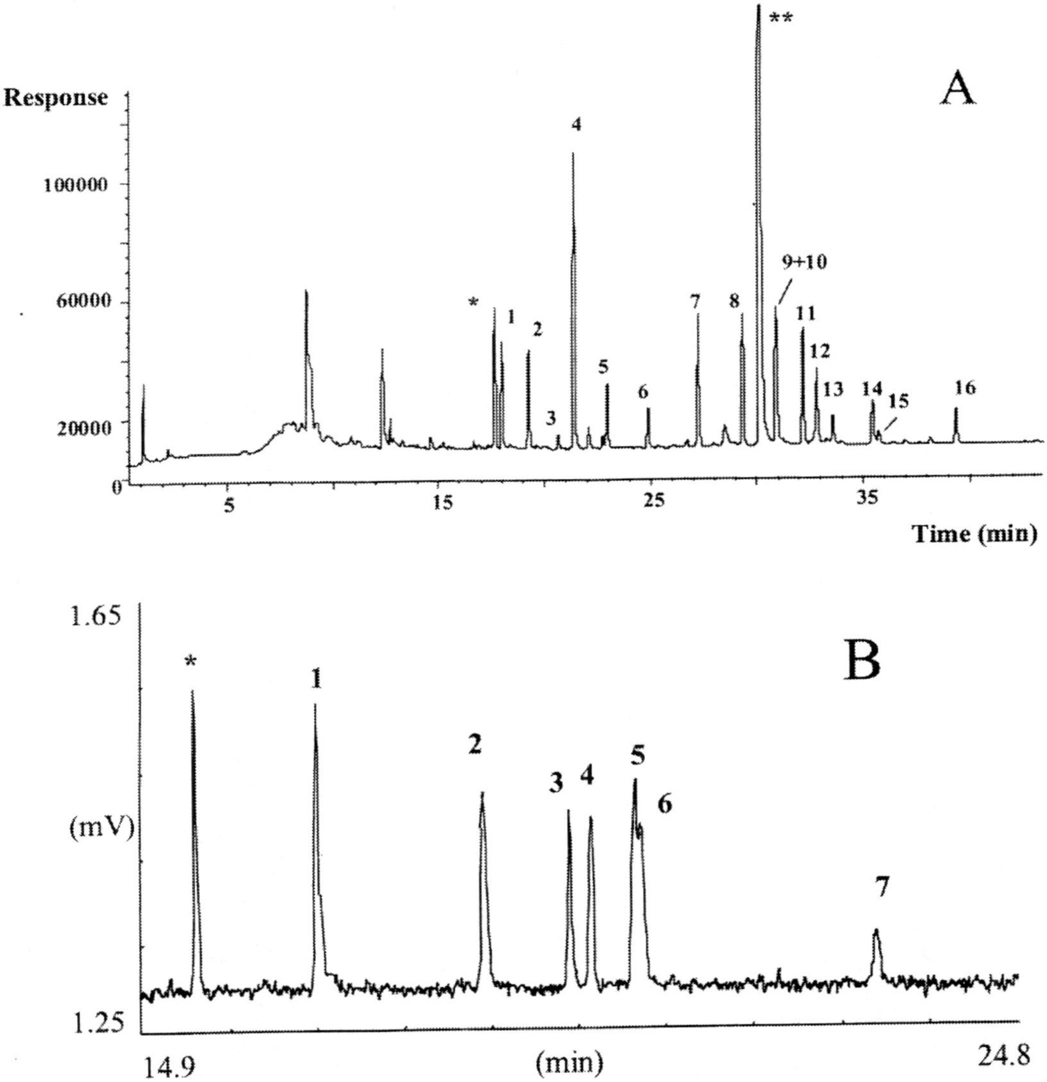

Figure 2. Chromatograms obtained by GC/ECD or GC/FPD after SPME over spiked serum samples. (A) 50 μg/L of organochlorine pesticides (ECD): (1) HCB (2) lindane, (3) δ-hexachlorocyclohexane (δ-HCH), (4) endosulfan-ether, (5) heptachlor, (6) aldrin, (7) heptachlor epoxide, (8) α-endosulfan, (9) 1,1-dichloro-2,2-bis(4-chlorophenyl)ethylene (p-p′-DDE)+dieldrin (10) endrin, (11) β-endosulfan, (12) 1,1-dichloro-2,2-bis(4-chlorophenyl)ethane (p-p′-DDD), (13) endosulfan sulphate, (14) 1,1,-trichloro-2,2-bis(4-chlorophenyl)ethane (p-p′-DDT), (15) methoxychlor. Internal standards: (*) α –HCH, (**) chlorfenson. (B) 10 μg/L of organophosphorus pesticides (FPD): (1) diazinon, (2) parathion methyl, (3) fenitrothion, (4) malathion, (5) fenthion, (6) chlorpyrifos, (7) methidathion. Internal standard: (*) phorate. Reprinted from [96] with permission from Elsevier.

5. Analysis of Fungicide Residues in Food Samples

The use of fungicides at various stages of cultivation and during post-harvest storage plays an important role in food protection and quality preservation. However, due to their biocidal activity and potential risk to the consumer, the control of fungicide residues in foods is a growing source of concern for the general population. Governments and international organizations are regulating the use of fungicides, setting the acceptable MRLs in foods; for example, the EU Commission imposes MRLs between 0.1 and 10.0 mg/kg, depending on the specific fungicide and the crop type [98]. When these compounds are applied according to good agricultural practices, MRLs are not exceeded, but their incorrect application may leave harmful residues, which involve possible health risk and environmental pollution. Therefore, thorough monitoring of fungicide residues is crucial for proper assessment of human exposure to fungicides through foods.

The analysis of fungicide residues represents a basic instrument not only for the protection of human health, through risk assessment studies and prevention strategies, but also for trade and official control purposes. Analytical methodologies employed must be capable of residue measurement at very low levels and must also provide unambiguous evidence to confirm both the identity and the quantity of any residues detected. Therefore, any instrumental technique that is to be used successfully in food analysis should achieve the separation of the matrix compounds and the identification of the fungicides at trace levels. Monitoring of fungicide residues in foods, mainly in fruits, vegetables and processed foods (i.e. fruit juices and wine) is imperative, especially in processed foods, for which there is few data in the literature. Table 3 summarizes some recent works of fungicide residue analysis in food samples.

The analysis of fungicides in wine is of special importance due to the widespread consumption of wine around the world and because winegrowers use this kind of pesticides to control fungi attacks which are very frequent in this cultivars. In fact, molds are between the principal parasites of vine; therefore, to obtain a good quality wine, vine must be protected from these parasites. However, the need of these phytosanitary treatments in vineyards has the disadvantage of potential appearance of fungicide residues in grapes that can pass into must and may remain in wine, affecting not only the wine-making process but also the wine quality and, thereby, entering the food chain [99, 100]. From a legal point of view, MRLs for grapes gave been established by the national guidelines of residues. However, no uniform limits have been set for wine (except in few counties around the world) and they are generally regulated through the various national standards for foodstuffs, as a MRL on wine grapes (although today there is a worldwide trend to lower the MRL to be separated strictly for wine and the legislation is reducing the maximum permitted quantity of pesticides, with a clear intention to reach "zero tolerance" [101, 102]).

Clean-up and extraction techniques are mandatory for the development of efficient analytical methods for the analysis of fungicides in a complex matrix as must or wine. Among the different sample extraction procedures that have been used, despite the fact that LLE with different solvents is frequently recommended [103, 104], nowadays, SPE [50, 105] and SPME [56, 106] are preferred although others like SBSE [62, 107] have also provided interesting results. Most of the SPE methods used for the extraction and preconcentration of fungicides from wine samples involve the use of polymeric cartridges (mainly Oasis HLB). As an example, Nozal *et al.* [50] developed an HPLC-APCI-MS method to analyze eight azolic fungicides (cyproconazole, diniconazole, tetraconazole, thiabendazole, flusilazole, triadimenol, triadimefon, carbendazim and the degradation product 2-aminobenzimidazole) in rose, red and white wines. In this article, Oasis HLB was used as a sorbent for SPE of these fungicides, finding that the benzimidazolic compounds (carbendazime, 2-aminobenzimidazole and thiabendazole) were the least retained analytes on the cartridges. The obtained recoveries were ranging from 83 to 109%.

Table 3. Some examples of the analysis of fungicide residues in food samples

Fungicide	Matrix	Analytical method and detection system	Sample pretreatment	Obser-vations	Ref.
Wines					
Captan, chłozolinate, dichlofuanid, fenarimol, folpet, hexaconazole, myclobutanil, nuarimol, penconazole, procymidone, triadimefon, vinclozolin, benalaxyl, cyprodinil, fludioxonil, metalaxyl, pyrimethanil	Grapes, must and wine	GC-ECD and GC-NPD	Micro on-line extraction (acetone-dichloro-methane mixture as extraction solvents)	LODs: 0.02-0.1 ng/g Recoveries: 78-107%	[144]
Pyrimethanil, nuarimol, procymidone, cyprodinil	White wine	MEKC-UV	SPME (on PDMS/DVB fiber)	Simultaneous determination with other type of pesticides. LODs: 17.6-32.3 μg/L Recoveries: 5-25%	[145]
Carbendazim, metalaxyl, pyrimethanil, procymidone, nuarimol, azoxystrobin, fenarimol, benalaxyl, penconazole	White wine	MEKC-DAD	SPME (on PDMS/DVB fiber)	Simultaneous determination with other type of pesticides. LODs: 0.054-0.113 mg/L -	[56]
Vinclozolin, iprodione, procymidone	Wine	TD-cGC-MS	SBSE (on PDMS)	LODs: 0.2–2 μg/L Recoveries: 7-35%	[62]

Table 3. Continued

Fungicide	Matrix	Analytical method and detection system	Sample pretreatment	Observations	Ref.
Metalaxyl, pyrimethanil, procymidone, nuarimol, azoxystrobin, fenarimol, benalaxyl, penconazole	Rose wine	MEKC-DAD	SPME (on PDMS/DVB fiber)	Simultaneous determination with other type of pesticides. LODs: 0.040-0.096 mg/L -	[57]
Cyproconazole, diniconazole, tetraconazole, thiabendazole, flusilazole, triadimenol, triadimefon, carbendazim, 2-aminobenzimidazole (degradation product)	Rose, red and white wine	HPLC-MS	SPE (on Oasis HLB)	LODs: 2.0-8.0 µg/L Recoveries: 83-109%	[50]
Metalaxyl, pyrimethanil, procymidone, nuarimol, azoxystrobin, fenarimol, benalaxyl, penconazole	Red wine	MEKC-DAD	SPME (on PDMS/DVB fiber)	Simultaneous determination with other type of pesticides. LODs: 0.063-0.157 mg/L Apparent recoveries: 90-107%	[58]
Fruits and vegetables					
Azoxystrobin, cymoxanil, fenhexamid, flusilazole, folpet, metalaxyl, ofurace, oxadixyl, procymidone, pyrimethanil, tebuconazole, trifloxystrobin, vinclozolin	Grape skin and whole grape	HPLC-DAD	SPE (on C_8)	Simultaneous determination with other type of pesticides. LOD: 10.3 µg/kg (grape skin) 30.8 µg/kg (whole grape). Recoveries: 79% (grape skin) and 57% (whole grape). Comparison between the	[146]

				pesticide residues found in grape skin and in the whole grape	
Bitertanol, carboxin, flutriafol, pyrimethanil, tebuconazole, triadimefon	Grapes	HPLC-MS	SPE (on C_{18}) and SBSE (on PDMS)	LODs: 0.25-125 ng/g Recoveries: 60-107% (SPE) and 15-101% (SBSE)	[65]
Thiabendazole, prochloraz and procymidone	Grapes	CZE-UV	SPE (on C_8)	LODs: 0.05-0.10 mg/kg Recoveries: 79-109%	[111]
Propiconazole, tebuconazole, fenbuconazole	Grapes	CD-MEKC-DAD	SPE (on C_{18})	LODs: 0.09-0.1 μg/mL Recoveries: 73-109% Chiral separation with hydroxypropyl-γ-CD as chiral selector	[112]
Azoxystrobin	Grapes and raisins	GC-ECD	SPE (on Celite and activated charcoal)	- Recoveries: 86% (grapes) and 99% (raisins) Study of the loss of residues on processing from grapes to raisins	[113]
Pyrimethanil, kresoxim-methyl	Grapes, strawberries, tomatoes and ketchup	GC-MS	SPME (on PA fiber)	LODs: 1.8-3.1 ng/g Recoveries: 90-107%	[115]
Pyrifenox, cyprodinil, pyrimethanil	Grapes and orange juice	CE-ESI-MS	SPME (on PDMS/DVB fiber)	Simultaneous determination with other type of pesticides. LODs: 0.09-0.12 μg/mL Recoveries: 45-66%	[14]

Table 3. Continued

Fungicide	Matrix	Analytical method and detection system	Sample pretreatment	Obser-vations	Ref.
Pyrimethanil, procymidone, nuarimol, fenarimol, benalaxyl, penconazole	Tomatoes	MEKC-DAD	SPME (on PDMS/DVB fiber)	Simultaneous determination with other type of pesticides. LODs: 0.134-0.373 mg/kg Apparent Recoveries: 94-102%	[59]
Azoxystrobin, carbendazim, cyprodinil, diethofencarb, difenconazole, dimoxystrobin, dodine, fenpropimorph, furmecyclox, imazalil, imidacloprid, kresoxim-methyl, metalaxyl, nuarimol, propamocarb, pyraclostrobin, spiroxamine, thiabendazole, tolyfluanid, triadimefon, triadimenol, trifloxystrobin	Apples, lettuces and oranges	HPLC-MS/MS	Extraction with acetonitrile	Simultaneous determination with other type of pesticides. - Recoveries: 77-124%	[147]
Diethofencarb	Oranges, grapes, onions and tomatoes	HPLC-MS	MSPD (on C_8)	Simultaneous determination with other type of pesticides. LOD: 0.001 mg/kg Recoveries: 67-878%	[67]
Pyrifenox, cyprodinil, pyrimethanil	Water, apples and orange juice	CE-UV	SPME (on PDMS/DVB)	Simultaneous determination with other type of pesticides. LODs: 2.5-47 µg/L Recoveries: 5-46%	[116]
Folpet, chlorothalonil, quinomethionat	Apples, cherry and	HPLC-DAD	SPE (on C_{18})	Simultaneous determination with	[114]

	peach juice			other type of pesticides. LODs: 0.5 µg/kg Recoveries: 94-100%	
Isoprothiolane	Spinach, komatsuna, qing geng cai, broccoli, cauliflower, green pepper and okra	GC-MS	PLE (ethyl acetate)	Simultaneous determination with other type of pesticides. LOD: 3 µg/kg Recoveries: 79-99%	[117]
Other food samples					
Hexaconazole	Black tea	GC-NPD	LLE (n-hexane: acetone)	LOD: 0.05 mg/kg Recoveries: 81-96%	[127]
Carbendazim	Wheat grains	HPLC-PDA	MSPD (on silica gel)	LOD: 3 µg/kg Recovery (%): 87%	[128]
Chlorothalonil, tolclofos-methyl, dichlofluanid, triadimefon, procymidone, cyproconazole, ofurace, benalaxyl, nuarimol, fenarimol	Honey	GC-MS	SPE (on C_{18})	Simultaneous determination with other type of pesticides. LODs: 0.1-5.4 µg/kg Recoveries: 89-99%	[54]
ETU, ethylenebis [isothiocyanate] sulphide	Almonds	HPLC-DAD/UV	MSPD (on washed sand)	- Recoveries: 76-85%	[148]
Tebuconazole, hexaconazole, flutriafol, penconazole	Cabbage, pannage, shrimp, orange juice and tap water	HPLC-UV	MIP-SPE (tebuconazole as the template molecule)	Simultaneous determination with other analytes. - Recoveries: 62-94%	[68]
Quinoxyfen, tebuconazole, fenarimol, *E*-dimethomorph, *Z*-dimethomorph	Hops, trub, wort, and beer	GC-MS	SPE (on Oasis HLB)	Simultaneous determination with other type of pesticides. LOD: 0.023 mg/L Recoveries: 73-136%	[126]
Isoprothiolane	Rice	GC-ECD and GC-MS	ASE (acetone and n-hexane)	Simultaneous determination with other type of pesticides. LOD: 0.023 mg/L Recoveries: 73-136%	[60]

SPME has also been used as extraction technique of fungicides from wine samples before their analysis by GC [106], HPLC [108] or CE [57]. The SPME fibers more employed are PA and PDMS/DVB [106, 108], although in some cases, different stationary phases are used and compared with them. As an example, Ravelo-Pérez *et al.* [56] optimized by means of an experimental design an off-line SPME procedure for the selective extraction of a group of twelve pesticides (i.e., nine fungicides (carbendazim, metalaxyl, pyrimethanil, procymidone, nuarimol, azoxystrobin, fenarimol, benalaxyl and penconazole), two insecticides (pirimicarb and tebufenozide) and one acaricide (tetradifon)) from white wine samples prior to their REPSM-MEKC-DAD separation. After testing different SPME fibers (PA, PDMS, PDMS/DVB and cabowax/templated resin (CW/TPR)), they found that PDMS/DVB stationary phase provided the best results, although carbendazim and metalaxyl could not be extracted from the wine samples by the SPME fiber. LODs achieved for the whole procedure ranged between 0.054 and 0.113 mg/L. The same procedure was also later applied to the analysis of rose [57] and red wines [58].

SBSE constitutes a relatively new extraction technique which is a variation of SPME (in this case, the stationary phase is thicker than in SPME and is located on the surface of a stir bar). This technique has also been applied to the extraction of fungicides from wine samples, but in a low number of occasions (mainly because there only exists one stationary phase commercialized, PDMS). An example of the application of SBSE in the extraction of fungicides from wine samples is the work of Sandra *et al.* [62], who analyzed three dicarboximide fungicides (vinclozolin, iprodione and procymidone) in white wines using SBSE (on PDMS) in combination with thermal desorption capillary-gas chromatograpy (TD-cGC). LODs obtained were between 0.2 and 2.0 μg/L.

Concerning fungicide residue determination in fruits and vegetables most of the published methods use the following samples preparation steps: solvent extraction and partitioning, preconcentration, clean-up and determination. Acetone, acetonitrile, methanol and ethyl acetate are the most used organic solvents for the solvent extraction [109], by means of procedures such as UAE [49] or MAE [110]. Regarding the preconcentration procedures, SPE [111-114], SPME [14, 59, 115, 116], MSPD [67], PLE [117] and SBSE [63, 65, 107] are the most common. As an example, Juan-García *et al.* [63] compared two procedures based on SPE (on C_{18}) and SBSE (on PDMS) in combination with MEKC-DAD for the simultaneous extraction of eight pesticides (i.e. two insecticides (acrinathrin and pyriproxyfen) and six fungicides (bitertanol, cyproconazole, fludioxonil, flutriafol, myclobutanil, and tebuconazole)) in lettuce, tomato, grape and strawberry. Results showed that comparing the SPE with SBSE, the first one is more sensitive, robust, and rapid than SBSE, as well as it provides higher extraction efficiencies and sample throughput. The recoveries obtained by SPE ranged from 40 to 106%, whereas by the SBSE method, the recoveries were between 12 and 47%.

The QuEChERS method (standing for quick, easy, cheap, effective, rugged and safe) is a sample preparation approach also used for the extraction of multiple fungicides in fruits and vegetables [118-120]. When compared with other sample preparation methods, it is clear that it is extremely fast and inexpensive. Wang *et al.* [121] compared the analytical characteristics of MSPD with those found for the QuEChERS method for the analysis of fifteen fungicide residues (thiabendazole, imazalil, thiophanate-methyl, pyrimethanil, procymidone, triadimefon, myclobutanil, triadimenol, fenarimol, dichlofluanid, epoxiconazole, iprodione, kresoxim-methyl, prochloraz, diniconazole) in apple, orange, banana, lettuce, grape and tomato samples. Results showed that the recoveries of most of the fungicides were higher when the QuEChERS method was used rather than MSPD.

Regarding fruit juices, these samples can be extracted directly by LLE [122], sometimes after dilution with distilled water to reduce or eliminate matrix interference [109]. Similar to the extraction and preconcentration of fungicides from fruits and vegetables, SPE [114], SPME [78], MSPD [123] and SBSE [107] are used in the analysis of fruit juices. Even the QuEChERS method has recently been applied [124]. Viñas *et al.* [107] compared two sample preparation methods, SBSE and membrane-assisted solvent extraction (MASE), coupled to the novel technique of ultra performance liquid chromatography (UPLC)-DAD for the sensitive, selective and solvent-free determination of six oxazole fungicide residues (hymexazol, drazoxolon, vinclozolin, chlozolinate, oxadixyl and famoxadone) in four fruit juices (peach, grape, strawberry and multifruits), wine and must, finding that SBSE-based method gave better results for sensitivity, repeatability and analyte recovery than MASE. UPLC uses short columns packed with sub-2 μm particles and high linear velocities, together with instrumentation that operates at higher pressures than are used in HPLC. The result is an improvement in resolution, sensitivity and speed of analysis [125]. Figure 3 shows the chromatographic profiles obtained using SBSE-UPLC-DAD for a wine sample (A) and the same sample fortified with the fungicides (B). Hymexazol and oxadixyl were not extracted. Another application of UPLC-MS/MS is the work of Romero-González *et al.* [124], who developed an analytical method to the simultaneous determination of 90 pesticides (some of them fungicides) in five fruit juices (apple, peach, pineapple, orange and multifruits) using the QuEChERS approach. Pesticides were quantified using matrix-matched calibration with recoveries between 70.4 and 108.5% and LOQs lower than 5 μg/L in all cases. The developed procedure was applied to commercial fruit juices, detecting carbendazim, cyprodinil and thiabendazole in a few samples. Figure 4 shows some UPLC-MS/MS chromatograms for cabendazim, thiabendazole and cyprodinil in different fruit juices.

Other food samples (e.g. cereals, tea, honey, nuts, beer, etc.) have also been analyzed by GC, HPLC or CE using mainly SPE [126], LLE [127] and MSPD [128] preconcentration procedures. Albero *et al.* [54] developed a SPE (on C_{18})-GC-MS method for the simultaneous determination of 10 fungicides (chlorothalonil, tolclofos-methyl, dichlofluanid, triadimefon, procymidone, cyproconazole, ofurace, benalaxyl, nuarimol and fenarimol) and other 41 pesticides in commercial honeys. LODs of the method ranged from 0.1 to 6.1 μg/kg for the different pesticides studied.

6. Conclusions and Future Trends

Analytical methods developed for the analysis of fungicides must be able to accurately determine the low levels at which these compounds are found in either environmental (i.e. soils and waters), food (i.e. fruits and vegetables) and biological samples (i.e. human urine and blood) which is very frequently the low μg/L or low μg/kg level. These methods might be used for a wide variety of purposes including regulatory monitoring and enforcement, risk assessment, field-application trials, import/export certification, organic food verification and marketing to consumers and thus, their importance, is more than proved. In this sense, an important application of fungicide analytical methods is to ensure the safety and quality of foods because of the growing demands of the society: good agricultural practices, tolerance-zero residues, traceability of the products, etc.

The number of fungicides used worldwide is continuously being changed: new ones appear and old ones with high persistence or lower effects on the pests are being eliminated (for example, annex I of European council directive 91/414/CEE related with those pesticides currently authorized in Europe is constantly being modified) and, as a result, new analytical methods for the determination of the new fungicides/pesticides are highly necessary/recommended and should come out in a relative low period of time. In fact, there are many new fungicides that are being introduced/studied and which persistence/distribution in the environment and food has not been fully characterized or analyzed (especially in processed foods, which are the ones that reach the consumer directly and which information is not fully known). Deserving of special mention is the analysis of metabolites and enantiomers (which can also have a negative effect) which are not always taken into account as well as the development of interdisciplinary studies.

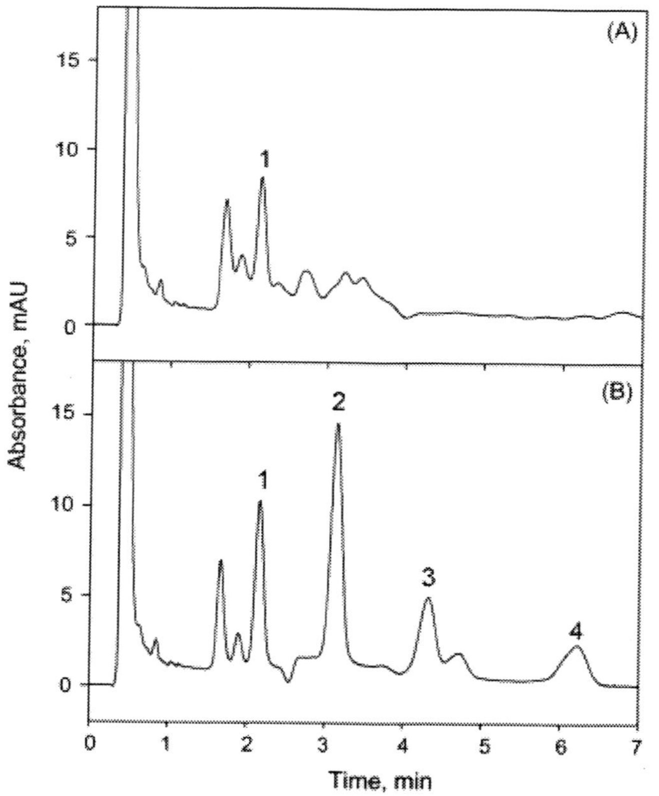

Figure 3. Elution profile obtained for a red wine (A) and the spiked wine (B) by SBSE-UPLC-DAD. Sample volume, 10 mL; extraction time, 30 min; extraction temperature, 60 °C; desorption time, 15 min. Peaks correspond to: (1) chlozolinate (50 μg/L); (2) drazoxolon (1 μg/L); (3) vinclozolin (0.5 μg/L) and (4) famoxadone (1 μg/L). Reprinted from [107] with permission from Elsevier.

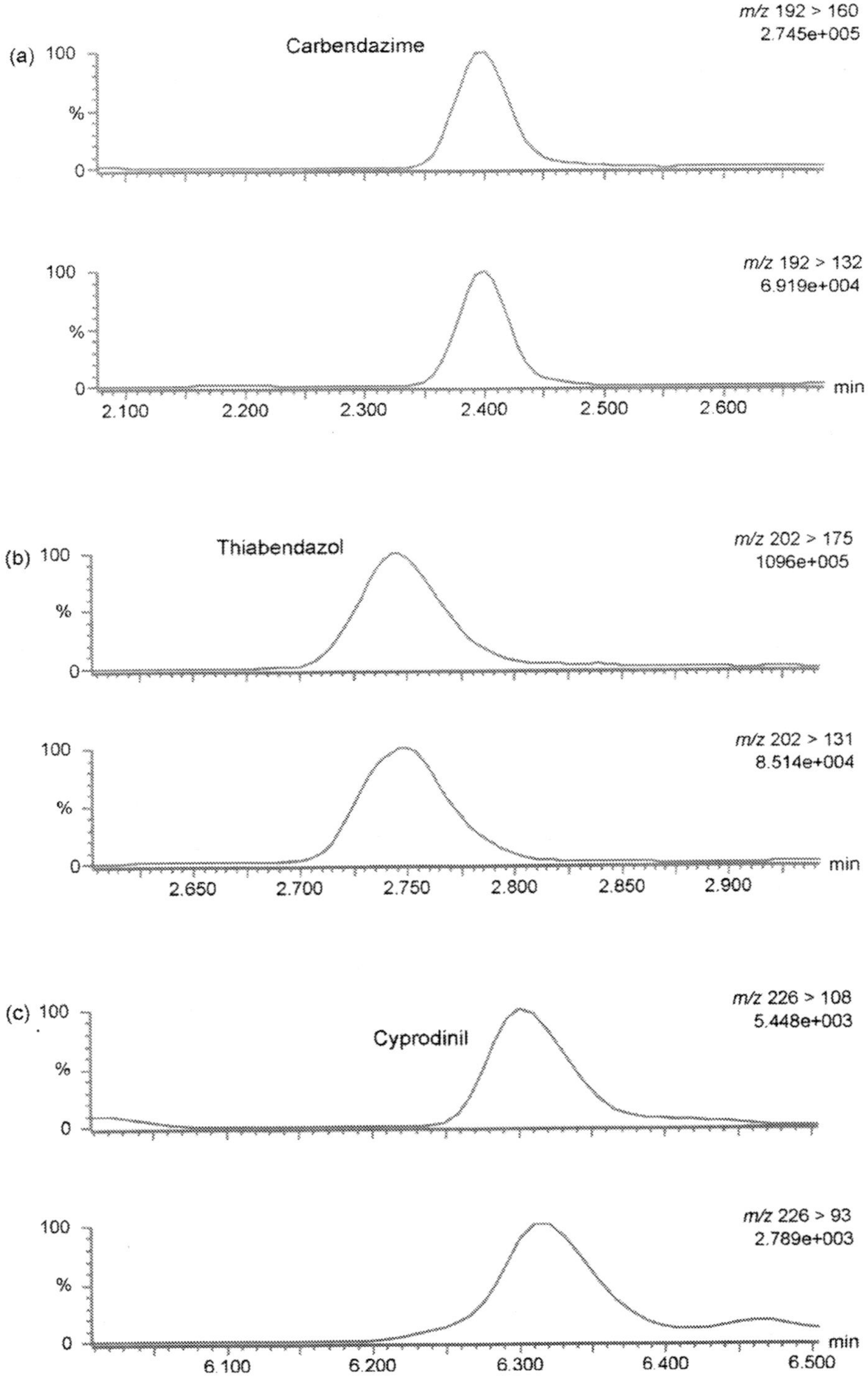

Figure 4. UPLC-MS/MS chromatograms for: (a) multifruit juice containing carbendazim at 33.6 µg/L; (b) orange juice containing thiabendazole (9.6 µg/L) and (c) peach juice containing cyprodinil at 5.1 µg/L. Quantification and confirmation transitions were shown for the 3 positive samples. Reprinted from [124] with permission from Elsevier.

Concerning the separation techniques used in fungicide residue analysis either GC and HPLC are the most commonly used, however, a higher number of works in which CE is being applied are also continuously coming out. In the case of liquid chromatography, the relative recent introduction of UPLC has expanded the application and importance of the technique in this field and it will surely expand its application in this field in which low analysis times with high peak efficiencies and sensitivity is particularly important.

In some cases, especially when dealing with complex samples such as foods or biological matrices suitable extraction methods as well as extensive cleanup of the extracts should be developed in order to eliminate the matrix components that interfere in the analysis. New trends in sample pretreatments, for the analysis of pesticides in general, is the need for fast and easy extraction methods, with high extraction efficiency and enrichment, low consumption of samples and reagents, and which also are environmentally friendly. Many of the current procedures developed up to now meet many of these requirements (i.e. SPE and SPME). However, among all, the QuEChERS method is probably the one that is gaining more and more importance because of its simplicity and easy applicability in governmental and private laboratories. New applications of the method to other matrices rather than fruits or vegetables will surely come out, however, new applications of techniques like SPME or SBSE are also expected.

New strategies in sample pretreatment involve as well the use of new extraction materials (like MWCNTs which are providing good results), but also the use of automated sample preparation steps and the integration of this step together with the chemical analysis under a single format (miniaturization) that may allow a rapid and sensitive analysis of the target analytes, especially in complex samples. In this sense, microchip technology and miniaturized techniques (nano and capillary-LC, CE, etc.), which is currently being studied and developed, might also play an important role in this important field.

REFERENCES

[1] Krol, WJ; Arsenault, TL; Pylypiw, HM; Mattina, MJI. Reduction of pesticide residues on produce by rinsing. *J. Agric. Food Chem.*, 2000, 48, 4666–4670.

[2] Agrios, H. Fitopatología. II Edition. Ed. Limusa, Grupo Noriega Editores, 2002, México, DF.

[3] Aubertot, JN; West, JS; Bousset-Vaslin, L; Salam, MU; Barbetti, MJ; Diggle, AJ. Improved resistance management for durable disease control: A case study of phoma stem canker of oilseed rape (Brassica napus). *European J. Plant Pathol.,* 2006, 114, 91–106.

[4] Ragsdale, NN; Hylin, JW; Sisler, HD; Witt, J. Health and environmental factors associated with agricultural use of fungicides. National Agricultural Pesticide Impact Assessment Program, 1991.

[5] Womac, AR; Mulrooney, JE; Scott, WP; Williford, JR. Influence of oil droplet size on the transfer of bifenthrin from cotton to tobacco budworm. *Pest. Sci.,* 1994, 40, 77-83.

[6] Ebert, TA; Taylor, RA; Downer, RA; Hall, FR. Deposit structure and efficacy of pesticide application. Interactions between deposit size, toxicant concentration and deposit number. *Pest. Sci.,* 1999, 55, 783-792.

[7] Schwack, W; Hartmann, M. Fungicides and photochemistry: Photodegradation of the azole fungicide penconazole. *Z. Lebensm. Unters. Forsch.* 1994, 198, 11-14.

[8] Sur, N; Pal, S; Banerjee, H; Adityachaudhury, N; Bhattacharyya, A. Photodegradation of fenarimol. *Pest Manag. Sci.*, 2000, 56, 289-292.

[9] Geerdink, RB; Niessen, WMA; Brinkman, UAT. Trace-level determination of pesticides in waters by means of liquid and gas chromatography. *J. Chromatogr. A,* 2002, 970, 65-93.

[10] Fillion, J; Sauvé, F; Selwyn, J. Multiresidue method for the determination of residues of 251 pesticides in fruits and vegetables by gas chromatography/mass spectrometry and liquid chromatography with fluorescence detection. *J. AOAC Int.,* 2000, 83, 698-713.

[11] Irace-Guigand, S; Aaron, JJ; Scribe, P; Barcelo, D. A comparison of the environmental impact of pesticide multiresidues and their occurrence in river waters surveyed by liquid chromatography coupled in tandem with UV diode array detection and mass spectrometry. *Chemosphere*, 2004, 55, 973-981.

[12] Picó, Y; Andreu, V. Determination of pesticides and their degradation products in soil: critical review and comparison of methods. *Trends Anal. Chem.*, 2004, 23, 772-789.

[13] Picó, Y; Rodríguez, R; Mañes, J. Capillary electrophoresis for the determination of pesticide residues. *Trends Anal. Chem.,* 2003, 22, 133-151.

[14] Hernández-Borges, J; Rodríguez-Delgado, MA; García-Montelongo, FJ; Cifuentes, A. Highly sensitive analysis of multiple pesticides in foods combining solid-phase microextraction, capillary electrophoresis-mass spectrometry and chemometrics. *Electrophoresis*, 2004, 25, 2065-2076.

[15] http://ec.europa.eu/food/plant/protection/resources/publications_en.htm.

[16] Benfenati, E; Natangelo, M; Tavazzi, S. Gas chromatography/mass spectrometry methods in pesticide analysis. Encyclopedia of Analytical Chemistry, Meyers, RA, Ed. Wiley and Sons, Ltd, 2000, New York.

[17] Barr, DB; Needham, LL. Analytical methods for biological monitoring of exposure to pesticides: a review. *J. Chromatogr. B,* 2002, 778, 5-29.

[18] Sheridan, RS; Meola, JR. Analysis of pesticide residues in fruits, vegetables and milk by gas chromatography/tandem mass spectrometry. *J. AOAC Int.,* 1999, 82, 982-990.

[19] Lehotay, SJ. Analysis of pesticide residues in mixed fruit and vegetable extracts by direct sample introduction-gas chromatography-tandem mass spectrometry. *J. AOAC Int.,* 2000, 83, 680-697.

[20] Wittke, K; Hajimiragha, H; Dunemann, L; Begerow, J. Determination of dichloroanilines in human urine by GC-MS, GC-MS-MS, and GC-ECD as markers of low-level pesticide exposure. *J. Chromatogr. B*, 2001, 755, 215-228.

[21] Bailey, R; Belzer, W. Large volume cold on-column injection for gas chromatography-negative chemical ionization-mass spectrometry analysis of selected pesticides in air samples. *J. Agric. Food Chem.*, 2007, 968, 55, 1150-1155.

[22] Navarro, M; Picó, Y; Marín, R; Mañes, J. Application of matrix solid-phase dispersion to the determination of a new generation of fungicides in fruits and vegetables. *J. Chromatogr. A,* 2002, 201-209.

[23] Vrizas, Z; Papadakis, EN; Papadopolou-Mourkidou, E. Microwave-assisted extraction-acid hydrolysis of dithiocarbamates for trace analysis in tobacco and peaches. *J. Agric. Food Chem.,* 2002, 50, 2220-2226.

[24] Liu, D; Wang, P; Zhou, W; Gu, X; Chen, Z; Zhou, Z. Direct chiral resolution and its application to the determination of fungicide benalaxyl in soil and water by high-performance liquid chromatography. *Anal. Chim. Acta.,* 2006, 555, 210-216.

[25] Carlucci, G; Di Pasquale, D; Ruggieri, F; Mazzeo, P. Determination and validation of a simple high-performance liquid chromatographic method for simultaneous assay of iprodione and vinclozolin in human urine. *J. Chromatogr. B*, 2005, 828, 108-112.

[26] Saad, B; Haniff, NH; Saleh, MI; Hashim, NH; Abu, A; Ali, N. Determination of *o*-phenylphenol, diphenyl and diphenylamine in apples and oranges using HPLC with fluorescence detection. *Food Chem.*, 2004, 84, 313-317.

[27] Hu, Y; Yang, X; Wang, C; Zhao, J; Li, W; Wang, Z. A sensitive determination of carbendazim and thiabendazole in apples by solid-phase microextraction-high performance liquid chromatography with fluorescence detection. *Food Addit. Contam.* 2008, 25, 314-319.

[28] Coli, A; Aaron, JJ. Fluorimetric analysis of pesticides: Methods, recent developments and applications. *Talanta*, 1998, 46, 815-843.

[29] Alder, L; Greulich, K; Kempe, G; Vieth, B. Residue analysis of 500 high priority pesticides: Better by GC-MS or LC-MS/MS. *Mass Spectrom. Rev.,* 2006, 25, 838-865.

[30] Picó, Y; Font, G; Ruiz, MJ; Fernández, M. Control of pesticide residues by liquid chromatography-mass spectrometry to ensure food safety. *Mass Spectrom. Rev.,* 2006, 25, 917-960.

[31] Lehotay, SJ; de Kok, A; Hiemstra, M; van Bodegraven, P. Validation of a fast and easy method for the determination of residues from 229 pesticides in fruits and vegetables using gas and liquid chromatography and mass spectrometric detection. *J. AOAC Int.*, 2005, 88, 595-614.

[32] Hernández, F; Pozo, OJ; Sancho, JV; Bijlsma, R; Barreda, M; Pitarch, E. Multiresidue liquid chromatography tandem mass spectrometry determination of 52 non gas chromatography-amenable pesticides and metabolites in different food commodities. *J. Chromatogr. A*, 2006, 1109, 242-252.

[33] Trösken, ER; Bittne, N; Völkel, W. Quantitation of 13 azole fungicides in wine samples by liquid chromatography-tandem mass spectrometry. *J. Chromatogr. A,* 2005, 1083, 113-119.

[34] Sagratini, G; Mañes, J; Giardiná, D; Damiani, P; Picó, Y. Analysis of carbamate and phenylurea pesticide residues in fruit juices by solid-phase microextraction and liquid chromatography-mass spectrometry. *J. Chromatogr. A,* 2007, 1147, 135-143.

[35] Blasco, C; Font, G; Picó, Y. Determination of dithiocarbamates and metabolites in plants by liquid chromatography-mass spectrometry. *J. Chromatogr. A,* 2004, 1028, 267-276.

[36] Mezinger, F; Schmitt-Kopplin, Ph; Freitag, D; Kettrup, A. Analysis of agrochemicals by capillary electrophoresis. *J. Chromatogr. A,* 2000, 891, 45-67.

[37] Ravelo-Pérez, LM; Hernández-Borges, J; Rodríguez-Delgado, MA. Pesticide analysis by liquid chromatography and capillary electrophoresis. *J. Sep. Sci.*, 2006, 29, 2557-2577.

[38] Hernández-Borges, J; Frías-García, S; Cifuentes, A; Rodríguez-Delgado, MA. Pesticide analysis by capillary electrophoresis. *J. Sep. Sci.*, 2004, 27, 947-963.

[39] El Rassi, Z. Capillary electrophoresis and electrochromatography of pesticides and metabolites. *Electrophoresis,* 1999, 20, 3280-3296.

[40] Rodríguez, R; Mañes, J; Picó, Y. Off-line solid-phase microextraction and capillary electrophoresis mass spectrometry to determine acidic pesticides in fruits. *Anal. Chem.*, 2004, 75, 452-459.

[41] Khrolenko, M; Dzygiel, P; Wieczorek, P. Combination of supported liquid membrane and solid-phase extraction for sample pretreatment of triazine herbicides in juice prior to capillary electrophoresis determination. *J. Chromatogr. A,* 2002, 975, 219-227.

[42] Hooijschuur, EWK; Kientz, CE; Dijksman, J; Brinkman, UATh. Potential of microcolumn liquid chromatography and capillary electrophoresis with flame photometric detection for determination of polar phosphorus-containing pesticides. *Chromatographia,* 2001, 54, 295-301.

[43] Kaltsonoudis, CK; Lamari, N; Prousalis, KP; Karamanos, NK; Tsegenidis, T. Analysis of carbendazim and thiabendazole in lemons by CE-DAD. *Chromatographia,* 2003, 57, 181-184.

[44] Molina, M; Silva, M. Rapid determination of fungicides in fruit juices by micellar electrokinetic chromatography: Use of organic modifiers to enhance selectivity and on-column high-salt stacking to improve sensibility. *Electrophoresis,* 2000, 21, 3625-3633.

[45] Eash, DT; Bushway, RJ. Herbicide and plant growth regulator analysis by capillary electrophoresis. *J. Chromatogr. A,* 2000, 880, 281-294.

[46] Frazier, RA; Ames, JM; Nursten, HE. The development and application of capillary electrophoresis methods for food analysis. *Electrophoresis,* 1999, 20, 3156-3180.

[47] Riu, J; Eichhorn, P; Guerrero, JA; Knepper, ThP; Barceló. D. Determination of linear alkylbenzenesulfonates in wastewater treatment plants and coastal waters by automated solid-phase extraction followed by capillary electrophoresis–UV detection and confirmation by capillary electrophoresis–mass spectrometry. *J. Chromatogr. A,* 2000, 889, 221-229.

[48] Martínez, D; Cugat, MJ; Borrull, F; Callull, M. Solid-phase extraction coupling to capillary electrophoresis with emphasis on environmental analysis. *J. Chromatogr. A,* 2000, 902, 65-89.

[49] Rodríguez, R; Picó, Y; Font, G; Mañes, J. Analysis of thiabendazole and procymidone in fruits and vegetables by capillary electrophoresis-electrospray mass spectrometry. *J. Chromatogr. A,* 2002, 949, 359-366.

[50] Nozal, MJ; Bernal, JL; Jiménez, JJ; Martín, MT; Bernal, J. Determination of azolic fungicides in wine by solid-phase extraction and high-performance liquid

chromatography-atmospheric pressure chemical ionization–mass spectrometry. *J. Chromatogr. A*, 2005, 1076, 90-96.

[51] Ravelo-Pérez, LM; Hernández-Borges, J; Cifuentes, A; Rodríguez-Delgado, MA. MEKC combined with SPE and sample stacking for multiple analysis of pesticides in water samples at the ng/L level. *Electrophoresis,* 2007, 28, 1805-1814.

[52] Kazos, EA; Stalikas, CD; Nanos, CG; Konidari, CN. Determination of dithiocarbamate fungicide propineb and its main metabolite propylenethiourea in airborne samples. *Chemosphere,* 2007, 68, 2104-2110.

[53] Belmonte-Vega, A; Garrido-Frenich, J; Martínez-Vidal, JL. Monitoring of pesticides in agricultural water and soils samples from Andalusia by liquid chromatography coupled to mass spectrometry. *Anal. Chim. Acta*, 2005, 538, 117-127.

[54] Albero, B; Sánchez-Brunete, C; Tadeo, JL. Analysis of pesticides in honey by solid-phase extraction and gas chromatography-mass spectrometry. *J. Agric. Food Chem.,* 2004, 52, 5828-5835.

[55] Ferrari, F; Sanusi, A; Millet, M; Montury, M. Multiresidue method using SPME for the determination of various pesticides with different volatility in confined atmospheres. *Anal. Bioanal. Chem.,* 2004, 379, 476-483.

[56] Ravelo-Pérez, LM; Hernández-Borges, J; Borges-Miquel, TM; Rodríguez-Delgado, MA. Multiple pesticide analysis in wine by MEKC combined with solid-phase microextraction and sample stacking. *Electrophoresis,* 2007, 28, 4072-4081.

[57] Ravelo-Pérez, LM; Hernández-Borges, J; Borges-Miquel, TM; Rodríguez-Delgado, MA. Pesticide analysis in rose wines by micellar electrokinetic chromatography. *J. Sep. Sci.,* 2007, 30, 3240-3246.

[58] Ravelo-Pérez, LM; Hernández-Borges, J; Borges-Miquel, TM; Rodríguez-Delgado, MA. Solid-phase microextraction and sample stacking micellar electrokinetic chromatography for the analysis of pesticide residues in red wines. *Food Chem.* 2008, 111, 764-770.

[59] Ravelo-Pérez, LM; Hernández-Borges, J; Borges-Miquel, TM; Rodríguez-Delgado, MA. Pesticide analysis in tomatoes by solid-phase microextraction and micellar electrokinetic chromatography. *J. Chromatogr. A*, 2008, 1185, 151-154.

[60] Cho, SK; El-Aty, AMA; Park, YS; Choi, JH; Khay, S; Kang, CA; Park, BJ; Kim, SJ; Shim, JH. A multiresidue method for the analysis of pesticide residues in polished rice (*Oryza sativa* L.) using accelerated solvent extraction and gas chromatography and confirmation by mass spectrometry. *Biomed. Chromatogr.,* 2007, 21, 602-609.

[61] Liu, Y; Zhao, E; Zhou, Z. Single-drop microextraction and gas chromatographic Determination of Fungicide in Water and Wine Sample. *Anal. Lett.,* 2006, 39, 2333-2344.

[62] Sandra, P; Tienpont, B; Vercammen, J; Tredoux, A; Sandra, T; David, F. Stir bar sorptive extraction applied to the determination of dicarboximide fungicides in wine. *J. Chromatogr. A,* 2001, 928, 117-126.

[63] Juan-García, A; Picó, Y; Font, G. Capillary electrophoresis for analyzing pesticides in fruits and vegetables using solid-phase extraction and stir-bar sorptive extraction. *J. Chromatogr. A,* 2005, 1073, 229-236.

[64] Durán-Guerrero; E; Castro-Mejías, R; Natera-Marín, R; García-Barroso, C. Optimization of stir bar sorptive extraction applied to the determination of pesticides in vinegars. *J. Chromatogr. A,* 2007, 1165, 144-150.

[65] Juan-García, A; Mañes, J; Font, G; Picó, Y. Evaluation of solid-phase extraction and stir-bar sorptive extraction for the determination of fungicide residues at low-µg/kg levels in grapes by liquid chromatography-mass spectrometry. *J. Chromatogr. A*, 2004, 1050, 119-127.

[66] Blasco, C; Font, G; Picó, Y. Comparison of microextraction procedures to determine pesticides in oranges by liquid chromatography–mass spectrometry. *J. Chromatogr. A,* 2002, 970, 201-212.

[67] Fernández, M; Picó, Y; Mañes, J. Determination of carbamate residues in fruits and vegetables by matrix solid-phase dispersion and liquid chromatography-mass spectrometry. *J. Chromatogr. A,* 2000, 871, 43-56.

[68] Hu, ML; Jiang, M; Wang, P; Mei, SR; Lin, YF; Hu, XZ; Shi, Y; Lu, B; Dai, K. Selective solid-phase extraction of tebuconazole in biological and environmental samples using molecularly imprinted polymers. *Anal. Bioanal. Chem.,* 2007, 387, 1007-1016.

[69] Pan, HJ; Ho, WH. Determination of fungicides in water using liquid phase microextraction and gas chromatography with electron capture detection. *Anal. Chim. Acta*, 2004, 527, 61-67.

[70] Picón-Zamora, D; Martínez-Galera, M; Garrido-Frenich, A; Martínez-Vidal, JL. Trace determination of carbendazim, fuberidazole and thiabendazole in water by application of multivariate calibration to cross-sections of three-dimensional excitation-emission matrix fluorescence. *Analyst,* 2000, 125, 1167-1174.

[71] Tsiropoulo, NG; Bakeas, EB; Raptis, V; Batistatou, SS. Evaluation of solid sorbents for the determination of fenhexamid, metalaxyl-M, pyrimethanil, malathion and myclobutanil residues in air samples. Application to monitoring malathion and fenhexamid dissipation in greenhouse air using C-18 or Supelpak-2 for sampling. *Anal. Chim. Acta,* 2006, 573, 209-215.

[72] López-Roldán, P; López de Alda, MJ; Barceló, D. Simultaneous determination of selected endocrine disrupters (pesticides, phenols and phthalates) in water by in-field solid-phase extraction (SPE) using the prototype PROFEXS followed by on-line SPE (PROSPEKT) and analysis by liquid chromatography-atmospheric pressure chemical ionisation-mass spectrometry. *Anal. Bional. Chem.,* 2004, 378, 599-609.

[73] D`Archivio, AA; Faneli, M; Mazzeo, P; Ruggieri, F. Comparison of different sorbents for multiresidue solid-phase extraction of 16 pesticides from groundwater coupled with high-performance liquid chromatography. *Talanta,* 2007, 71, 25-30.

[74] Bagheri, H; Saraji, M; Barceló, D. Evaluation of polyaniline as sorbent for SPE of a variety of polar pesticides from water followed by CD-MEKC-DAD. *Chromatographia*, 2004, 59, 283-289.

[75] Wang, S; Zhao, P; Min, G; Fang, G. Multi-residue determination of pesticides in water using multi-walled carbon nanotubes solid-phase extraction and gas chromatography–mass spectrometry. *J. Chromatogr. A,* 2007, 1165, 166-171.

[76] Lambropoulou, DA; Konstantinou, IK; Albanis, TA. Determination of fungicides in natural waters using solid-phase microextraction and gas chromatography coupled with electron-capture and mass spectrometric detection. *J. Chromatogr. A,* 2000, 893, 143-156.

[77] Gonçalves, C; Alpendurada, MF. Comparison of three different poly(dimethylsiloxane)-divinylbenzene fibers for the analysis of pesticide multiresidues in water samples: structure and efficiency. *J. Chromatogr. A,* 2002, 963, 19-26.

[78] Natangelo, M; Tavazzi, S; Benfenati, E. Evaluation of solid phase microextraction-gas chromatography in the analysis of some pesticides with different mass spectrometric techniques: application to environmental waters and food samples. *Anal. Lett.,* 2002, 35, 327-338.

[79] Lambropoulou, DA; Albanis, TA. Liquid-phase microextraction techniques in pesticide residue analysis. *J. Biochem. Biophys. Methods,* 2007, 70, 195-228.

[80] Lambropoulou, DA; Albanis, TA. Sensitive trace enrichment of environmental andiandrogen vinclozolin from natural waters and sediment samples using hollow-fiber liquid-phase microextraction. *J. Chromatogr. A,* 2004, 1061, 11-18.

[81] Sandahl, M; Úlfsson, E; Mathiasson, L. Automated determination of vinclozolin at the ppb level in aqueous samples by a combination of microporous membrane liquid-liquid extraction and adsorption chromatography. *Anal. Chim. Acta*, 2000, 424, 1-5.

[82] Sandahl, M; Mathiasson, L; Jönsson, JA. Determination of thiophanate-methyl and its metabolites at trace level in spiked natural water using the supported liquid membrane extraction and the microporous membrane liquid-liquid extraction techniques combined on-line with high-performance liquid chromatography. *J. Chromatogr. A,* 2000, 893, 123-131.

[83] Fenoll, J; Hellín, P; Marín, C; Martínez, CM; Flores, P. Multiresidue analysis of pesticides in soil by gas chromatography with nitrogen-phosphorus detection and gas chromatography mass Spectrometry. *J. Agric. Food Chem.*, 2005, 53, 7661-7666.

[84] Navalón, A; Prieto, A; Araujo, L; Vílchez, JL. Determination of pyrimethanil and kresoxim-methyl in soils by headspace solid-phase microextraction and gas chromatography-mass spectrometry. *Anal. Bioanal. Chem.,* 2004, 379, 1100-1105.

[85] Chu, BL; Guo, BY; Peng, Z; Wang, Z; Guo, G; Lin, JM. Studies on degradation of imazalil enantiomers in soil using capillary electrophoresis. *J. Sep. Sci.*, 2007, 30, 923-929.

[86] Sánchez-Brunete, C; Miguel, E; Tadeo, JL. Multiresidue analysis of fungicides in soil by sonication-assisted extraction in small columns and gas chromatography. *J. Chromatogr. A,* 2002, 976, 319-327.

[87] Lambropoulou, DA; Albanis, TA. Determination of the fungicides vinclozolin and dicloran in soils using ultrasonic extraction coupled with solid-phase microextracion. *Anal. Chim. Acta,* 2004, 514, 125-130.

[88] Borga, K; Gabrielsen, GW; Skaare, JU. Biomagnification of organochlorines along a Barents Sea food chain. *Environ. Pollut.*, 2001, 113, 187-198.

[89] Strandberg, B; Strandberg, L; Bergqvist, PA; Falandysz, J; Rappe, C. Concentrations and biomagnification of 17 chlordane compounds and other organochlorines in harbour

porpoise (Phocoena phocoena) and herring from the southern Baltic Sea. *Chemosphere,* 1998, 37, 2513-2523.

[90] Strandberg, B; Bandh, C; van Bavel, B; Bergqvist, PA; Broman, D; Naf, C; Pettersen, H; Rappe, C. *Sci. Total Environ.*, 1998, 217, 143-154.

[91] Colosio, C; Harari, R; Birindelli, S; Campo, L; Fustinoni, S; Harari, H; Somaruga, C; Tiramani, M; Visentin, S; Maroni, M. Occupational exposure to fungicides in floriculture in Ecuador. *G. Ital. Med. Lav. Ergon.*, 2003, 25, 107-108.

[92] He, FS. Biological monitoring of exposure to pesticides: current issues. *Toxicol. Lett.,* 1999, 108, 277-283.

[93] Kumazawa, T; Suzuki, O. Separation methods for amino group-possessing pesticides in biological samples. *J. Chromatogr. B,* 2000, 747, 241-254.

[94] Fustinoni, S; Campo, L; Colosio, C; Birindelli, S; Foà, V. Application of gas chromatography-mass spectrometry for the determination of urinary ethylenethiourea in humans. *J. Chromatogr. B*, 2005, 814, 251-258.

[95] Weiss, T; Hardt, J; Angerer, J. Determination of urinary 2-thiazolidinethione-4-carboxylic acid after exposure to alkylene bisdithiocarbamates using gas chromatography-mass spectrometry. *J. Chromatogr. B*, 1999, 726, 85-94.

[96] López, FJ; Pitarch, E; Egea, S; Beltrán, J; Hernández, F. Gas chromatographic determination of organochlorine and organophosphorus pesticides in human fluids using solid phase microextraction. *Anal. Chim. Acta*, 2001, 433, 217-226.

[97] Barr, DB; Barr, JR; Maggio, VL; Whitehead Jr, RD; Sadowski, MA; Whyatt, RM; Needham, LL. A multi-analyte method for the quantification of contemporary pesticides in human serum and plasma using high-resolution mass spectrometry. *J. Chromatogr. B*, 2002, 778, 99-111.

[98] Community Directive 93/38/CE. Official Journal of the European Community, 1993, L211/6, Brussels, Belgium.

[99] Oliva, J; Navarro, S; Barba, A; Navarro, G; Salinas, MR. Effect of pesticide residues on the aromatic composition of red wines. *J. Agric. Food Chem.,* 1999, 47, 2830-2836.

[100] Stavropoulos, P; Athanasopoulos, PE; Kyriakidis, NB. Degradation of pyrazophos and methidathion in fortified red and white wine under conditions of light and darkness. *Food Chem.,* 2001, 72, 473-477.

[101] Cooney, CM. New pesticide law drops "zero-tolerance" standard, focuses on exposures to children. *Environ. Sci. Technol.*, 1996, 30, A380-A380.

[102] Pascual, JA; Ros, M; Fernández, P; Bernal, A; Lacasa, A. Future of compost as an alternative to chemical compounds in ecological agriculture. In Waste Management and the Environment II, vol. 78, United Kingdom: Wit Press; 2004; 251-262.

[103] De Melo-Abreu, S; Caboni, P; Cabras, P; Alves, A; Garau, VL. A comparison of a gas chromatographic with electron-capture detection and gas chromatographic with mass spectrometric detection screening methods for the analysis of famoxadone in grapes and wines. *J. Chromatogr. A,* 2006, 1103, 362-367.

[104] Cabras, P; Angioni, A; Garau, VL; Pirisi, FM; Cabitza, F; Pala, M; Farris, GA. Fenhexamid residues in grapes and wine. *Food Add. Contam.,* 2001, 18, 625-629.

[105] Wong, JW; Webster, MG, Halverson, CEA, Hengel, MJ; Ngim, KK; Ebeler, SE. Multiresidue pesticide analysis in wines by solid-phase extraction and capillary gas

chromatography-mass spectrometric detection with selective ion monitoring. *J. Agric. Food Chem.,* 2003, 51, 1148-1161.

[106] Zambonin, CG; Cilenti, A; Palmisano, F. Solid-phase microextraction and gas chromatography-mass spectrometry for the rapid screening of triazole residues in wine and strawberries. *J. Chromatogr. A,* 2002, 967, 255-260.

[107] Viñas, P; Aguinaga, N; Campillo, N; Hernández-Córdoba, M. Comparison of stir bar sorptive extration and membrane-assisted solvent extraction for the ultra-performance liquid chromatographic determination of oxazole fungicide residues in wines and juices. *J. Chromatogr. A,* 2008, 1194, 178-183.

[108] Millán, S; Sampedro, MC; Unceta, N; Goicolea, MA; Rodríguez, E; Barrio, RJ. Coupling solid-phase microextraction and high-performance liquid chromatography for direct and sensitive determination of halogenated fungicides in wine. *J. Chromatogr. A,* 2003, 995, 135-142.

[109] Ahmed, FE. Analysis of pesticides and their metabolites in food and drinks. *Trends Anal. Chem.,* 2001, 20, 649-661.

[110] Singh, SB; Foster, GD; Khan, SU. Determination of thiophanate methyl and carbendazim residues in vegetable samples using microwave-assisted extraction. *J. Chromatogr. A,* 2007, 1148, 152-157.

[111] Rodríguez, R; Boyer, I; Font, G; Picó, Y. Capillary zone electrophoresis for the determination of thiabendazole, prochloraz and procymidone in grapes. *Analyst*, 2001, 126, 2134-2138.

[112] Ibrahim, WAW; Hermawan, D; Sanagi, MM. On-line preconcentration and chiral separation of propiconazole by cyclodextrin-modified micellar electrokinetic chromatography. *J. Chromatogr. A*, 2007, 1170, 107-113.

[113] Lentza-Rizos, C; Avramides, EJ; Kokkinaki, K. Residues of azoxystrobin from grapes to raisins. *J. Agric. Food Chem.,* 2006, 54, 138-141.

[114] Topuz, S; Özhan, G; Alpertunga, B. Simultaneous determination of various pesticides in fruit juices by HPLC-DAD. *Food Control*, 2005, 16, 87-92.

[115] Navalón, A; Prieto, A; Araujo, L; Vílchez, JL. Determination of pyrimethanil and kresoxym-methyl in green groceries by headspace solid-phase microextraction and gas chromatography-mass spectrometry. *J. Chromatogr. A*, 2002, 975, 355-360.

[116] Hernández-Borges, J; Cifuentes, A; García-Montelongo, FJ; Rodríguez-Delgado, MA. Combining solid-phase microextraction and on-line preconcentration-capillary electrophoresis for sensitive analysis of pesticides in foods. *Electrophoresis*, 2005, 26, 980-989.

[117] Tanaka, T; Hori, T; Asada, T; Oikawa, K; Kawata, K. Simple one-step extraction and cleanup by pressurized liquid extraction for gas chromatographic–mass spectrometric determination of pesticides in green leafy vegetables. *J. Chromatogr. A*, 2007, 1175, 181-186.

[118] Anastassiades, M; Mastovská, K; Lehotay, S. Evaluation of analyte protectants to improve gas chromatographic analysis of pesticides. *J. Chromatogr. A,* 2003, 1015, 163-184.

[119] Payá, P; Anastassiades, M; Mack, D; Sigalova, I; Tasdelen, B; Oliva, J; Barba, A. Analysis of pesticide residues using the Quick Easy Cheap Effective Rugged and Safe

(QuEChERS) pesticide multiresidue method in combination with gas and liquid chromatography and tandem mass spectrometric detection. *Anal. Bioanal. Chem.*, 2007, 389, 1697-1714.

[120] Anastassiades, M; Lehotay, S. Fast, and easy multiresidue method employing acetonitrile extraction/partitioning and "dispersive solid-phase extraction" for the determination of pesticide residues in produce. *J. AOAC Int.*, 2003, 86, 412-431.

[121] Wang, S; Xu, Y; Pan, C; Jiang, S; Liu, F. Application of matrix solid-phase dispersion and liquid chromatography-mass spectrometry to fungicide residue analysis in fruits and vegetables. *Anal. Bioanal. Chem.*, 2007, 387, 673-685.

[122] Pose-Juan, E; Cancho-Grande, B; Rial-Otero, R; Simal-Gándara, J. The dissipation rates of cyprodinil, fludioxonil, procymidone and vinclozolin during storage of grape juice. *Food Control*, 2006, 17, 1012-1017.

[123] Tadeo, JL; Sánchez-Brunete, C. Analysis of pesticide residues in fruit juices by matrix-solid phase dispersion and gas chromatographic determination. *Chromatographia*, 2003, 57, 793-798.

[124] Romero-González, R; Garrido-Frenich, A; Martínez-Vidal, JL. Multiresidue method for fast determination of pesticides in fruit juices by ultra performance liquid chromatography coupled to tandem mass spectrometry. *Talanta*, 2008, 76, 211-225.

[125] Swartz, ME. UPLC™. An introduction and review. *J. Liq. Chromatogr. Relat. Technol.*, 2005, 28, 1253-1263.

[126] Hengel, MJ; Shibamoto, T. Method development and fate determination of pesticide-treated hops and their subsequent usage in the production of beer. *J. Agric. Food Chem.*, 2002, 50, 3412-3418.

[127] Karthika, C; Sachin, PJ. Gas chromatographic method for the determination of hexaconazole residues in black tea. *J. Zhejiang Univ. Sci. B*, 2008, 9, 160-164.

[128] Michel, M; Buszewski, B. Isolation and determination of carbendazim residue from wheat grain by matrix solid-phase dispersion and HPLC. *J. Sep. Sci.*, 2003, 26, 1269-1272.

[129] Baugros, JB; Giroud, B; Dessalces, G; Grenier-Loustalot, MF; Cren-Olivé, C. Multiresidue analytical methods for the ultra-trace quantification of 33 priority substances present in the list of REACH in real water samples. *Anal. Chim. Acta*, 2008, 607, 191-203.

[130] Zhou, Q; Xiao, J; Ding, Y. Sensitive determination of fungicides and prometryn in environmental water samples using multiwalled carbon nanotubes solid-phase extraction cartridge. *Anal. Chim. Acta*, 2007, 602, 223-228.

[131] Fidente, P; Di Giovanni, C; Seccia, S; Morrica, P. Determination of cymoxanil in drinking water and soil using high-performance liquid chromatography. *Biomed. Chrom.*, 2005, 19, 766-770.

[132] Rial-Otero, R; González-Rodríguez, RM; Cancho-Grande, B; Simal-Gándara, J. Parameters Affecting Extraction of Selected Fungicides from Vineyard Soils. *J. Agric. Food Chem.*, 2004, 52, 7227-7234.

[133] Rybár, I; Góra, R; Hutta, M. Method of fast trace microanalysis of the chiral pesticides epoxiconazole and novaluron in soil samples using off-line flow-through extraction

and on-column direct large volume injection in reversed phase high performance liquid chromatography. *J. Sep. Sci.*, 2007, 30, 3164-3173.

[134] Kawata, K; Asada, T; Oikawa, K. Determination of pesticides in compost by pressurized liquid extraction and gas chromatography–mass spectrometry. *J. Chromatogr. A*, 2005, 1090, 10-15.

[135] Sunyer, J; Herrero, C; Ozalla, D; Sala, M; Ribas-Fitó, N; Grimalt, J, Basagaña, X. Serum organochlorines and urinary porphyrin pattern in a population highly exposed to hexachlorobenzene. *Environ. Health: A Global Access Sci. Source*, 2002, 1, 1-8.

[136] Hanaoka, T; Takahashi, Y; Kobayashi, M; Sasaki, S; Usuda, M; Okubo, S; Hayashi, M; Tsugane, S. Residuals of beta-hexachlorocyclohexane, dichlorodiphenyl-trichloroethane, and hexachlorobenzene in serum, and relations with consumption of dietary components in rural residents in Japan. *Sci. Total Environ.*, 2002, 286, 119-127.

[137] Bhatnagar, VK; Kashyap, S; Zaidi, SA; Kulkarni, PD; Saiyed, HN. Levels of DDT, HCH, HCB residues in human blood in Ahmedabad, India. *Bull. Environ. Contam. Toxicol.,* 2004, 72, 261-265.

[138] Proença, P; Pinho-Marques, E; Teixeira, H; Castanheira, F; Barroso, M; Ávila, S; Vieira, DN. A fatal forensic intoxication with fenarimol: analysis by HPLC/DAD/MSD. *Forensic Sci. Int.,* 2003, 133, 95-100.

[139] Barkatina, EN; Pertsovsky, AL; Murokh, VI; Kolomiets, ND; Shulyakovskaya, OV; Veretennikova, ND; Venger, ON. Determination of organochlorine pesticides in human adipose tissue in Minsk, Republic of Belarus. *Bull. Environ. Contam. Toxicol.,* 2002, 69, 30-34.

[140] Canal-Raffin, M; Receveur, M; Martínez, B; Titier, K; Ohayon, C; Baldi, I; Molimard, M; Moore, N; Brochard, P. Quantification methods of folpet degradation products in plasma with HPLC-UV/DAD: Application to an *in vitro* toxicokinetic study in rats. *J. Chromatogr. B,* 2008, 865, 106-113.

[141] Kavser, A; Voigt, F; Stubbe, M. First results on the concentrations of some persistent organochlorines in the common hamster *Cricetus cricetus* (L.) in Saxony-Anhalt. *Bull. Environ. Contam. Toxicol.,* 2001, 67, 712-720.

[142] Qiu, J; Wang, QX; Wang, P; Jia, GF; Li, JL; Zhou, ZQ. Enantioselective degradation kinetics of metalaxyl in rabbits. *Pest. Biochem. Physiol.*, 2005, 83, 1-8.

[143] Naso, B; Perrone, D; Ferrante, MC; Bilancione, M; Lucisano, A. Persistent organic pollutants in edible marine species from the Gulf of Naples, Southern Italy. *Sci. Total Environ.,* 2005, 343, 83-95.

[144] Navarro, S; Barba, G; Navarro, G; Vela, N; Oliva, J. Multiresidue method for the rapid determination –in grape, must and wine- of fungicides frequently used on vineyards. *J. Chromatogr. A*, 2000, 882, 221-229.

[145] Molina-Mayo, C; Hernández-Borges, J; Borges-Miquel, TM; Rodríguez-Delgado, MA. Determination of pesticides in wine using micellar electrokinetic chromatography with UV detection and sample stacking. *J. Chromatogr.* A, 2007, 1150, 348-355.

[146] Teixeira, MJ; Aguiar, A; Afonso, CMM; Alves, A; Bastos, MMSM. Comparison of pesticides levels in grape skin and in the whole grape by a new liquid chromatographic multiresidue methodology. *Anal. Chim. Acta*, 2004, 513, 333-340.

[147] Hetherton, CL; Sykes, MD; Fussell, RJ; Goodall, DM. A multi-residue screening method for the determination of 73 pesticides and metabolites in fruits and vegetables using high-performance liquid chromatography/tandem mass spectrometry. *Rapid Comm. Mass Spectrom.,* 2004, 18, 2443-2450.

[148] Garcinuño, RM; Ramos, L; Fernández-Hernando; Cámara, C. Optimization of a matrix solid-phase dispersion method with subsequent clean-up for the determination of ethylene bisdithiocarbamate residues in almond samples. *J. Chromatogr. A,* 2004, 1041, 35-41.

In: Fungicides
Editors: P. De Costa and P. Bezerra

ISBN: 978-1-60692-631-4

Chapter X

DETERMINATION OF BENZIMIDAZOLE COMPOUNDS IN FOOD AND ENVIRONMENTAL SAMPLES: A REVIEW

C. Cacho and C. Perez-Conde*

Analytical Chemistry Department, Faculty of Chemistry, Universidad Complutense de Madrid, Ciudad Universitaria s/n, 28040, Madrid, Spain

ABSTRACT

Benzimidazole compounds can be used both as anthelmintic agents for the prevention and treatment of parasitic infections in animals or humans and as fungicidal agents to prevent spoilage of crops during their storage and transport. It has been repeatedly demonstrated that benzimidazole parent compounds, as well as their metabolites, are capable of reaching the edible parts of food, thus entering the trophic chain. Consequently, an increasing public concern about their massive use in recent years has led to a continuously evolving legislation that restricts their maximum residue limits (MRLs) in milk, meat or crops to a few mg/Kg. Additionally, their massive use has led to their accumulation in the environment, where a maximum contamination level of 0.1 μg/L has been legislated for ground or drinking waters.

A considerable effort has been invested in recent years in the development of new analytical methodologies for the determination of benzimidazole compounds in several kinds of samples. The present review comprises a thorough description of the currently available methodologies for the analysis of benzimidazole compounds in milk, meat, vegetables, fruits or drinking water samples.

Different extraction methodologies such as Soxhlet extraction, microwave and ultrasound assisted extraction procedures, accelerated solvent extraction and solid phase extraction will be compared. Similarly, the techniques most commonly used for the quantification of benzimidazole compounds (immunoassays, GC, HPLC or capillary electrophoresis or chemical sensors) in the aforementioned samples will be discussed in

* Corresponding author. E-mail: cpconde@quim.ucm.es

detail. Additionally, special attention will be paid to aspects such as sample clean-up and enrichment procedures.

INTRODUCTION

The use of benzimidazole compounds (Figure 1) as anthelmintic drugs in the treatment and prevention of parasitic infections or as fungicides to prevent crop spoilage has undoubtedly pushed forward both livestock and agricultural productivities up to levels unbelievable just a few years ago. In this sense, benomyl and thiabendazole have widely been applied as fungicides, while albendazole, mebendazole, oxfendazole and thiabendazole are widely used as anthelmintic drugs.

The most common degradation pathways of pesticides in the environment include their hydrolysis, photochemical and microbe-mediated degradations. However, the high stability of most benzimidazole compounds towards any of these mechanisms makes them extremely persistent, as they can only be hydrolysed in strong acidic or basic media, which are scarcely found in the environment. Benzimidazole chemicals have also proven to be quite resistant to microbial degradation in the environment. Their high persistence, together with their massive use in recent years have led to the accumulation of these compounds in the environment and living organisms.

Although many public benefits have been realized by the use of benzimidazole compounds, their potential impact on both the environment and public health cannot be disregarded. Even if acute toxic effects of benzimidazole compounds are scarce due to the high LD_{50} values (Table 1), several toxic effects have been associated with a chronic exposure to benzimidazole compounds, the most important of them being their teratogenicity [1]. In this sense, the Committee for Veterinary Medicinal Products of the European's Medicine Agency (EMEA) has recently evaluated the teratogenic effect of the most commonly used benzimidazole anthelmintic drugs. An acceptable diary intake (ADI) of 2.5 μg/kg bw per day was estimated for the oral administration of oxfendazole, fenbendazole or febantel in sheep, which corresponded to a non-observed effect limit (NOEL) of 7.5 mg/kg bw per day [2].

Other toxic effects commonly found after a chronic exposure to benzimidazole compounds include congenic malformations [3-5], polyploidy [6], diarrhea [7], anaemia [8], pulmonary oedemas [9] or necrotic lymphoadenopathy [9]. What's even more, some benzimidazole metabolites and degradation products have been reported to be more toxic than the corresponding parent compounds, and thus should also be considered [1,10]. Figure 2 shows the degradation pathways of the most commonly used benzimidazole compounds in animals and humans.

Table 1. LD_{50} values of benzimidazole compounds in rats (mg/kg)

Benzimidazole	LD_{50} (mg/kg)
Albendazole	> 10000
Benomyl	9590
Cambendazole	> 10000
Carbendazim	> 10000
Fenbendazole	> 10000
Flubendazole	2560
Mebendazole	40
Oxfendazole	6400
Oxibendazole	> 10000
Thiabendazole	3100
Triclabendazole	> 10000

In order to control the amount of benzimidazole derivatives that can be used under certain circumstances and the maximum residue limits (MRLs) that can be tolerated in water or food, legislation is under continuous revision by environmental protection agencies worldwide, so that exposure to benzimidazole compounds can be minimized as much as possible. Table 2 shows the nowadays legislated MRLs for the most commonly used benzimidazole compounds and their major metabolites in various matrices.

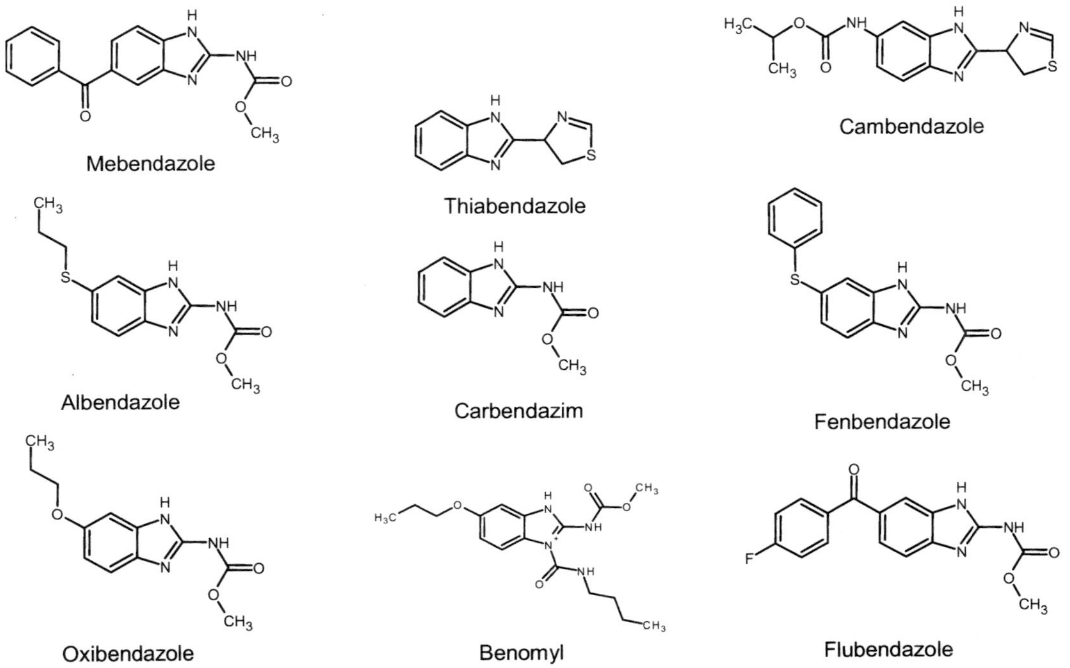

Figure 1. Chemical structures of the most widely used benzimidazole compounds.

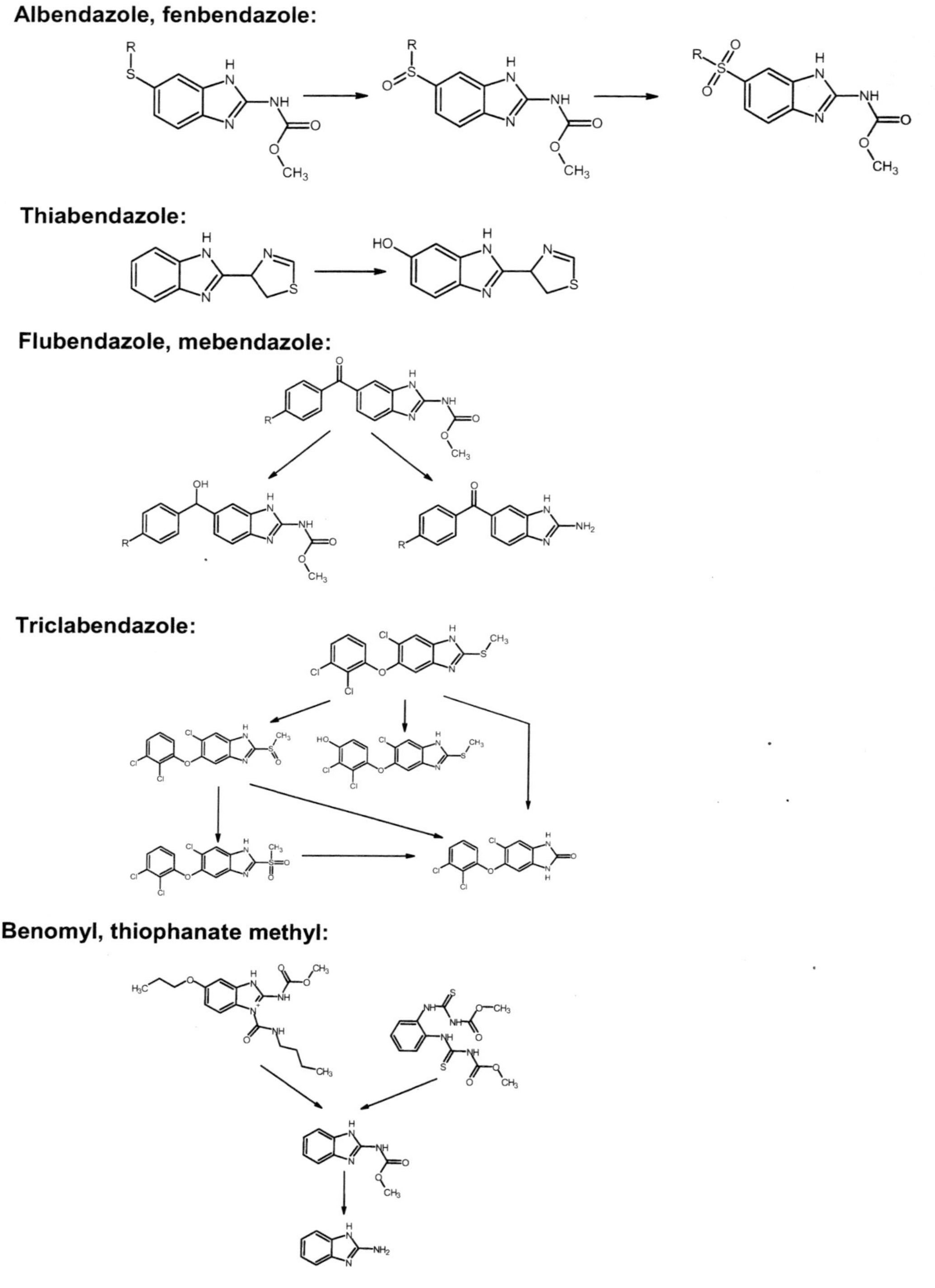

Figure 2. Degradation pathways of the most widely used benzimidazole compounds.

Table 2. Maximum residue limits of benzimidazole compounds in food and environmental samples

Sample	MRL, mg/Kg
Apple	5
Avocado	15
Banana	5
Chestnut	0,10
Citrus samples	5
Hazelnut	0,10
Mushroom	10
Nuts	0,10
Papaya	10
Pear	5
Potato	15
Other vegetable samples	0,05
Kidney	0,1
Liver	0,1
Meat	0,1
Milk	0,1
Water	0,1 µg/L

A high effort has been invested in the last decades in order to develop and validate analytical methodologies capable of quantification of benzimidazole compounds and their metabolites in environmental or food samples at concentration levels below the legislated MRLs. As can be observed in data shown in Figure 3, publication of original papers on the analysis of benzimidazole compounds has experienced an exponential expansion since the 1980s. These manuscripts deal either with the improvement of the analytical methodologies or with the application of existing analytical methods to the quantification of benzimidazole compounds in food samples. In this sense, manuscripts describing new analytical methodologies are commonly published in journals as *Journal of Chromatography A*, *Analytica Chimica Acta* or *Journal of Separation Science*, while purely applied manuscripts are generally published in *Journal of Agricultural and Food Chemistry*, *Journal of AOAC International*, *Food Chemistry* or *Food Control*.

Analysis of food samples usually requires several clean-up and enrichment procedures in order to isolate benzimidazole compounds from interfering matrix components and diminish the detection limit of the analytical method. Even if several papers describe the development of an analytical methodology able of quantifying one or two benzimidazole compounds in water, vegetable, milk and meat samples, multiresidual determination of benzimidazole compounds within a single analytical run has proven to be an extremely difficult task.

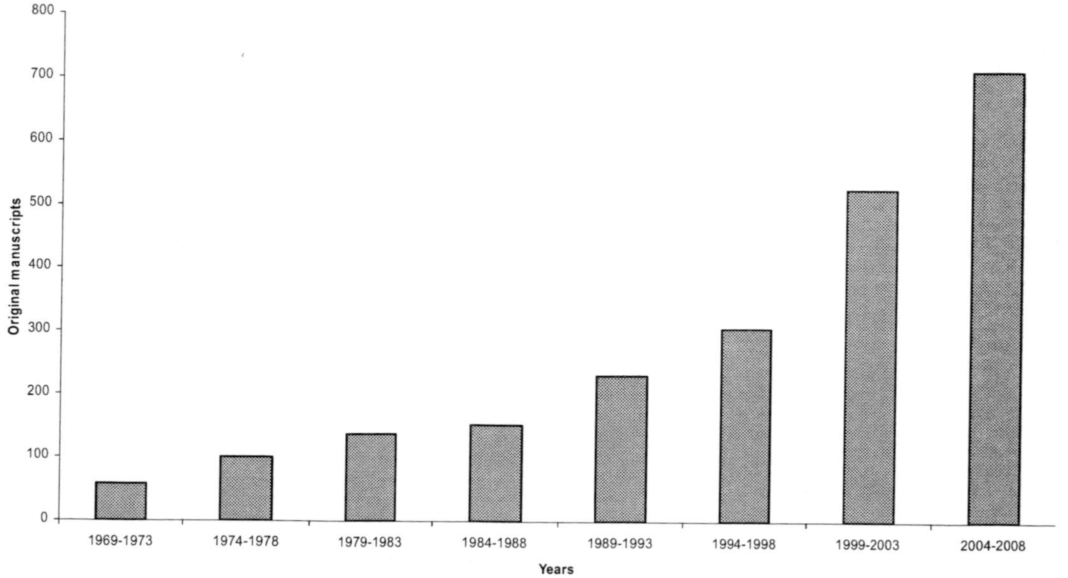

Figure 3. Original papers published dealing with the analysis of benzimidazole compounds in food and environmental samples.

Table 3. pKa values of the most commonly used benzimidazole compounds and their major metabolites

Benzimidazole	pKa_1	pKa_2
Albendazole (ABZ)	5,54	13,11
ABZ-SO	5,69	13,25
ABZ-SO_2	3,50	11,20
ABZ-NH_2-SO_2	5,98	13,30
Fenbendazole (FBZ)	5,12	12,72
Oxfendazole	4,13	11,79
FBZ-SO_2	3,41	11,12
Flubendazole (FLU)	4,10	11,76
FLU-HMET	6,58	13,87
FLU-RMET	5,57	13,14
Mebendazole (MBZ)	4,13	11,79
MBZ-OH	5,60	13,16
MBZ-NH_2	6,61	13,89
Oxibendazole	6,26	13,78
Thiabendazole (TBZ)	5,22	12,83
5-OH-TBZ	7,65	5,46
Triclabendazole (TCB)	5,31	12,91
TCB-SO	1,82	10,95
TCB-SO_2	1,82	9,99
Cambendazole	5,44	13,04
Carbendazim	5,52	13,09

In this sense, as solubility of most benzimidazole compounds in aqueous media considerably increases at low pH values, the strict control of pH on both samples and solutions used for its clean-up or enrichment has proven to be a crucial step in order to quantitatively recover benzimidazole compounds. As can be observed in Table 3, it can be very difficult to find a pH range where a wide range of benzimidazole compounds are in the neutral state.

ANALYTICAL METHODOLOGIES USED FOR SAMPLE TREATMENT

1. Extraction of Benzimidazole Compounds

Methods used for the extraction of benzimidazole compounds and their metabolites from solid samples do not differ much from those commonly employed in the extraction of other organic pollutants. In this sense, the extraction with either pure polar organic solvents (i.e. ethyl acetate, acetonitrile, methanol or dimethylsulfoxide) seems a very valuable starting point [11]. As most benzimidazole compounds are much more soluble in an acidic media, a mixture of an acidic solution and any of these organic solvents can sometimes provide better extraction efficiencies. In this sense, the addition of an acidic solution to the extractant has proven crucial to quantitatively extract benzimidazole compounds from citrus samples [12].

Several extraction techniques have been successfully employed for quantitative extraction of benzimidazole compounds from environmental and food samples. In this sense, Soxhlet extraction of the samples with any of the above mentioned solvents was traditionally carried out for a period of time of up to 24 hours in order to quantitatively extract benzimidazole compounds from vegetables, fruits or meat samples [11,13]. In recent years, the introduction of more efficient extraction techniques such as microwave assisted extraction [13-16], ultrasonic assisted extraction [17,18], accelerated solvent extraction [19-21], matrix solid phase dispersion [22] or supercritical fluid extraction [23,24] have considerably diminished the extraction time, without sacrifying benzimidazole recoveries.

Generally, lack of selectivity during the extraction of benzimidazole compounds from the different samples leads into the co-extraction of several matrix components which can thus interfere in the analysis. In order to remove most co-extracted matrix interferents, a clean-up procedure of the extracts is usually required. In this sense, both liquid-liquid extraction and solid phase extraction have been successfully applied for sample clean-up and enrichment.

2. Sample Clean-up and Enrichment

The analysis of organic pollutants in food or environmental samples represents a challenge. As most extraction procedures and commonly used detection systems are non-selective, a clean-up step of the extracts prior to their analysis must usually be carried out, in order to isolate the analytes from matrix components that could otherwise interfere in the analysis. As has been previously stated, the selection of the optimum clean-up procedure for the determination of benzimidazole compounds within these matrices can sometimes be a very difficult task. Next paragraphs enclose a thorough description of the most common clean-up procedures used in the multiresidual determination of benzimidazole compounds in environmental and food samples.

On the other hand, an enrichment step of the sample extracts can sometimes be necessary in order to diminish the detection limits of the analytical method, thus enabling the quantification of benzimidazole compounds at concentration levels below the legislated maximum residue limits. In this sense, solid phase extraction has proven to be a very valuable tool whenever high enrichment factors are mandatory.

2.1. Liquid-liquid Extraction (LLE)

Even if liquid-liquid extraction techniques have almost been disregarded nowadays due to the high consumption of toxic organic solvents, it renders very satisfactory results, and is thus considered a very good starting point when treatment an unknown sample. Isolation of benzimidazole compounds from complex samples, however, usually requires of several extraction steps, in order to completely remove matrix interferents.

The first liquid-liquid extraction procedure which satisfactorily removed most interferents, was described by Pease et al. [25] in 1969. These authors described a clean-up procedure based on several liquid-liquid extraction techniques with ethyl acetate and different buffered solutions. Benomyl was initially extracted from vegetable samples by blending with ethyl acetate.

The extracts were then submitted to three liquid-liquid extraction steps in order to isolate it from matrix interfering compounds. In this sense, a first extraction technique with a basic buffer solution removed polar compounds soluble in this media, while benzimidazole compounds remained in the organic phase. These were subsequently extracted into diluted HCl, thus eliminating apolar compounds which remained in ethyl acetate phase. Finally, the HCl extract was neutralized by the addition of diluted NaOH and benzimidazole compounds were re-extracted into ethyl acetate. Figure 4 shows a schematic diagram of the different liquid-liquid extraction steps involved in the isolation of benzimidazole compounds from a complex matrix.

These authors demonstrated that, even if benomyl could directly be determined by fluorescence spectrometry, a much higher sensitivity could be afforded if it was previously derivatized into 2-aminobenzimidazole. In this sense, hydrolysis of the sample extracts after their clean-up procedure rendered a much higher recovery. For this purpose, two hydrolysis steps were carried out in order to transform benomyl into 2-aminobenzimidazole. Thus, carbendazim was initially formed by an acid hydrolysis, and was subsequently hydrolysed into 2-aminobenzimidazole in a highly basic media. Recoveries obtained in this case were higher than 75% for all the vegetable samples under study. Similar results were obtained when 2-aminobenzimidazole was determined by colorimetric analysis following bromination [26].

A few years later, this procedure was adapted to the determination of benomyl, carbendazim and 2-aminobenzimidazole in vegetable [27,28], fruit [28] and soil samples [27]. Quantification of benomyl, carbendazim and 2-aminobenzimidazole by cation exchange liquid chromatography yielded detection limits of 50 μg/kg [27]. Derivatization into the corresponding carbendazim and 2-aminobenzimidazole acetates and their quantification by gas liquid chromatography proved to be a much more sensible method, with detection limits below 0.01 μg/kg [28]. Recoveries were higher than 70% in all cases.

As has been previously stated, control of pH of the samples must sometimes be taken into account in order to ensure a robust extraction method. In this sense, the addition of an acidic media to the extractant can considerably improve the extraction efficiency of benzimidazole compounds from acidic samples. Thus, HCl has successfully been used in order to increase the extraction efficiency of benzimidazole compounds from citrus samples. The extracts must be subsequently neutralized prior to their clean-up by liquid-liquid extraction procedures.

In 1979, Tjan and Jansen [29] extracted benomyl, carbendazim and thiabendazole from crop samples by blending with ethyl acetate containing 0.1 N HCl. The addition of HCl was proven necessary to ensure a robust extraction of thiabendazole from most crop samples. The extracts were neutralized (pH 7.5) by the addition of a dilute NaOH solution, and benzimidazole compounds were subsequently extracted into ethyl acetate. Benzimidazole compounds were finally derivatized with pentafluorobenzyl bromide in K_2CO_3 and determined by gas chromatography. Recoveries obtained were higher than 90% for all samples.

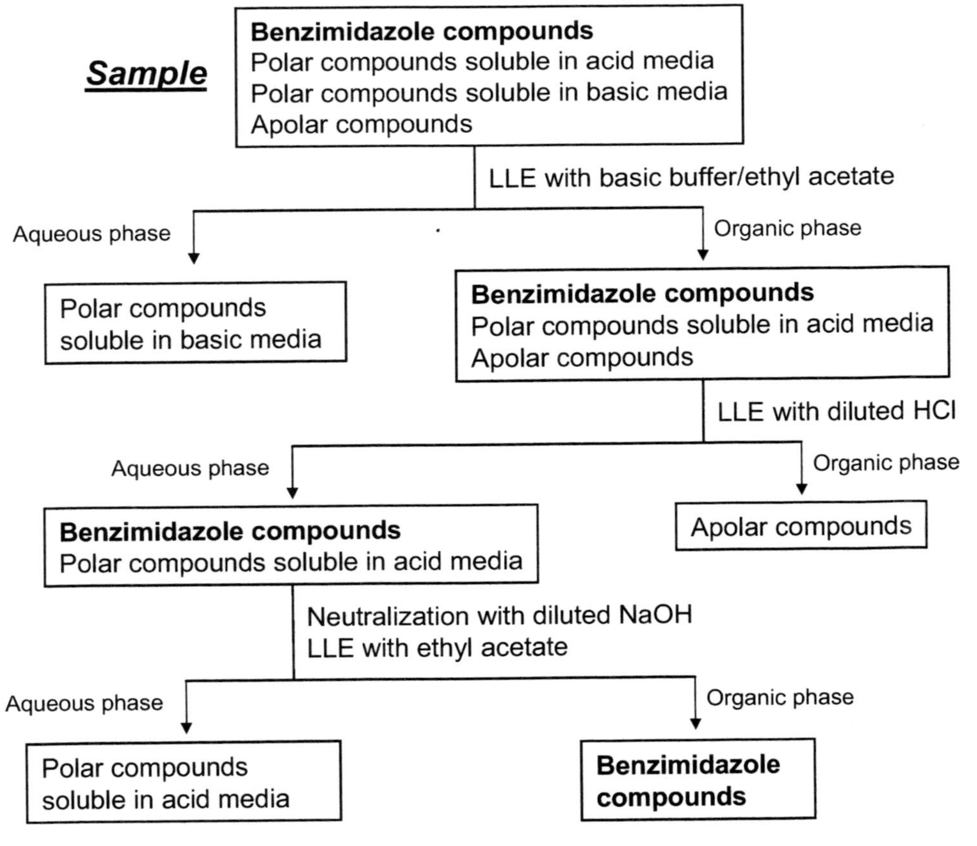

Figure 4. LLE steps involved in the isolation of benzimidazole compounds in food samples [25].

In 1994, liquid-liquid extraction with mixtures of ethyl acetate and buffered aqueous solutions was successfully applied to the isolation of benzimidazole compounds from more complex samples. In this sense, Blanchflower et al. [30] applied a clean-up procedure similar to that initially developed by Pease [25] to the purification of muscle and liver animal samples. In this case, extraction of fenbendazole and oxfendazole from the samples was carried out by sonication with a methanol:water (20:7, v/v) mixture in an ultrasonic bath. The extracts were then washed with light petroleum, diluted with phosphate and extracted into a diethyl ether-ethyl acetate (60:40, v/v) mixture. This extract was cleaned-up by different liquid-liquid extraction steps with basic and acid buffer solutions. Recoveries of the overall process ranged from 86 to 91%, being the detection limits of 50 μg/kg for fenbendazole and 100 μg/kg for oxfendazole.

Fletouris et al. [31] described the use of liquid-liquid extraction using a highly basic buffer solution (pH 10) and ethyl acetate for the successful isolation of benzimidazole compounds present in milk samples. The extracts were subsequently evaporated to dryness and reconstituted in mobile phase prior to their analysis by HPLC. Overall recoveries obtained for the determination of albendazole and its major metabolites (albendazole sulfoxide, albendazole sulfone and albendazole 2-aminosulfone), mebendazole, oxibendazole, fenbendazole and its major metabolites (oxfendazole and fenbendazole sulfone) ranged from 79 to 100%. Detection limits were below 5 μg/L in all cases.

In 2000, De Ruyck et al. [32] developed a fast chromatographic method for the determination of albendazole, fenbendazole, oxibendazole, tetramisole, levamisole and thiabendazole in milk samples. Extraction of these compounds from milk samples was carried out by shaking the samples in the presence of an acetonitrile:ethyl acetate (50:50, v/v) mixture and defatting by the addition of iso-octane. A clean-up procedure of the extract by liquid-liquid extraction with methylene chloride enabled isolation of benzimidazole compounds. The extract obtained by this manner was evaporated to dryness and redissolved in mobile phase for HPLC analysis. Extraction recoveries of the different anthelmintics ranged from 68 to 86%, being the detection limits below 4 μg/L in all cases.

Even if ethyl acetate – aqueous buffer solution mixtures have been by far the most commonly used for liquid-liquid purification of different matrices for the isolation of benzimidazole compounds since the work developed by Pease et al in 1969 [25], other combinations have also shown satisfactory results. In this sense, extraction by using ethanol – dichlorometane [33], hexane – ethyl acetate [34] or water – dichlorometane [35] have successfully been applied to the isolation of the most polar benzimidazole compounds. These purification steps enable the isolation of thiophanate methyl, which cannot be analysed by using a purification methodology based on mixtures of aqueous buffers and ethyl acetate, as it will always be in the ionised state and thus be soluble in the aqueous layer.

The first work describing the analysis of thiophanate methyl together with other benzimidazole compounds dates from 1977, when Farrow et al. [36] adapted the methodology initially developed by Pease [25] to the analysis of benzimidazole compounds in citrus samples. After extraction by reflux in the presence of 2M HCl, the extracts were purified by several liquid-liquid extractions steps using different buffered solutions and chloroform. Recoveries obtained ranged from 32 % of thiophanate methyl to 84% of thiabendazole. Even if such a low recovery was obtained for thiophanate methyl, it was quantified directly for the first time, without the need of hydrolysing it into carbendazim.

Gilvydis et al. [37] demonstrated that the "salting-out" effect played a very important role in further increasing the recoveries obtained for the determination of thiophanate methyl. These authors considerably improved the methodology developed by Farrow et al. [36], by the saturation of the aqueous phases used in the purification step. For this purpose, these authors evaluated the effect that adding different salts to aqueous phases used in the liquid-liquid purification steps had on the recoveries obtained for the determination of thiophanate methyl, obtaining the best results for solutions saturated with NaCl. Under these conditions, a recovery as high as 63% was obtained for the determination of thiophanate methyl in crop samples. Quantitative recoveries for benomyl, carbendazim and thiabendazole were also obtained.

2.2. Solid Phase Extraction (SPE)

In recent years, solid phase extraction has proven to be a very valuable technique for the enrichment and clean-up of several samples, having been successfully applied to the determination of benzimidazole compounds present in water and food samples.

In 1996, JunkerBuchheit et al. [38] compared different sorbents for the enrichment of water samples by a solid phase extraction process. The enrichment factors achievable by a new polymeric ethylvinylbenzene-divinylbenzene sorbent and C_{18} in order to preconcentrate water samples were thus evaluated. The authors concluded that the highest enrichment factor was obtained for a mixture of the new polymeric sorbent and C_{18}, since this mixture enabled a higher retention of carbendazim present in the water samples. A 97% recovery was obtained for the determination of carbendazim in spiked drinking and surface water samples. The detection limit obtained was of 7 μg/L.

A few years later, Shimamura et al. [39] used a polystyrene PS-2 cartridge for the enrichment of water samples prior to the quantification by LC/MS. Water samples were spiked with 10-30 μg/L of a mixture of 22 pesticides. After enrichment on the polystyrene cartridge, detection limits of 0.02-0.3 μg/L and recoveries of 71-127% were obtained, depending on the pesticide.

In 2000, Jeannot et al. [40] compared different enrichment procedures for the quantification of benzimidazole compounds in water samples. In this sense, they evaluated the enrichment factors achievable by liquid-liquid extraction and solid phase extraction procedures on C_{18} and active carbon cartridges. Quantification of the different pesticides was carried out by HPLC, using both UV radiation and mass spectrometry as detection systems. The most appropriate method for the analysis of carbendazim consisted in the enrichment of the water samples on a C_{18} cartridge. Detection limits obtained under these conditions were of 6 ng/L. Zamora et al. [41,42] extended the methodology developed by Jeannot to the quantification of fuberidazole, thiabendazole and benomyl in water samples.

Hogendoorn et al. [17] applied a polystyrene-divinylbenzene (PS-DVB) cartridge as sorbent for the enrichment of water samples. The developed methodology enabled the determination of carbendazim present in groundwater samples with mean recoveries ranging from 71 to 101%. Detection limits obtained by this methodology was below 0.1 μg/L.

The addition of surfactants to the water samples has proven to be a very valuable way to enhance the achievable enrichment factors. In this sense, Halko et al. [43] evaluated the effect of adding oligoethyleneglycol monoalkylether (Genapol X-080) and polyoxyethylenelauryl esther (POLE) as surfactants for the enrichment of groundwater samples containing carbendazim, benomyl, thiabendazole and fuberidazole. Detection limits obtained by using these micelles decreased 3-fold, ranging from 0.01 to 7 μg/L. A few years later, Moral et al. [44] used sodium dodecylsulphate (SDS) enabling a much higher breakthrough volume to be achieved. The detection limits obtained under these conditions were below 5 ng/L.

First application of solid phase extraction for purification of food samples dates from 1993, when Steenbaar et al. [45] successfully determined mebendazole in eel muscle samples. For this purpose, mebendazole was initially extracted with ethyl acetate. After addition of hexane, the extract was purified on a silica gel sorbent. The acidified methanolic extract was evaporated to dryness and reconstituted in the mobile phase for HPLC analysis on a C_8 column. A recovery higher than 70% was obtained in all cases, with a detection limit below 10 μg/kg. The developed methodology was successfully applied to the determination of fenbendazole [46], mebendazole [47] and their metabolites in eel and trout muscle samples.

Cooper et al. [48] evaluated different sorbents for the SPE clean-up of animal tissues. For this purpose, these authors compared the performance of both polar (silica gel) and apolar (C_{18}, C_8, PS-DVB) sorbents for the isolation of sulfonamides, benzimidazoles, nitroimidazoles and nitrofurans in pig kidney samples. Optimum results were obtained when utilising a two-step SPE clean-up procedure of the sample extracts, first on a silica gel column, followed by the clean-up of the extracts on a C_{18} cartridge. Recoveries obtained for the different veterinary drugs ranged from 40 to 70%, with detection limits of 2-18 μg/kg.

A few years later, Sorensen et al. [49] used chloride and cyanide based polymeric matrices as sorbents for the clean-up of trout muscle and skin samples by solid phase extraction. Mean overall recoveries higher than 81% were obtained in all cases. The method's detection limits ranged from 3.8 to 4.5 μg/kg. The developed methodology has been applied to the determination of fenbendazole and its major metabolites in trout treated with fenbendazole. Fenbendazole, fenbendazole sulfone and fenbendazole sulfoxide were detected in both muscle and skin tissues shortly after administration, being concentrations higher in skin samples.

In 2003, Danaher et al. [24] evaluated different sample clean-up procedures for the determination of a mixture of benzimidazole compounds in chicken, cow and pig liver samples. For this purpose, purification of the samples by both liquid-liquid extraction and solid phase extraction procedures has been compared. By using different sorbents, these authors evaluated the responsible mechanism for the retention of benzimidazole compounds in a SPE process within the sample matrix. In this sense, materials based solely on reversed-phase retention mode (C_{18}), ion exchange (a strong cation exchange resin) or a mixture of both mechanisms (Oasis®), were evaluated.

Recoveries of benzimidazole compounds obtained by liquid-liquid extraction were rather low. Additionally, brownish extracts of different intensities were obtained for most liquid-liquid extraction procedures, thus hampering detection of benzimidazole compounds. On the other hand, sample clean-up on either C_{18} or Oasis® SPE sorbents lead to the co-extraction of several matrix components which interfered in the analysis of benzimidazole compounds. Optimum results for sample clean-up were obtained when using a strong cation exchange resin as sorbent in a SPE process. Under these conditions, quantitative recoveries were obtained for all the evaluated benzimidazole compounds, except for mebendazole which could not be analyzed by this procedure.

In recent years, a new technology based on molecular imprinting has strongly come into scene. Molecularly imprinted polymers (MIPs) are highly cross-linked polymers capable of selectively rebinding the target molecule and structurally related compounds [50]. Briefly, MIPs are synthetic polymers prepared in the presence of the analyte which acts as template guiding the polymerization step. Removal of the template molecule after polymerization leaves cavities complementary to the analyte in chemical functionality, size and shape. These cavities are responsible for the characteristic molecular recognition of these materials. Acting in a similar manner to that of antibodies, these imprinted materials have sometimes been denoted as "*plastic antibodies*".

De Prada et al. [51] developed an imprinted polymer against fenbendazole. This imprinted polymer was proven to be able of selectively rebinding fenbendazole from beef liver samples. Fenbendazole was analyzed by square wave voltammetry being the recoveries higher than 95% in all cases.

Solid phase extraction has been successfully applied to the purification of vegetable samples, in order to isolate the benzimidazole compounds. In this sense, Aharonson et al. [52] developed a solid phase extraction procedure for the determination of benomyl, carbendazim and thiabendazole in vegetable samples. The sample extracts were cleaned-up by three consecutive SPE procedures using magnesia, zeolite and alumina as polar sorbents. Final quantification of the benzimidazole compounds was carried out by fluorescence spectrometry. Overall recoveries ranged from 60 to 70%. Use of apolar sorbents as polyethylene (Extrelut^{TM}) and control of the pH of the citrus samples prior to the extraction of benzimidazole compounds enabled higher concentrations to be achieved [53].

A few years later, Hiemstra et al. [54] developed an automated solid phase extraction procedure for the clean-up of fruit and vegetable samples. These authors compared the traditional liquid-liquid partition steps and the developed automated solid phase extraction procedure for the isolation of carbendazim and thiabendazole present in lettuce and citrus samples. A much higher sample throughput (50 samples/day) could be achieved by the developed methodology, compared to that achievable by purification by liquid-liquid extraction steps using mixtures of acetone, dichloromethane and petroleum ether. Quantitative recoveries for both carbendazim and thiabendazole were obtained by the developed automated methodology.

The introduction of ion exchange materials as sorbents in solid phase extraction, either independently or in combination with other polymeric materials, enabled a considerable improvement in the sample clean-up of vegetable samples for the determination of benzimidazole compounds. In this sense, several procedures describe the development of purification methodologies of extracts of citrus, banana, apple and grape samples by ion exchange solid phase extraction.

In this sense, Arenas et al. [55] developed a method for the quantification of thiabendazole present in banana samples. Thiabendazole was extracted from bananas by sonication in ethyl acetate. The sample extract was percolated through a strong cation exchange resin and thiabendazole was eluted with 0.1M KH_2PO_4 in acetonitrile. Final determination of thiabendazole by HPLC-fluorescence spectrometry enabled a recovery of 94%. Control of the sample's pH enabled the applicability of the developed methodology to the determination of thiabendazole in citrus samples [56].

A few years later, Young et al. [57,58] analysed thiabendazole and carbendazim in orange, apple and grape juice samples by using an Oasis® cartridge as sorbent for the solid-phase extraction purification. As has been previously stated, this sorbent presents a mixed sorption mechanism, both as cation exchange resin and reversed phase sorbent. These authors evaluated the mechanism responsible of the interaction of benzimidazole compounds. In this sense, optimum performance was obtained when the Oasis® sorbent operated sequentially in a cation exchange and reversed phase retention modes. Recoveries obtained for the determination of thiabendazole and carbendazim in fruit juice samples ranged from 74 to 90%.

ANALYTICAL METHODOLOGIES USED FOR THE DETECTION OF BENZIMIDAZOLE COMPOUNDS

1. Immunoassays

Immunochemical techniques have widely been applied to the determination of biological macromolecules in clinical analysis. In order to extent the applicability of immunochemical techniques to the analysis of small molecules (haptenes), it is necessary to bind them to a carrier macromolecule, generally a protein, which provides immunogenic activity. Owing to the antigenic activity of the haptene molecules, they are able of selectively rebinding the raised antibodies, and thus can be determined by an immunochemical technique.

Immunoassays are recognized as promising methods for the determination of a wide range of environmental pollutants. Their most important advantages are their high selectivity, rapidity and sensitivity. Taking these into account, numerous immunoassays have been developed for the determination of benzimidazole compounds in a wide range of matrices (i.e. fruits, vegetables, cattle, milk or plasma).

In 1978, Nerenberg et al. [59] determined oxfendazole in plasma and serum samples by means of a radioimmunoassay. However, as benzimidazole compounds do not present immunogenic activity by themselves, coupling of oxfendazole to a polylysine carrier was necessary prior to their inoculation in rabbits. The developed antibodies were successfully applied to the quantification of oxfendazole in bovine, equine and canine plasma and serum samples. The developed methodology was further applied to quantification of oxfendazole in sheep fat tissue [60].

A few years later, Newsome et al. [61] raised a polyclonal antibody against carbendazim by coupling 2-succinaminobenzimidazole to human serum albumin as carrier biomolecule. The antibody was able of selectively rebinding carbendazim in crop samples without the need of any sample clean-up. In order to quantify the amount of benomyl present in these samples, a hydrolysis step of the extracts was performed in an acidic media. Thus, benomyl was quantitatively transformed into carbendazim, and the total amount (benomyl+carbendazim) was analysed by the developed immunoassay. Benomyl content in the samples can further be calculated from the difference between the results obtained after and before acidic hydrolysis of the sample extracts.

Nowadays, the most commonly used immunoassay methods for the determination of benzimidazole compounds in different matrices are based on competitive immunoassays between free and labelled antibodies. Among them, those based on enzyme tracers have provided the most promising results, and thus *enzyme linked immunosorbent assays* (ELISA) have largely taken over radioimmunoassays [11]. In this sense, there have been a number of significant applications of ELISA technology in the area of benzimidazole analysis in recent years. Even if some authors describe the use of polyclonal antibodies for the determination of benzimidazole compounds in vegetable [62] or bovine liver [63] samples, the higher selectivity of most monoclonal antibodies make them a preferable choice, and have thus been used to a much higher extent.

In 1992, Brandon et al. [64] developed a set of monoclonal antibodies able of selectively rebinding thiabendazole and other thiazolyl compounds, i.e. 5-hydroxyhiabendazole and cambendazole. Depending on the antibody's selectivity, thiabendazole alone or the group of thiazolyl benzimidazole compounds could be successfully quantified in bovine liver samples, with a detection limit of 20 ppb by an ELISA competitive immunoassay. Results were validated by comparison with those obtained by HPLC-UV. The stability of the assay materials enabled the preparation of a kit with a shelf life of at least 6 months.

Although initially developed for the analysis of bovine liver samples, these ELISA kits have been successfully applied to the quantification of thiabendazole in vegetable samples. In this sense, quantitative recoveries were obtained in the analysis of several fruits (i.e. orange, grapefruit, banana and apple) [65], potatoes [66], or fruit juices and bulk juice concentrates [67].

In 1994 [68], the same authors prepared a monoclonal antibody which recognised the major benzimidazole compounds and several of their metabolites. The antibody, raised in mice using methyl 5(6)-[carboxypentyl-thio]-2-benzimidazolecarbamate as hapten, was used to develop an ELISA method able of detecting albendazole, fenbendazole, oxfendazole, mebendazole, flubendazole, carbendazim and their metabolites in bovine liver aqueous extracts at concentrations ranging from 1 to 8 ppb.

It was not until 2002 that Brandon et al. [69] developed the first ELISA methodology for the determination of benzimidazole compounds in milk samples. For this purpose, two monoclonal antibodies (MAb 587 and MAb 591), known for their ability to selectively rebind several benzimidazole anthelmintic drugs, were compared for the selectivity of the recognition of fenbendazole, but only MAb 591 proved to be highly selective, with only a 13% cross-reactivity against fenbendazole sulfone. Thus, this antibody was selected as optimum for the determination of fenbendazole in milk samples with a detection limit of 3 μg/L, while MAb 587 was used for the quantification of its major metabolites, with a detection limit of 7 μg/L.

The developed methodology was applied to the pharmacokinetic study of the depletion of fenbendazole and its major metabolites in milk samples. For this purpose, fenbendazole was administered in the forms of feed, drench and paste to three groups of dairy cattle, and milk was collected and analysed immediately after the administration and every 12 hours for the following 5 days. Results obtained by the ELISA methodology using MAb 591 antibody proved that fenbendazole residues were maximum 12-24 hours after its administration, and declined rapidly thereafter. On the other hand, the major metabolites (fenbendazole sulfone and fenbendazole sulfoxide) were successfully quantified by an ELISA methodology using MAb 587 antibody. In this case, maximum concentrations of fenbendazole metabolites in milk samples occurred 24-36 h after exposure to the parent compound and declined gradually. After 72 hours from the administration of fenbendazole to the different groups of dairy cattle, residues of either the parent compound or its metabolites were undetected in the milk samples.

2. Gas Chromatography (GC)

The determination of benzimidazole compounds by gas chromatography generally requires of their derivatization into more volatile compounds prior to their injection in the gas chromatograph. In this sense, only thiabendazole and triclabendazole can be determined by gas chromatography without a previous derivatization step. Depending on the derivatizing reagent used and the kinetics of the process, derivatization can be done either on batch by heating the samples for 30-180 minutes or on-column. It has repeatedly been reported than in most cases a complex mixture of derivatized benzimidazole compounds can be formed [70].

As several variables might influence the selectivity of the derivatization process (reagents involved, benzimidazole type, sample matrix, temperature, time, injection conditions in the gas chromatograph...), the selection of an appropriate derivatization protocol can sometimes be an extremely difficult task. Thus, several procedures should be given a try in order to determine which one fits best for the desired purpose. A brief description of the most commonly used derivatization protocols will be given in the following paragraphs.

In general, most commonly used derivatization mechanisms involve either the methylation or the acylation of the amino and hydroxyl groups, which in some cases must be done after a hydrolysis step of the carbamate residue.

In 1987, Lafuente et al. [34] directly determined thiabendazole in fruits by gas chromatography using both a nitrogen-phosphorus detector and an electron capture detector. Separation on a widebore capillary column (10 m x 0.53 mm) with a silicone bonded phase and detection by NPD enabled a detection limit of 10 μg/kg to be achieved. Similar results were obtained for the determination of thiabendazole in fruits on a fused silica capillary column (25 m x 0.2 mm) [53].

In 1996, Amijee et al. [71] compared different methylating agents for the on-column derivatization of albendazole and oxfendazole. In this sense, different phenyltrimethyl-ammonium and trimethylsulfonium salts were evaluated for the selectivity and efficiency of the methylation process. These authors observed the formation of up to five methylated derivatives when using these methylating agents. Chemical structures of these methylated derivatives are shown in Figure 5.

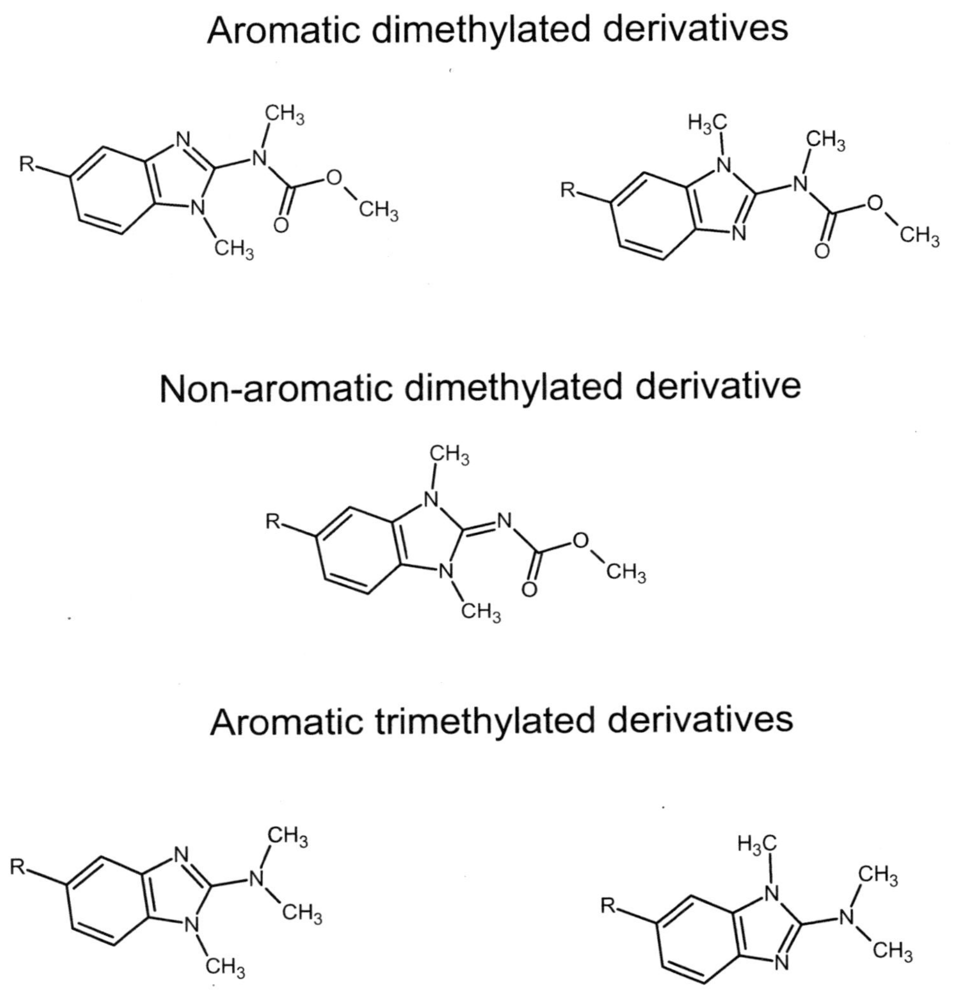

Figure 5. Methylated derivatives of albendazole and oxbendazole [71].

As can be observed from data shown on Table 4, the amount formed of these methylated derivatives depends on several factors, including both the methylating cation and the corresponding counter ion. Thus, highest methylating selectivity for the derivatization of albendazole and oxfendazole was obtained when phenyltrimethylammonium acetate was used as methylating reagent. In this case, yield of the aromatic dimethylated products was higher than 80% for the methylation of both albendazole and oxfendazole. In this case, around 20% of the non-aromatic dimethylated derivative was formed. The use of trimethylsulfonium acetate as methylating reagent also provided satisfactory results in the derivatization of albendazole. This reagent wasn't suitable for the methylation of oxfendazole, as the obtained selectivity in this case was rather poor.

Table 4. Amount formed of methylated derivatives with various methylating reagents

Benzimidazole compound	Methylating reagent	% Aromatic dimethylated derivatives	% Non-aromatic dimethylated derivatives	% Trimethylated derivatives
Albendazole	Methprep	36.81	29.17	34.03
	PTMA-OH	19.63	35.62	44.75
	PTMA-F	50.86	17.14	32.00
	PTMA-CN	59.11	40.89	0.00
	PTMA-OAc	80.65	19.35	0.00
	TMSu-CN	69.36	30.64	0.00
	TMSu-OAc	58.82	41.18	0.00
	TMSuO-OH	79.80	20.20	0.00
	TMSuO-F	82.02	17.98	0.00
	TMSuO-OAc	87.21	12.79	0.00
Oxibendazole	PTMA-F	50.86	17.14	32.00
	PTMA-CN	59.11	40.89	0.00
	PTMA-OAc	80.65	19.35	0.00
	TMSu-CN	60.36	30.64	0.00
	TMSu-OAc	58.82	41.18	0.00

Acylation of benzimidazole compounds is commonly carried out by heating the samples in the presence of pentafluorobenzyl bromide in a basic media. In 1998, Anastassiades et al. [23] successfully used pentafluorobenzyl bromide (PFB-Br) as derivatizing reagent of carbendazim using K_2CO_3 as catalyst. After the addition of PFB-Br, samples were heated at 60°C for three hours. The developed methodology was successfully applied to the quantification of carbendazim in orange juice samples.

Benomyl and thiophanate methyl could also be analysed by this methodology, as long as they are conveniently hydrolysed prior to their extraction from the samples. In this sense, benomyl was transformed into carbendazim by heating the sample at 60°C for 20 minutes at pH 3, while transformation of thiophanate methyl required of the heating of the samples with a saturated solution of K_2CO_3 in acetonitrile. Overall recoveries ranged from 85 to 93%.

In 2007, Liu et al. [72] compared both derivatization mechanisms for the determination of 2-mercaptobenzimidazole in animal tissues by gas chromatography. For this purpose, pentafluorobenzyl bromide and N-methyl-N-(trimethylsilyl)trifluoroacetamide were used as derivatizing reagents. None of them were able of quantitatively derivatize 2-mercaptobenzimidazole on their own, but satisfactory results were obtained for a derivatizing protocol using both reagents. In this sense, a first derivatization step was carried out in the presence of pentafluorobenzyl bromide under strong basic conditions. The acylated 2-mercaptobenzimidazole was subsequently methylated by N-methyl-N-(trimethylsilyl)-trifluoroacetamide. The final product was quantitatively determined by gas chromatography/mass spectrometry, being the detection limit 10 μg/kg.

3. High Performance Liquid Chromatography (HPLC)

HPLC is currently the most widely used technique for the separation and quantification of benzimidazole compounds in environmental and food samples. However, multiresidual separation of a wide range of benzimidazole compounds within a single chromatographic run can be a challenge.

A wide range of detectors have been successfully applied to the quantification of benzimidazole compounds after their chromatographic separation. Among them, UV spectrophotometry and mass spectrometry (MS) are the most commonly used for the analysis of all the benzimidazole compounds. Fluorescent detectors are also suitable for the quantification of albendazole, cambendazole, fenbendazole, thiabendazole, triclabendazole and their metabolites. Additionally, a few papers describe the detection of benzimidazole compounds by amperometric and photometric techniques [11].

Most LC methods for the determination of benzimidazole compounds have been developed using reversed phase columns. For this purpose, mixtures of polar organic solvents such as methanol or acetonitrile with water or buffered solutions can be used in order to separate benzimidazole compounds. Both isocratic and gradient elution modes have been successfully applied to the quantification of benzimidazole compounds in food and environmental samples by reversed phase chromatography.

3.1. Reversed Phase Liquid Chromatography

3.1.1. Isocratic Elution

In 1980, Bogan et al. [73] applied isocratic elution reversed phase chromatography to the quantification of eight benzimidazole compounds for the first time. For this purpose, a C_{18} column was used as stationary phase which enabled the separation of albendazole, fenbendazole and oxfendazole compounds and their major metabolites with a mobile phase consisting on a methanol:ammonium carbonate mixture. A detection limit of 20 μg/L was obtained for the determination of the different benzimidazole compounds in both plasma and blood samples.

In 2002 isocratic elution was applied to the analysis of benzimidazole fungicides in food samples by reversed phase chromatography for the first time. For this purpose, Brito et al. [74] separated carbendazim from other pesticides (captan, chlorotalonil, lufenuron and diafenthurion) by means of a LiChrospher C_{18} column (125x4,6 mm I.D.; 5 μm) with a mobile phase consisting on a methanol:water (70:30 v/v) mixture. Under these conditions, carbendazim eluted from the column in 7.6 min. The recoveries obtained for carbendazim in samples spiked with 0.5-1 mg/kg ranged from 70 to 103 %. The obtained detection limit (0.2 mg/kg) was below the legislated maximum residue limit for coconut samples.

In 2003, Takeba et al. [75] successfully applied isocratic elution reversed phase chromatography to the determination of twelve benzimidazole anthelmintics in livestock food (cattle, pig and chicken muscle, milk and eggs). For this purpose, a Capcell Pak C_{18} column (150x4,6 mm I.D.; 5 μm) was used as stationary phase. A mobile phase consisting in an acetonitrile:0.5 M ammonium acetate (20:80, v/v) was used in the separation of albendazole, mebendazole, oxfendazole, oxibendazole, thiabendazole and 5-hydroxythiabendazole, while an acetonitrile:0.5 M ammonium acetate (40:60, v/v) mobile phase enabled the separation of fenbendazole, flubendazole, parbendazole, triclabendazole and its major metabolites. The mean recoveries obtained for samples spiked with 0.1-0.5 mg/kg ranged from 72.6 to 97.2%, with RSD values below 9%. The detection limits were 0.01-0.05 mg/kg.

3.1.2. Gradient Elution

In 1980, Allan et al. [76] compared isocratic and gradient elution chromatography for the separation of mebendazole and its major metabolites in human plasma by using a SEP PAK C_{18} column. These authors concluded that gradient elution chromatography provided a better resolution, thus minimizing detection limits.

A few years later, Marvin et al. [77] successfully employed gradient elution chromatography to the separation of benomyl, carbendazim, aldicarb and its metabolites in drinking waters. After an on-line preconcentration of the samples by means of a C_8 pre-column, the analytes were eluted and separated in a C_8 column by an acetonitrile:water gradient. Detection limits obtained by the developed methodology ranged from 2.5 to 11 μg/L.

In 2007, Ozhan et al. [78] determined benomyl and carbendazim in the presence of other fungicides (chlorotalonil, folpel, quinomethionate and tetradifon) in surface water. A Luna C_{18} column (250 x 46 mm I.D.; 5 μm) was used for their separation under a gradient elution profile from an aqueous solution of 0.6% ammonia to acetonitrile, after the preconcentration of the samples on a C_{18} cartridge. The mean recoveries obtained for samples ranged from 64 to 97%, with detection limits of 5-25 ng/L.

First application of gradient elution reversed phase chromatography to the determination of benzimidazole compounds in food samples dates from 1997, when LeBoulaire et al. [22] successfully determined thiabendazole and mebendazole in the presence of other veterinary drugs (chloramphenicol, nicarbazin and virginiamycin) in meat samples. A mixture of ammonium acetate (0.01 M, pH 5.2), acetonitrile and methanol was selected as optimum mobile phase. In this sense, a gradient elution from 56:30.8:13.2 (v/v/v) to 36:44.8:19.2 (v/v/v) enabled the baseline separation of the different drugs on a Spherisorb C_{18} column (250x4.6 mm I.D.; 5 μm). Mean recoveries obtained for the quantification of thiabendazole and mebendazole in samples spiked with 0.1-8 ppm ranged from 69 to 102%. Detection limits ranged from 1-2 μg/kg for mebendazole and 9-9.5 for thiabendazole.

Sorensen et al. [49] successfully applied a C_{18} column to the determination of fenbendazole and its major metabolites in trout. In this sense, a gradient elution profile from phosphoric acid (17.5 mM, pH 3):acetonitrile (78.5:21.5 v/v) to phosphoric acid (17.5 mM, pH 3):acetonitrile (20:80, v/v). Mean recoveries obtained for samples fortified with 50-150 mg/kg ranged from 81 to 94%. Detection limits were about 4 μg/kg, thus enabling the determination of fenbendazole and its metabolites in trout samples at concentrations level well below the legislated MRLs.

In 2000, Chonan et al. [79] determined albendazole, thiabendazole and its major metabolite (5-hydroxythiabendazole) in the presence of other veterinary drugs in meat, liver, kidney and milk samples. The analytes were separated in a CapCell Pak C_{18} column (150 x 4.6 mm; 5 μm) by using a mobile phase consisting on a mixture of an aqueous phosphate buffer (0.1% pH 7.0) (mobile phase A) and acetonitrile (mobile phase B). In order to achieve baseline resolution of all the analyzed veterinary drugs, a gradient elution profile from 90:10 (A:B, v/v) to 50:50 (A:B, v/v) was performed. Under these conditions, mean recoveries for samples fortified at the 0.1 mg/kg level ranged from 72 to 100%. Detection limits achieved by the developed methodology were of 5-50 μg/kg.

A few years later, Su et al. [80] analysed albendazole, thiabendazole, mebendazole and their major metabolites in muscle, liver and milk samples by gradient reversed phase chromatography. For this purpose, a Cosmosil 5-C_{18} M-II column (250 x 4.6 mm I.D.; 5 μm) was used as stationary phase and a mobile phase consisting on a mixture of 0.02 M sodium dihydrogen phosphate (pH 3.3, mobile phase A) and acetonitrile (mobile phase B). A gradient from 90:10 (A:B, v/v) to 30:70 (A:B, v/v) in 19 minutes enabled the baseline separation of all the benzimidazole compounds. Average recoveries for samples fortified at 0.05-2.50 mg/L were of 71.4-104.3%, depending on the analyte. A detection limit of 5-30 ng/L was obtained.

De Ruyck et al. [81] used a C_{18} column (150 x 2.1 mm I.D.; 5 μm) for the determination of thiabendazole, oxfendazole, oxibendazole, albendazole, fenbendazole, febantel, triclabendazole, levamisole and tetrahydroimidazole in milk samples. A gradient from 0.1% formic acid:acetonitrile (65:35, v/v) to (25:75, v/v) enabled the baseline separation of all the benzimidazole anthelmintics in 11 minutes. Mean recoveries for samples fortified with 5-150 μg/L ranged from 79.9 to 109.3%, with detection limits of 1.1-1.4 μg/L.

3.2. Ionic Pair Liquid Chromatography

The addition of ion pair forming agents as octane sulphonate or tetrabutylammonium to the mobile phase can sometimes render satisfactory results in the separation of benzimidazole compounds within a C_{18} reversed phase LC column [11].

First application of ion pair liquid chromatography to the separation of benzimidazole compounds dates from 1992, when Negro et al. [82] determined triclabendazole's metabolites in plasma and urine samples. For this purpose, 1 mM sodium decanesulphonate was added as ion pair forming agent to a 0.05 phosphate buffer (pH 7.0):acetonitrile (55:45, v/v) mobile phase. Under these conditions, baseline separation of triclabendazole sulfone and triclabendazole sulfoxide was achieved in a C_{18} column. Mean recoveries for samples spiked with 0.1-9 mg/L of both triclabendazole sulfone and triclabendazole sulfoxide ranged from 90.2 to 91.7%. The detection limit in both plasma and urine samples was of 10 μg/L.

A few years later, Botsoglou et al. [83] investigated the effect of the addition of different ion-pair agents to the separation of fenbendazole and oxfendazole by using C_{18} as stationary phase and 0.01 phosphoric acid:acetonitrile (75:25, v/v) mobile phase. In this sense, the addition of an anionic pair forming agent as octane sulphonate increased the retention times in a very high acidic media (pH < 3.7), while the use of a cationic pair forming agent as tetrabutyl ammonium decreased the retention times in a very high acidic media (pH < 3.7). No changes in retention times were observed for higher pH values. Optimum results were obtained when adding octane sulphonate pH 2.2.

In 1996, Fletouris et al. [31] extended the afore optimized conditions to the screening analysis of benzimidazole residues in milk samples. The developed methodology enabled the separation of albendazole and its metabolites (albendazole 2-aminosulfone, albendazole sulfoxide and albendazole sulfone), fenbendazole and its metabolites (oxfendazole, p-hydroxyfenbendazole and fenbendazole sulfone), mebendazole and oxibendazole in milk samples, with overall recoveries ranging from 79 to 100%.

The method was further improved by the simultaneous addition of octane sulfonate and tetrabutyl ammonium to the mobile phase. In this sense, Fletouris et al. [84] used a Nucleosil C_{18} stationary phase for the separation of albendazole's major metabolites in animal tissues (muscle, fat, liver and kidney). 2.5 mM tetrabutylammonium and 5 mM octane sulfonate were added as ion-pairing agents to a 0.01 M phosphoric acid:acetonitrile (75:25, v/v) mobile phase. Under these conditions, albendazole sulfone, albendazole-2-aminosulfone and albendazole sulfoxide could be baseline separated in less than 12 minutes. Mean recoveries obtained for samples fortified at 0.5-1280 μg/kg ranged from 76.8 to 109.6%. Detection limits obtained were 6-14 μg/kg for albendazole sulfoxide, 0.2-0.4 μg/kg for albendazole 2-aminosulfone and 0.10-0.15 μg/kg for albendazole sulfone.

In 2000, de Ruyck et al. [32] employed gradient elution for the ion-pair liquid chromatographic separation of fenbendazole, thiabendazole, albendazole, oxibendazole and levamisole in milk samples on a C_{18} column. In this case, the mobile phase consisted on a mixture of a phosphoric acid buffer solution (pH 3.5) containing 0.01 M octane sulphonate (mobile phase A), acetonitrile (mobile phase B) and water (mobile phase C). Gradient elution from 80:20 (A:B, v/v) to 50:50 (A:B, v/v) and then to 50:50 (C:B, v/v) enabled the baseline separation of all the evaluated benzimidazole compounds in milk samples with recoveries ranging from 68 to 85%. Detection limits obtained were of 1.4-6.9 μg/L.

In 2004, Prousalis et al. [85] determined carbendazim, thiabendazole and o-phenylphenol residues in lemon samples by ion pair HPLC. Baseline separation of the analytes was performed on a Supelcosil C_{18} (250 x 4.6 mm I.D.; 5 μm) with a mobile phase consisting on acetonitrile:water:ammonia (39:60.5:0.5 v/v/v). Average recoveries obtained for lemon samples fortified at the 1-5 mg/kg ranged from 81.1 to 106%. Detection limits obtained were below 50 μg/kg, thus enabling the quantification of carbendazim, thiabendazole and o-phenylphenol residues at concentration levels below the legislated MRLs.

3.3. Normal Phase Liquid Chromatography

Most apolar benzimidazole compounds can successfully be separated on a silica stationary phase. In this sense, Karlaganis et al. applied normal phase LC to the determination of mebendazole and its metabolites in plasma samples [86] in 1979 using a mixture of acetonitrile, chloroform-saturated water and formic acid (44.7:55.1:0.2, v/v/v) as mobile phase.

In 1984, Alvinerie et al. [87] separated albendazole from its major metabolites on a silica column using an hexane:ethanol (89:11, v/v) mixture as mobile phase. The method was successfully applied to the determination of albendazole, albendazole-sulfone and albendazole-sulfoxide in sheep plasma samples.

3.4. Cation Exchange Chromatography

A strong cation exchanger resin has sometimes been successfully applied to the separation of benzimidazole compounds in an acidic media. In this sense, Kirkland et al. [27]

determined benomyl, carbendazim and 2-aminobenzimidazole in soil and plant tissues. The separation by strong cation exchange chromatography in a Zipax SCX (100 x 2.1 mm; 5 μm) column using a 0.025 M tetramethylammonium nitrate solution as mobile phase at 60°C enabled the analysis of benomyl and its major metabolites in a single analytical run for the first time.

A few years later, Arenas et al. [88] separated thiabendazole and 5-hydroxythiabendazole in raw milk samples by means of strong cation exchange chromatography. Recoveries ranged from 96-115% for samples fortified at 0.5-2 mg/L level.

3.5. Liquid Chromatography on Selective Stationary Phases

A considerable effort has been invested in recent years in the development of new stationary phases able of selectively interacting with the target analytes. In this sense, the introduction of crown ether modified silica stationary phases, cyclodextrins, immobilized antibodies or molecularly imprinted polymers (MIPs), has considerable facilitated the analysis of pesticides in complex samples, since the higher selectivity of these materials doesn't require of such an extensive clean-up step of the sample's extracts prior to their analysis.

Turiel et al. developed an imprinted material towards thiabendazole [89] using methacrylic acid as functional monomer, divinylbenzene as cross-linker, azo-bis-isobutyronitrile as initiator and an acetonitrile:toluene (3:1, v/v) mixture as porogenic solvent. Batch rebinding studies were initially performed in order to confirm if the polymer had conveniently been imprinted. In this sense, comparison of the results obtained for the rebinding of thiabendazole on the imprinted polymer and a non-imprinted polymer prepared in a similar manner but in absence of the template molecule (thiabendazole), showed a very high degree of selectivity in the rebinding of thiabendazole by the MIP, thus demonstrating the efficiency of the imprinting process.

The imprinted polymer particles were then packed in a LC stainless steel column (40 x 4.6 mm). After removal of the template molecule by flushing a methanol:acetic acid (1:1, v/v) mixture overnight, different mobile phases were evaluated in order to achieve a selective retention of thiabendazole within the imprinted polymer. In this sense, even if both methanol and acetonitrile successfully separated thiabendazole from matrix components, retention times were much lower in case of using methanol, and thus this solvent was selected. In order to minimize peak tailing commonly observed when using high affinity stationary phases as MIPs in a liquid chromatographic system, the addition of increasing amounts of acetic acid was subsequently evaluated. The optimum conditions for the separation of thiabendazole from matrix interfering component were the elution with 100% MeOH, and a switch to a MeOH:HAc (80:20, v/v) after 2.4 minutes.

The developed methodology was successfully applied to the quantification of thiabendazole in citrus, strawberry and grape samples, with recoveries ranging from 88.7 to 102.4% and detection limits of 0.01 mg/kg. As no previous sample clean-up was required, a very high sample throughput could easily be achieved.

4. Capillary Electrophoresis (CE)

Capillary electrophoretic techniques are very promising tools for the determination of pesticide residues in food and environmental samples because of the high separation efficiencies, the short analysis time and the very low consumption of both reagents and hazardous solvents. Also, its capability to conduct analysis in a miniaturized format enables the development of microchips that can be easily adapted to the routine analysis of a wide range of hazardous pesticides.

In principle, capillary electrophoresis was restricted to the separation of charged analytes within an electrostatic field. The development of micellar electrokinetic chromatography in 1984 [90] and capillary electrochromatography in 1987 [91], enabled the separation of neutral compounds, thus considerably pushing forward the application of capillary electrophoretic techniques.

Even if most benzimidazole compounds can be protonated in a very high acidic media (pH < 4), most of their separations by capillary electrophoretic techniques have been carried out by micellar electrokinetic chromatography in a neutral buffered solution. In this sense, MEKC has been successfully applied to the quantification of benzimidazole fungicides in vegetables, fruits and fruit juices, or in water samples.

First determination of a benzimidazole compound by capillary electrophoresis dates from 1997, when Wu et al. [92] quantitatively analyzed carbendazim present in grain samples with a 40 mM phosphate buffer (pH 7.0) containing 60 mM sodium dodecyl sulfate. Obtained recoveries for samples fortified with 0.1-1.0 mg/kg carbendazim ranged from 82.6 to 94.6%, with detection limits of 0.05 mg/kg.

In the same year, Penmetsa et al. [93] compared the performance of capillary zone electrophoresis and micellar electrokinetic chromatography for the separation of carbendazim, metalaxyl, propiconazole and vinclozolin in lake water samples. The analysed fungicides could only be conveniently separated by means of MEKC using a 10 mM sodium phosphate:methanol (90:10, v/v) buffer containing 100 mM sodium cholate. Average recoveries obtained for a lake water sample spiked with 4 μg/L of each fungicide ranged from 42 to 87%.

In 2000, Molina et al. [94] developed an analytical methodology based on micellar electrokinetic chromatography for the determination of carbendazim in fruit juices in the presence of other commonly used fungicides (metalaxyl, captan, procymidone, folpet, captafol, vinclozolin and iprodione) at trace levels. Sensitivity of the method is considerably enhanced by using an on-column enrichment by high-salt stacking, thus enabling detection limits in the range of a few μg/L. The developed methodology enables quantitative recovery of all the analysed fungicides in fruit juices, and is thus proposed for routine analysis of these samples.

A few years later, Segura et al. [95] applied micellar electrokinetic chromatography to the analysis of neutral pesticides of environmental impact. In this sense, separation of thiabendazole, carbendazim, naphthalene acetamide, carbaryl and 1-naphthol were baseline separated in less than 10 minutes using a 30 mM ammonium chloride/ammonia buffer (pH 9.0) electrolyte containing 15 mM sodium dodecyl sulphate. The developed methodology was successfully applied to the determination of the afore mentioned pesticides in cucumber samples with recoveries ranging from 90.1 to 110.2%. Detection limits obtained under these conditions were of 0.2-1.1 mg/L.

In 2003, da Silva et al. [96] developed a MEKC methodology for the separation of carbendazim from other commonly used pesticides as atrazine, simazine, propazine, ametryn, diuron, linuron, carbaryl and propoxur. In this sense, an electrolyte composed of 20 mM phosphate buffer (pH 2.5):methanol (90:10, v/v) containing 25 mM sodium dodecyl sulphate enabled the baseline separation of the pesticides in less than 6 minutes. The developed methodology was successfully applied to the quantification of several pesticides in drinking water and carrot samples, with detection limits of 2-46 μg/L.

Kaltsonoudis et al. [97] developed a capillary zone electrophoretic method for the quantification of carbendazim and thiabendazole in citrus samples. For this purpose, the authors used an electrolyte consisting on 50 mM phosphate (pH 3.0) buffer:acetonitrile (1:2, v/v). The developed methodology enabled the quantitative recovery of both benzimidazole fungicides from lemon samples, being the detection limits below 2.3 mg/L.

In 2004, Takeda et al. [98] developed a capillary zone electrophoretic technique for the simultaneous separation and on-line enrichment of amitrole, carbendazim, 2-aminobenzimidazole, thiabendazole and 1,2-diaminobenzene in distilled water and acid samples by using different formic acid/ammonium formate (pH 4.0) electrolytes. The concentration factors achievable by sample stacking in the presence of formic acid were in the range of 7.6-27 fold.

In capillary electrochromatography, the mobile phase is moved through a stationary phase by means of an electric field, thus combining the principles of HPLC and capillary electrophoresis. In this sense, separation of charged compounds within the capillary is due to both their different electrophoretic mobility in a strong electric field and their different partition between the mobile and the stationary phases. On the other hand, separation of neutral compounds in an electric field is made possible due to their different affinities for both the mobile and stationary phases.

In 2008, Cacho et al. [18] developed a non-aqueous capillary electrochromatographic methodology for the determination of benzimidazole compounds in citrus samples. The high selectivity inherent to imprinted materials was exploited to prepare different monolithic stationary phases capable of selectively rebinding thiabendazole in lemon and orange samples by using an acetonitrile mobile phase containing 4% (w/v) citric acid. The developed methodology enabled the determination of thiabendazole in crude sample extracts, without the need for any previous sample clean-up. Mean recoveries obtained for samples spiked in the 1–15 mg/kg ranged from 85 to 105%. The detection limits achieved by this method ranged from 0.04 to 0.05 mg/Kg.

SUMMARY

As can be observed, a wide range of analytical methodologies have been successfully applied to the determination of benzimidazole compounds in environmental and food samples. Tables 5–7 comprise the extraction, clean-up, enrichment and determination methods used for the determination of benzimidazole compounds in these samples.

Table 5. Analytical methodologies used for the determination of benzimidazole compounds in water samples

Benzimidazole	Clean-up & enrichment	Determination	Reference
Carbendazim	Solid phase extraction	HPLC	[17]
Carbendazim	Solid phase extraction	HPLC	[38]
Carbendazim	Liquid-liquid extraction Solid phase extraction	HPLC	[40]
Benomyl, fuberidazole, thiabendazole	Solid phase extraction	HPLC Fluorescence	[41,42]
Benomyl, carbendazim, fuberidazole, thiabendazole	Solid phase extraction	HPLC	[43]
Benomyl, carbendazim, fuberidazole, thiabendazole	Solid phase extraction	HPLC	[44]
Benomyl, carbendazim	Solid phase extraction	HPLC	[77,78]
Carbendazim	On-line stacking	CE	[96]
Carbendazim, thiabendazole	On-line stacking	CE	[98]

Table 6. Analytical methodologies used for the determination of benzimidazole compounds in fruit and vegetable samples

Benzimidazole	Extraction method	Clean-up & enrichment	Determination	Reference
Thiabendazole	Sonication with acetonitrile	None	CE	[18]
Benomyl, carbendazim, thiophanate methyl	Supercritical fluid extraction	None	GC HPLC	[23]
Benomyl	Blend with ethyl acetate	Liquid-liquid extraction	Fluorescence	[25]
Benomyl	Blend with ethyl acetate	Liquid-liquid extraction	Colorimetric analysis	[26]
Benomyl, carbendazim, 2-aminobenzimidazole	Blend with ethyl acetate	Liquid-liquid extraction	HPLC	[27]
Benomyl, carbendazim, 2-aminobenzimidazole	Blend with ethyl acetate	Liquid-liquid extraction	GC	[28]
Benomyl, carbendazim, thiabendazole	Blend with acidified ethyl acetate	Liquid-liquid extraction	GC	[29]

Table 6. Continued

Benzimidazole	Extraction method	Clean-up & enrichment	Determination	Reference
Thiabendazole	Extraction in hexane-ethyl acetate	Solid phase extraction	GC	[34]
Benomyl, carbendazim, thiabendazole, thiopahante methyl	Reflux in HCl	Liquid-liquid extraction	HPLC	[36]
Benomyl, carbendazim, thiabendazole, thiopahante methyl	Reflux in HCl	Liquid-liquid extraction	HPLC	[37]
Thiabendazole	Extraction in NaOH	Solid phase extraction	GC	[53]
Carbendazim, thiabendazole	Blending with acetone	Liquid-liquid extraction Solid phase extraction	HPLC	[54]
Thiabendazole	Sonication with ethyl acetate	Solid phase extraction	HPLC	[55,56]
Thiabendazole	Soxhlet with methanol	None	Immunoassay	[65-67]
Carbendazim	Solid phase extraction	Solid phase extraction	HPLC	[74]
Carbendazim, thiabendazole	Extraction with acidified acetonitrile	Solid phase extraction	HPLC	[85]
Thiabendazole	Sonication with acetonitrile	None	HPLC	[89]
Carbendazim	Solid phase extraction	Solid phase extraction On-line stacking	CE	[94]
Thiabendazole, carbendazim	Homogenized with acetone	Liquid-liquid extraction	CE	[95]
Carbendazim, thiabendazole	Extraction in ethyl acetate	Liquid-liquid extraction	CE	[97]

Table 7. Analytical methodologies used for the determination of benzimidazole compounds in meat, liver and milk samples

Benzimidazole	Extraction method	Clean-up & enrichment	Determination	Reference
Mebendazole, thiabendazole	Matrix solid phase dispersion	None	HPLC	[22]
Albendazole, fenbendazole, mebendazole, flubendazole, oxibendazole, thiabendazole, metabolites	Supercritical fluid extraction	Liquid-liquid extraction Solid phase extraction	HPLC	[24]
Fenbendazole, oxfendazole	Sonication with methanol:water	Liquid-liquid extraction	HPLC	[30]
Albendazole, fenbendazole, mebendazole, oxibendazole	Shake with ethyl acetate	Liquid-liquid extraction	HPLC	[31]
Albendazole, fenbendazole, oxibendazole, thiabendazole	Shake with acetonitrile: Ethyl acetate	Liquid-liquid extraction	HPLC	[32]
Mebendazole	Blend in ethyl acetate	Solid phase extraction	HPLC	[45,47]
Fenbendazole, metabolites	Blend in ethyl acetate	Solid phase extraction	HPLC	[46]
Fenbendazole, metabolites	Blend in acetonitrile-hexane	Solid phase extraction	HPLC	[49]
Fenbendazole	Extraction in ethyl acetate	Solid phase extraction	Voltammetry	[51]
Thiabendazole, cambendazole, metabolites	Extraction in dimethyl sulfoxide:H_2O	None	Immunoassay	[64]
Albendazole, carbendazim, fenbendazole, flubendazole, mebendazole, oxfendazole	Extraction in dimethyl formamide:H_2O	None	Immunoassay	[68]
Fenbendazole, metabolites	Sonication with water	None	Immunoassay	[69]
Albendazole, fenbendazole, mebendazole, oxfendazole, thiabendazole, metabolites	Extraction in acetonitrile-hexane	Solid phase extraction	HPLC	[75]

Table 7. Continued

Benzimidazole	Extraction method	Clean-up & enrichment	Determination	Reference
Albendazole, thiabendazole, metabolites	Homogenize with acetonitrile	Solid phase extraction	HPLC	[79]
Albendazole, mebendazole, thiabendazole, metabolites	Extracted with acetonitrile	Liquid-liquid extraction Solid phase extraction	HPLC	[80]
Albendazole, fenbendazole, oxfendazole, thiabendazole, triclabendazole, metabolites	Extraction with ethyl acetate	Liquid-liquid extraction	HPLC	[81]
Albendazole, metabolites	Shake with ethyl acetate	Liquid-liquid extraction	HPLC	[84]
Thiabendàzole, metabolites	Extraction with ethyl acetate	Solid phase extraction	HPLC	[88]

REFERENCES

[1] McKellar, QA; Scott, EW. The benzimidazole anthelmintic agents-A review. *Journal of Veterinary Pharmacology and Therapeutics*, 1990, 13, 223-247.

[2] http://www.emea.europa.eu/pdfs/vet/mrls/Oxfendazole1.pdf, available on-line on July 2008.

[3] Delatour, P; Lorgue, G; Courtot, D; Lapras, M. Embryotoxic and antimitotic properties of parbendazole, mebendazole and cambendazole. *Comptes Rendus Herbomadaires des Seances de L Academie des Sciences Serie D*, 1976, 282, 517-518.

[4] Delatour, P; Debroye, J; Lorgue, G; Courtot, D. Experimental embryotoxicity of oxfendazole in rat and sheep. *Recueil de Medicine Veterinarie*, 1977, 133, 639-645.

[5] Bogan, JA; Marriner SE. *Albendazole in helminthiasis*. 1st edition. London: Royal Society of Medicine; 1984.

[6] http://www.emea.europa.eu/pdfs/vet/mrls/026897en.pdf, available on-line on July 2008

[7] Froyman, R; de Keyser, H. Flubendazole – Safety regarding egg production and reproductive performance on breeder chickens. *Avian Diseases*, 1983, 27, 43-48.

[8] Seiler, JP. Toxicology and genetic effects of benzimidazole compounds. *Mutation Research*, 1975, 32, 151-167.

[9] Main, DC; Vass, DE. Cambendazole toxicity in calves. *Australian Veterinary Journal*, 1980, 56, 237-238.

[10] Delatur, P; Parish R. *Drug residues in animals*. 1st edition. Orlando: Academic Press Inc.; 1989.

[11] Danaher, M; De Ruyck, H; Crooks, S.R.H.; Dowling, G; O'Keeffe, M. Review of methodology for the determination of benzimidazole compounds in biological matrices. *Journal of Chromatography B – Analytical Technologies in the Biomedical and Life Sciences*, 2007, 845, 1-37.
[12] Nose, N; Kobayashi, A; Tanaka, A; Hirose, A; Watanabe, A. Determination of thiabendazole by electron capture gas – liquid chromatography after reaction with pentafluorobenzyl chloride. *Journal of Chromatography*, 1977, 130, 410-413.
[13] Halko, R; Sanz, CP; Ferrera, ZS; Rodriguez, JJS. Determination of benzimidazole fungicides in soil samples using microwave assisted micellar extraction and liquid chromatography with fluorescence detection. *Journal of AOAC International*, 2006, 89, 1403-1409.
[14] Singh, SB; Foster, GD; Khan, SU. Determination of thiophanate methyl and carbendazim residues in vegetable samples using microwave assisted extraction. *Journal of Chromatography A*, 2007, 1148, 152-157.
[15] Singh, SB; Foster, GD; Khan, SU. Microwave assisted extraction for the simultaneous determination of thiamethoxam, imidacloprid and carbendazim residues in fresh and cooked vegetable samples. *Journal of Agricultural and Food Chemistry*, 2004, 52, 105-109.
[16] Zhang, W; Tempest, P. Highly efficient microwave assisted fluorous Ugi and post-condensation reactions for benzimidazoles and quinoxalinones. *Tetrahedron Letters*, 2004, 45, 6757-6760.
[17] Hogendoorn, EA; Westhuis, K; Dijkman, E; Heusinkveld, EAG; Chamkrasul, P; Biadul, P; Baumann, RA; Cornelese, AA; van der Linden, MA. Determination of carbendazim in water, soil and sediment samples by RPLC with and without column switching and various spectrophotometric detection modes. *International Journal of Environmental Analytical Chemistry*, 2000, 78, 67-85.
[18] Cacho, C; Schweitz, L; Turiel, E; Perez-Conde C. Molecularly imprinted capillary electrochromatography for selective determination of thiabendazole in citrus samples. *Journal of Chromatography A*, 2008, 1179, 216-223.
[19] Blasco, C; Font, G; Pico, Y. Analysis of pesticides in fruits by pressurized liquid extraction and liquid chromatography – ion trap – triple stage mass spectrometry. *Journal of Chromatography A*, 2005, 1098, 37-43.
[20] Pawlowski, TM; Poole, CF. Extraction of thiabendazole and carbendazim from foods using pressurized hot (subcritical) water for extraction. A feasibility study. *Journal of Agricultural and Food Chemistry*, 1998, 46, 3124-3132.
[21] Lehotay, SJ; Lee, CH. Evaluation of fibrous cellulose drying agent in supercritical fluid extraction of diverse pesticides. *Journal of Chromatography A*, 1997, 785, 313-327.
[22] LeBoulaire, S; Bauduret, JC; Andre, F. Veterinary drug residues survey in meat: An HPLC method with a matrix solid phase dispersion extraction. *Journal of Agricultural and Food Chemistry*, 1997, 45, 2134-2142.
[23] Anastassiades, M; Schwack, W. Analysis of carbendazim, benomyl, thiophanate methyl and 2,4-dichlorophenoxyacetic acid in fruits and vegetables after supercritical fluid extraction. *Journal of Chromatography A*, 1998, 825, 45-54.

[24] Danaher, M; O'Keefe, M; Glennon, D. Development and optimisation of a method for the extraction of benzimidazoles from animal liver using supercritical carbon dioxide. *Analytica Chimica Acta*, 2003, 483, 313-324.

[25] Pease, HL; Gardiner, JA. Fluorometric and colorimetric procedures for determining residues of benomyl. *Journal of Agricultural and Food Chemistry*, 1969, 17, 267-270.

[26] Pease, HL; Holt, RF. Improved method for determining benomyl residues. *Journal of the Association of Official Analytical Chemists*, 1971, 54, 1399.

[27] Kirkland, JJ; Holt, RF; Pease, HL. Determination of benomyl residues in soils and plant tissues by high speed cation exchange liquid chromatography. *Journal of Agricultural and Food Chemistry*, 1973, 21, 368-371.

[28] Pyysalo, H. A rapid gas – liquid chromatographic method for determining benomyl residues in foods. *Journal of Agricultural and Food Chemistry*, 1977, 25, 995-997.

[29] Tjan, GH; Jansen, JTA. Gas-liquid chromatographic determination of thiabendazole and methyl-2-benzimidazole carbamate in fruits and crops. *Journal of the Association of Official Analytical Chemists*, 1979, 62, 769-773.

[30] Blanchflower, Cannavan, A; Kennedy, DG. Determination of fenbendazole and oxfendazole in liver and muscle using liquid chromatography – mass spectrometry. *Analyst*, 1994, 119, 1325-1328.

[31] Fletouris, DJ; Botsoglou, Psomas, IE. Mantis, AI. Rapid quantitative screening assay of trace benzimidazole residues in milk by liquid chromatography. *Journal of AOAC International*, 1996, 79, 1281-1287.

[32] De Ruyck; van Renterghem, R; de Ridder, H.; de Brabander, D. Determination of anthelmintic residues in milk by high performance liquid chromatography. *Food Control*, 2000, 11, 165-173.

[33] Bushway, J; Young, BES; Paradis, LR; Perkins, LB. Determination of methyl-2-benzimidazolecarbamate in bulk fruit juice concentrates by competitive inhibition enzyme immunoassay. *Journal of AOAC International*, 1994, 77, 1237-1243.

[34] Lafuente, MT; Tadeo, JL; Tuset, JJ. GCL analysis of thiabendazole in citrus fruit. *Journal of Chromatographic Science*, 1987, 25, 84-87.

[35] Corti, P; Dreassi, E; Politi, N; Aprea, C. Comparison of an HPTLC and HPLC procedure for the determination of chloroprofam, propham and thiabendazole residues in potatoes. *Food Additives and Contaminants*, 1991, 8, 607-616.

[36] Farrow, JE; Hoodless, RA; Sargent, M; Sidwell, JA. Fungicide residues 6: Determination of residues of post – harvest fungicides on citrus fruit by high performance liquid chromatography. *Analyst*, 1977, 102, 752-758.

[37] Gilvydis, DM; Walters, SM. Ion – pairing liquid chromatographic determination of benzimidazole fungicides in foods. *Journal of the Association of Official Analytical Chemists*, 1990, 73, 753-761.

[38] JunkerBuchheit, A; Witzenbacher, M. Pesticide monitoring of drinking water with the help of solid phase extraction and high performance liquid chromatography. *Journal of Chromatography A*, 1996, 737, 67-74.

[39] Shimamura, Y; Tomiyama, N; Murakoshi, M; Kobayashi, H.; Matano, O. Multiresidue method of pesticides in water using automated solid phase extraction and liquid

chromatography atmospheric pressure chemical ionization mass spectrometry. *Journal of Pesticide Science*, 1998, 23, 241-249.

[40] Jeannot, R; Sabik, H; Sauvard, E; Gessin, E. Application of liquid chromatography with mass spectrometry combined with photodiode array detection and tandem mass spectrometry for monitoring pesticides in surface waters. *Journal of Chromatography A*, 2000, 879, 51-71.

[41] Zamora, DP; Vidal, JLM; Galera, MM; Frenich, AG; Gonzalez, JLL; Arahal, MR. Correction of predicted concentration in the use of solvent – based calibration lines for determining carbendazim, fueridazole and thiabendazole in water after a SPE step. *Talanta*, 2003, 60, 335-344.

[42] Frenich, AG; Zamora, DP; Vidal, JLM; Galera, MM. Standardization of SPE signals in multicomponent analysis of three benzimidazolic pesticides by spectrofluorimetry. *Analytica Chimica Acta*, 2003, 477, 211-222.

[43] Halko, R; Sanz, CP; Ferrera, Z.S.; Rodriguez, JJS. Determination of benzimidazole fungicides by HPLC with fluorescence detection after micellar extraction. *Chromatographia*, 2004, 60, 151-156.

[44] Moral, A; Sicilia, MD; Rubio, S; Perez-Bendito, D. Sodium dodecyl sulphate – coated alumina for extraction / preconcentration of benzimidazolic fungicides from natural waters prior to their quantification by liquid chromatography / fluorimetry. *Analytica Chimica Acta*, 2006, 569, 132-138.

[45] Steenbaar, JG; Hajee, CAJ. High performance liquid chromatographic determination of the anthelmintic mebendazole in eel muscle tissue. *Journal of Chromatography – Biomedical Applications*, 1993, 615, 186-190.

[46] Iosifidou, EG; Haagsma, N. High performance liquid chromatographic determination of fenbendazole and its metabolites, sulphoxide and sulphone, in fish muscle tissue. *Journal of Liquid Chromatography & Related Technologies*, 1996, 19, 1819-1830.

[47] Hajee, CAJ; Haagsma, N. Liquid chromatographic determination of mebendazole and its metabolites, aminomebendazole and hydroxymebendazole, in eel muscle tissue. *Journal of AOAC International*, 1996, 79, 645-651.

[48] Cooper, AD; Creaser, CS; Farrington, WHH; Tarbin, JA; Shearer, G. Development of multi-residue methodology for the HPLC determination of veterinary drugs in animal tissues. *Food Additives and Contaminants*, 1995, 12, 167-176.

[49] Sorensen, LK; Hansen, H. Determination of fenbendazole and its metabolites in trout by a high performance liquid chromatographic method. *Analyst*, 1998, 123, 2559-2562.

[50] B. Sellergren, *Molecularly Imprinted Polymers: Man-Made Mimics of Antibodies and their Application in Analytical Chemistry,* 1st edition, Amsterdam: Elsevier, 2001.

[51] De Prada, AGV; Loaiza, OA; Serra, B; Morales, D; Martinez-Ruiz, P; Reviejo, AJ; Pingarron, JM. Molecularly imprinted polymer solid phase extraction coupled to square wave voltammetry at carbon fibre microelectrodes for the determination of fenbendazole in beef liver. *Analytical and Bioanalytical Chemistry*, 2007, 388, 227-234.

[52] Aharonson, N; Ben-Aziz, A. Determination of residues of benomyl, its hydrolysis product and thiabendazole in various crops. *Journal of the Association of Official Analytical Chemists*, 1973, 56, 1330-1334.

[53] Oishi, M; Onishi, K; Kano, I; Nahazawa, H. Capillary gas chromatographic determination of thiabendazole in citrus and apple juices. *Journal of AOAC International*, 1994, 77, 1293-1296.

[54] Hiemstra, M; Joosten, JA; DeKok, A. Fully automated solid phase extraction clean-up and on-line liquid chromatographic determination of benzimidazole fungicides in fruit and vegetables. *Journal of AOAC International*, 1995, 78, 1267-1274.

[55] Arenas, RV; Johnson, NA. Liquid chromatographic fluorescence method for the determination of thiabendazole residues in green bananas and banana pulp. *Journal of AOAC International*, 1994, 77, 710-713.

[56] Arenas, RV; Rahman, H; Johnson, NA. Determination of thiabendazole residues in whole citrus fruits by liquid chromatography with fluorescence detection. *Journal of AOAC International*, 1996, 79, 579-582.

[57] Young, MS; Philips, DJ; Iraneta, PC; Krol, J. Mixed – mode solid phase extraction and clean-up procedures for the liquid chromatographic determination of thiabendazole and carbendazim in fruit juices. *Journal of AOAC International*, 2001, 84, 556-561.

[58] Young, MS; Early, MF; Mallet, CR; Krol, J. Application of a mixed – mode solid phase extraction and clean-up procedure for LC/MS determination of thiabendazole and carbendazim in apple juice. *Journal of AOAC International*, 2001, 84, 1608-1613.

[59] Nerenberg, C; Bunkel, RA; Matin, SB. Radioimmunoassay of oxfendazole in bovine, equine or canine plasma or serum. *Journal of Pharmaceutical Sciences*, 1978, 67, 1553-1557.

[60] Nerenberg, C; Tsina, I; Matin, SB. Radioimmunoassay of oxfendazole in sheep fat. *Journal of Association of Official Analytical Chemists*, 1982, 65, 635-639.

[61] Newsome, WH; Shields, JB. A radioimmunoassay for benomyl and methyl-2-benzimidazolecarbamate on food crops. *Journal of Agricultural and Food Chemistry*, 1981, 29, 220-222.

[62] Newsome, WH; Collins, PG. Enzyme linked immunosorbent assay of benomyl and thiabendazole in some foods. *Journal of Association of Official Analytical Chemists*, 1987, 70, 1025-1027.

[63] Johnson, L; Baster, GA; Crooks, SRH; Brandon, DL; Elliot, CT. Reduction of sample matrix effects – The analysis of benzimidazole residues in serum by immunobiosensor. *Food and Agricultural Immunology*, 2002, 14, 209-216.

[64] Brandon, DL; Binder, RG; Bates, AH; Montague, WC. A monoclonal antibody – based ELISA for thiabendazole in liver. *Journal of Agricultural and Food Chemistry*, 1992, 40, 1722-1726.

[65] Brandon, DL; Binder, RG; Bates, AH; Montague, WC. Competitive ELISA of thiabendazole residues in produce using indirectly immobilized monoclonal antibodies. *Food and Agricultural Immunology*, 1995, 7, 99-108.

[66] Brandon, DL; Binder, RG; Wilson, RE; Montague, WC. Analysis of thiabendazole in potatoes and apples by ELISA using monoclonal antibodies. *Journal of Agricultural and Food Chemistry*, 1993, 41, 996-999.

[67] Bushway, RJ; Brandon, DL; Bates, AH; Li, L; Larkin, KA; Young, BS. Quantitative determination of thiabendazole in fruit juices and bulk juice concentrates using a

thiabendazole monoclonal antibody. *Journal of Agricultural and Food Chemistry*, 1995, 43, 1407-1412.

[68] Brandon, DL; Binder, RG; Bates, AH; Montague, WC. Monoclonal antibody for multiresidue ELISA of benzimidazole anhelmintics in liver. *Journal of Agricultural and Food Chemistry*, 1994, 42, 1588-1594.

[69] Brandon, DL; Bates, AH; Binder, RG; Montague, WC. Analysis of fenbendazole residues in bovine milk by ELISA. *Journal of Agricultural and Food Chemistry*, 2002, 50, 5791-5796.

[70] Knapp, DR; *Handbook of Analytical Derivatization Reactions*. 1st edition. New York: Wiley, 1979.

[71] Amijee, M; Cheung, J; Wells, RJ. Direct on – column derivatization in gas chromatography II. Comparison of various on – line methylation reagents and the development of a new selective methylation reagent. *Journal of Chromatography A*, 1996, 738, 43-55.

[72] Liu, Y; Zou, QH; Xie, MX; Han, J. A novel approach for simultaneous determination of 2-mercaptobenzimidazole and derivatives of 2-thiouracyl in animal tissue by gas chromatography / mass spectrometry. *Rapid Communications in Mass Spectrometry*, 2007, 21, 1504-1510.

[73] Bogan, JA; Marriner, S. Analysis of benzimidazoles in body fluids by high performance liquid chromatography. *Journal of Pharmaceutical Sciences*, 1980, 69, 422-423.

[74] Brito, NM; Navickiene, S; Polese, L; Jardim, EFG; Abakerli, RB; Ribeiro, ML. Determination of pesticide residues in coconut water by liquid – liquid extraction and gas chromatography with electron – capture plus thermoionic specific detection and solid phase extraction and high performance liquid chromatography with ultraviolet detection. *Journal of Chromatography A*, 2002, 957, 201-209.

[75] Takeba, K; Fujimuna, K; Sakamoto, M; Jimbo, K; Oka, H; Ito, Y; Nakazawa, H. Determination of benzimidazole anthelmintics, in livestock foods by HPLC. *Journal of the Food Hygienic Society of Japan*, 2003, 44, 246-252.

[76] Allan, RJ; Goodman, HT; Watson, TR. Two high performance liquid chromatographic determinations for mebendazole and its metabolites in human plasma using a rapid Sep Pak C_{18} extraction. *Journal of Chromatography*, 1980, 183, 311-319.

[77] Marvin, CH; Brindle, ID; Hall, CD; Chiba, M. Rapid on – line precolumn high performance liquid chromatographic method for the determination of benomyl, carbendazim and aldicarb species in drinking water. *Journal of Chromatography*, 1991, 555, 147-154.

[78] Ozhan, G; Alpertunga, B. Determination of various fungicides in water by LC-DAD analysis. *Fresenius Environmental Bulletin*, 2007, 16, 880-886.

[79] Chonan, T; Nishimura, K.; Hirama, Y. Rapid determination of residues of five kinds of veterinary drugs in livestock products by HPLC. *Journal of the Food Hygienic Society of Japan*, 2000, 41, 326-329.

[80] Su, SC; Chang, CL; Chang, PC; Chou, SS. Simultaneous determination of albendazole, thiabendazole, mebendazole and their metabolites in livestock by high performance liquid chromatography. *Journal of Food and Drug Analysis*, 2003, 11, 307-319.

[81] De Ruyck, H; Daeseleire, E; de Ridder, H; van Renterghem, R. Development and validation of a liquid chromatographic – electrospray tandem mass spectrometry multiresidue method for anthelmintics in milk. *Journal of Chromatography A*, 2002, 976, 181-194.

[82] Negro, A; Alvarez-Bujidos, ML; Ortiz, AI; Cubria, JC; Mendez, R; Ordonez, D. Reverse phase ion – pair high performance liquid chromatographic determination of triclabendazole metabolites in serum and urine. *Journal of Chromatography*, 1992, 576, 135-141.

[83] Botsoglou, NA; Fletouris, DJ; Psomas, IE; Vassilopoulos, VN. Chromatographic behaviour of the anthelmintic fenbendazole and its major metabolite oxfendazole in various ion – pair liquid chromatographic systems. *Journal of Liquid Chromatography*, 1994, 17, 4229-4243.

[84] Fletouris, DJ; Papapanagioutou, EP; Nakos, DS; Psomas, IE. Highly sensitive ion pair liquid chromatographic determination of albendazole marker residue in animal tissues. *Journal of Agricultural and Food Chemistry*, 2005, 53, 893-898.

[85] Prousalis, KP; Polygenis, DA; Syrokou, A; Lamari, FN; Tsegenidis, T. Determination of carbendazim, thiabendazole, and o-phenylphenol residues in lemons by HPLC following sample clean-up by ion – pairing. *Analytical and Bioanalytical Chemistry*, 2004, 379, 458-463.

[86] Karlaganis, G; Munst, GJ; Bircher, J; Burkhardt, B; Eckert, J. Determination of the anthelmintic drug mebendazole in plasma. *Experientia*, 1979, 35, 950.

[87] Alvinerie, M; Galtier, P. Simultaneous determination of albendazole and its principal metabolites in plasma by normal phase high performance liquid chromatography. *Journal of Pharmaceutical and Biomedical Analysis*, 1984, 2, 73-79.

[88] Arenas, RV; Johson, NA. Liquid chromatographic fluorescence method for multiresidue determination of thiabendazole and 5-hydroxythiabendazole in milk. *Journal of AOAC International*, 1995, 78, 642-646.

[89] Turiel, E; Tadeo, JL; Cormakc, PAG; Martin-Esteban, A. HPLC – imprinted stationary phase prepared by precipitation polymerisation for the determination of thiabendazole in fruit. *Analyst*, 2005, 130, 1601-1607.

[90] Terabe, S.; Otsuka, K. Ichikawa, K; Tsuchiya, A; Ando, T. Electrokinetic separations with micellar solutions and open – tubular capillaries. *Analytical Chemistry*, 1984, 56, 111-113.

[91] Knox, JH; Grant, IH. Miniaturisation in pressure and electroendoosmotically driven liquid chromatography: Some theoretical considerations. *Chromatographia*, 1987, 24, 135-143.

[92] Wu, YS; Lee, HK; Li, SFY. Determination of carbendazim residues in grains by solid phase extraction and micellar electrokinetic chromatography with ultraviolet detection. *Journal of Chromatographic Science*, 1997, 35, 513-518.

[93] Penmetsa, KV; Leidy, RB; Shea, D. Separation of fungicides by micellar electrokinetic capillary chromatography. *Electrophoresis*, 1997, 18, 235-240.

[94] Molina, M; Silva, M. Rapid determination of fungicides in fruit juices by micellar electrokinetic capillary chromatography: Use of organic modifiers to enhance

selectivity and on – column high – salt stacking to improve sensitivity. *Electrophoresis*, 2000, 21, 3625-3633.

[95] Segura, A; Cruces-Blanco, C; Cortacero, S; Carrasco, A. Application of micellar electrokinetic capillary chromatography to the analysis of uncharged pesticides of environmental impact. *Journal of Agricultural and Food Chemistry*, 2004, 52, 5791-5795.

[96] Da Silva, CL; de Lima, EC; Tavares, MFM. Investigation of preconcentration strategies for the trace analysis of multi-residue pesticides in real samples by capillary electrophoresis. *Journal of Chromatography A*, 2003, 1014, 109-116.

[97] Kaltsonoudis, CK; Lamari, FN; Prousalis, KP; Karamanos, NK; Tsegenidis, T. Analysis of carbendazim and thiabendazole in lemons by CE-DAD. *Chromatographia*, 2003, 57, 181-184.

[98] Takeda, S; Fukushi, K; Chayama, K; Nakayama, Y; Tanaka, Y; Wakida, S. Simultaneous separation and on-line concentration of amitrole and benzimidazole pesticides by capillary electrophoresis with a volatile migration buffer applicable to mass spectrometric detection. *Journal of Chromatography A*, 2004, 1051, 297-301.

In: Fungicides
Editors: P. De Costa and P. Bezerra

ISBN: 978-1-60692-631-4

Chapter XI

DISAPPEARANCE OF FUNGICIDES IN FRESH AND PROCESSED AGRICULTURAL PRODUCTS. INFLUENCE OF THE ELABORATION TECHNIQUES

Paula Payá*[*]*, José Oliva and Alberto Barba

Dpt. Agricultural Chemistry, Geology and Pedology, Faculty of Chemistry, University of Murcia. Campus Espinardo, 30100 Murcia, Spain

ABSTRACT

The use of fungicides on vegetable and fruit crops has reached significant levels in areas of intensive agriculture, both for consumption as fresh and those aimed at processed foods (chilled, frozen, canned, beer and wine).

From an environmental point of view, there are numerous studies in order to ascertain specific concentration levels of pesticide residues in different ecosystems, as well as their degradation, metabolism, mobility, etc. However, the field studies, designed specifically to meet their dynamics of disappearance in habitual conditions of farming, are made only for registration purposes and are less known.

The persistence of pesticides in field is directly influenced by weather conditions (temperature and solar radiation) and these are of great importance in the dissipation of residues in the case of raw vegetable ingestion. However, it should be pointed that there are manipulation and manufacturing processes that can suppose positive effects on the dissipation of pesticide residues, such as washing and blanching in the freezing process, peeling and sterilization in the can manufacture; fermentation and filtering in the beer and wine elaboration, etc.

In this chapter, we will present data on the field dissipation and influence of the manufacturing processes in the disappearance of fungicides belonging to different classes (penconazole, procymidone, metalaxyl, thiram, mancozeb, cyprodinil, fludioxinil,

[*] E-mail: paulapp@um.es; Tel.: 0034968367473; Fax: 0034968364148

quinoxyfen, azoxystrobin, etc.) present at food agricultural products. These studies were carried out on vegetables matrices such as pepper, tomato, celery, broccoli, lettuce, apricot, peach, grape, barley, etc.

The studies analyzed show that basic processes in the manufacture of plant origin foods decrease the initial concentration in the treated crop. Thus, washing and blanching in the freezing of leafy vegetables and *Solanaceae* decrease the concentration of the fungicides studied. The peeling and thermal treatment to obtain canned stone fruit and fruit juices produce considerable elimination of the initial residues. And last, oenotechnological processes made during the wine-making manage the total elimination of fungicides residues initially present in the grapes in some cases.

The data obtained from these studies allow the determination of the so-called "transfer factor", regarded as the percentage of increase or decrease in the residue concentration in processed foods. These factors would provide significant data for inclusion in the annexes of Regulation 396/2003 of the European Union which states that when no maximum residue levels are established for processed foods, those for raw foods must be applied, considering the specific factors of concentration or dilution in the transformation processes.

INTRODUCTION

In spite of the fact that pesticide use has declined in recent years, today it is the only effective means to combat pests and diseases and thus ensure the quantity, quality and regularity of agricultural production. As a result of their use, consumers show their great concern over the risk to health that can be leaded by the presence of residues of these products in foods of plant origin that they consume daily. Besides that, the environmental education of today's society involves increasing awareness of contamination particularly in soils and waters and generally in ecosystems caused by the misuse of pesticides [Berry, 1991; Hamilton, 2002].

The maximum residue level (MRL) for each crop and pesticide defines the maximum amount permitted so that the residue presence does not suppose health hazards to consumers. Therefore, its establishment by the competent authorities, the conducting of surveillance plans and the estimated intake calculations are means of control that ensures the health quality and hygiene of agricultural production. However, one of the possible causes of alarm in consuming population of agricultural products are the results of evaluations carried out in specific cases that illustrate MRL violation as direct consequence of pesticide application [Johnston, 1991].

Currently, the modernization of farming systems and consequently the best training of farmers and agricultural technicians coupled with the widespread use of Good Agricultural Practices (GAP), alongside the rise of alternative pest and disease control (useful fauna, pheromones, growth regulators and biotechnology) have meant more rational use of plant protection within the concept of sustainable agriculture [Bellapart, 1996; Jimenez Diaz and Lamo de Espina, 1998].

The presence of pesticide residues in agricultural products derived solely from the treatment plant made during its growing season producing an initial deposit which depends on the dose used, pesticide nature [Roberts and Hudson, 1999], formulation type [Liu et al.,

1996], application system [Henrieta et al., 2006; Cabizza et al., 2007] and plant morphology and type (surface/weight relation and surface type) [Reynolds et al., 2005], harvest position on plant and weather conditions. Once the application is practiced and the deposit produced on the plant, the amount of pesticide is decreasing gradually over time. Its greater or lesser disappearance rate is influenced by the plant substrate, the number of treatments [Ebbert et al., 1999], application time [Henrieta et al., 2005] and pesticide physicochemical properties. But also, pesticide deposited on the plant may be subjected to dissipation processes due to mechanical causes (rain and wind), physical ones (volatilization, temperature and wind), chemical ones (chemical stability of the molecule, light, temperature and pH) or metabolic own plant factors (hydrolysis, redox reactions, etc.) [Seib, 1985; South et al., 2000; Sckidmore and Ambrus, 2004].

This disappearance in field is associated with pseudo first-order kinetics represented by a curve with two distinct stages. The first one, which usually runs for the first few days, corresponds to the stage of physical and chemical degradation, and the second one, which is slower than the other, is the persistence stage where the metabolic degradation prevails [Timme et al, 1986; Morton et al., 2001]. Although this kinetic model remains in most cases, we can find differences in behavior since this process is intimately related to pesticide-plant duality.

An important factor in reducing pesticide residues in agricultural products once collected is the manipulation to which can be subjected during industrial processes of fresh marketing, processing and preservation as well as in domestic handling or cooking. Processes such as washing, peeling, blanching, sterilization, freezing and conservation in modified atmosphere can significantly reduce the residue levels present in the original products. But we must also bear in mind that the transformation process can affect the nature of residues, changing their identity and forming new chemical substances called neo-residues, of which we must know their toxicological significance. Normally, the mechanical processes (washing, peeling, squeezing and mechanical extraction by pressing) do not produce changes in the chemical nature of the fungicide active molecules. Nevertheless, fermentation and thermal processes can cause alterations in the active molecules. In the latter, chemical reactions of hydrolysis and pyrolysis mainly occur. Also, there could be some enzymatic reactions but they are unlikely because the heat treatments inactivate enzymes. In general, though some isolated cases of more toxic neo-residue formation than the original active substance have been reported during the heat processing, substances that may occur are harmless or less toxic in most cases [Holland et al., 1994; Timme and Walz-Tylla, 2004; Chavarri et al., 2005; Coscollá and Coscollá, 2006].

Another problem that we can find in plant food processing is that there is a concentration of residues and not reduction. This can happen in processing when taking certain parts of the plant product where residues are or where the highest residue concentration is, i.e. products from citrus peel, olive oil or essential oils from citrus fruit, where affinity between the physical-chemical substance extracted and lipophilic fungicides takes place during the extraction [Somogyi et al., 1996; Cabras et al., 1997].

The study of greater or lesser reduction intensity of pesticide residues in these processes takes on greater importance in the manufacture of baby foods because of the increased sensitivity of children to the presence of these toxics. An important evidence of this issue are the restrictive European Union Directives relating to baby foods such as 91/321 and 96/5 which indicate that food for infants and young children must not contain any substance in such quantity as to may pose a threat to children health. Other subsequent Directives (99/39 and 99/50) establish a provisional MRL at 0.01 mg/kg for any food product prepared for babies. Lastly recent Directives (2003/14 and 2003/13) set specific MRLs for various pesticides ranging between 0.003 and 0.008 mg/kg. As far as we are increasingly reaching limits claiming that baby food is completely free of pesticide residues. This is the case of the Directive 2006/125 which regulates the pesticides that cannot be used in crops intended for children's products.

Also important is the influence that the processes of fermentation, clarification, filtration and chemical and microbiological stabilization have on the disappearance of pesticides present in raw materials led to the manufacture of fermented alcoholic beverages (wine and beer) [Oliva and Beard, 2002; Ruediger et al., 2004; Fernandez et al., 2005a and 2005b; Miyake et al., 1999 and 2002].

However, currently there is no legislation on the MRLs allowed for these processed products and we must use those established for the fresh product. Therefore, it is extremely interesting to know the percentages that each elimination process can produce in the various pesticide-crop combinations. These percentages express the term known as transfer factor which can be defined as the ratio between the residue concentration in the processed food and that in the original product.

Most studies, which have been conducted on this field, have been aimed at knowing the behavior of the group of insecticides due to the most toxicological risk to consumers. The use of these synthetic chemical pesticides is constantly decreasing, while there is an increase in the use and the emergence of new molecules with antifungal activity. For these reasons we consider the field and processing dissipation study of the most widely used fungicides in different crops absolutely interesting. This chapter presents the results obtained in these work lines by different research groups including ours.

Dissipation of Fungicides in Crops

The large number of factors affecting the dissipation of pesticides in crops has been amply highlighted by several authors who have studied the behavior of these products in field experiences. Specially, there is no common pattern of behavior in the case of fungicides finding different dissipation kinetics depending on the chemical family to which the studied fungicide belongs and the crop to which it is applied on.

In a study of the degradation of triazolic fungicides (cyproconazole, hexaconazole, penconazole, propiconazole and tebuconazole) in peach during the time period defined by its pre-harvest interval, all with the exception of propiconazole reached levels exceeding the MRLs and showing high stability in this fruit. The fruit weight increase during growing was considered as the main factor in the apparent elimination of residues. The experimental models show that the codistillation and photodegradation are the main mechanisms in the disappearance of the triazols studied [Angioni et al., 2003].

Penconazole, which is a fungicide widely used to combat powdery mildew, presents different behavior on vegetables and fruits. It maintained levels 2.5 times below the MRL in pepper (0.20 mg/kg) from the first day of application, marking a total persistence but at this so low level throughout the experience (12 days), with no degradation stage and a final value of 0.04 mg/kg [Barba et al., 2000a]. However, it does not reach values below their MRL in the case of zucchini, (0.10 mg/kg) even when the pre-harvest interval (PHI) time is over, introducing also first order kinetics with linear regression, which does not conform to an exponential equation (without stage of degradation). The residue value is 0.24 mg/kg at 21 days [Barba et al., 2000a]. The differences observed for both crops may be due mainly to the characteristics of the crop and the application because the zucchini is uncovered at soil level and its initial charge is higher, despite having used the same rate of application. In tomato, the residue was twice its MRL at the day of its application (0.1 mg/kg) but it was already below the MRL 3 days after the treatment and it maintained residue levels below its limit of determination (0.05 mg/kg) at the 14th day. Its kinetics presents a clear stage of degradation during the first 3 days (70% decreasing from baseline) [Barba, 2001]. When used in fruit, particularly in apricot, it left residues below its MRL (0.1 mg/kg) at the application day, displaying exponential kinetics with strong persistence in a range of less than 0.01 mg/kg. By contrast, it maintained levels slightly above the MRL (0.1 mg/kg) in peach during the first 3 days of the trial (latency period) and then presents exponential kinetics for dissipation, virtually disappearing when the PHI finishes (14 days) [Barba et al., 2000b]. Finally, it remains above its MRL (0.2 mg/kg) in table grapes until the end of its PHI (21 days) [Barba, 2001]. When used in wine grapes, penconazole has an initial value below the MRL, 0.14 versus 0.20 mg/kg, having 79% dissipation at 28 days with a half-life time of 12 days [Navarro et al., 2001]. Other studies on this and other fungicides of the family of triazols report that the residue values were about 0.02 mg/kg after 6 days of its application because its susceptibility to photodegradation, among other factors [Schwack and Hartman, 1994]. However, there are differences in half-life time for cyproconazole and penconazole because both are systemic and are quickly absorbed by the grape tissues but cyproconazole has a half-life time of 4 days [Papadopoulou-Mourkidou et al, 1995] and penconazole of 12 days.

Metalaxyl, phenylamide with systemic action and widely used in controlling mildew, left initial residues 7 times higher than its MRL in a field experience conducted on broccoli (0.1 mg/kg) reaching the MRL after 7 days of application and presenting kinetics with two distinct stages but not very pronounced. On the first 14 days further degradation appeared but slower degradation or persistence phenomenon took place from that time until the end of the experience [Barba et al., 2000c]. In zucchini, this fungicide is coming to its MRL (0.1 mg/kg) within the PHI reaching levels 19 times higher than this limit on the day of its application [Barba et al., 2000c]. Its behavior is similar to penconazole in tomato, though being from different families, reaching values lower than its limit of determination after 7 days (0.05 mg / kg) [Barba, 2001]. Finally, in the case of table grapes, only sample from the first day exceeded the MRL (2 mg / kg) [Barba, 2001].

Metalaxyl had a half-life time of 8.3 days and a reduction percentage of 89% at 28 days in a study supervised on wine grapes, reaching residue levels of 0.10 ± 0.04 mg/kg at that time, well below its MRL (1 mg/kg) allowed under the law [Navarro et al., 2001]. In other studies conducted over 6 years in several countries in various doses, the intervals and the number of applications indicate that these fungicide residues in wine grapes ranged between 0.06 and 4.40 mg/kg after 4 weeks, while were among 0,032 and 2.60 mg/kg at 6 weeks. This great variability in the content of residues is due mainly to climatic conditions and usually the lowest values are found in drier areas. Experimental values showed that residues found after 3 weeks of treatment ranged between 0.06 and 1.3 mg/kg in countries like Spain, Italy and Australia, whereas they varied between 0.34 and 6.8 mg/kg in Germany [Cabras et al, 1987]. This corroborates the idea that the degradation is higher in areas of low and warm water regime as the Mediterranean countries [Coscollá, 1996a]. Degradation of some products cause rapid decline of their residues in grapes. In this sense, we find that cymoxamil residue concentration is 0.23 mg/kg and declines to 0.05 mg/kg after 8 days when 8 applications have been carried out and sample taken immediately after the last one [Belasco et al., 1981].

Within the family of dicarboximidic fungicides we have the use of procymidone in pepper, widely accepted to control *Botrytis*. This presents a level of 18% of its MRL after the first day of application and only 10% of its initial value after its PHI, then having degradation just over 75% in the first 3 days of experience [Barba et al., 2000a].

Another dicarboximidic fungicide is vinclozolin. It was studied in wine grapes showing that the residue level was below the MRL allowed in the legislation 7 days after the treatment being the residue level approximately 10% of its MRL (5 mg/kg) at the end of its PHI (21 days) [Navarro et al., 2001]. This residue value is intermediate between those found by researchers in various other studies for the same application rate and the same length of time elapsed since treatment. Thus, Lemperle et al. when studying the degradation of vinclozolin and two other dicarboximidic fungicides (iprodione and procymidone) over three years (1978-1980) found values in the range of 0.6-1.5 mg/kg for vinclozolin and slightly higher for iprodione (0.7-2.0 mg/kg) and procymidone (1.7-3.8 mg/kg) [Lemperle et al., 1982]. However, Gennari et al. in a study conducted in four Italian regions found that the levels ranged between 0.11 and 0.70 mg/kg at the 26th day of the treatment [Gennari et al., 1985]. In Spain but especially in Catalonia, the degradation of this anti-*Botrytis* has also been studied well by Giralt et al. In 1991 and 1992, they observed that 1 month after its application, the levels were respectively 0.87 and 0.59 mg/kg for vinclozolin reaching dissipation rates of the order of 85.3% in the first year and 84.9% in the second one [Giralt et al., 1991, 1992]. Lastly, Garcia Cazorla and Xirau conducted a study in the vineyards in Penedés (Northeastern Spain) to determine what concentrations of vinclozolin and other anti-*Botrytis* fungicides were accumulated in grapes 30 days after the treatment and found that the level was 0.37 ± 0.06 mg/kg for vinclozolin [García Cazorla and Xirau, 1994].

Data obtained in different European countries and in New Zealand and South Africa indicate that, the levels of vinclozolin can range between 0.6 and 9.3 mg/kg after 14 days of treatment and decline to 0.4-5.1 mg/kg after 30 days [WHO / FAO, 1982]. The half-life time of vinclozolin ranges 1.2 to 4.6 days [Gennari et al, 1985]. From the available data, it appears to be strong influence of external factors (weather, grape variety, number of treatments, etc.) on the decline percentage and residue levels found and especially the lowest residue concentrations are found in the warmer and dried areas [Cabras et al, 1987].

Other experiments with dichlofuanid or dicarboximidic fungicides show the low residue levels found in grapes when the product is applied correctly and PHI observed [Brandolini et al, 1979; Cabras, 1995]. Studies on the accumulation of iprodione, procymidone and vinclozolin in grapes, found concentrations of 1.01, 0.78 and 0.37 mg/kg, respectively, after 3 treatments made at intervals of 1 month with the corresponding trade formulations [García Cazorla and Xirau, 1994]. Other works showed the rapid dissipation of pesticides in grapes even when higher doses than the recommended were used. For example, the half-life time of cyproconazole ranged 3-4 days [Papadopoulos et al., 1995].

Thiram, which belongs to the family of dithiocarbamates, presents certain similarity in the late residue levels in stone fruits such us apricot and peach and lemon fruit, although there are differences between their dissipation kinetics. Studying this in depth, its MRL (3 mg/kg) was exceeded in apricot even at the PHI (14 days) and the dissipation kinetics were linear with two distinct stages as a latency period of 4 days and degradation until the PHI was over [Barba et al., 2000a]. In peach, this fungicide presented levels more than twice its MRL (3 mg/kg) during the first two days after treatment, remaining thereafter below its MRL until the end of the PHI. Its kinetics followed the classic exponential model there [Barba et al., 2000b]. Finally, the level of thiram exceeded 30 times its MRL in lemon on the day of application (0.1 mg/kg) but dropped 50% on the following day and reaching levels 7 times higher than its MRL at the end of the PHI time [Barba, 2001]. In tomato, the level of the fungicide product was less than its MRL (0.1 mg/kg) 21 days after the application [Barba, 2001].

Another dithiocarbamate widely used in wine grapes is mancozeb. It is one which suffers minor degradation and presents longer half-life time (13.5 days), although this value is less than the range of 28-35 days cited in other studies [Ripley et al., 1978]. Anyway, the residue levels found were 0.22 mg/kg at 28 days of treatment and were well below its MRL (5 mg/kg expressed as S_2C) [Navarro et al., 2001]. In this same crop and after the use of maneb, the residue concentration exceeded this limit in some countries like Germany and reached levels between 6.1-6.8 mg/kg in France. By contrast, the highest level of residues found in Spain for the same fungicide is of 2.1 mg/kg [Coscollá, 1996b].

Another fungicide widely used on vegetables is chlorothalonil which is commonly applied to celery causing residue levels below its MRL (10 mg/kg) from the first day of treatment and presenting almost linear kinetics with two-day latency period [Barba et al., 2000c].

Cyprodinil and fludioxonil, which are usually applied in the same formulation, presented residue values below their MRLs since the first day of application in table grapes [Barba, 2001]. When these two fungicides were studied in tomatoes, greenhouse crops together with azoxystrobin and pyrimethanil was found that their residues were below the MRLs during the time period corresponding to their PHI except for cyprodinil. The mechanism of disapperearance studied with model system showed that decrease in residues was due to photodegradation and codistillation in pyrimethanil, to fotodegradation in fludioxonil, and to evaporation and codistillation in cyprodinil. Azoxystrobin residues were stable during all experiments [Garau et al., 2002].

The evolution of cyprodinil and fludioxonil in lettuce indicated that residues of both were between 9-10 times below its MRL (2 mg/kg for both products) under conditions of GAP. Similar behaviors appeared in the table grape crop [Marin et al., 2003].

Fenarimol, belonging to the pyrimidinyl carbinol fungicides with systemic action and effects of prevention, treatment and eradication against powdery mildew in wine grapes, showed a residue level of 0.06 mg/kg after 28 days representing 33% of the value of its MRL (0.2 mg/kg) [Navarro et al., 2001]. The value of 0.06 mg/kg is similar to that obtained in other studies [Dagne et al, 1991] on Barbera grapes in the area of Piedmont in Italy. The reduction percentage throughout the study was 91%, this being higher in the final stage and much smaller in the first one. Its half-life time was 7.8 days [Navarro et al., 2001].

Kresoxim-methyl and tetraconazole, both fungicides newly marketing and used in viticulture, did not leave detectable residue in berries 21 days after their application. Others like azoxystrobin, fluazinam and mepanipyrim did appear in grape sample [Cabras et al., 1998]. Kresoxim-methyl, cyprodinil, difenoconazole and thiram were not detected since the time of their application in apples var. Golden [Ticha et al., 2007].

In an experience where pyrimethanil was applied in table grapes var. Italy, it was found that its levels were below the MRL immediately after treatment. The fungicide presented a half-life time of 12 days according to pseudo first-order kinetics [Angoini et al., 2006]. Another study, conducted with this fungicide but on tomato crop showed that residues of pyrimethanil decreased by half and reached its limit of detection at 5.7 and 13.7 days after application, respectively [Sadler, 2002].

Azoxystrobin, which is within the group of strobilurin fungicides, when applied to table grapes showed levels below the MRL (2 mg/kg) at 0, 15 and 21 days after the application [Lentz-riz et al., 2006].

Under field conditions, spiroxamine dissipation on grapes var. Roditis and Cabernet Sauvignon was master during the first 2 weeks and then slower to the sixth week. About 7 days alter application, half of the initial concentration spiroxamine remained on the grapes being the respective proportion about 10% at the 42nd day. At the 14 and 35 days, the residues levels were 0.44 and 0.22 mg/kg, respectively, both below the MRL set by the European Union (1 mg/kg) [Tsiropoulos et al., 2005].

When the field treatment is made with quinoxyfen, which is a very novel fungicide in controlling powdery mildew, a concentration of 0.38 mg/kg (less than its MRL established at 0.5 mg/kg) was found in grapes collected after applying the product. Fourteen days later, the residue levels fell to 0.09 mg/kg [Cabras et al., 2000].

It can be ensured that the agricultural use of fungicides, conducted under criteria of good agricultural practice or GAP usually does not cause the presence of residues exceeding the MRLs in fruits or vegetables. In the cases discussed in this chapter in which residue values exceeded these limits, application under critical conditions (no observation of PHIs, non-recommended doses, etc.) have been used in. The disappearance kinetics of the referred fungicides followed models experimentally reviewed in supervised field trials aimed at contrasting the pesticide dissipation in plant products.

Elimination of Pesticides in Industrial Processes

The washing is usually the first operation carried out in any industrial processing of fruits and/or vegetables. This so simple operation can produce significant removals of plant protection products generally and fungicides particularly. The greater or lesser elimination depends on several factors [Holland et al., 1994; Timme and Walz-Tylla, 2004]:

a) The nature or type of fungicide. The contact action ones suffer higher removal because the pesticide is found on the surface of the plant product, while the elimination is low or zero in the penetrating and/or systemic action ones because the product is inside the fruit. Also important is the polarity of the fungicide and its solubility in water. The higher the values of these characteristics, the easier their elimination is. But, we must remember that most fungicides are not very water-soluble.
b) Features of the formulation. The presence of adherents diminishes the elimination of the active ingredient.
c) Morphology of the plant product. Because of morphological characteristics such as the fruit surface, there is a greater removal in plant products with a smooth surface rather than rough. The shape of fruit (leaves, bracts, stems, etc.) is crucial in eliminating by washing as well because the entire surface of the fruit can be accessed or not depending on its form, i.e. more elimination in apples, nectarines and peaches than in artichokes, lettuce, etc. Also, the presence of chemical compounds on the surface as essential oils or waxes decreases the elimination because of the non-polar nature of pesticides.
d) Period since the application. The percentage of elimination is less by the increasing time since the treatment as it will eventually produce partial penetration of residues in the plant tissues.
e) Type and intensity of the washing. The use of detergents, the increase of water temperature and changes in pH levels below or above 7 produce more elimination of fungicide residues that the drinking water at room temperature. Another factor to consider is the length of washing and whether it occurs in continuous or discontinuous manner. The longer duration and continually, the greater elimination of residues is. Adding mechanical agitation to the washing and even brushing the fruit are also important for removing higher percentage of plant protection products. Although, we must bear in mind that commonly used fungicides are mainly eliminated by mechanical effect towed by water, since they are low water soluble.

As we note, there are several factors influencing the elimination of fungicides by washing the plant product. Thus, it is very difficult to determine an average rate of elimination and we find in various studies that levels of declining may be different because it is very complicated that two studies use the same conditions, both in the pattern of water used and the intensity of mechanical drag and processing time. As examples and guidance indications of the quantitative importance that this industrial process can have on the disappearance of fungicide residues from different families, sets of the values of dissipation found for different processes in washing are shown in Table 1 and 2 for vegetables and fruits, respectively.

Some studies under GAP and most unfavourable conditions called as CAP by us, in which harvest is at the same day of treatment, have been conducted for certain fungicides.

Another basic operation in obtaining lots of processed vegetables is the peeling of the fresh product. The peeling can be manually or through chemical peeling. The last consists of removing the skin of the fruit by the use of chemicals, especially NaOH in low concentrations. Also, the consumption of some fresh products without industrial processing is usually a result of peeling, although the uptake of that product unpeeled can provide nutrients and fiber that are very essential to the daily diet.

During the manual peeling, contact fungicides are removed together with the peel. In the case of pervasive and systemic ones, the elimination is much lower, since greater proportion is inside the fruit. When performing a chemical peeling, the highest percentage of elimination is produced by altering the active molecule by changing the pH and also by the effect of temperature, since this kind of process is carried out at temperatures between 60-80 °C.

Table 1. Elimination of fungicides in the washing process of vegetables

Vegetable	Fungicide	% of elimination	Reference
Tomato	Chlorothalonil	89	Sances et al., 1992
	Chlorothalonil	94	Holland et al., 1994
	Thiram	13 (CAP)	Barba, 2001
	Penconazole	16 (CAP)	Barba, 2001
	Metalaxyl	16 (CAP)	Barba, 2001
	Dithiocarbamates	57	Chavarri et al., 2005
Pepper	Penconazole	100 (GAP)-50(CAP)	Barba et al., 2000a
	Procymidone	25 (GAP)-8 (CAP)	Barba et al., 2000a
Celery	Chlorothalonil	85(GAP)-95(CAP)	Barba et al., 2000c
Broccoli	Metalaxyl	25 (CAP)	Barba et al., 2000c
Potato	Thiabendazole	90	Petersen et al., 1996
	Thiabendazole	75-90	JMPR, 1977
Lettuce	Fludioxonil	81-86	Gamón et al., 2006a
	Cyprodinil	19-51	Gamón et al., 2006a
	Procymidone	59-63	Gamón et al., 2006a
	Folpet	85-95	Gamón et al., 2006a
	Iprodione	60	Gamón et al., 2006a
	Metalaxyl	38	Gamón et al., 2006a
Zucchini	Metalaxyl	20 (GAP)-18 (CAP)	Barba et al., 2000a
	Penconazole	25 (GAP)-70 (CAP)	Barba et al., 2000a
Asparagus	Dithiocarbamates	47	Chavarri et al., 2005
Spinach	Dithiocarbamates	100	Chavarri et al., 2205
Cauliflower	Captan	0	Fernández et al., 2006

In the case of fruits for fresh consumption that have a thick peel, which is not traditionally edible, there is nearly complete elimination of pesticide residues. In consequence, the peeling of citrus fruits eliminate fungicides residues totally, since most penetrate into the cells of essential oils because of its lipid solubility and are found in the peel and are not transferred to the pulp. Other fruits with high elimination can be bananas, pineapples, kiwi, mangoes, avocados etc. [Holland et al., 1994] and various fruiting vegetables which are usually peeled (melon, watermelon, cucumbers and pumpkins).

Table 2. Elimination of fungicides in the washing process of fruits

Fruit	Fungicide	% of elimination	Reference
Orange	2-phenylphenol	0	Reynolds, 1996
	Imazalil	20-40	Reynolds, 1996
	Thiabendazole	10-30	Reynolds, 1996
Strawberry	Captan	28	Drieghe et al., 1996
	Carbendazim	60	Drieghe et al., 1996
	Dithiocarbamates	33	Drieghe et al., 1996
	Folpet	55	Drieghe et al., 1996
	Procymidone	45	Drieghe et al., 1996
	Vinclozolin	23	Drieghe et al., 1996
	Tolyfluanid	37	Christensen y Granby. 2002
	Fenhexamid	34	Christensen y Granby. 2002
	Pyrimethanil	19	Christensen y Granby. 2002
	Azoxystrobin	45	Angioni et al., 2004
	Fenhexamid	60	Angioni et al., 2004
	Pyrimethanil	45	Angioni et al., 2004
Table grapes	Metalaxyl	51 (GAP)-25(CAP)	Barba, 2001
	Penconazole	71 (GAP)-50 (CAP)	Barba, 2001
	Cyprodinil	100 (CAP)	Barba, 2001
	Fludioxonil	54 (GAP)-70 (CAP)	Barba, 2001
	Iprodione	50	Poulsen et al., 2004
	Procymidone	25	Poulsen et al., 2004
	Dithiocarbamates	40	Poulsen et al., 2004
	Phthalimides	90	Poulsen et al., 2004
	Triazoles	10	Poulsen et al., 2004
	Famoxadone	36-42	Gamón et al., 2006b
	Fludioxonil	34-78	Gamón et al., 2006b
	Iprodione	56-63	Gamón et al., 2006b
	Azoxystrobin	75	Lentza-Rizos et al., 2006
Peach	Myclobutanil	0	Barba et al., 2001
	Chlorothalonil	97	Holland et al., 1994
	Thiram	17	Chavarri et al., 2205
Nectarine	Myclobutanil	26.4	Barba et al., 2001
Apricot	Penconazole	25 (CAP)	Barba et al., 2000b
	Thiram	0 (GAP)-72 (CAP)	Barba et al., 2000b
Apple	Miclobutanil	53	Kaya et al., 2006
Lemon	Thiram	37 (GAP)-45 (CAP)	Barba, 2001
Plum	Captan	100	Barba et al., 2001
	Folpet	33.5	Barba et al., 2001
	Captan+ Folpet	45.4	Barba et al., 2001

In the case of leafy vegetables (lettuce, escarole, spinach, chicory, cabbage, etc.), the elimination of outer leaves represents a decrease of fungicide residues accumulated in the plant. In addition, this elimination is very usual because superficial leaves are usually withered with soil rests.

In the case of the stem fruits like celery, the removal of leaves and top part of the stem produce high elimination of fungicide residues as these usually have higher content than the central part of the stem. The peeling of root vegetables and tubers and removing the outer layers of the bulbs (onions and garlic) also produce high eliminations of fungicides. Lastly, we must not forget either fresh consumption or industrial processing of edible grain legumes (beans, peas and beans) where the removal of the pod produces a decrease in the residual content of fungicides in the product collected.

When wishing to get processed foods of fresh vegetables, manual peeling (i.e. tangerines, oranges, lemons, peas, onions, beans, garlic) or chemical peeling (i.e. stone fruits and pome fruits) is performed depending on the type of plant.

The values of elimination achieved by this process depend on several factors: type of pesticide and crop, depth of the layer removed and possible cross-contamination with the peeled part. In the case of chemical peeling, it depends on the concentration of the chemical used, the final pH reached by the dissolution, the contact time to totally eliminate the skin and the temperature at which the dissolution is, besides the type of pesticide. One factor to consider in the case of using the peel as a by-product addressed to the cosmetics or food industry and the preparation of cattle feed is the possible presence of residues of fungicides in these products and therefore their entry into the consumer well by skin absorption or ingestion through the food chain.

Table 3 shows some indicative figures for the elimination of fungicides by manual or chemical peeling both in fruits as vegetables.

In the usual process of industrial development and conservation of plant foods, heat treatments are carried out after the washing and peeling that can accommodate from blanching to sterilization or pasteurization to lengthen the product's shelf life.

This kind of treatments is very effective in the dissipation of fungicide residues as it dramatically accelerates the degradation of their molecules by thermal lability producing degradation in less complex compounds that are normally harmless or less toxic. But also, some active substances may give most toxic metabolites such as the dithiocarbamates that degrade to ethylenethiourea (ETU), more toxic than the product where it comes from. In this sense, a study of Fournier and Bonderf in 1983 on spinach containing residues of mancozeb and maneb revealed that when they applied a heat treatment, it produced an increase in the content of ETU [Fournier and Bonderf, 1983]. The same applies to the degradation of daminozide in UDMH (1.1-dimethylhidrazine) that is more toxic than the original substance [Laperulo-Loftus et al., 1992]. Therefore, the European Union have recently required studies on the nature and possible toxicity of metabolites that can be originated in the degradation of the active substance and that finally the processed product may contain in order to authorize the use of pesticides in food to be cooked or transformed.

The elimination of residues by the heat treatment is usually a chemical process due to the effect of high temperatures on the rate of chemical reactions of decomposition of the active substance and its metabolites. Although, it is possible to find physical processes implied as the residue volatilization by the temperature effect. When the heat treatment is performed in the presence of water, the processes that normally occur in the degradation of the active substance are hydrolysis reactions.

The heat treatments used in industry are very varied, i.e. initial blanching to inactivate enzymes that can cause alterations in the plant by activity of other enzymes (browning), roast of peppers, sterilization for canned vegetables (peach, apricot, mandarin segments, pears, tomatoes, etc.) or pasteurization of a juice or nectar. Also many treatments for domestic processed foods use heat as a source of preparation of vegetable products, i.e. boiling in water at 100 °C, cooking in pressure cookers at temperatures above 100 °C, frying in oil, roasted products, cooking or heating in microprobe, etc. Therefore, processes and factors involved in the possible degradation of the fungicide contained in the fresh product can be quite varied. In addition, we should take into account that the effectiveness depends on the conditions of heat processing.

Among the most relevant factors related to higher or lower elimination of fungicide residues in a plant product by heat treatment, we can highlight:

Table 3. Elimination of fungicides in the peeling of fruits and vegetables

Plant product	Fungicide	% of elimination	Reference
Peeling			
Apple	Myclobutanil	76	Kaya et al., 2006
Peach	Myclobutanil	69-100	Coscolla et al., 2006
	Tebuconazole	76-100	Coscolla et al., 2006
	Thiophanate-methyl	71-100	Coscolla et al., 2006
Orange	Imazalil	97	Coscollá et al., 2001
	Thiabendazole	97	Coscolla et al., 2001
	2-phenylphenol	99	Coscolla et al., 2001
Asparagus	Dithiocarbamates	52	Chavarri et al., 2005
Persimmon	Captan	90	Fernández et al., 2006
Chemical peeling			
Peach	Penconazole	100	Barba et al., 2000b
	Thiram	100	Barba et al., 2000b
	Thiram	30	Chavarri et al., 2005

a) Type of process
b) Temperature reached and duration. The higher temperature and longer time, the greater the residue elimination is [Holland et al., 1994; Hamilton and Crossley, 2004].
c) Open or closed cooking system. Doing it in open allows greater volatilization of the product.
d) Addition of water. It facilitates the hydrolysis and may dilute the resulting residue. This last one depends on the residue's water solubility, which is marked by the value

of the partition coefficient in n-octanol/water as an indication of his hydrophilic or lipophilic character.

e) Physico-chemical characteristics of the fungicide. Some examples are volatility, stability, type and system of the applied formulation and nature of the plant product.

Table 4. Elimination of fungicides in the thermal treatment of fruits and vegetables

Plant product	Fungicide	% of elimination	Reference
Blanching			
Pepper	Penconazole	100 CAP	Barba et al., 2000a
	Procymidone	9 GAP-17 CAP	Barba et al., 2000a
Celery	Chlorothalonil	100 GAP-100CAP	Barba et al., 2000c
Broccoli	Metalxyl	85 CAP	Barba et al., 2000c
Zucchini	Penconazole	100 GAP-100 CAP	Barba et al., 2000a
	Metalaxyl	69 CAP	Barba et al., 2000a
Apricot	Penconazole	4 CAP	Barba et al., 2000b
	Thiram	53 GAP-62 CAP	Barba et al., 2000b
Tomato	Metalaxyl	100 CAP	Barba, 2001
	Penconazole	100 CAP	Barba, 2001
	Thiram	65 CAP	Barba, 2001
	Dithiocarbamates	100	Barba, 2001
Asparagus	Dithiocarbamates	100	Chavarri et al., 2005
Other thermal treatments (Sterilization, cooking, pasteurization, etc)			
Apricot	Penconazole	34-39 CAP	Barba et al., 2000b
	Thiram	46-47 GAP	Barba et al., 2000b
	Thiram	32-71 CAP	Barba et al., 2000b
Lemon	Thiram	100 CAP	Barba, 2001
Beans	Benomyl	50	JMPR, 1978
Potato	Thiabendazole	0	JMPR, 1977
Peach	Thiram	25	Chavarri et al, 2005
Orange	2-phenylphenol	10-50	Reynolds, 1996
	Thiabendazole	0-20	Reynolds, 1996
Apple	Tolyfluanid	81	Rasmussen et al., 2003
Persimmon	Captan	100	Fernández et al., 2006
Tomato	Maneb	74	Kontou et al., 2004
Cauliflower	Captan	100	Fernández et al., 2006

In general, fungicides with low volatility and stable to hydrolysis are those with lower dissipation during a heat treatment.

Table IV presents some examples illustrating the levels of elimination produced by the various thermal processes that can be carried out both in industry and in home processing.

But normally, industrially processed foodstuffs imply the performance of more than one of the operations described. And also, to obtain an industrial product suppose the use of different raw materials (fruits with cereals, vegetables with meat products, fruit or varied vegetable salads, etc.). In the manufacture of canned vegetables, studies with radiolabelled carbon atoms reported by Farrow confirmed total or nearly total dissipation of most of the studied fungicides [Carles, 1988]. In the tomato canning, it was observed that the elimination percentage of benomyl was 67%, though it was 30% in another study.

In the case of citrus juice, the only case where there is total elimination of the fungicide used is when the fruits suffer treatment in postharvest. In this sense, a study conducted in the Community of Valencia (Spain) showed that there was a elimination in the juice producing of 97% for imazalil and thiabendazole and 99% for 2-phenylphenol.

For other non-citrus juices, both fruit (peach, apple, apricot, grape, etc.) and vegetables ones (carrot and tomato) there was high elimination but not as sharply as in citrus. Table V shows some evidence for the elimination produced by the combination of different operations to obtain juice.

To obtain marmalades, fruit compotes and jams also produce significant removal of fungicides that may be in fresh fruit. A study on strawberry compote showed a reduction for tolyfluanid of 91% and 33% and 25% for pyrimethanil and fenhexamid, respectively, in relation with the initial concentration in strawberries [Christensen, Granby, 2002]. Another study showed as captan underwent 99% reduction in compote of plums [Koivistoinen, 1965].

Table 5. Elimination de fungicides in the obtaining of juices

Plant product	Fungicide	% Elimination	Reference
Apple	Captan	70-90	FAO, 1994
	Fenarimol	90	FAO, 1995
	Metiram	90	FAO, 1995
	Thiram	70	FAO,1996
	Bitertanol	90	Holland et al., 1994
	Myclobutanil	61	Kaya et al., 2006
Grapes	Tebuconazole	60	FAO, 1994
	Cyprodinil	100	Barba, 2001
	Fludioxonil	100	Barba, 2001
	Metalaxyl	100	Barba, 2001
	Penconazole	100	Barba, 2001
Tomato	Chlorothalonil	100	Chrysayi-Tokousbaides et al., 2000
	Metalaxyl	100	Barba, 2001
	Penconazole	100	Barba, 2001
	Thiram	100	Barba, 2001

Finally, procedures for food conservation at low temperatures (cold and/or freezing) are widely used in plant products of usual consumption observing increasing practice in recent years due to changes in eating habits of society.

The use of low temperatures in food preservation seeks to extend its life by minimizing the reactions of degradation and limiting microbial growth. A large number of physiological phenomena and processes of chemical and biochemical nature have shown that the rate of these reactions is reduced by half for every 10 degrees drop in temperature of the product to keep.

The study of the evolution of cyprodinil and fludioxonil residues in table grapes under refrigeration into refrigerator (4 ºC) showed elimination of cyprodinil residues of 38% in 25 days for grapes treated in critical conditions, i.e. same day for collection and introduction into the refrigerator. Fludioxonil elimination was 64% in the same conditions. Also for both products and under the conditions mentioned above, we studied their behavior in lettuce obtaining that the cyprodinil ramainig percentage was 11% and there was 100% elimination of fludioxonil up to 21 days after the trial [Marin et al., 2003].

Another system of food preservation is freezing. This procedure consists not only of maintaining temperatures below zero for the original product but also of subjecting it to various pre-frozen operations (washing, peeling and heat treatment). These operations are the leading cause of the disappearance of residues, as one would expect that fungicide residues should remain virtually the same during the period stored at a low temperature. Indicative examples include that penconazole disappears completely in a frozen pepper product; procymidone has similar behavior as this of penconzaole under GAP while in CAP the reduction is 62% over the fresh product. Chlorothalonil disappears in celery completely. Metalaxyl is eliminated in broccoli completely when the trial takes place on the plant that has been treated with GAP and in the case of CAP there is remaining percentage of 7%. To grow zucchini note that there is a total elimination of penconazole. Metalaxyl disappearance is only 86% in CAP conditions but the elimination is total in GAP conditions [Barba et al., 2000a].

Regarding the influence of the type and storage time on the elimination of fungicide residues from the processed products, we can state there are no significant variations in 6-12 months after keeping a product frozen [Barba et al. 2000a; Garrido et al., 1998].

The mechanical processes (washing and peeling) and thermal ones (blanching, sterilization, pasteurization, etc.) are the main causes of the disappearance of fungicide residues in the elaboration of both domestic and industrial processed plant foods. Mostly, the elimination levels range between 30-100% relating the initial residues. If using GAP already get residue levels below those established MRLs, the implementation of conservation and cooking processes further ensure further the health quality and hygiene of the plant foods produced with these techniques.

Elimination of Fungicide Residues in Products Obtained by Fermentative Processes

In wine production, harvested grape bunches are transported to the wine cellar, where the preparation begins including oenotechnological processes such as crushing, draining, maceration, pressing, clearing, alcoholic fermentation, racking, clarification, stabilization and filtration. The type of wine and proper use of these processes can be a decisive factor in the disappearance or elimination of pesticide residues [Garcia and Xirau, 1994; Navarro et al., 1997, 1999 and 200; Flore et al., 2000; Goats and Angioni, 2000; Fernandez et al., 2005a and 2005b; Oliva et al., 2006, 2007a and 2007b].

Both clearing and clarification of musts seem to be compulsory practices to eliminate potential residues. For example, when removing lees in suspension from must either by dynamic (centrifuge) or statically (with or without clarifying agents), 90% of S, 70% of phthalimides and 40% dicarboximidic fungicides are lost, whereas water soluble products soluble remain in the must [Cabras et al., 1987]. Anyway, we should have in mind that the water solubility of most pesticides is low. Other products such as benzimidazols are not eliminated by the clearing but they are indeed by a clarification treatment with bentonite [Molina et al., 1995]. Along with this one, others are used as clarifying agents: silica gel, gelatin or activated charcoal [Flori and Zironi, 1984; Gnaegi and Aerny, 1984]. Finally, filtering the wine before bottling has some effect on the residue elimination, although it is minimal.

In studies conducted by our research group on the disappearance of the fungicides benalaxyl, metalaxyl, cyproconazole, fenarimol, penconazole, vinclozolin and mancozeb in traditional winemaking processes compared to that made by carbonic maceration, it is clear that the remaining residues in wines, obtained by the latter technique, are between 5 and 10 times lower than those achieved in the traditional process. In both cases, the product with the lowest rate of dissipation was metalaxyl [Navarro et al., 1999 and 2000].

In the case of traditional winemaking, remaining percentages are held between 67-95% (for fenarimol and metalaxyl, respectively) in the process of maceration. In the pressing, the first significant decrease of residue levels occurs having mean values equal to 30% of the initial amount in pomace and it should be pointed out that the pesticide presenting greater disappearance is mancozeb. In the fermentation, the changes are minor and remainders between 8 -17% are kept in the lees. Finally, the clarification and filtration just help to make residues disappear [Navarro et al., 1999].

Much lower remaining percentages are obtained in the carbonic maceration than in the previous case and consequently the percentages are higher in the pomace, possibly because the grapes remain virtually intact in the maceration process itself on the first few days. For this case, the remaining percentages of the products surveyed were also lower in the final wine [Navarro et al., 2000].

The evolution of the residue levels of four fungicides (cyprodinil, fludioxonil, pyrimethanil and quinoxyfen) during elaboration of three types of wine with maceration (traditional red wine, carbonic maceration red wine and red wine of long maceration and prefermentation at low temperature) and two types of wine without maceration (pink and white) has been studied. The disappearance curves of each fungicide have been analyzed during the period of time of each wine-making process (21 days) and during the different steps involved in the oenological elaborations. Fludioxonil was the fastest fungicide to reduce its residual levels during the time and steps of wine-making procedures without maceration, while pyrimethanil was the lowest in practically all the cases (with and without maceration). During carbonic maceration wine-making, the decay constant of cyprodinil was greater than that of the rest pesticides in all assays (time and steps) [Fernandez et al., 2005b].

Azoxystrobin, fluazinan and mepanipyrim got their residue levels reduced in the process from the grapes to the musts, much more in those obtained in the winemaking with maceration (0.12 versus 0.20 mg/kg for azoxystrobin in must with and without maceration, respectively) [Goats et al., 1998]. Another study on the elimination of quinoxyfen by oenotechnological processes showed that after the grape pressing, only 45% of the residues were found in must compared to the amount in the berries. If it is submitted to centrifuge, 8% of its residue concentration disappears and nothing is detected in wine at the end of the fermentative process [Cabras et al., 2000].

The beer is a full drink included in the diet of many citizens in much of the world for hundreds of years. His influence on health.is based on the absence of negative attributes and presence of antioxidants, vitamins, minerals, etc. However, taking into account the need to protect crops of barley and hops by pesticides, the study of the transfer of pesticide residues from barley or hops to beer across the different stage of its development (germination, drying and roasting, soaking, cooking, fermentation, maturation, filtration and stabilization) is essential as well.

An important factor on the transfer of pesticide residues between barley and malta during the malting process is the octanol-water partition coefficient of a pesticide (Kow). So, coefficient values greater than 2 allow their transference to malt [Miyake et al., 2002; Uygun et al., 2007]. This physical-chemical feature along with others like vapour pressure and Henry's constant influences the tendency of some fungicide residues to pass from the malt to must in the stages of maceration and cooking [Hack et al., 1997; Miyake et al., 1999]. Finally, if fungicide residues remain in the must, they could be transferred to beer during the fermentation causing not only possible toxic effects for consumer but also changes in the beer because of their influence on yeast [Jones et al., 1998].

Possible residues of fungicides that can be found in beer are mostly contributed by barley, as those in the hops do not reach the end of the process because there is a dilution factor in the beer over 250 [Hengel and Shibamato, 2002]. A work carried out by FAO and WHO showed that hops with high content of triadimenol led to beers in which no residue of this fungicide was detected and this also happened to fenarimol and iprodione [WHO/FAO, 1982, FAO, 1994 and 1995].

In a study on the decline of pesticide residues from barley to malt in the manufacture of beer, it was found that the disappearance of fungicide residues on barley grains (after steeping) reached values between 30 and 41%, depending on their K_{ow} ratios. The remaining percentages during the malting showed similar patterns for myclobutanil and propiconazole and similar percentages for them. Nuarimol introduced slightly higher remaining percentages. The steeped grains make disappear between 41 and 35.9% of the original values in the barley grains. The sleeping water removes between 14 and 25% more and the cured dried green malt causes remaining residues ranging between 40 and 50% having greater elimination when malt is dried and cured. It can be seen that the average reduction percentages of various pesticides tested (globally assessed) are in the range of 50% for the sleeping, 25% for the germination, 15% in the drying and 8% in the curing [Navarro et al., 2007].

When studying the behavior of the fungicides myclobutanil, propiconazole and nuarimol during the 4-month brewing process, only myclobutanil exceeded its MRL in barley after the mashing step although the phases of spent grain, brewer wort and final beer were also examined. In all cases, a substantial fraction (26-42%) is lost in the spent grain. The half-life time of the fungicides during the storage of spent grain ranged between 82 and 187 days and the order of the disappearance rate was myclobutanil > nuarimol > propiconazole. The phases that had more influence on the disappearance of fungicides were the mashing and boiling. In the storage of finished beer, there is also disappearance of residues, though less important than in the elaboration [Navarro et al., 2005].

A study on the evolution of pesticides from hops to beer showed that the fungicide fenarimol when added to hops, it remained at levels of 45% compared with its original concentration after cooking (1.1 mg/kg) remaining at slightly lower levels until the final beer. This is not toxicologically relevant since its MRL is 5 mg/kg in hops [Navarro et al., 2006].

Overall and seeing the high dilution provoked for the raw material, physical and chemical characteristics of pesticides, heat treatment and the fermentation process, it is very difficult to find beers containing residues of fungicides. In positive cases for residue levels, these were so low that present no toxicological hazard to consumers.

The fermentation processes along with the operations of pressing, clarification, filtration and bottle storage or the cooking in the case of brewing are the root causes of the disappearance of fungicides that may be present in grapes and barley. The most important oenotechnological process having effect on the elimination of residues in wine-making is the separation of the solid parts of grapes (i.e. pomace and lees).

REFERENCES

Angioni, A; Aguilera del Real, A; Russo, M; Melis, M; Cavitas, F; Cabras, P. Triazole fungicide degradation in peaches in the field and in model systems. *Food Additives & Contaminants*, 2003 20(4), 368-374.

Angoini, A; Schirra, M; Garau, VL; Melis, M; Tuberoso, CIG; Cabras, P. Residues of Azoxystrobin, fenhexamid and pyrimethanil in strawberry following field treatments and the effect on domestic washing. *Food Additives & Contaminants*, 2004 21(11), 1065-1070.

Angoini, A; Sarais, G; Dedola, F; Caboni, P. Pyrimethanil residues on table grapes Italia after field treatment. *Journal of Environmental Science and Health, Part B*, 2006 41(6), 833-841.

Barba, A. Residuos de plaguicidas en elaborados de origen vegetal. Influencia del proceso de fabricación en su desaparición y aspectos toxicológicos. Informe Final Proyecto Investigación PB/3FS/97, Fundación Séneca, Comunidad Autónoma de la Región de Murcia (Spain). 2001, 31 pp.

Barba, A; Navarro, S; Oliva, J; Cámara, MA, Vera, N. Disappearance of several pesticide during freezing of pepper and marrow. First Mediterranean Workshop Research and European Policy on Pesticide Residues in Mediterranean Countries (Athens), 2000a, 72-73.

Barba, A; Navarro, S; Oliva, J; Cámara, MA, Vera, N. Disappearance of insecticides during canning of apricot and peach fruits. 3rd European Pesticide Residue Workshop (York, UK), 2000b, 45.

Barba, A; Oliva, J; Navarro, S; Cámara, MA, Vera, N. Disappearance of several pesticides during freezing of celery and broccoli. 3rd European Pesticide Residue Workshop (York, UK), 2000c, 44.

Barba, A; Oliva, J; San Nicolás, FT; Cámara, MA. Influence of washing and brushing procedures in the desappearance of different pesticide residues in stone fruits (prunus). 2nd MGPR "International Symposium of Pesticide in Food and the Environment in Mediterranean Countries" (Valencia, Spain), 2001, 53.

Belasco, IJ; Han, JL; Charzanowski, RL. Metabolism of (14C) cymoxanil in grapes and potatoes. *Pesticide Science*, 1981 12, 355-364.

Bellapart, C. Nueva agricultura biológica en equilibrio con la agricultura química. Madrid: Ed. Mundi-Prensa; 1996.

Berry, YC. The hazards of healthy living; pesticide risks in perspective. *Shell Agriculture*, 1991 9, 18-20.

Brandolini, V; Flori, P; Musacci, P. Residui di antibotritici sull´uva en el vino: esperenze condotte in Emilia Romagna. *Vitivinicoltura*, 1979 11, 29-32.

Cabizza, M; Satta, M; Falcón, S; Onano, M; Uccheddu, G. Degradation of cyprodinil, fludioxonil, cyfluthrin and pymetrozine on lettuce alter different application methods. *Journal of Environmental Science and Healt, Part B*, 2007 42, 761-766.

Cabras, P. Residui di fitofarmaci nella practica agrícola. *Informazione Fitopatologiche*, 1995 9, 22-29.

Cabras, P; Angioni, A. Pesticide residues in grapes, wine and their processing products. *Journal of Agricultural and Food Chemistry*, 2000 48, 967-973.

Cabras, P; Angioni, A; Garau, VL; Melis, M; Pirisi, FM; Karim, M; Minelli, EV. Persistence of insecticide residues in olives and olive oil. *Journal of Agricultural and Food Chemistry*, 1997 45, 2244-2247.

Cabras, P; Angioni, A; Garau, VL; Pirisi, F; Cabitza, F; Pala, M; Farris, GA. Fate of quinoxyfen residues in grapes, wine and their processing products. *Journal of Agricultural and Food Chemistry*, 2000 48, 6128-6131.

Cabras, P; Angioni, A; Garau, VL; Pirisi, F; Espinoza, J; Mendoza, A; Cabitza, F; Pala, M; Brandolini, V. Fate of azoxystrobin, fluazinam, kresoxim-methyl, mepanipyrim and tetraconazole. *Journal of Agricultural and Food Chemistry*, 1998 46, 3249-3251.

Cabras, P; Meloni, M; Pirisi, FM. Pesicide fate from vine to wine. *Reviews of Environmental Contamination and Toxicology*, 1987 99, 83-117.

Carles, L. Résidus de pesticides, quel risqué pour les consummateurs. *Arboriculture Fruitiere*, 1988 405, 48-49.

Chavarri, MJ; Herrera, A; Ariño, A. The decrease in pesticides in fruit and vegetables during commercial processing. *International Journal of Food Science &Technology*, 2005 40, 205-211.

Christensen, HB; Granby, K. Processing factors and variability of pyrimethanil, fenhexamid and tolyfluanid in strawberries. 4th European Pesticide Residue Workshop (Rome, Italy), 2002, 124.

Chrysayi-Tkousbalides, M; Karayianni-Christou, M. Determination of buprofezin, deltamethrin, dicofol and chlorotalonil residues in field processing tomato. First Mediterranean Workshop Research and European Policy on Pesticide Residues in Mediterranean Countries (Athens), 2000, 45.

Coscollá R; Coscollá C. Cómo disminuir o eliminar los residuos de plaguicidas en frutas, hortalizas y alimentos transformados. Valencia (Spain): Phytoma-España SL; 2006.

Coscollá, R. Algunas consideraciones sobre la problemática de los residuos de plaguicidas en productos vegetales. *Fruticultura Profesional*, 1996a 83, 64-76.

Coscollá, R. Problemática de los residuos de plaguicidas en uva de mesa y vinificación. *Phytoma,* 1996b 83, 192-198.

Coscollá, R; Gadea, A; Cervera, L; Gamóm, M; Fabado, F; Saez, A; Pelegrí, R; Peris, I. Pesticida residues transference from citrus fruit to jueces. 2nd MGPR "International Symposium of Pesticide in Food and the Environment in Mediterranean Countries" (Valencia, Spain), 2001, 61.

Coscollá, R; Gamón, M; García, B; Ten, A; Mir, L. Ensayo sobre la reducción del contenido en residuos de plaguicidas en frutos de melocotón por pelado. *Agrícola Vergel,* 20006 296, 370-371.

Dagna, L; Gasparini, G; Icardi, ML; Sesia, E. Recerca finalizzata sull destino di alcuni fitofarmaci nell´uva, nell mosto in vino. *L'Enotecnico*, 1991 27 (11), 59-69.

Drieghe, S; Dejonckheere, W; Steubaur, W. Pesticide residue concentrations in a Belgian total diet study 1991-1993. Poster P001. 1er European Pesticide Residue Workshop (Alkmaar, NL), 1996.

Ebbert, TA; Taylor, RAJ; Downer, RA; Hall, FR. Deposit structure and efficacy of pesticide application. I: Interaction between deposit size, toxicant concentration and deposit number. *Pesticide Science*, 1999 55, 783-792.

FAO. Pesticide residues in food. 1994. Evaluations Part I and II, residues. Rome (Italy): FAO Plant Production and Protection Paper 131/1 131/2, Food and Agriculture Organization of the United Nations; 1994.

FAO. Pesticide residues in food. 1995. Evaluations Part I, residues. Rome (Italy): FAO Plant Production and Protection Paper 137, Food and Agriculture Organization of the United Nations; 1995.

FAO. Pesticide residues in food. 1996. Evaluations Part I, residues. Rome (Italy): FAO Plant Production and Protection Paper 142, Food and Agriculture Organization of the United Nations; 1996.

Fernández, MJ; Oliva, J; Barba, A; Cámara, MA. Effects of clarification and filtration processes on the removal of fungicide residues in red wines (var. Monastrell). *Journal of Agricultural and Food Chemistry*, 2005a 53, 6156-6161.

Fernández, MJ; Oliva, J; Barba, A; Cámara, MA. Fungicide dissipation curves in wine-making process with and without maceration step. *Journal of Agricultural and Food Chemistry*, 2005b 53, 804-811.

Fernández-Cruz, ML; Barreda, M; Villaroya, M; Peruga, A; Llanos, S; García-Baudín, JM. Captan and fenitrothion dissipation in field-treated cauliflowers and effect of household processing. *Pest Management Science*, 2006 62, 637-645.

Flori, P; Zironi, R. Residui antibotritici e tecnologie enologiche. *Ricerca Viticola ed Enologica,* 1984 1-2, 47-50.

Flori, P; Frabboni, B; Cesari, A. Pesticide decay models in wine-making process and wine storage. *Italian Journal of Food Science*, 2000 12, 279-289.

Fournier, E; Bonderf, J. Les produits antiparasitaires a usage agricole; conditions d'utilisation et toxicologie. París (France): Technique et Documentation; 1983.

Gamón, M; García, B; Ten, A; Mir, L; Coscollá, R. Experiencia sobre la reducción del contenido en residuos de plaguicidas en lechuga por lavado. *Agrícola Vergel,* 2006a 296, 368-370.

Gamón, M; Badía, V; Serena, G; Coscollá, R. Disminución del contenido en residuos de plaguicidas por lavado y pelado de productos vegetales. Experiencia sobre reducción del contenido en residuos de plaguicidas por lavado en uva de mesa.-Valencia-2005. *Agrícola Vergel,* 2006b 296, 365-367.

Garau, VL; Angioni, A; Aguilera del Real, A; Russo, M; Cabras, P. Dissappearance of azoxystrobin, pyrimethanil, cyprodinil and fludioxonil on tomatoes in a greenhouse. *Journal of Agricultural and Food Chemistry*, 2002 50, 1929-1932.

García Cazorla, J; Xirau, M. Persistence of dicarboximidic fungicide residues in grapes, must and wine. *American Journal of Enology and Viticulture*, 1994 45(3), 338-340.

Garrido, JA; Casado, E, Jiménez, I; Toledano, R; De Alba, M. Degradation of several pesticides during freezing in strawberry. 2nd European Pesticide Residue Workshop (Almería, Spain), 1998, 190.

Gennari, M; Zanini, E; Cignetti, A; Bicchi, C; D´Amato, A; Tacheo, MB; Spessotto, M; Flori, P;

Imbroglini, G; Leandro, A; Conte, L. Vinclozolin decay on different grape vines in four differing Italiana reas. *Journal of Agricultural and Food Chemistry*, 1985 33 (6), 1231-1237.

Giralt, LL; Reyes, J; Casadevall, M; García, J. Determinación de los residuos antibotritis específicos en uva. *Informe Serveis de Protecció des Vegetals Generalitat de Catalunya,* 1991, 331-337.

Giralt, LL; Reyes, J; Casadevall, M; García, J. Determinación de los residuos antibotritis específicos en uva. Finca de St. Jaume Seroliveres. *Informe Serveis de Protecció des Vegetals Generalitat de Catalunya*, 1992, 216-220.

Gnaegi, F; Aerny, J. Influence des fongicides inhibileurs de la biosynthesé des sterols sur la fermentation alcoolique et al qualité du vin. *Bulletin l`OIV,* 1984 646, 996-1005.

Hack, M; Nitz, S; Parlar, H. Behavior of [^{14}C] atrazine, [^{14}C] terbutylazine, and their major metabolites in the brewing process. *Journal of Agricultural and Food Chemistry*, 1997 45, 1375-1380.

Hamilton, DJ. Food contamination with pesticide residues. In: Pimentel, editor. Encyclopedia of Pest Management. New Cork: Marcel Dekker Inc.; 2002; 4.

Hengel, MT; Shibamato, T. Method development and fate determination of pesticide-treated hops and their subsequent usage in the production of beer. *Journal of Agricultural and Food Chemistry,* 2002 50, 3412-3418.

Henriet, F; Deloy, S; Pigeon, O; Moreau, JM. Fate of epoxiconazole and Kresoxim-methyl in wheat according to time of application. *Communications in Agricultural and Applied Biological Sciences*, 2005 70(4), 1013-1022.

Henriet, F; Pigeon, O; Moreau, JM. Influence of the spraying system on fungicides distribution on wheat plants. *Communications in Agricultural and Applied Biological Sciences*, 2006 71(2-pt-A), 193-195.

Holland, PT; Hamilton, D; Ohlin, B; Skidmore, MW. Effects of storage and processing on pesticide residues in plant products. *Pure Applied Chemistry*, 1994 66, 335-356.

Jiménez Díaz, RM; Lamo de Espinosa, J. Agricultura Sostenible. Madrid; Ed. Mundi-Prensa; 1998.

JMPR (Joint Meeting Pesticide Residues). Pesticide residues in food evaluations. Part I. Rome. FAO Plant Production and Production Paper Series; 1977.

JMPR (Joint Meeting Pesticide Residues). Pesticide residues in food evaluations. Part I. Rome. FAO Plant Production and Production Paper Series; 1978.

Johnston, J. Pesticide: Public responsibilities. *Chemistry in Britain*, 1991 27, 111-112.

Jones, RD; Kavanagh, TE; Vlarke, BJ. Determination of carbaryl residues in malt and beer and their impact on beer quality. *Journal of the American Society of Brewing Chemists,* 1988 46, 43-50.

Kaya, U; Ugur, A; Okner, H. Processing factors of some pesticides in apple. 6th European Pesticide Residue Workshop (Corfu, Greeke), 2006, 221.

Koivistoinen, P; Karinpi, A; Kononen, M; Roine, P. Magnitude and stability of captan residues in fresh and preserved plant products. *Journal of Agricultural and Food Chemistry*, 1965 13, 468-472.

Kontou S; Tsipi, D; Tzia, C. Stability of the dithiocarbamate pesticide maneb in tomato homogenates during cold storage and thermal processing. *Food Additives & Contaminants*, 2004 21 (11), 183-189.

Lemperle, E; Emmanoulidis, N; Kerner, E. Das abbauverhalten der fungizide Ronilan, Rovral und Sumisclex auf Weintrauben. *Deutsche Lebensmittel-Rundschau*, 1982 2, 51-68.

Lentza-Rizos, C; Avramides, AJ; Kokkinaki, K. Residues of azoxystrobin from grapes to raisins. *Journal of Agricultural and Food Chemistry*, 2006 54, 138-141.

Leparulo-Loftus, M; Peterseb, BJ; Chaisson, CF; Tomerlin, JR. Dietary exposure assessment in the analysis of risk from pesticides in foods. In: Finley JW, Robinson SF, Armstrong, DJ editors. Food safety assessment. Washington DC USA: American Chemical Society; 1992; 214-229.

Liu, SH; Campbel, RA; Studens, JA; Waner, RG. Adsortion and traslocation of glyphosate in aspen as influenced by droplet size, droplet number and herbicide concentration. *Weed Science*, 1996 44, 482-488.

Marín, A; Oliva, J; García, C; Navarro, S; Barba, A. Dissipation rates of cyprodinil and fludioxonil, in lettuce and table grape under cold storage condition. *Journal of Agriculture and Food Chemistry,* 2003 51, 4708-4711.

Miyake, Y; Hashimoto, K; Matsuki, H; Ono, M; Tajima, R. Fate of insecticide and fungicide residues on barley during storage and malting. *Journal of the American Society of Brewing Chemists*, 2002 60, 110-115.

Miyake, Y; Koji, K; Matsuki, H; Tajima, R; Ono, M; Mine, T. Fate of agrochemicals residues associates with malt and hops, during brewing. *Journal of the American Society of Brewing Chemists*, 1999 57, 46-54.

Molina, R; Mingot, J, Manrique de Lara, A; Martin, G. Oenological aspects of bentonite. I. *Alimentación, Equipos y Tecnología,* 1995 14 (8), 61-65.

Morton, R; Bryan, JG; Desmarchelier, JM; Dilli, S; Haddad, PR; Sharp, GJ. Statistical analysis of decay of organophosphorus and pyrethroids insecticides and carbaryl on paddy rice, maize sunflower and field peas. *Journal of Stored Products Research*, 2001 37, 277-285.

Navarro, S; Oliva, J; Navarro, G; Barba, A. Dissipation of chlorpyrifos, fenarimol, metalaxyl, penconazole and vinclozolin in grapes. *American Journal of Enology and Viticulture*, 2001 52(1), 35-40.

Navarro, S; García, B; Navarro, G; Oliva, J; Barba, A. Effect of wine-making practices on the concentrations of fenarimol and penconazole in rose wines. *Journal o Food Protection*, 1997 60, 1120-1124.

Navarro, S; Barba, A; Oliva, J; Navarro, G; Pardo, F. Evolution of residual levels of six pesticides during elaboration of red wines. Effect of winemaking process in their disappearance. *Journal of Agricultural and Food Chemistry*, 1999 47, 264-270.

Navarro, S; Oliva, J; Barba, A; Navarro, G; García, MA; Zamorano, M. Evolution of chlorpyrifos, fenarimol, metalaxyl, penconazole and vinclozolin in red wines elaborated by carbonic maceration of Monastrell grapes. *Journal of Agricultural and Food Chemistry*, 2000 48, 3537-3541.

Navarro, S; Pérez, G; Vela, N; MENA, L; Navarro, G. Behavior of myclobutanil, propiconazole and nuarimol residues during lager beer brewing. *Journal of Agricultural and Food Chemistry,* 2005, 53, 8572-8579.

Navarro, S; Pérez, G; Navarro, G; Mena, L; Vela, N. Fate of fungicide residues from barley to malt. 6th European Pesticide Residue Workshop (Corfu, Greeke), 2006, 225.

Navarro, S, Pérez, G; Navarro, G, Vela , N. Decline of pesticide residues from barley to malt. *Food Additives & Contaminants,* 2007 24 (8), 851-859.

Oliva, J; Barba, A. Elaboración de vino en presencia de residuos de plaguicidas. Alteraciones, control y desaparición. *Tecnología del vino*, 2002 4, 45-49

Oliva, J; Barba, A; Payá, P; Cámara, MA. Disappearance of fenhexamid residues during wine-making process. *Communications in Agricultural and Applied Biological Sciences*, 2006 71/2, 65-74

Oliva, J; Payá, P; Cámara, MA; Barba, A. Removal of famoxadone, fluquinconazole and trifloxystrobin residues in red wines: Effects of clarification and filtration processes. *Journal of Environmental Science and Health, Part B*, 2007a 42, 775 -781

Oliva, J; Payá, P, Cámara, MA; Barba, A. Removal of pesticides from white wine by the use of fining agents and filtration. *Communications in Agricultural and Applied Biological Sciences*, 2007b 72/2, 171-180.

Papadopoulos-Mourkidou, E; Kotopoulou, A; Papadopoulos, G. Dissipation of cyproconazole and quinalphos on/in grapes. *Pesticide Science*, 1995 45(2), 111-116.

Petersen, B; Tomerlin, RJ; Barraj, L. Pesticide degradation: exceptions to the rule. *Food Technology*, 1996 50, 221-223.

Poulsen, E; Andersen, JM; Hansen, HK. Pesticide residues in grapes: Processing factors and variations in among countries in 2001-2003. 5th European Pesticide Residue Workshop (Stockholm, Sweden), 2004, 207.

Rasmussen RR; Poulsen, ME; Hansen, HC. Distribution of multiple pesticide residues in a segments after home processing. *Food Additives & Contaminants*, 2003 20 (11), 1044-1063.

Reynolds, SL. Effect of processing on pesticide residues. SCI Lecture Papers Series; Paper nº 0081; London; Society of Chemical Industry; 1996.

Reynolds, SL; Fussell, RJ; Mcarthur, R. Investigation into the validity of extrapolation in setting maximum residue levels for pesticides in crop of similar morphology. *Food Additives & Contaminants*, 2005 22, 31-38.

Ripley, BD; Cox, DF; Wiebe, J; Frank, R. Residues of dikar and ethilenthiourea in treated grapes and commercial grape products. *Journal of Agricultural and Food Chemistry*, 1978 26, 134-142.

Roberts, T; Hudson, D. Metabolic Pathways of agrochemicals. Part two: Insecticides and fungicides. Cambrige: The Royal Society of Chemistry; 1999.

Ruediger, GA; Pardon, KH; Sas, AN; Godden, PW; Pollnitz, AP. Removal of pesticides from red and white wine by the use of fining and filter agents. *Australian Journal of Grape and Wine Research*, 2004 10, 8-16.

Sadlo, S. Disappearance of pyrimethanil residues on tomato plants. *Journal of Agricultural and Food Chemistry*, 2002 50, 1089-1091.

Sances, F; Toscano, Z; Gaston, L. Bush tomatoes show very low levels of pesticide residues. *California Agriculture*, 1992 46(5), 17-20.

Sckidmore, MW; Ambus, A. Pesticide metabolism in crops and livestock. In Hamilton D and Crossley S, editor. Pesticide residuesin food and drinking water: Human exposure and risks. Chichester, West Sussex, England: Wiley and Sons; 2004; 63-120.

Seiber, JN. General principles governing the fate of chemicals in the environment. In: Hilton JL, editor. Agricultural chemical on the future. Belltsville Symp. Agric. Resch. nº 8; 1985.

Somogyi, LP; Ramaswamy, HS; Hiu YH. Processing Fruits: Science and Technology. Vol 1. Biology, Principles and Application. Boca Raton, London, New York and Washington DC: CRC Press; 1996.

Sur, N; Pal, S; Banerjee, H; Adityachaudhury, N; Bhattacharyya, A. Communication to the editor photodegradation of fenarimol. *Pest Management Science*, 2000 56, 289-292.

Ticha, J; Hajslova, J; Kovalczuk, T; Jech, M; Honzicek, J; Kocourek, V; Lansky, M; Kloutvorova, J; Falta, V. Safe apples for baby-food production: Survey of pesticide treatment regimes leaving minimum residues. *Food Additives & Contaminants*, 2007 24(6),.605-620.

Timme, G; Frehse, G; Laska, V. Statistical interpretation and graphic representation of degradation behaviour of pesticide residues. II. *Planzenschutz Nachrictel Bayer*, 1986 39,187-203.

Timme, G; Walz-Tylla, B. Effects of food preparation and processing on pesticide residues in commodities of plant origin. In Hamilton D and Crossley S, editor. Pesticide residuesin food and drinking water: Human exposure and risks. Chichester, West Sussex, England: Wiley and Sons; 2004; 121-148.

Tsiropoulos, NG; Miliadis, GE; Likas, DT; Liapis, K. Residues of spiroxamine in grapes following field application and their fate from vine to wine. *Journal of Agricultural and Food Chemistry*, 2005 53, 10091-10096.

Uygun, U; Özkara, R; Özbey, A; Koksel, H. Residue levels of malathion and fenitrothion and their metabolites in postharvest treated barley during storage and malting. *Food Chemistry,* 2007 100, 1165-1169.

WHO/FAO. Pesticide residues in food: 1981 evaluations. Rome: FAO, 1982.

Reviewed by:

Prof. Dr. Jorge Mataix (Dpt. Agrochemistry and Environment, University Miguel Hernández, Elche, Spain).

Prof. Dr. Antonio Valverde (Dpt. Physical Chemistry, Biochemistry and Inorganic Chemistry, University of Almería, Almería, Spain).

In: Fungicides
Editors: P. De Costa and P. Bezerra

ISBN: 978-1-60692-631-4

Chapter XII

APPLE SCAB AND POWDERY MILDEW DEMETHYLATION INHIBITOR (DMI) FUNGICIDE RESISTANCE IN APPLE, CHERRY, AND ROSE

Peter L. Sholberg and Julie Boulé
Agriculture and Agri-Food Canada, Pacific Agri-Food Research Centre, British Columbia, Canada

ABSTRACT

Fungicide resistance is an important concern to growers of horticultural crops in British Columbia, Canada. In the past, *Venturia inaequalis,* found in several orchards with an apple scab problem, were resistant to benomyl, a fungicide commonly used at the time. More recently, harvested apples decayed by *Penicillium expansum* or *Botrytis cinerea* were found to be resistant to thiabendazole. Because of this history of fungicide resistance it was decided that a survey to identify resistance to Demethylation Inhibitors (DMI-fungicides) in apple, cherry, and rose was needed now that these fungicides had been used for more than 10 years. Relative growth of 72 *V. inaequalis* isolates from 27 orchard blocks were tested for resistance to myclobutanil. Two isolates, 2445-3 and 2451-3, were found with resistance to myclobutanil at 0.05 g/L and qualify as being field resistant according to standard criteria. DMI resistance to powdery mildew fungi is difficult to quantify because conidia can only be accurately tested on living tissue of the host plant. Contamination of the host tissue and poor viability of the test fungus also makes evaluation difficult. Quantification of myclobutanil resistance by *Podosphaera leucotricha* (apple powdery mildew), *P. clandestina* (cherry powdery mildew) and *Sphaerotheca pannosa* (rose powdery mildew) were based on assaying conidia from samples collected from infected orchards and testing them for germination on leaf disks sprayed with myclobutanil. Five out of 10 apple, 13 out of 14 cherry, and 9 out of 10 rose powdery mildew samples showed some resistance to myclobutanil because the number of germinated spores on treated leaves did not differ significantly from the number of germinated spores on untreated leaves. Apple scab resistance to myclobutanil does not appear to be widespread in BC because it only occurred in one area of the provinces. On the other hand powdery mildew resistance appears to be widespread and could be responsible for ineffective control experienced by apple, cherry, and rose growers. The implications of DMI-resistance and strategies to mitigate DMI resistance are discussed.

Keywords: Sterol-inhibiting fungicides; *Podosphaera leucotricha*; *P. clandestina; Sphaerotheca pannosa*; *Venturia inaequalis*; myclobutanil

INTRODUCTION

Fungicide resistance became a major concern to the agricultural industry after several failures of benzimidazole and metalaxyl-containing fungicides in the late 1970s and early 1980s (Delp, 1988). Due to this crisis the large manufactures of fungicides banded together to form the "Fungicide Resistance Action Committee" (FRAC). It exists to promote effective use of fungicides, reduce the risk of resistance developing, and to manage resistance when it occurs. Additional information on resistance management not included in this chapter is readily available from this source.

Fungicide resistance develops in a pathogen population in at least two different ways. Resistance characterized by sudden and marked loss of effectiveness and by the presence of sensitive and resistant pathogen populations is referred to as 'single-step' or 'discontinuous' resistance (Brent, 1995). This type of resistance occurred less than three years after benomyl became widely available in France (Smith, 1988). In contrast to 'single-step' resistance is 'multi-step' or continuous resistance (Brent, 1995). Resistance to DMI fungicides develops gradually and is more difficult to detect (Deising et al., 2002). This chapter will be restricted to detection of DMI resistance in *Venturia inaequalis,* and *Podosphaera leucotricha* in apple, *Podosphaera clandestina* in cherry, and *Sphaerotheca pannosa* in rose.

An important component of resistance management is monitoring for its presence in the fungal pathogen population. For DMI resistance it is important to be able to detect the presence of less tolerant isolates in the population and determine what percentage of the population they constitute. This requires obtaining base-line data on the typical pathogen population before the pathogen is exposed to widespread use of a new fungicide (Brent, 1995). Köller et al. (1991) determined baseline sensitivity of *V. inaequalis* to be 0.07 $\mu g \cdot ml^{-1}$ for myclobutanil, the DMI fungicide used exclusively in this study. The first report of DMI resistant *V. inaequalis* came from an experimental orchard in Nova Scotia, Canada where 10 years of continuous use of the DMI, bitertanol, led to resistance (Hildebrand et al., 1988). The results indicated that DMI fungicides could become ineffective for the control of apple scab when used exclusively for several years. Braun and McRae (1992) showed that a population of *V. inaequalis* exposed to various DMI's over 12 years developed a bimodal lognormal distribution with a mean of 0.045 $\mu g \cdot ml^{-1}$ for the sensitive population and 0.46 $\mu g \cdot ml^{-1}$ for the resistant population. This development is consistent with the expectation of a direction selection process resulting in a slowly developing resistant population (Georgopoulos, 1987). Stanis and Jones (1985) stated that genetic analysis of nine isolates with reduced sensitivity was determined by a single gene. However in crossing studies of monoascosporic isolates with different DMI sensitivities, Sholberg and Haag (1993) did not always obtain less sensitive progeny. This suggests that several genes may be involved in determining DMI resistance. Fungicide resistance was recently monitored in Quebec, Canada where 238 *V. inaequalis* monoconidial isolates from 48 apple orchards were tested for myclobutanil DMI resistance (Jobin and Carisse, 2007). This was the first time it was done in Quebec since 1994 and the results showed a high level of resistance to myclobutanil prompting the authors to conclude that DMI use should be discontinued or significantly reduced. A similar state of affairs could be the case in British Columbia (BC), Canada because DMI resistance has not been monitored since 1991 (Sholberg and Haag, 1993).

DMI fungicides are also used extensively for the control of powdery mildew in apple, cherry, and rose. Fungicide resistance by the powdery mildew fungi develops most quickly on cucurbit plants and most slowly on apple according to Hollomon and Wheeler (2002). Grape powdery mildew caused by *Uncinula necator* is the most important disease of wine grapes and is almost exclusively controlled by the use of fungicides (Sholberg, 2004). Many of the characteristics of grape powdery mildew are shared by apple, cherry, and rose powdery mildew and these diseases would be expected to develop resistance to DMI fungicides in a similar fashion (Jarvis et al., 2002). Poor control of grape powdery mildew by DMI fungicides has been reported from vineyards in California (Gubler et al., 1996; Ypema et al., 1997), New York (Erickson and Wilcox, 1997), and Ontario, Canada (Northover and Homeyer, 2001). The Ontario authors speculate that the DMI resistant isolates were blown in from a neighboring vineyard, came on nursery stock infected by DMI resistant *U. necator*, selected by overuse of DMI fungicides in the vineyard, or blown in from outside the vineyard where it was selected in vineyards in Canada or across the border in the United States. Studies on apple, cherry, and rose powdery mildew DMI resistance are much less common than grape. Grove et al. (2000) reported that DMI-related control failures occurred in cherry orchards in the state of Washington. Similar failures have been reported on cherry and rose in BC but have not been documented. Control failures by DMI fungicides in apple are strongly suspected especially since it is believed that *P. leucotricha* produces viable ascospores and thus has a functioning sexual stage (Grove, 1999).

Testing for fungicide resistance in fungi that cause powdery mildew requires the use of living plant tissue because these fungi are obligate parasites (Green et al. 2002). Dose response relationships are usually measured as infection levels; sometimes colony numbers are counted or microscopic assessments are made of early infection events and colony growth (Hollomon and Wheeler, 2002). The sample size of any survey is limited by the need to maintain powdery mildew through repeated sub-culturing on leaf material. Techniques that have been developed for monitoring DMI resistance in powdery mildew are time consuming and expensive and likely will be replaced by molecular methods in the future such as those developed by Délye et al. (1997;1998) for grape and barley powdery mildew.

The objectives of this study were to 1) adapt and apply techniques for monitoring resistance to DMI fungicides; 2) survey samples of infected apple and cherry for resistance to DMI fungicides in commercial orchards; and 3) survey samples of infected roses for resistance to DMI fungicides in commercial greenhouses. The samples used in these studies were mostly from the BC interior and most of them were collected in the spring and summer of 2007.

Materials and Methods

Apple Scab Survey

Infected apple leaves with distinct sporulating apple scab lesions (*Venturia inaequalis)* were collected from 11 commercial fruit growers located across British Columbia (BC), Canada (Table 1). In addition, nine isolates used in the Pacific Agri-Food Research Centre (PARC) apple breeding program and a pear scab isolate were also tested. A total of 71 isolates collected from 27 apple blocks were evaluated for DMI-resistance. The leaves were placed in plastic bags and kept at 2°C until they were needed. The method used was adapted from Smith et al. (1991). One lesion was wet with sterile distilled water and a loopful of conidia was streaked across 2% water agar plate. Plates were incubated overnight at room temperature, and five individual germinated conidia were transferred to a 20 mL potato dextrose agar (PDA) plate. Colonies of *V. inaequalis* were incubated for 4 weeks at 20°C. Only one of the monoconidial colonies per lesion was used for sensitivity tests. A 1% stock solution of myclobutanil (Nova® 40W, Dow Agrosciences, Calgary, Alberta, Canada) was used to amend PDA cooled to 50°C at concentrations of 0.05 and 0.1 g/L. Agar plugs (6 mm diameter) were cut from each monoconidial colony and transferred to four plates containing 10 ml of amended or nonamended PDA. Inoculated plates were sealed with parafilm and incubated in the dark for 4 weeks at 20°C. Colony diameters were measured and recorded without including plug diameters. The relative growth (RG) was calculated by dividing the colony diameter on myclobutanil-amended medium by the diameter on unamended medium x 100 (Hsiang 1997). The isolates with a relative growth of 10% or more were tested a second time and the results averaged.

Table 1. Location in British Columbia, Canada of the apple scab blocks tested with date collected and cultivar

Isolate	Date	Apple cultivar	Orchard Location
1843	6-Nov-00	Spartan/Summerred	Agassiz
1845	6-Nov-00	Gala/Discovery	Agassiz
1969	3-Jan-02	Spartan/Summerred	Agassiz
1971	3-Jan-02	Antonovka.D/ M	Agassiz
2107	26-Nov-02	8S-49-40/Jonagfree	Agassiz
2193	4-Nov-03	8S-26-50/Katjk	Agassiz
2196	4-Nov-03	8S-26-50/Akane	Agassiz
2332	14-Jul-05	Spartan/Alkemene	Agassiz
2338	14-Jul-05	8S-26-50/Carola	Agassiz
2437	8-May-07	Pacific Gala	Agassiz
2439	6-Jun-07	Spartan	Penticton
2440	6-Jun-07	McIntosh	Penticton

2441	6-Jun-07	Imperial Gala	Penticton
2442	6-Jun-07	Red Delicious	Penticton
2445	6-Jun-07	Ambrosia	Penticton
2447	13-Jun-07	Gala	Penticton
2449	13-Jun-07	Spartan	Penticton
2451	13-Jun-07	Spartan	Penticton
2452	13-Jun-07	Spartan	Penticton
2454	13-Jun-07	Golden Delicious	Penticton
2457	12-Jun-07	Pacific Gala	Agassiz
2465	3-Jul-07	Fuji	Penticton
2467	5-Jul-07	McIntosh	Winfield
2468	5-Jul-07	McIntosh	Winfield
2473	17-Jul-07	McIntosh	Erickson
2474	17-Jul-07	McIntosh	Wynndel
2497	31-Aug-07	pear	Ainsworth

Powdery Mildew Survey

Leaves infected with apple powdery mildew (*Podosphaera leucotricha)* displaying visible lesions were found in eight commercial fruit grower blocks (Table 2). The apple powdery mildew present in the greenhouse on apple seedlings was also tested. A total of 10 apple powdery mildew isolates were evaluated for DMI-resistance.

Leaves infected with cherry powdery mildew (*Podosphaera clandestina)* displaying visible lesions were found in nine commercial fruit grower blocks (Table 3). In addition, the cherry powdery mildew present in the greenhouse on rootstocks acquired from a commercial nursery was tested. The total number of cherry powdery mildew isolates evaluated for DMI-resistance was 13.

Table 2. Location in British Columbia, Canada of *P. leucotricha* isolates tested with date collected (2007) and apple cultivar

Isolate	Date	Apple cultivar	Orchard Location
2455	13-Jun	Golden Del.	Penticton
2469	5-Jul	Gala	Winfield
2470	5-Jul	McIntosh	Winfield
2475	24-Jul	McIntosh	Winfield
2500	13-Sep	Nicholas	Oliver
2501	13-Sep	Gala	Oliver
2507	13-Sep	Honeycrisp	Cawston
2509	13-Sep	Smoothy Gold	Cawston
2510	13-Sep	Granny Smith	Keremeos
2537	15-Jun	Cameo	Summerland

Table 3. Location in British Columbia, Canada of *P. clandestina* isolates tested with date collected (2007) and cultivar

Isolate	Date	Cherry cultivar	Location
2476	24-Jul	Lapins	Winfield
2478	24-Jul	Lapins	Winfield
2479	24-Jul	Cherry mix	Oyama
2480	24-Jul	Lapins	Winfield
2499	13-Sep	(young)	Oliver
2504	13-Sep	Lapins	Keremeos
2506	13-Sep	Sweetheart	Cawston
2523	6-Nov	Sweetheart	Canyon
2524	6-Nov	Staccato	Erickson
2525	6-Nov	Sweetheart	Erickson
2534	30-Jul	Lapins	Summerland
2536	6-Jul	Lapins	Summerland
2535	28-Jun	Mazzard	Summerland

Table 4. Location in British Columbia, Canada of *S. pannosa* isolates tested with date collected (2007) and cultivar

Isolate	Date	Rose cultivar	Location
2466	5-Jul	April	Rutland
2487	3-Aug	Decora	Lavington
2489	3-Aug	Prestige	Lavington
2491	3-Aug	Happy Hour	Langley
2526	4-Oct	Torero	Rutland
2527	4-Oct	Gotcha	Rutland
2528	4-Oct	Tropical Amazon	Rutland
2529	4-Oct	Ballet	Rutland
2530	4-Oct	Explosion	Rutland
2533	18-Jun	Hope for Humanity	Kelowna

Leaves infected with rose powdery mildew (*Sphaerotheca pannosa*) displaying visible lesions were found in four commercial rose greenhouses (Table 4). The total number of isolates evaluated for DMI-resistance was 10.

Infected apple, cherry, or rose leaves were divided into two equal parts with half placed in a plastic bag and the other half flattened between two layers of water absorbent paper, placed in a flat closed envelop, and stored at 2°C until needed.

Powdery mildew DMI-resistance was evaluated by assessing spore germination on foliage sprayed with myclobutanil. Apple seedlings ('Cameo') grown in flats at the PARC greenhouse (22°C with a 16-h photoperiod) until the two-leaf stage were potted in peat moss growth medium (Promix, Premiere Horticulture, Riviere-du-Loup, Que.) in 85 mm diameter 'Durapots'. Similarly, 100 bare root cherry rootstocks ('Mazzard') and 50 roses ('Hope for Humanity') were potted in 4.8 L pots. The seedlings were fertilized weekly with 2 $g{\cdot}L^{-1}$ of

15-15-18 fertilizer for the duration of the experiment. Thirty grams of 14-14-14 fertilizer was added to both cherry and rose seedlings. The crops were kept free of powdery mildew by leaf removal and weekly fall applications of a 1% soap (Palmolive®) solution.

Each treatment consisted of four single leaf replicates. Leaves were inspected visually and those showing powdery mildew symptoms were discarded. Young tender leaves were collected, disinfested by spraying with 70% ethanol for 30 s (Olmstead et al., 2000), rinsed with sterile distilled water (SDW) and air dried before treatment with myclobutanil from a hand atomizer.

Inoculation with dry conidia of each pathogen (*Podosphaera leucotricha* for apple; *Podosphaera clandestina* for cherry; and *Sphaerotheca pannosa* for rose) was conducted in the greenhouse on selected leaves of each host. Conidia from 10-20 infected leaves were dislodged and scattered with a fine paintbrush (Nicot et al., 2002) onto the adaxial side of the test leaves 20-22 h following fungicide application. Inoculated, detached leaves were floated individually in sterile 90 mm-disposable plastic petri dishes, adaxial side up in 1% sucrose solution (Olmstead et al., 2000). The plates were placed in a high relative humidity environment on the greenhouse bench (22°C with a 15-h photoperiod) for three days. Leaf sections (1 cm^2) were cut from inoculated leaves with a scalpel, fixed to a slide with clear nail polish, adaxial side up, and stained with two drops of aqueous 0.1 $mg \cdot ml^{-1}$ acridine orange (AC/CN Pharmaceutical Inc., Plainview, NY), for 1 min. The slides were rinsed with SDW and examined with a fluorescent microscope (Carl Zeiss Canada, Inc., Don Mills, Ontario, Canada) with standard blue florescent light excitation – green emission using a 20X objective. Conidia with germ tubes one third the length of the spore or longer were counted as germinated (Figure 1).

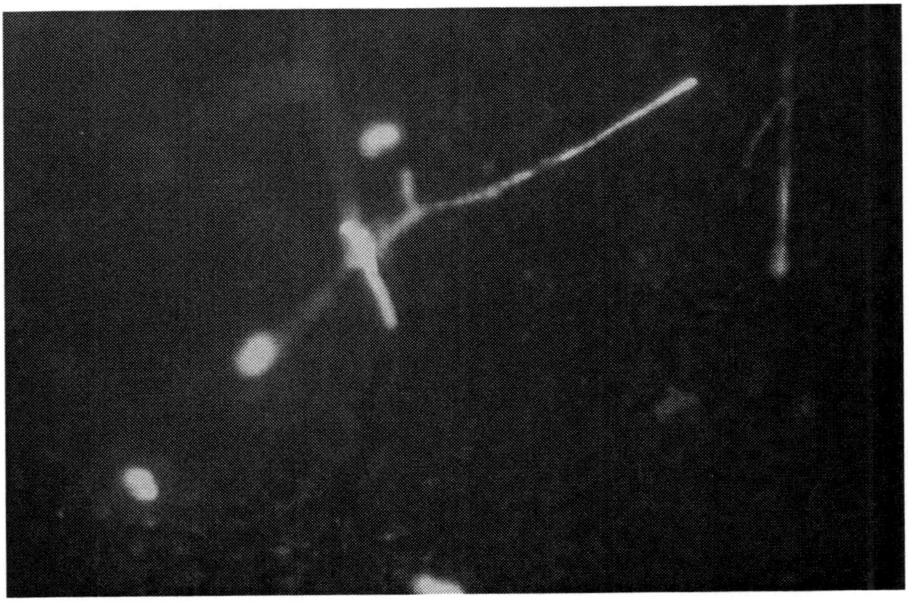

Figure 1. Germinated conidia of *Podosphaera leucotricha* (apple powdery mildew) fluorescing green at 20X magnification.

RESULTS AND DISCUSSION

Apple Scab

Quantification of *V. inaequalis* sensitivity to myclobutanil is based on inhibition of mycelial growth. Köller et al. (1991) determined that the baseline sensitivity for myclobutanil was 0.07 $\mu g{\cdot}ml^{-1}$ after studying 13 baseline isolates on a frequency distribution of ED_{50} values determined for 300 wild type phenotypes. These results compared well with those found by Ficcadori et al. (1987) for fenarimol, bitertanol, and penconazole. In this study 72 isolates were screened for resistance to myclobutanil at 0.05 and 0.1 $\mu g{\cdot}ml^{-1}$ (Table 5). A sample size of 50 is sufficient to detect DMI-resistance according to Smith et al. (1991) and larger sample sizes do not greatly improve the precision of the test. The sensitivity distribution chart showed that approximately 40% of the BC isolates were very sensitive to 0.05 $\mu g{\cdot}ml^{-1}$ and when the rate was doubled to 0.1$\mu g{\cdot}ml^{-1}$ an additional 20% were sensitive to myclobutanil (Figure 2). Less sensitive isolates were found but they were relatively rare indicating that the BC population was still generally sensitive to myclobutanil. When comparing the sensitivities of these isolates to those given by Smith et al. (1991) they most closely resembled the wild-type population with a high percentage of isolates with RG values less than 30%. However, two isolates were found with RG values greater than 80% which means that they are DMI resistant according to Köller et al. (1997) (Figure 3). These particular isolates were collected from 'Ambrosia' and 'Spartan' apples, respectively, from two adjacent Penticton, BC apple orchards that either did not use myclobutanil or only used it once a season. The two isolates were not typical of the *V. inaequalis* population in BC in contrast to what was found in Quebec where 71.4% of the Quebec isolates were above the threshold level (Jobin and Carisse, 2007). Therefore we can speculate that these isolates did not originate here but came from another location. Another possibility is that these isolates were dodine-resistant and thus predisposed to DMI- resistance (Köller and Wilcox, 2001). DMI-resistance is speeded up in *V. inaequalis* isolates that are already resistant to an unrelated fungicide. Widespread resistance to both benomyl and dodine has been reported for some BC apple orchards (Sholberg et al., 1989). For this reason and the fact that DMI fungicides have been used for many years in BC, strategies that reduce the likelihood of fungicide resistance should be practiced. Monitoring for resistance should be conducted more often in the future because of the possibility of finding isolated areas of resistance. Growers with fungicide resistance need to know as soon as possible so they do not spread DMI-resistant isolates to adjacent orchards and use appropriate fungicides for disease control.

Apple Powdery Mildew

Myclobutanil was first registered in Canada in 1992 for control of apple scab and powdery mildew. Therefore it had been in use for 15 years before local isolates of *P. leucotricha* were monitored for resistance. In BC, apple cultivars sensitive to powdery mildew are treated with at least one spray of myclobutanil per season (Sholberg et al., 2001). A population of *V. inaequalis* isolates developed resistance over a period of 12 years when exposed to various DMIs (Braun and McRae, 1992). It was expected that resistance to apple powdery mildew likely would be found if enough samples could be obtained and tested. The sample size of any powdery mildew survey is limited by the need to maintain it through repeated sub-culturing on leaf material, and difficulties associated with collection and transfer to the laboratory (Hollomon and Wheeler, 2002).

Table 5. Relative growth (RG) of *V. inaequalis* isolates on myclobutanil

Isolate	0.05 μg·ml^{-1}	0.1 μg·ml^{-1}	Isolate	0.05 μg·ml^{-1}	0.1 μg·ml^{-1}
	RG	RG		RG	RG
1843	0.00%	0.00%	2447-4	61.55%	19.00%
1845	0.00%	0.00%	2449-1	39.85%	6.50%
1969	0.00%	0.00%	2449-2	70.15%	28.20%
2107	1.00%	0.00%	2451-1	65.55%	51.95%
2193	1.30%	6.30%	2451-2	46.00%	12.00%
2196	4.20%	0.00%	**2451-3**	83.95%	33.30%
2332	4.40%	0.00%	2451-4	70.45%	37.10%
2338	0.00%	0.00%	2452-1	62.00%	42.80%
1971	1.70%	0.00%	2452-2	52.05%	32.80%
2437-2	0.00%	0.00%	2452-3	33.30%	23.60%
2437-5	0.00%	0.00%	2452-4	56.60%	41.75%
2437-6	0.00%	0.00%	2454-1	8.95%	6.85%
2437-4	1.20%	0.00%	2454-3	49.05%	45.00%
2439-1	2.40%	1.59%	2454-4	50.10%	15.15%
2439-3	5.20%	0.00%	2454-2	45.70%	37.55%
2439-5	0.00%	0.00%	2457-1	24.30%	14.80%
2439-4	12.40%	2.94%	2457-2	49.00%	21.50%
2440-1	11.30%	2.35%	2457-3	9.00%	6.60%
2440-2	49.60%	0.85%	2457-4	3.40%	34.95%
2440-3	38.15%	7.11%	2465-1-3	2.60%	0.00%
2440-4	51.70%	18.90%	2465-1-4	8.10%	0.00%
2441-1	54.00%	30.29%	2465-3	27.30%	21.80%
2441-4	39.45%	0.00%	2465-4	30.75%	20.90%
2441-2	34.00%	7.49%	2465-5	27.90%	6.70%
2441-5	11.90%	5.00%	2467-2	5.70%	0.00%
2442-1	12.30%	14.40%	2467-3	2.95%	0.00%
2442-2	51.25%	38.50%	2467-4	1.80%	0.00%
2442-4	69.10%	25.30%	2468-1	28.60%	11.20%
2442-3	11.20%	0.00%	2473-1	0.00%	0.00%
2445-1	0.00%	7.15%	2473-3	12.15%	2.05%
2445-3[1]	89.10%	78.50%	2473-4-1	27.00%	1.80%
2445-4	69.20%	72.00%	2473-4-4	9.00%	2.20%
2445-5	27.80%	18.80%	2473-5	21.30%	2.95%
2447-1	64.40%	33.65%	2474-2	9.20%	0.00%
2447-2	64.40%	37.50%	2474-3	0.00%	0.00%
2447-3	67.70%	29.30%	2497-1	0.00%	0.00%

[1] In bold, isolates with RG > 80%.

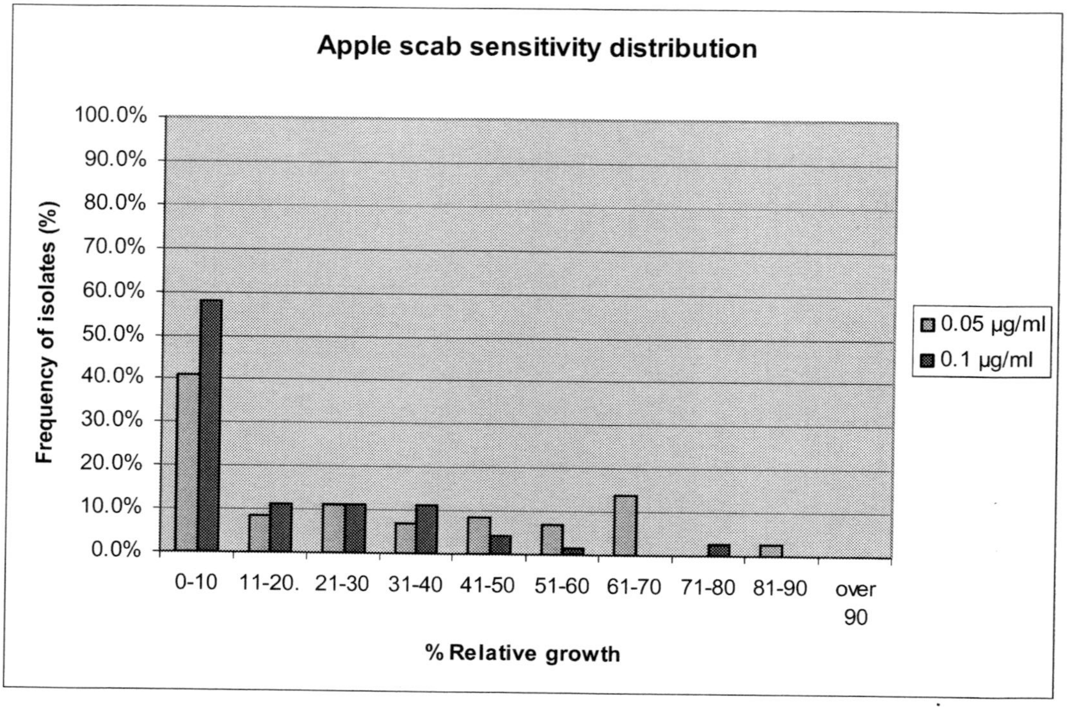

Figure 2. Sensitivity distribution of *V. inaequalis* isolates at 0.05 and 0.1 $\mu g \cdot ml^{-1}$ myclobutanil. Note that two isolates are over 80% which indicates field resistance.

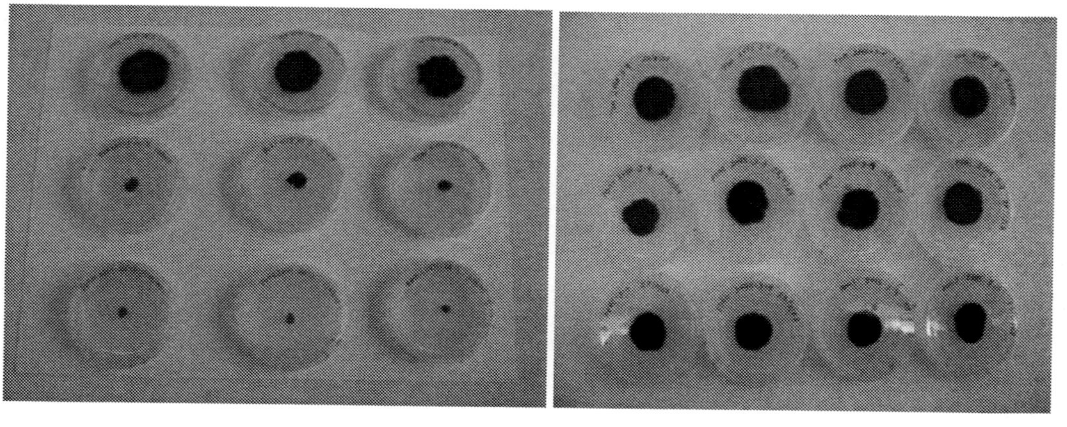

Figure 3. DMI-sensitve and DMI-resistant apple scab. The plates in the top rows contain unamended PDA, the middle rows contains 0.05 myclobutanil, and the lower rows contains 0.1 $mg \cdot l^{-1}$ myclobutanil. Note the unrestricted growth of the DMI-resistant *V. inaequalis* isolate (#2445-3) on the middle and lower plates in the picture on the right.

Five isolates were sensitive to myclobutanil because a significantly higher number of spores germinated on the untreated leaves (Table 6). On the otherhand, five isolates were resistant because a similar number of conidia as the control germinated on treated leaves. Resistance was found in Penticton, BC on 'Golden Delicious', in Keremeos, BC on 'Granny Smith' and in Winfield, BC on 'McIntosh' apple cultivars. Two myclobutanil sprays had been applied in June 2007 where the DMI-resistant *P. leucotricha* was found in Winfield, BC. Resistance was also identified in the powdery mildew present in the greenhouse at PARC where no myclobutanil had been applied. Resistance to DMI fungicides develops gradually (Deising et al., 2002). Specific information on DMI resistance for apple powdery mildew is lacking although Hollomon and Wheeler (2002) thought *P. leucotricha* was slow to develop resistance.

Table 6. Percent spore germination of *P. leucotricha* on leaves treated at 0.05 and 0.1 g·L^{-1} myclobutanil

Isolate	Untreated	0.05	0.1
2501	41.8 a[1]	17.3 b	0.5 b
2507	27.4 a	11.3 b	14 b
2470	11.2 a	6.2 b	3.6 b
2509	32.3 a	24.5 ab	12.5 b
2500	29.8 a	12.6 ab	8.1 b
2455[2]	9.0 a	12.3 a	6.5 a
2469	15.7 a	9.3 a	5.5 a
2537	5.3 a	3.3 a	3.1 a
2510	28.0 a	17.8 a	20.3 a
2475	4.2 a	3.2 a	2.8 a

[1] These values are means of three replications. Numbers in each row followed by the same letter are not significantly different at $p \leq 0.05$ as decided by Waller-Duncan k-ratio (k = 100) test.

[2] Isolates in bold are resistant to myclobutanil.

Cherry Powdery Mildew

Until recently cherry powdery mildew was not considered a major problem in BC and targeted sprays for its control were rare. With the release of new cherry cultivars and extension of the cherry growing season powdery mildew has become an important problem. Myclobutanil was used by growers occasionally for the control of brown rot shortly after it was registered in Canada but much less than it is now used for control of powdery mildew. A concern expressed by growers that DMI fungicides gave poor control of cherry powdery mildew was one of the reasons for this survey. Furthermore reports from the state of Washington indicated that resistance had developed to DMI fungicides (Grove et al., 2000). Based on this information there was a strong possibility that *P. clandestina* had developed resistance to myclobutanil in BC. As discussed above for apple monitoring, cherry powdery mildew is difficult to evaluate for DMI resistance thus the number of samples was limited to 14 samples.

Only one isolate was found to be sensitive to myclobutanil because a higher number of spores germinated on untreated leaves than on treated leaves (Table 7). The rest of the isolates showed a high level of resistance to myclobutanil germinating in equal numbers on treated or untreated leaves. Myclobutanil resistance was found on 'Lapins' in Winfield and Keremeos, BC and on 'Sweetheart' in Cawston, Oyama and Oliver, BC. Spray records were not available for these blocks. Interestingly an isolate collected from 'Lapins' in Summerland, BC in early July was sensitive to myclobutanil but an isolate collected from the same block in late July was not. The resistant isolates may be spreading from locations where DMI-resistance has developed to DMI-sensitive orchards. *Podosphaera clandestina* conidia and ascospores are capable of being dispersed long distances by wind, water, insects, or on seeds (Jarvis et al., 2002).

Rose Powdery Mildew

As discussed above for apple and cherry, monitoring rose powdery mildew resistance is also difficult so only 10 samples were evaluated. Information on DMI-resistance by *S. pannosa* in roses is limited. Our own experience with myclobutanil on a susceptible rose cultivar indicated that *S. pannosa* might be DMI-resistant in Kelowna, BC.

Table 7. Percent spore germination of cherry powdery mildew on leaves treated with 0.05 and 0.1 g·L^{-1} myclobutanil

Isolate	Untreated	0.05	0.1
2536	13.2 a[1]	2.1 b	5.0 b
2534[2]	4.9 a	2.3 a	2.5 a
2506	52.9 a	58.3 a	29.2 a
2480	59.7 a	81.4 a	81.5 a
2479	32.4 a	39.4 a	75.8 a
2523-1	67.8 a	71.0 a	63.4 a
2478	31.5 a	34.3 a	63.6 a
2499	65.2 a	34.4 a	33.8 a
2525	83 a	68.8 a	74.6 a
2535	11.6 a	6.6 a	8.7 a
2476	55.5 a	57.3 a	43.5 a
2524	60.0 a	36.4 a	71.4 a
2504	53.5 a	44.4 a	33.2 a
2523-2	75.2 a	68.9 a	37.0 a

[1] These values are means of three replications. Numbers in each row followed by the same letter are not significantly different at $p \leq 0.05$ as decided by Waller-Duncan k-ratio (k = 100) test.
[2] Isolates in bold are resistant to myclobutanil.

As was the case with cherry only one isolate was sensitive to myclobutanil (Table 8). Nine out of the 10 isolates showed some resistance to myclobutanil since the number of germinated spores on treated leaves was very close to the number of germinated spores on untreated leaves. Resistance was found on 'Happy Hour'and 'Hope for Humanity' from Langley and Kelowna, BC, respectively. Resistance was also identified in the powdery mildew present on 'April', 'Torero', 'Gotcha', 'Tropical Amazon', 'Ballet' and 'Explosion' cultivars from Rutland, BC. This particular rose grower had stopped using myclobutanil for lack of efficacy and is now using a potassium bicarbonate based product. In Lavington, BC where myclobutanil was not being used 'Decora' was sensitive although 'Prestige' was resistant.

Table 8. Percent spore germination of rose powdery mildew on leaves treated at 0.05 and 0.1 g/L myclobutanil

Isolate	Untreated	0.05 g/L	0.1 g/L
2487	84.9 a[1]	40 b	57.5 ab
2491[2]	50.5 a	61.4 a	32.3 a
2533	2.1 a	1.8 a	1.4 a
2527	27.6 a	31.7 a	50.6 a
2528	58.2 a	39.2 a	41.5 a
2466	11.4 a	9.2 a	11.8 a
2526	54.3 a	40.7 a	46.7 a
2489	35.3 a	30.2 a	27.2 a
2529	40.1 a	37.9 a	39.0 a
2530	29.9 a	29.7 a	25.8 a

[1] These values are means of three replications. Numbers in each row followed by the same letter are not significantly different at $p \leq 0.05$ as decided by Waller-Duncan k-ratio (k = 100) test.

[2] Isolates in bold are resistant to myclobutanil.

CONCLUSION

Resistance of *V. inaequalis* to myclobutanil was sporadic. Monitoring 72 isolates for DMI resistance indicated that most isolates were sensitive. Although two isolates displayed practical resistance to myclobutanil, this resistance did not appear to correspond with overuse of DMI fungicides.

DMI resistance in the apple powdery mildew population was well established and found in half the isolates that were examined. It is possible that anti-resistance strategies will be sufficient to prolong use of DMI fungicides for apple powdery mildew. The use of QoI fungicides in a mixture has been suggested but resistance developed within two seasons in wheat powdery mildew in northern Germany despite the use of a QoI/DMI mixture (Hollomon and Wheeler, 2002). So far, anti-resistance strategies based on FRAC recommendations have only worked for grape powdery mildew with QoI fungicides. If apple, cherry and rose powdery mildew is similar to the cereal powdery mildews, the QoI fungicides will not remain effective for very long. The use of a multi-site partner like sulfur is an important anti-resistance strategy for apple and cherry powdery mildew but sulfur is phytotoxic in warm weather, which limits its use. The introduction of new chemistries effective against resistant powdery mildew fungi is needed. Quinoxyfen represents a new chemistry that has a novel mode of action against the powdery mildew fungi. It would provide an important alternative to DMI-fungicides for use in an anti-resistance strategy.

When it was first introduced for wheat powdery mildew, it provided season-long protection from a single early season spray and was thought to be a low risk for resistance (Hollomon et al., 1997). More recently, resistance to quinoxyfen by *Blumeria graminis* has been found but subsequent tests indicate that the leaf disc sporulation assay used to determine resistance may have overestimated resistance to quinoxyfen (Green and Gustafson, 2006). This could also be the case with DMI resistance in cherry populations where outright crop failures have not been recorded as far as we are aware in contrast to rose where myclobutanil is completely ineffective. Thus, further testing of cherry populations should be done using a molecular technique such as the method described by Hollomon and Wheeler (2002) where a single PCR product, representative of DMI resistance, is detected by linking the PCR test to a fluorescent dye (picoGreen). If DMI resistance were confirmed, then a recommendation should be made to stop using DMI fungicides for cherry powdery mildew.

According to Jutsum et al. (1998) for effective resistance management an assessment of genetic, ecological and operation risk factors is required, which must then be translated into meaningful local strategies that can be implemented through appropriate labelling of products and education of end users. An important part of this strategy includes establishment of baselines before a new fungicide is introduced. However these strategies do not deal with resistance from a source outside the region. All precautions may be taken by growers in a certain region but if the resistant isolates were developed outside the region and are brought in on nursery stock or possibly blown in, they have no control over resistance development. Therefore, the most important thing for them is to know if fungicide resistance is present so steps could be taken to mitigate the problem. Regular monitoring for fungicide resistance would be their most important anti-resistance strategy.

REFERENCES

Braun, P.G., and McRae, K.B. (1992). Composition of a population of *Venturia inaequalis* resistant to myclobutanil. *Can J. Plant Pathol. 14:* 215-220.

Brent, K.J. Fungicide Resistance in Crop Pathogens: How can it be Managed? Brussels, International Group of National Associations of Manufacturers of Agrochemical Products. 1995.

Delp, C.J. Fungicide Resistance in North America. St. Paul, MN, The American Phytopathological Society. 1988.

Délye, C., Bousset, L., and Corio-Costet, M-F. (1998). PCR cloning and detection of point mutations in the eburicol 14α-demethylase (CYP51) gene from *Erysiphe graminis* f. sp. *hordei,* a "recalcitrant" fungus. *Curr. Genet. 34:* 399-403.

Délye, C., Laigret, F., Corio-Costet, M-F. (1997). A mutation in the 14α-demethylase gene of *Uncinula necator* that correlates with resistance to a sterol biosynthesis inhibitor. *Appl. Environ. Microbiol. 63:* 2966-2970.

Deising, H.B., Reimann, S., Peil, A., and Weber, W.E. (2002). Disease management of rusts and powdery mildews. In K. Esser & J.W. Bennett (Eds.), *The Mycota: a Comprehensive Treatise on Fungi as Experimental Systems for Basic and Applied Research* (XI Agricutural Applications, pp. 243-269). Berlin: Springer Verlag.

Erickson, E.O. and Wilcox, W.F. (1997). Distribution of sensitivities to three sterol demethylation inhibitor fungicides among populations of *Uncinula necator* sensitive and resistant to triadimefon. *Phytopathology 87:* 784-791

Fiaccadori, R., Gielink, A.J., and Dekker, J. (1987). Sensitivity to inhibitors of sterol biosynthesis in isolates of *Venturia inaequalis* from Italian and Dutch orchards. *Neth. J. Pl. Path. 93:* 285-287.

Georgopoulos, S.G. (1987). The development of fungicide resistance. In M.S. Wolfe & C.E. Caten, (Eds.) *Populations of Plant Pathogens: their Dynamics and Genetics* (pp. 239-251). Oxford, UK:Blackwell Scientific Publications.

Green, E.A., and Gustafson, G.D. (2006). Sensitivity of *Uncinula necator* to quinoxyfen: evaluation of isolates selected using a discriminatory dose screen. *Pest Manag. Sci. 62:* 492-497.

Green, J.R., Carver, T.L., and Gurr, S.J. (2002). The formation and function of infection and feeding structures. In R. R. Bélanger, W.R. Bushnell, A.J. Dik, & T.L. Carver (Eds.), *The Powdery Mildews: a Comprehensive Treatise* (pp. 66-82). St. Paul, MN: American Phytopathological Society Press.

Grove, G.G., Boal, J., and Bennett, L.H. (2000). Managing powdery mildew of cherry in Washington orchards and nurseries with spray oils. Plant Health Progress: DOI: 10.1094/PHP-2000-0628-01-RS.

Grove, G.G. (1999). New angles on apple powdery mildew. *Good Fruit Grower*, April 15, pp.45.

Gubler, W.D., Ypema, H.L., Ouimette, D.G., and Bettiga, L.J. (1996). Occurrence of resistance in *Uncinula necator* to triadimefon, myclobutanil, and fenarimol in California grapevines. *Plant Dis. 80:* 902-909.

Hildebrand, P.D., Lockhart, C.L., Newbery, R.J., and Ross, R.G. (1988). Resistance of *Venturia inaequalis* to bitertanol and other demethylation-inhibiting fungicides. *Can. J. Plant Pathol. 10:* 311-316.

Hollomon, D.W., and Wheeler, I.E. (2002). Controlling powdery mildews with chemistry. In R. R. Bélanger, W.R. Bushnell, A.J. Dik, & T.L. Carver (Eds.), *The Powdery Mildews: a Comprehensive Treatise* (pp. 249-255). St. Paul, MN: American Phytopathological Society Press.

Hollomon, D.W., Wheeler, I., Dixon, K., Longhurst, C., and Skylakakis, G. (1997). Defining the resistance risk of the new powdery mildew fungicide quinoxyfen. *Pestic. Sci. 51:* 347-351.

Hsiang, T., Yang, L., and Barton, W. (1997). Baseline sensitivity and cross-resistance to demethylation-inhibiting fungicides in Ontario isolates of *Sclerotinia homoeocarpa. Eur. J. Plant Pathol. 103:* 409-416.

Jarvis, W.R., Gubler, W.D., and Grove, G.G. (2002). Epidemiology of powdery mildews in agricultural pathosystems. In R.R. Belanger, W.R. Bushnell, A.J. Dik & T.W. Carver (Eds.), *The Powdery Mildews: a Comprehensive Treatise* (pp. 169-199). St Paul, MN: American Phytopathological Society Press.

Jobin, T., and Carisse, O. (2007). Incidence of myclobutanil- and kresoxim-methyl-insensitive isolates of *Venturia inaequalis* in Quebec orchards. *Plant Dis. 91:*1351-1358.

Justum, A.R., Heaney, S.P., Perrin, B.M., and Wege, P.J. 1998. Pesticide resistance: assessment of risk and the development and implementation of effective management strategies. *Pestic. Sci.* 54:435-446.

Köller, W., Wilcox, W.F. (2001). Evidence fpr the predisposition of fungicide-resistant phenotypes of *Venturia inaequalis* to a preferential selection for resistance to other fungicides. *Phytopathology 91:* 776-781.

Köller, W., Wilcox, W.F., Barnard, J., Jones, A.L., and Braun, P. G. (1997). Detection and quantification of resistance of *Venturia inaequalis* populations to sterol demethylation inhibitors. *Phytopathology 87:*184-190.

Köller, W., Parker, D.M., and Reynolds, K. L. (1991). Baseline sensitivities of *Venturia inaequalis* to sterol demethylation inhibitiors. *Plant Dis. 75:*726-728.

Nicot, P.C., Bardin, M. and Dik, A.J. (2002). Basic methods for epidemiological studies of powdery mildews: Culture and preservation of isolates, production and delivery of inoculum, and disease assessment. In R. R. Bélanger, W.R. Bushnell, A.J. Dik, & T.L. Carver (Eds.), *The Powdery Mildews: a Comprehensive Treatise* (pp. 83-99). St. Paul, MN: American Phytopathological Society Press.

Northover, J., and Homeyer, C.A. (2001). Detection and management of myclobutanil-resistant grapevine powdery mildew (*Uncinula necator)* in Ontario. *Can. J. Plant Pathol. 23:* 337-345.

Olmstead, J. W., Lang, G.A. and Grove, G.G. (2000). A leaf disk assay for screening sweet cherry genotypes for susceptibility to powdery mildew. *HortScience 35:* 274-277.

Sholberg, P.L. (2004). Management of grape diseases in arid climates. In S.A.M.H. Naqvi, Editor, *Diseases of Fruits and Vegetables*, (Volume II, pp. 53-80). Dordrecht, The Netherlands: Kluwer Academic Publishers.

Sholberg, P.L., Lane, W.D., Haag, P., Bedford, K., and Lashuk, L. (2001). A novel technique for evaluation of apple (*Malus* x *domestica* Borkh.) cultivars for susceptibility of powdery mildew. *Can. J. Plant Sci. 81:* 289-296.

Sholberg, P.L., and Haag, P.D. (1993). Sensitivity of *Venturia inaequalis* isolates from British Columbia to flusilazole and myclobutanil. *Can. J. Plant Pathol. 15:* 102-106.

Sholberg, P.L., and Haag, P.D. (1993). Sensitivity of *Venturia inaequalis* isolates from British Columbia to flusilazole and myclobutanil. *Can. J. Plant Pathol. 15:*102-106.

Sholberg, P.L and Yorston, J. M. (1991). Phenotype patterns of benomyl-resistant isolates of *Venturia inaequalis* in eight orchards in BC, Canada. *Plant Disease 75:*616-619.

Sholberg, P.L., Yorston, J. M. and Warnock, D. (1989). Resistance of *Venturia inaequalis* to Benomyl and Dodine in BC, Canada. *Plant Disease 73:*667-669.

Smith, C. M. (1988). History of benzimidazole use and resistance. In Charles J. Delp Editor, *Fungicide Resistance in North America* (pp. 23-24). St. Paul, MN: APS Press.

Smith, F. D., Parker, D. M. and Köller, W. (1991). Sensitivity distribution of *Venturia inaequalis* to the sterol of demethylation inhibitor flusilazole: Baseline sensitivity and implications for resistance monitoring. *Phytopathology 81:*392-396.

Stanis, V.F., and Jones, A.L. (1985). Reduced sensitivity to sterol-inhibiting fungicides in field isolates of *Venturia inaequalis. Phytopathology 75:*1098-1101.

Wurms, K., Labbé, C. Benhamou, N. And Bélanger, R. R. (1999). Effects of Milsana and benzotiadiazole on the ultrastructure of powdery mildew haustoria on cucumber. *Phytopathology 89:*728-736.

Ypema, H.L., Ypema, M., and Gubler, W.D. (1997). Sensitivity of *Uncinula necator* to benomyl, triadimefon, myclobutanil, and fenarimol in California. *Plant Dis. 81:* 293-297.

In: Fungicides
Editors: P. De Costa and P. Bezerra

ISBN: 978-1-60692-631-4

Chapter XIII

OCCURRENCE, PROBLEMS, ANALYSIS AND REMOVAL OF FILAMENTOUS FUNGI IN DRINKING WATER

***R. Russell M. Paterson*[1], *Gunhild Hageskal*[2], *Ida Skaar*[2], *Nelson Lima*[1]**

[1]IBB-Institute for Biotechnology and Bioengineering, Centre of Biological Engineering, Universidade do Minho, Campus de Gualtar, 4710-057 Braga, Portugal

[2]National Veterinary Institute, Section of Mycology, PO Box 8156 Dep, 0033 Oslo, Norway

ABSTRACT

The occurrence of filamentous fungi in drinking water has been known for many years. However, the quantity of scientific literature on the subject is only beginning to increase. Filamentous fungi have been considered only as annoying contaminants of agar plates used to count bacteria from water. There are various potential issues associated with the fungi-in-drinking-water phenomenon, including blockage of water pipes, organoleptic problems such as odour and taste, biofilm formation, spread of pathogenic fungi, and mycotoxins production. Drinking water raises issues of biosecurity in relation to mycotoxin production. This chapter presents a review of fungi in drinking water, with emphases on (a) methods of isolation, (b) fungi detected, (c) problems which occur, (d) avoidance or removal, and (e) methods to detect biochemicals such as mycotoxins. The literature on bottled will be assessed because it is being returned increasingly due to the presence of filamentous fungi. Domestic tap water will be considered. Suggestions for future collaborative work will be made which will include the use of standardised methodology for isolation and identification of filamentous fungi, the use of "ring tests", standard biochemical analysis, and the need for international research projects. Also, sound methods for the removal and control of filamentous fungi will be devised in the longer term. It is intended that standardised methodology will be the major output of such research equivalent to those that exist for bacteria.

INTRODUCTION

Filamentous fungi have received increased focus as drinking water contaminants. It is gratifying that investigations regarding this potential hazard are increasing. These organisms are accepted as common in water, although the extent of the problems they create remains unresolved. The following chapter considers the issue on the basis of the work of two research groups who individually have produced some of the most relevant work and the present monograph updates previous reviews (e.g. Paterson and Lima 2005; Hageskal *et al.* 2009).

Fungi are a ubiquitous and diverse group of unique organisms sometimes naively referred to as the "fifth kingdom". The (under) estimated number of fungal species is 1.5 x 10^6 (Hawksworth 2001) of which only a small number have been identified (ca. 5%). The fungi range in size from species with massive underground structures to microscopic single-celled yeasts. A large group is characterized by hyphal growth (i.e. the mycelium) which absorbs nutrients and supports spores (i.e. conidia). The sexuality of filamentous fungi is complex (see Paterson et al. 2006) with some species being represented only by an asexual (anamorph) stage, whereas a sexual stage (teleomorph) is recognised in others. Together these form the holomorph. The asexual reproduction stage is the one usually obtained in culture.

Several filamentous fungi have commercial applications such as in the production of antibiotics (e.g. penicillin), organic acids (e.g. citric acid), industrial alcohol (e.g. biofuel) and enzymes (e.g. amylases). The organisms are also abundant sources of potential pharmaceuticals such as enzyme inhibitors (Paterson 2008a). They are used as foodstuff directly in the form of mushrooms and "Quorn", the *Fusarium* biomass produced in bioreactors. In addition, the organisms are employed in the production of a diverse range of important food products (e.g. cheese, wine, meats, and soya sauce). Traditional Chinese medicines, which have huge worldwide markets, include fungi (e.g. *Ganoderma* and *Cordyceps*) and these are investigated increasingly as novel conventional medicines (Paterson 2006a; 2008b). One of the most important roles of fungi is in the biodegradation of organic materials in the environment. In this respect, they are observed on decaying foodstuff in which some fungi produce toxins (mycotoxins) (Venâncio and Paterson 2007). Many are notorious plant pathogens and others are reported as human pathogens, particularly in immunocompromised patients in hospitals.

The problems for which filamentous fungi are responsible include organoleptic (taste, odour, colour), infections, allergic reactions and mycotoxin production. The reason why fungi have not been examined more fully as drinking water contaminants is that they have not been associated with acute disease or rapid poisonings of humans (or other animals). However, consumption of mycotoxins in foodstuffs may have fatal effects on animals and humans, although the predominant effects are probably chronic. In addition, contaminated water may act as inocula of fungi into food. The sources of fungi and fungal products in drinking water are predominately natural, but they could conceivably be deliberately spread in water by nefarious actions (Paterson 2006b).

Natural Contamination

This concept represents the fungal equivalent of the well-recognised bacterial contamination of drinking water. Fungi are eukaryotic organisms that grow by heterotrophic absorption of nutrients. (The heterotrophy implies inclusion in heterotrophic plate counts of water, although this does not occur routinely.) Filamentous fungi are present in the environment in large amounts. They are in soil, organic material, water and air, and can also enter drinking water from various locations. Furthermore, fungi can become established in many ways in water distribution systems, such as via sediments, plant debris and biofilms. Soft deposits in pipelines have been reported as key sites for fungi (Zacheus et al. 2001). Particular common fungal genera, such as *Penicillium*, *Aspergillus* and *Fusarium* are likely to be present in significant numbers in water. Incidentally the *Oomycetes* will not be discussed in this entry since they are no longer considered to be fungi, and, in any case, are not associated with the problems described, except perhaps as occasional growth.

Occurrence of Filamentous Fungi in Drinking Water

Fungal contamination of water has been reported for decades, although investigations have been inadequate compared with those for bacteria. Confirmed reports of fungal contamination of drinking water are sporadic. Hageskal *et al.* (2009) provided a comprehensive review of filamentous fungi in drinking water: Portuguese water has been investigated recently (Gonçalves et al. 2006a), and studies of Norwegian drinking water provided important additional knowledge (Hageskal *et al.* 2006; 2007). The data is growing continuously, although systematic studies are lacking in general. Indeed, most of the fungal water studies are undertaken in response to an isolated contamination problem. There have been only a few reports from distribution systems (*ca.* 15) from approximately 10 countries, and virtually none from developing countries (Kelley *et al.* 2003). Various fungal isolation methods have been used, making direct comparisons impossible. Fungal identifications have often been to the genus rather than species level. This may be problematic because of the potential health hazards and water quality problems associated with particular fungal species. Colony counts of total fungi alone are not sufficient for the fungal analyses of water, and identification to genus also gives limited information on the fungal diversity. The species identity should be established, especially in clinical settings, although this can be difficult due to inadequacies in fungal taxonomy in general (Paterson et al. 2004; 2006).

Penicillium and *Acremonium* were isolated most frequently in an EU project conducted in order to control the mycological quality of tap water in Portugal. These genera demonstrated an inverse relationship with respect to isolation frequency (i.e. when one was high, the other was low throughout the test period). *Penicillium expansum* and *P. brevicompactum* were isolated often, with *P. expansum* being the well-known patulin producer. The other potential mycotoxin producers, *Alternaria* and *Chaetomium*, were isolated at low frequency, and *Claviceps* were not detected (Gonçlaves et al. 2006a). *Penicillium* has been demonstrated to be common in previous studies (Kelley et al. 2003; Hageskal *et al.* 2006). It was moderately unexpected that *Aspergillus*, especially, and

Fusarium were not more common in Portuguese water systems. A rather wide range of other genera were identified, perhaps reflecting the variety of methods used. Nevertheless, many taxa were also isolated from the distribution systems examined in Kelley et al. (2003), where methods were more standardized, and fungi were identified to species. Results from the US distribution systems demonstrated that the fusaria were well represented, while the aspergilli were less frequent. Several of the isolated fungal species were potential toxin producers: Interestingly, the oestrogenic and carcinogenic mycotoxin zearalenone was produced *in vitro* in water by a *Fusarium graminearum* strain isolation from the US distribution system indicating the potential for problems (Paterson 2007a): The production of mycotoxins from fusaria is now recognized as an issue in water (Bucheli *et al* 2008). Strains in Kelley et al. (2003) were assessed for variation in nucleic acids in order to determine the similarity of the species detected throughout the systems. However, natural variation within the general population was unexamined making interpretation difficult.

A 12-month survey was performed in Germany on drinking water from 29 groundwater-derived supplies to assess the dissemination of ''hygienically'' relevant fungi (Göttlich et al. 2002). Importantly, a correlation with standard hygiene bacterial indicators was not found. Common allergenic *Aspergillus* were encountered rarely while *Acremonium, Exophiala, Penicillium* and *Phialophora* dominated the fungal diversity. Some were encountered throughout the drinking water systems and constituted a residual mycobiota, and it was interesting that nucleic acid analysis for strain variation was considered unnecessary.

A more recent Norwegian study investigated water from 14 drinking water distribution systems including surface- and groundwater-derived supplies (Hageskal *et al.* 2006; 2007). Fungi were common in both water supplies, although they were three times more likely to be recovered from surface-derived, compared to ground-derived, water. *Trichoderma, Penicillium* and *Aspergillus* were the most frequent. Nearly all fungi were identified to species, and *Trichoderma viride* was the most frequent species throughout Norwegian distribution systems. *Aspergillus* species were isolated frequently from Norwegian water in contrast to the results from the US and German distribution systems (Kelley et al. 2003; Göttlich et al. 2002). Similar results were reported from Greek water (Arvanitidou *et al.* 1999; 2000). *Aspergillus ustus* was one of the species most commonly isolated from Norwegian water. The fungus was isolated throughout the distribution systems, especially in ground-derived systems, and this species appears to have the ability to survive and adapt to high temperatures, since it was often isolated from hot water installations. A wide diversity of filamentous fungi was identified, and species of pathogenic, allergenic and toxigenic potential were among the most common.

Relevance of Filamentous Fungi in Water

Distributed Water

The issue of the significance of filamentous fungi in water is complex, and the contribution of waterborne fungi to health and water quality problems are not yet determined completely. Fungal contaminated water will be of most importance in hospitals or other health care institutions, where immunocompromised patients undergo treatment. One theory is that hospital water systems may be the source of nosocomial mycoses (Anaissie and Costa 2001). Fungi can be aerosolized when water passes through installations such as taps or showers, and consequently may be inhaled. Fungal diseases of humans usually originate from an exogenous source in the environment and are acquired through inhalation, ingestion or traumatic implantation. Filamentous fungi can be implicated in three categories of disease in humans and animals: infections (mycoses), allergies and/or toxicoses.

Human Mycoses

A dramatic increase in the numbers of invasive diseases caused by filamentous fungi has occurred recently (Sheppard et al. 2004) which can be attributed to the large numbers of patients undergoing immunosuppressive therapies, chemotherapy, and organ and bone marrow transplantations. Patient suffering from immunoincompetent conditions such as AIDS are also at risk. Pathogenic yeasts (e.g. *Candida albicans* and *Cryptococcus neofarmans*) remain very problematic. Among the filamentous fungi, *Aspergillus* is by far the most important genus, and *A. fumigatus* accounts for 90% of the cases. Additionally, *A. flavus* is now considered to be a major concern which perhaps has been underappreciated (Hedayati et al. 2007). *Fusarium* and *Zygomycetes* are common problems amongst the remainder, and several fungal species, such as *Aspergillus ustus*, have been characterized as emerging pathogens in immunocompromised patients. Problems with resistance against antifungal medicines are also increasing, making the focus on prevention of exposure to such fungi more important than ever. It is, of course, likely that at least some of these problematic fungal species will be present in water supplies at some stage and, consequently, pose a threat.

Allergic Responses

As many as 236 unique fungal allergic extract products representing 45 genera and 73 species of fungi have been produced (Esch 2004). All are available in an attempt to identify which fungi produce allergies, and this indicates the potential of drinking water to be a carrier of such fungi. Furthermore, a significant number of these fungi have been reported from water. A few cases have been connected directly to fungal contaminated water. Outbreaks of skin irritations associated with taking showers and baths (Åslund 1984), and hypersensitivity pneumonitis caused by elevated levels of filamentous fungi in water (Metzger *et al.* 1976) were reported. Also, these may have been involved in extrinsic allergic alveolitis in tap water (Muittari *et al.* 1980).

Mycotoxins

Secondary metabolites from fungi are those that are not involved directly in the universal biochemical processes, such as DNA replication, protein formation, glycolysis, etc. These are the fungal chemicals that can cause problems in water, i.e. mycotoxins, pigments, tastes and odours. It is likely that concentrations will be low under normal circumstances (see Paterson 2007a), although recent reports are concerned with the effects of low concentrations in water (Bucheli *et al.* 2008; Gromadzka *et al.* 2009). There are potentially thousands of mycotoxins (CAST 2003; Venâncio and Paterson 2007), although only a few are recognized as mycotoxins causing significant problems in food, feed and beverages. Mycotoxin contaminated food and drink may have severe effects on human and animal health ranging from chronic to acute disease, and death. The bioactivities include mutagenic, teratogenic, oestrogenic, and carcinogenic effects. Mycotoxins may damage (a) major organs such as the liver, kidney and lungs, and/or (b) the nervous, endocrine and immune systems. In this respect, it is important to realize that foetuses and infants are highly susceptible to even small amounts of mycotoxins. Nefarious acts of adding mycotoxins to water need to be appreciated as potential problems (Paterson 2006b). Finally, it is conceivable that liquid runoff from contaminated crops or agricultural waste products could contain mycotoxins and fungi that could subsequently enter the water system (Bucheli *et al.* 2008).

The economic costs resulting from mycotoxins in the United States alone exceed $1.4 $\times$ 10^9 per annum (CAST 2003). For aflatoxin, a figure of $500 x 10^6 has been given, although this does not take into account other factors which would increase the amount significantly (Bhatnagar *et al.* 2008). The importance of mycotoxins can be anticipated to increase as new regulations are assigned to them (e.g., recent European Union regulations on patulin), and as awareness grows in line with the general increased recognition of food safety issues. The most important mycotoxin producers are members of *Penicillium*, *Aspergillus*, *Fusarium* and *Claviceps*. However, different mycotoxins (and fungi) may be detected in commodities that are not considered conventionally from this perspective (e.g., water). The effects of fungi on animal drinking water require consideration, since it is likely to be of a poorer quality than human drinking water. This may affect animal productivity and mycotoxins in animals may be consumed by humans (i.e., ''secondary mycotoxicosis'').

Large volumes of water are used in the manufacture of foods, feeds, and beverages. Mycotoxins could be included in these commodities, especially if this water is stored (see Paterson *et al.* (1997). In addition, the water will often be partially or fully evaporated during food or beverage processing, hence concentrating any mycotoxins present in the water or causing them to crystallize out of solution. The *in vitro* studies of Kelley et al. (2003) indicated that fungi can produce mycotoxins and other secondary metabolites in water. Zearalenone, which has oestrogenic and carcinogenic properties, was detected from water inoculated with *F. graminearum* (Paterson 2007a) at 15 ng l^{-1} concentration, a level similar to those reported as potential problems in Gromadzka *et al.* (2009). Only trace amounts of aflatoxins were detected in domestic drinking water. Other fungal mycotoxins and metabolites were reported in solution from water *in vitro*, and secondary metabolites from fungi isolated from water were detected. Aflatoxins in stored water have also been reported (Paterson *et al.* 1997).

Tastes and Odours

The organoleptic problems that may develop in water are not associated conventionally with fungi. However, filamentous fungi can grow in waters to the extent that they are visible (Paterson 2007a), and produce the same volatile compounds as the actinomycetes, such as geosmin (Paterson et al. 2007). These eukaryotic organisms may reduce the disinfecting power of chemicals, although not necessarily to the extent as to make them ineffective. Water treatment plants can be affected, since fungi may contribute to the biological load of sand filters and perhaps make them less effective. A special case is stored water where fungi can accumulate and toxin concentrations could be high within the fungal cells and/or in the water.

For example, bottled water can be considered as stored. Many of the compounds produced by bacteria in relation to taste and odour are also produced by filamentous fungi. In addition, fungi produce their own battery of compounds with distinctive off-odours and tastes. Fungal isolates are capable of transforming 2,4,6-tricholorophenol to 2,4,6-trichloroanisol, which causes taste and odour problems in the distribution system. Canhoto and Magan (2003) suggested ''electronic nose'' technology to detect off-odours from fungi in potable water which could be of considerable utility. A musty smell in the Parisian water system was attributed to fungi (Monteil *et al.* 1999), while another survey indicated that the taste and odour problems were attributed to actinomycetes or algae, although the reasons why fungi were not implicated were not obvious (Kelley *et al.* 2003).

Pigments

Little information on the production of pigments by fungi in water exists, although they are likely to be responsible for the occurrence in some cases, since fungi produce a great deal of pigmentation in general. *In vitro* investigations have indicated the presence of a red pigment produced by *F. graminearum* in water (Kelley *et al.* 2003; Paterson (2007a).

Stored Water

Bottled Water

Bottled water has world sales of \$5.7 × 10^9 and are projected to increase (Rosenberg 2003). Fungal contamination of bottled water occurs (Cabra and Fernández Pinto 2002; Lima, unpublished results) and production of the mycotoxin citrinin has been demonstrated in bottled water (Criado *et al.* 2005) although experimental controls appeared to be inadequate in that study (e.g. uninoculated water was not tested). Filamentous fungi can be observed as visible clumps of growth inside the bottle, which is unacceptable to the consumer, resulting in significant financial loss due to product recall and ''downtime'' from the need for special sanitation treatments. However, the major loss may be the bad publicity created by such incidents.

In general, standardized methods to detect fungi are not employed currently by the bottling companies' quality control system. Analysis for fungi using conventional techniques are time-consuming (a minimum of two weeks are required for growth and identifications), meaning that contamination problems will persist for that period of time before remedial action is taken. However, little information exists in this area. Bottled water is often expected to be purer compared with tap water, although this is not necessarily the case. There are anecdotal reports of bottled water being returned to the manufacturer because of visual fungal growth. Finally, a most useful publication has been produced with respect to the microbiological safety of bottled water which includes mycological aspects (Food Standards Agency 2008).

Stored Water Tanks

Aflatoxins are the most significant mycotoxins, and were reported from stored water in the first reported natural occurrence of any mycotoxin (or fungal secondary metabolite) from water (Paterson et al. 1997; Paterson 2006b). It is also these compounds that are considered to be the most probable threat in terms of security of the water supply. Zearalenone or similar compounds were also detected in the stored water. People may drink water from storage tanks whether the water is intended for that purpose or not. In the United Kingdom, water is often stored in tanks for bathroom or potable purposes. Obviously, potable water is stored in certain specific situations, such as in cruise ships. Finally, bottled water is also a form of storage.

Control of Fungi in Water

Water utilities appear to have little expertise with filamentous fungi, largely because they have not been implicated directly in health or quality problems (in water at least). The control strategies and efficiency of water treatment against fungi is understood poorly in general, and the few studies conducted are inconsistent. Nevertheless, chemical coagulation was reported to be the most effective water treatment method (Niemi *et al.* 1982), while another study found that sand filtration gave better removal of fungi than coagulation with iron (Kelley *et al.* 2003). Chlorination used for disinfection of water was found to be insufficient (Franková and Horecka 1995; Nagy and Olson 1985), while the use of chlorine dioxide and ozone were reported as the most effective disinfectants against fungal spores by Kelley *et al.* (2003). Ultra violet (UV) radiation may have potential in the case of fungi with limited pigmentation, since the UV sensitivity of the fungi is related to pigmentation. Fungal species with pigmented conidia and hypha, such as *Aspergillus* and *Penicillium* species, are often more resistant to UV than unpigmented species (Waipara 1998). This was also experienced in the study by Kelley et al. (2003) where melanized thick-walled species predominated after treatment. Incidentally, fungal conidia appear to exhibit similar susceptibilities to disinfectants as *Giardia* cysts.

Several investigations have also reported fungi as residents of biofilms in water and waste-water pipe surfaces (Doggett 2000; Gonçalves *et al.* 2006b; Hendrickx *et al.* 2002; Kelley *et al.* 2003; Nagy and Olson 1982). Treatment of fungi established in biofilms in water distribution systems was investigated by Kelley *et al.* (2003). Although most cleaning techniques were found to be insufficient for the removal of fungi in biofilms, flow jetting was observed to offer the most effective treatment. Fungi are capable of attached and unattached growth in water. It is assumed that fungi scavenge nutrients from the environment to support growth in oligotrophic (very low nutrient) situations such as water. Filamentous fungi can survive water treatment and disinfection, and contaminate the water that reaches the consumers. It is probable that fungi do not behave in any particular manner that requires special procedures for control under normal circumstances. However, in certain settings, as for example in hospital environments, surveillance of the water distribution system may be appropriate, since species of clinical concern have been observed to colonize the water system.

In the case of water stored in tanks where *A. flavus* and mycotoxins were detected (Paterson et al. 1997; Paterson 2006b), the contaminated water was drained and thoroughly cleaned, including with the used of "bleach" at low concentration. The system was rinsed carefully with water. The whole system was checked and cleaned by professional on a regular contract basis (e.g. twice per year).

UNNATURAL CONTAMINATION

Biological Weapons (Nefarious Contamination)

"Security is one of the top priorities of large and small water utilities across the USA" (Mays 2004). Fungi may be considered as potential biological weapons, since they cause infections of animals, humans, and/or crops. In addition, the potential of fungi to produce toxins (which can be purified) is relevant. Aflatoxins are accepted as being a threat, although the induction of cancers in the long-term is the predominate effect of these mycotoxins. T-2 toxin is also recognized as a potential chemical weapon. The potential of using fungi and, particularly, mycotoxins as weapons require more thorough assessment (CAST 2003; Paterson 2006b). However, there is no obvious fungal equivalent to botulinum toxin for example. One could consider a more immediate threat from ergot alkaloids, or the LSD-like effect of toxins from the mushroom *Amanita* sp. Quantity is the issue of relevance if mycotoxins are to be considered as weapons. The fungus, or more specifically the toxin, will be at much higher concentrations than would occur normally, and may be capable of being measured readily. Water systems or bottled water would be obvious targets, and knowledge of fungi and mycotoxins in water is more essential than ever as a result. Mycotoxins would be difficult to remove generally when dissolved in the water supply. Boiling or autoclaving will not remove them, although the levels may be reduced in some cases. The effect of high concentrations of mycotoxins on water purifications systems is unknown, although it is likely that they would become less efficient at least. However, not all mycotoxins are water-soluble, but could be present as particles. Biosensors (e.g., protozoa) may be appropriate for detecting mycotoxins in these circumstances, as the higher concentrations would be more likely to have an effect on the test organisms. Also, biosensors are less specific and, theoretically, any toxicity could be detected with the same test, in an inexpensive and rapid manner (Paterson 2006b).

Fungal Biological Control Agents

These are natural fungal pathogens of insects or plants used to control insect or plant pests/diseases. The procedures tend to be experimental and generally do not compete with conventional control methods. However, commercial preparations exist and are apparently used frequently in Cuba, for example, and in some developing countries. These pathogenic fungi may be applied by spray, and enter the water systems in this manner. Also, infected target organisms could conceivably pollute the water supply (see Paterson 2006b). The production of toxins by these fungi could present an additional problem.

METHODS

Fungal Isolations

There is not an international standard method described for the analyses of filamentous fungi in water, hence several isolation procedures are used. Most studies performed use membrane filter techniques. Others perform direct plate spreading, and centrifugation of water to obtain the fungal propagules. Different isolation procedures result in various detection limits of fungi in the water samples and differences in fungal recovery. The incubation temperature is also crucial for which fungal species will be obtained, since high incubation temperatures may select for some species and loss of others (e.g. *A. fumigatus* is associated with high temperature).

The isolation media also varies among the investigations, which might result in selectivity towards some fungal genera and loss of others. Examples of media used for fungal analyses of water are: Sabouraud dextrose agar (SDA), malt extract agar (MEA), potato dextrose agar (PDA), Czapec Dox agar (CDA) and half-strength cornmeal agar (CMA/2). Dichloran rose bengal chloramphenicol agar (DRBC) (King *et al.* 1979) and dichloran 18% glycerol agar (DG18) (Hocking and Pitt 1980) are now recommended as general media for the purpose of isolation and enumeration of fungi in foods of high water activity ($a_w > 0.90$) (Samson *et al.* 2004), and may therefore also be suitable for water analyses. A recurring problem with isolating fungi is ensuring that they are not overgrown by faster growing species. Dichloran 18% glycerol agar has several advantages; the characteristic colony appearance on agar plates facilitates differentiation of species which makes secondary selection and re-isolation of pure cultures easier to accomplish, as compared to DRBC. DG18 also inhibits overgrowth of fast growing fungi such as *Mucorales* and *Trichoderma*, which facilitate colony counts. Finally, another advantage is that DG18 does not produce readily substances toxic to the fungus when exposed to light. Media containing rose bengal are light sensitive and produce inhibitory compounds in significant concentrations after two hours exposure to light (Samson *et al.* 2004). The use of media containing rose bengal could affect the results and may be inappropriate for studies of fungi in drinking water. Some researchers recommend a combination of low and high nutritional media to obtain the complete cross section of fungi present in water (Kelley *et al.* 2003; Kinsey *et al.* 1999). Employing a low-nutritional medium, such as CMA/2, in addition to DG18 may give supplementary knowledge about fungi in water.

Enumeration

In terms of assessing the contribution of fungi to problems in water, an overarching concern is quantification, which may have contributed to fungi being almost overlooked in the past. Filamentous fungi in water are often enumerated by counting the total number of visible colonies on agar plates, referred to as colony forming units (CFU) per volume water sample investigated (Mara and Horan 2006). Due to the nature of filamentous fungi, the data generated in this way may be difficult to interpret. Fungi have a tendency to be unevenly distributed in water which causes difficulty in ensuring samples are representative and which can particularly cause problems in diluted samples. The possibility that one fungal colony may originate from clusters of spores or hyphal fragments, is also a relevant problem in the analyses of fungi in water. On the other hand, one individual fungal colony can become separated into smaller pieces during sampling or filtration, so that one single fungal species could be over-represented. Another potential problem with the CFU count method is that not all fungal colonies are able to grow on agar media under laboratory conditions. If a fungus does not spore, or is at a stage in the lifecycle when conidia do not form, they cannot be isolated in a representative manner. Also, what is a single fungus? Is it one conidium, colony, conidiophore, or hyphal cell? In effect, the CFU counts of filamentous fungi in water samples are therefore not likely to give the precise number of individual fungi present, but are nevertheless helpful in providing an indication of the level of contamination in the samples. Interpretation of fungal count data requires caution and experience in the field.

Identification and Characterisation of Fungi in Water

The phenotypic identification of fungi to species level is based on (a) morphological characteristics such as septation of hypha; (b) formation and morphology of fruiting-bodies and conidiophores; (c) branching patterns and frequency of branching; and (d) size, form, colour and ornamentation of the conidia. Macroscopic characters such as colony form, structure, size and colour are also important. In addition, appearance and growth on different culture media is used for differentiation. There are only a few selective media available for the isolation of fungi. Selective media were first developed to inhibit bacterial growth and to reduce the colony size of fast growing fungi, but they are also useful in distinguishing between different groups of fungi and even between certain fungal species. Based on the aforementioned criteria, fungi are identified to species or even subspecies level by employing light microscopy according to conventional identification keys. Morphological identification of filamentous fungi is time consuming and difficult, and experience is required to ensure accurate identifications. The morphological approach to species identification may benefit from supplementation with chemical and molecular research tools, especially in cases where the morphological characters are variable leading to overlap among species, and when isolates are sterile or non viable. A polyphasic approach to identification is needed to cover all aspects of the species identity. Paterson et al. (2004; 2006) have recommended a novel identification system for mycotoxigenic fungi where a readily identifiable morphological character is employed (e.g. a conidiophore) together with analysis for the mycotoxin(s) of interest which may have utility with respect to water.

Molecular technology and phylogenetic studies have reformed the taxonomy of many fungal genera, and DNA technology makes it possible to identify fungi genetically. Genotypic identification of filamentous fungi to the species level is based on the principle of genetic variation in DNA sequences within species. Sequencing of the ribosomal DNA (rDNA) internal transcribed spacer (ITS) region, followed by similarity search in databases like EMBL/GenBank, is widely used among researchers in order to identify fungi. It is noteworthy, however, that the problem of erroneously identified species has lead to uncertainty with respect to the accuracy of fungal databases. For example, it has been estimated that approximately 40% of the *Trichoderma/Hypocrea* records in GenBank are either misidentified or unidentified at the species level (Druzhinina *et al.* 2006). To solve such problems, barcode-based identification programs and databases with vouchered sequences are being developed for several genera, such as for the genus *Trichoderma* (Druzhinina *et al.* 2005) and *Penicillium* (see Paterson and Lima 2009). These systems are based on defined combinations of absolute species-, clade- and genus-specific oligonucleotides allocated within DNA sequences. The barcode-based identification is supported by phylogenetic studies, and is reliable and useful as a compliment to traditional methods. In addition, microarray technology has the potential to achieve specific, sensitive, quantitative and high-throughput tools for detection, identification and characterisation of fungi in natural environments (Gentry *et al.* 2006). A wide range of specific gene markers and probes are now available that will, in time, be of use in drinking water (Haughland *et al.* 2004). These may avoid problems with fungal isolations and identifications in future surveys, although whether they have been tested adequately remains to be seen.

Furthermore, gene probes are becoming available for the detection of specific mycotoxin metabolic pathways in fungi (Edwards *et al.* 2002; Paterson *et al.* 2003; Paterson 2004a), or in environmental samples (Paterson *et al.* 2000; Paterson 2006c). For example, the novel use of a probe for the isoepoxydon dehydrogenase (*idh*) gene of the patulin biosynthetic pathway has demonstrated the potential for identifying patulin metabolic pathways. Consequently, it may be useful in water distribution system for identifying areas containing patulin-producing fungi. Such problem areas could then be subjected to control via an HACCP approach (Paterson 2006c). Other PCR-based methods are discussed in Paterson (2006d; 2007b). However, problems of enzyme inhibition require to be addressed as the use of internal amplification controls have not been employed with the PCR of fungi in general (Paterson 2007b; 2008a) leading to the possibility of false negative results. And the practice of growing fungi for diagnostic or phylogenetic nucleic acid analysis on media which support mutagenic and inhibitory secondary metabolite production (e.g. aflatoxins) needs to be revised (Paterson and Lima 2009).

The analysis of ergosterol is a effective method for quantification of total fungal biomass. Ergosterol is a near universal lipid of fungi that increases in concentration with growth. Ergosterol was detected readily in water and was correlated with visual growth (Kelley and Paterson 2003; Paterson 2007a). However, the problem of taking representative samples remains where the distribution of fungi is uneven.

Recommended Procedures

The following methods have been developed and tested by the authors, and may be used to analyse water distribution systems or bottled water for the occurrence of filamentous fungi.

Isolation Based on NS 4716 (Anon. 1991), with Modifications

1. Membrane filter 100 ml of the water sample through 0.45 μm filter
2. Place the filter on dichloran 18% glycerol agar (DG18) plates
3. Incubate the plates at 20°C for 1-2 weeks, the plates must be checked visually every week
4. Count colonies and present as colony forming units (CFU)/100 ml water.
5. To isolate pure single colonies for identification, subculture positive cultures on potato dextrose agar (PDA) or malt extract agar (MEA).

Total Filamentous Fungi

1. Filter the water sample through two 0.45 μm filters.
2. Place one of the filters onto neopeptone-glucose rose Bengal aureomycin agar (NGRBA) with 5 replicates for filamentous fungal isolation and colony counting,
3. Place the second filter onto half strength cornmeal agar (1/2 CMA) with 5 replicates for filamentous fungal isolation and colony counting.

Zoosporic Fungi

"Baiting'' methods are employed in order to isolate these fungi, although they are not generally considered to be a serious problem.

1. Add several 0.5 cm^2 pieces of autoclaved snake skin and grass to 200 ml aliquots of samples in shake flasks and incubate for a maximum of 1 week at 12°C and 22°C.
2. Remove fungal growth aseptically and plate out onto 1/2 CMA.
3. Count the colonies on the plates, and identify the individual colonies.

Water Pipes and Sediments

Use a swab to collect the samples and plate onto the above media.

Taste and Odour

Treat the samples as above.

It is important not to smell the cultures, as this is contrary to good health and safety practice.

Analysis of Isolated Fungi for Mycotoxins

Figure 1 demonstrates a flow diagram for (a) the determination of biomass by ergosterol and (b) mycotoxin analysis. These methods are in Paterson and Bridge (1994), although this book is out of print and source papers may be required. References to these are available in Paterson (2004b).

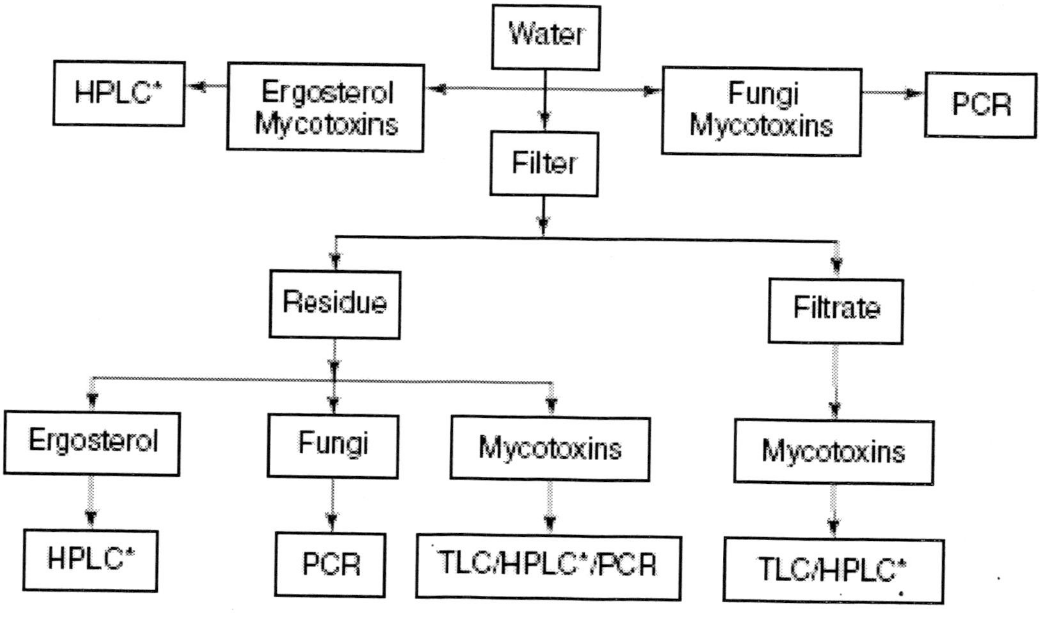

Figure 1. Flow diagram of the biochemical analysis of water for fungi and fungal metabolites. The use of commercial immunoaffinity columns is recommended for chromatographic mycotoxin analysis before or after filtration. Developments in NMR and mass spectroscopy mean that very low levels of metabolites will be able to be identified. HPLC, high-performance liquid chromatography; TLC, thin layer chromatography; PCR, polymerase chain reaction.

Thin Layer Chromatography: Extracellular Secondary Metabolites

1. Culture the fungus on yeast extract sucrose agar for 7 days.
2. Remove agar plugs (6 mm diameter) from the cultures by using a sterilized cork borer.
3. Place these at the origin of a TLC plate and then remove after 10 s.
4. Elute the TLC plate in toluene/ethyl acetate/90% formic acid (5:4:1; v/v/v).

Intracellular Secondary Metabolites

1. Grow the cultures on Czapecks yeast extract agar.
2. Place chloroform/methanol (2:1; v/v) onto the colony end of an agar plug.
3. Touched this briefly onto the origin of a TLC plate.
4. Elute the TLC plate in chloroform/acetic acid/propan-2-ol (85:15:20; v/v/v).
5. Observe spots in extracellular and intracellular modes by examination under white light and UV light.

Spray reagents:

1. Extracellular: *p*-anisaldehyde
2. Intracellular: Ceric sulphate

After spraying the TLC plates, repeat the white/UV light visualizations, and compare results with database in Paterson and Bridge (1994) or pure standards (e.g. from Sigma).

HPLC

1. Grow the cultures on YES and extract in chloroform.
2. Evaporate and resuspend the chloroform in a small volume of chloroform.
3. Inject an aliquot into an HPLC.
4. Use alkylphenone standards to standardize the runs so that retention indices could be calculated. The HPLC conditions involve a reversed phase column, gradient solvent system of acetonitrile water, with UV detection at 254 nm. Compare the retention indices of peaks obtained with those in databases (see Paterson 2004b).

PCR Mycotoxin Potential (e.g. the Isoepoxydon Dehydrogenase Gene for Patulin (Paterson et al. 2003)

1. Culture strains on malt extract agar and inoculate into 1 ml glucose yeast extract medium in Eppendorf tubes.
2. Grow these for 3 days at *ca.* 20∘C.
3. Decant the pellet.
4. Extract the DNA by standard methodology.
5. Amplify the IDH gene fragment by PCR.

Various other forms of analysis are possible in attempt to determine if identical isolates occur throughout a system. DNA fingerprinting of isolated strains in order to determine variation within particular species is one example. However, these are of limited value unless the variation within the natural population is known, thus one different isolate may actually represent a different taxon.

Biochemical Analysis of Water

No other authors have published methods for this form of analysis in water except those described in Kelley et al. (2003). The use of immunoaffinity columns is recommended for analyzing water as large volumes can be used, although the affect of large volumes of water on the integrity of the packing material must be considered and the procedure requires validation. Figure 1 demonstrates a flow diagram for the determination of (a) biomass by ergosterol and (b) mycotoxins. PCR for the detection of genes involved in mycotoxin production, and for identification of a particular taxa, is also illustrated the diagram. The diagram indicates how pigmentation could be tested. The sample could be analyzed directly or after filtration where the filtrate and the eluate can be analyzed separately. The method for the direct analysis of water by PCR is similar to that given for isolated fungi above and should be referred to.

Chromatographic Analysis

1. Direct injection: This is highly convenient as it simply involves injecting the water directly into a high-performance liquid chromatograph. HPLC Water 600 UV detector. Injection volume: 100 µl, solvent: actetonitrile/water.
2. Solvent extraction: Use liquid-liquid fractionation to concentrate the mycotoxins. Add chloroform to the water and remove in a separating funnel. Evaporate the solvent in a rotary evaporator until it is dry. Resuspend the extract in minimal volume for injection into HPLC.
3. Use the retention indices in the references in Paterson (2004) to identify the peaks.
4. Immunoaffinity columns for concentrating the target compound: Elute the water of interest through an immunoaffinity column using a peristaltic pump.

Volumes of 1 to 20 litres have been used by the current authors. The column can then be treated according to the manufacturer's instructions. This process has been used for aflatoxins and zearalenone. It is noted that the procedure requires validation.

Ergosterol

1. Filter the water.
2. Reflux the residue in 60 ml methanol/ethanol (5:1; v/v) with 10% (w/v) potassium hydroxide for 1 h.
3. Extract this with 60 ml petroleum ether and rotary evaporate at 40°C to dryness.
4. Rinse the residue in 15 ml of methanol filtered through a 0.45 µm filter (Millipore) and evaporate this using a sample concentrator.
5. Add HPLC methanol (250 µl) and inject 100 µl into a HPLC at 282 nm. Use a reversed phase Nova Pak C18 (3.9 × 150 mm) column, HPLC methanol as solvent, and the flow rate should be 2 ml min^{-1}.
6. Determine the concentration of the ergosterol standards by UV spectroscopy.

PCR

Do as above in section ''PCR Mycotoxin Potential (e.g. the Isoepoxydon Dehydrogenase Gene for Patulin *(Paterson et al. (2003)*'', except on an aliquot of water (Fig. 1). However, in all cases, internal amplification controls are required if false negative results are to be avoided (Paterson 2007b: 2008a).

REFERENCES

Anaissie, EJ; Costa, SF. Nosocomial aspergillosis is waterborne. *Clinical Infectious Diseases,* 2001 33, 1546-1548.

Anon. (1991) Norwegian standard for water analysis: Microfungi in water. *Determination with the membrane filter method* (In Norwegian). NS 4716. Oslo, Norway: The Standardization Organizations in Norway.

Arvanitidou, M; Kanellou, K; Constantinides, TC; Katsouyannopoulos, V. The occurrence of fungi in hospital and community potable waters. *Letters in Applied Microbiology,* 1999 29, 81-84.

Arvanitidou, M; Spaia, S; Velegraki, A; Pezarloglou, M; Kanetidis, D; Pangidis, P; Askepidis, N; Katsinas, Ch; Vayonas, G; Katsouyannopoulos, V. High level of recovery of fungi from water and dialysate in haemodialysis units. *Journal of Hospital Infection* 2000 45, 225-230.

Åslund, P. Hudirritasjoner förorsakade av mikrosvampar. *Vår Föda,* 1984 36, 327-336.

Bhatnagar, D; Rajasekaran, K; Payne, GA; Brown, RL; Yu, J; Cleveland, T.E. The 'omics' tools: genomics, proteomics, metabolomics and their potential for solving the aflatoxin contamination problem. *World Mycotoxin Journal,* 2008 1, 3-12.

Bucheli, TD; Wettstein, FE; Hartmann, N; Erbs, M; Vogelgsang, S; Forrer, H-R; Schwarzenbach, RP. *Fusarium* mycotoxins: overlooked aquatic micropollutants? *Journal of Agricultural and Food Chemistry,* 2008 56, 1029-1034.

Cabra, D; Fernández Pinto, VE. Fungal spoilage of bottled mineral water. *International Journal of Food Microbiology,* 2002 72, 73–76.

Canhoto, OF; Magan, N. Potential for detection of microorganisms and heavy metals in potable water using electronic nose technology. *Biosensors and Bioelectronics,* 2003 18, 751–754.

CAST. (2003) Mycotoxins: Risks in Plant, Animal, and Human Systems. Ames, IA, *Council for Agricultural Science and Technology.*

Criado, MV; Pinto, EVF; Badessari, A; Cabral, D. Conditions that regulate the growth of moulds inoculated into bottled water. *International Journal of Food Microbiology,* 2005 99, 343–349.

Doggett, MS. Characterization of fungal biofilms within a municipal water distribution system. *Applied and Environmental Microbiology,* 2000 66, 1249-1251.

Druzhinina, I; Kopchinskiy, AG; Komon, M; Bissett, J; Szakacs, G; Kubicek, CP. An oligonucleotide barcode for species identification in *Trichoderma* and *Hypocrea. Fungal Genetics and Biology,* 2005 42, 813-828.

Druzhinina, IS; Kopchinskiy, AG; Kubicek, CP. The first 100 *Trichoderma* species characterized by molecular data. *Mycoscience,* 2006 47, 55-64.

Edwards, SG; O'Callaghan, J; Dobson, ADW. PCR- based detection and quantification of mycotoxigenic fungi. *Mycological Research,* 2002 106, 1005–1025.

Esch, RE. Manufacturing and standardizing fungal allergen products. *Journal of Allergy and Clinical Immunology,* 2004 113, 210–215.

Food Standards Agency. (2008) Food industry guide to good hygiene practice: Bottled water. UK, TSO (The Stationery Office).

Franková, E; Horecka, M. Filamentous soil fungi and unidentified bacteria in drinking water from wells and water mains near Bratislava. *Microbiological Research,* 1995 150, 311-313.

Gentry, TJ; Wickham, GS; Schadt, CW; He, Z; Zhou, J. Microarray applications in microbial ecology research. *Microbial Ecology,* 2006 52, 159-175.

Gonçalves, AB; Paterson RRM; Lima N. Survey and significance of filamentous fungi from tap water. *International Journal of Hygiene and Environmental Health,* 2006a 209, 257-264.

Gonçalves, AB; Santos, IM; Paterson RRM; Lima N. FISH and Calcofluor staining techniques to detect *in situ* filamentous fungal biofilms in water. *Revista Iberoamericana de Micologia,* 2006b 23, 192-196.

Göttlich, E; van der Lubbe, W; Lange, B; Fiedler, S; Melchert, I; Reifenrath, M; Flemming, H-C; Hoog, S. Fungal flora in groundwater-derived public drinking water. *International Journal of Hygiene and Environmental Health,* 2002 205, 269–279.

Gromadzkaa, K; Was´kiewicza, A; Golin´skia, P; S´wietlikb, J. Occurrence of estrogenic mycotoxin – zearalenone in aqueous environmental samples with various NOM content *Water Research*, 2009, 1–9, doi:10.1016/j.watres.2008.11.042.

Hageskal, G; Gaustad, P; Heier, B.T; Skaar, I. Occurrence of moulds in drinking water. *Journal of Applied Microbiology,* 2007 102, 774-780.

Hageskal, G; Knutsen, AK; Gaustad, P; de Hoog, GS; Skaar, I. Diversity and significance of mold species in Norwegian drinking water. *Applied and Environmental Microbiology,* 2006 72, 7586-7593.

Hageskal, G; Lima N; Skaar, I. The study of fungi in drinking water. *Mycological Research,* 2009 133, 165-172.

Haughland, RA; Varma, MM; Wymer, LJ; Vesper, SJ. Quantitative PCR analysis of selected *Aspergillus, Penicillium* and *Paecilomyces* species. *Systematic and Applied Microbiology,* 2004 27, 198–210.

Hawksworth, DL. The magnitude of fungal diversity: the 1.5 million species estimate revisited. *Mycological Research,* 2001 105, 1422-1432.

Hedayati, MT; Pasqualotto, AC; Warn, PA; Bowyer, P; Denning DW. *Aspergillus flavus*: human pathogen, allergen and mycotoxin producer. *Microbiology,* 2007 153, 1677-1692.

Hendrickx, TLG; Meskus, E; Keiski, RL. Influence of the nutrient balance on biofilm composition in a fixed film process. *Water Science and Technology,* 2002 46, 7-12.

Hocking, AD; Pitt, JI. Dichloran-Glycerol medium for enumeration of xerophilic fungi from low-moisture foods. *Applied and Environmental Microbiology,* 1980 39, 488-492.

Kelley, J; Kinsey, G; Paterson, R; Brayford, D; Pitchers, R; Rossmore, H. (2003). *Identification and Control of Fungi in Distribution Systems*. Denver, CO. AWWA Research Foundation and American Water Works Association.

Kelley, J; Paterson, RRM. Comparisons of ergosterol to other methods for determinations of *Fusarium graminearum* biomass in water as a model system. In: Lima N, Smith D editors. *Biological Resource Centres and the use of Microbes,* European Culture Collections' Organisation XXII–Braga, September 17–19. Braga: Micoteca da Universidade do Minho; 2003; 235–239.

King, AD; Hocking, AD; Pitt, JI. Dichloran-rose bengal medium for enumeration and isolation of molds from foods. *Applied and Environmental Microbiology,* 1979 37, 959-964.

Kinsey, GC; Paterson, RR; Kelley, J. Methods for the determination of filamentous fungi in treated and untreated waters. *Journal of Applied Microbiology Symposium Supplement,* 1999 85, 214S-224S.

Mays, LW. (2004) *Water Supplies Systems Security*. Denver, CO: AWWA Products.

Mara, D; Horan, N. (2006) *The Handbook of Water and Wastewater Microbiology*. London, UK: Elsevier Academic Press.

Metzger, WJ; Patterson, R; Fink, J. Sauna takers disease. Hypersensitivity pneumonitis due to contaminated water in a home sauna. *Journal of the American Medical Association*, 1976 236, 2209-2211.

Monteil, A; Rigal, S; Welte, B. Study of the origin of musty taste in the drinking water supply. *Water Science and Technology,* 1999 40, 171–177.

Muittari, A; Kuusisto, P; Virtanen, P. An epidemic of extrinsic allergic alveolitis caused by tap water. Clinical Allergy, 1980 10, 77-90.

Nagy, LA; Olson, BH (1985) Occurrence and significance of bacteria, fungi and yeasts associated with distribution pipe surfaces. Proceedings of the American Water Works association, *Water quality technical conference.* Denver, Colorado: American Water Works Association, 213-238.

Nagy, LA; Olson, BH. The occurrence of filamentous fungi in drinking water distribution systems. *Canadian Journal of Microbiology,* 1982 28, 667-671.

Niemi, RM; Knuth, S; Lundström, K. Actinomycetes and fungi in surface waters and in potable water. *Applied and Environmental Microbiology,* 1982 43, 378-388.

Paterson, RRM. *Cordyceps* - a traditional Chinese medicine and another fungal therapeutic biofactory? *Phytochemistry,* 2008b, In Press.

Paterson, RRM. Fungal enzyme inhibitors as pharmaceuticals, toxins, and scourge of PCR. *Current Enzyme Inhibition,* 2008a 4, 46-59.

Paterson, RRM. Mycological Progress, 2007a 6, 115. Erratum for Robert, R; Paterson, M. Zearalenone production and growth in drinking water inoculated with *Fusarium graminearum*. *Mycological Progress,* 2007 6, 109-113.

Paterson, RRM. Internal amplification controls have not been employed in diagnostic fungal PCR hence potential false negative results. *Journal of Applied Microbiology,* 2007b 102, 1-10.

Paterson, RRM. Fungi and fungal toxins as weapons. *Mycological Research,* 2006b 110, 1003-1010.

Paterson, RRM. *Ganoderma* - a therapeutic fungal biofactory. *Phytochemistry,* 2006a 67, 1985-2001.

Paterson, RRM. Identification and quantification of mycotoxigenic fungi by PCR. *Process Biochemistry,* 2006d 41, 1467-1474.

Paterson RRM. Primers from the isoepoxydon dehydrogenase gene of the patulin biosynthetic pathway to indicate critical control points for patulin contamination of apples. *Food Control,* 2006c 17, 741-744.

Paterson, RRM. Standardized data on 474 fungal metabolites or ''extrolite''. *Mycological Research,* 2004b 108, 596–597.

Paterson, RRM. The isoepoxydon dehydrogenase gene of patulin biosynthesis in cultures and secondary metabolites as candidate PCR inhibitors. *Mycological Research,* 2004a 108, 1431–1437.

Paterson, RRM; Archer, S; Kozakiewicz, Z; Lea, A; Locke, T; O'Grady, E. A gene probe for the patulin metabolic pathway with potential use in novel disease control. *Biocontrol Science and Technology,* 2000 10, 509–512.

Paterson, RRM; Kozakiewicz, Z; Locke, T; Brayford, D; Jones, S.C.B. Novel use of the isoepoxydon dehydrogenase gene probe of the patulin metabolic pathway and chromatography to test penicillia isolated from apple production systems for the potential to contaminate apple juice with patulin. *Food Microbiology,* 2003 20, 359–364.

Paterson, RRM; Lima, N. (2005) *Fungal Contamination of Drinking Water.* In: Lehr J; Keeley, J; Lehr, J; Kingery III, TB. Editors. Water Encyclopedia. New York. John Wiley & Sons, Inc, 1-7. DOI: 10.1002/047147844X.wq1516.

Paterson, RRM; Lima, N. Mutagens manufactured in fungal culture may affect DNA/RNA of producing fungi. *Journal of Applied Microbiology,* 2009, doi:10.1111/j.1365-2672.2008.04024.x

Paterson, RRM; Vènâncio, A; Lima, N. Solutions to *Penicillium* taxonomy crucial to mycotoxin research and health. *Research in Microbiology,* 2004 155, 507–513.

Paterson, RRM; Kelley, J; Gallagher, M. Natural occurrence of aflatoxins and *Aspergillus flavus* (LINK) in water. *Letters in Applied Microbiology,* 1997 25, 435–436.

Paterson, RRM; Bridge, PD. (1994). *Biochemical Techniques for Filamentous Fungi.* IMI Techniques Series No. 1. Wallingford, UK. CAB International.

Paterson, RRM; Venâncio, A; Lima, N. A novel identification system based on 318 penicillia strains using the isoepoxydon dehydrogenase gene and patulin production. *Revista Iberoamericana de Micologia,* 2006 23, 155-159.

Paterson, RRM; Venâncio, A; Lima, N. Why do food and drink smell like earth? In: Méndez-Vilas, A. editor. *Communicating Current Research and Educational Topics and Trends in Applied Microbiology,* 2007 1, 120-128.

Rosenberg, FA. The microbiology of bottled water. *Clinical Microbiology Newsletter,* 2003 25, 41-44.

Samson, RA; Hoekstra, ES; Frisvad, JC. (2004). *Introduction to food- and airborne fungi. Utrecht,* The Netherlands: Centraalbureau voor Schimmelcultures.

Sheppard, DC; Ibrahim, AS; Edwards, JE Jr. (2004). Humanmycosis: The role of molecular biology. In: Tkacz, JS; Lange, L. editors. *Advances in Fungal Biotechnology for*

Industry, Agriculture and Medicine. New York. Kluwer Academic/Plenum Publishers, 361–384.

Venâncio, A; Paterson, R. (2007) The challenge of mycotoxins. In McElhatton, A; Marshall, R.J. editors. *Food Safety - A Practical and Case Study Approach.* Berlin, Springer, 24-47.

Waipara, NW. (1998). *A method to asses the lethal effect of UV-C irradiation of fungal spores on a dry surface.* Oslo, Norway: National Veterinary Institute.

Zacheus, OM; Lehtola, MJ; Korhonen, LK; Martikainen, PJ. Soft deposits, the key site for microbial growth in drinking water distribution networks. *Water Research,* 2001 35, 1757–1756.

INDEX

A

B

D

E

F

G

H

I

J

K

L

M

N

O

P

Q

R

S

T

U

V

W

X

Y

Z